a **LANGE** clinical manual

Neonatology

Management, Procedures, On-Call Problems, Diseases, Drugs

2nd Edition

Editor

Tricia Lacy Gomella, MD
Attending in Neonatology
Francis Scott Key Medical Center
Part-Time Instructor in Pediatrics
The Johns Hopkins University School of Medicine
Baltimore, Maryland

Associate Editor

M. Douglas Cunningham, MD
Director, Infant Special Care
Women's Hospital, Saddleback Memorial Medical Center
Laguna Hills, California
Professor of Clinical Pediatrics and Neonatology
University of California, Irvine
California College of Medicine

Consulting Editor

Fabian G. Eyal, MD
Director, Division of Neonatology
Francis Scott Key Medical Center
Assistant Professor of Pediatrics
The Johns Hopkins University School of Medicine
Baltimore, Maryland

APPLETON & LANGE
Norwalk, Connecticut/San Mateo, California

0-8385-1284-4

Copyright © 1992 by Appleton & Lange
A Publishing Division of Prentice Hall
Previous edition copyright © 1988 by Appleton & Lange
A Publishing Division of Prentice Hall.

93 94 95 96 / 10 9 8 7 6 5 4 3

Prentice Hall International (UK) Limited, *London*
Prentice Hall of Australia Pty. Limited, *Sydney*
Prentice Hall Canada, Inc., *Toronto*
Prentice Hall Hispanoamericana, S.A., *Mexico*
Prentice Hall of India Private Limited, *New Delhi*
Prentice Hall of Japan, Inc., *Tokyo*
Simon & Schuster Asia Pte. Ltd., *Singapore*
Editora Prentice Hall do Brasil Ltda., *Rio de Janeiro*
Prentice Hall, *Englewood Cliffs, New Jersey*

ISBN 0-8385-1284-4
ISSN 0697-6295

PRINTED IN THE UNITED STATES OF AMERICA   printed on recycled paper

To my twin sons, Leonard and Patrick, and singleton, Andrew

Contents

Contributors

Marilee C. Allen, MD
[Follow-up of High-Risk Infants]
Assistant Professor of Pediatrics, Division of Neonatology, The Johns Hopkins University School of Medicine, Baltimore, Maryland

Michael R. Barsotti, MD
[Fluids and Electrolytes]
Assistant Clinical Professor and Neonatal/Perinatal Fellow, Division of Neonatal/Perinatal Medicine, Department of Pediatrics, University of California, Irvine, California College of Medicine

Gordon Bingham, CRTT, RTT
[Respiratory Management]
Neonatal Supervisor, Department of Respiratory Care and Supervisor, Neonatal Intensive Care Unit, A. B. Chandler Medical Center, Lexington, Kentucky

Richard N. Broaddus, RRT, MBA
[Respiratory Management]
Senior Therapist, Department of Respiratory Care, A. B. Chandler Medical Center, Lexington, Kentucky

E. B. Cartaya, MD
[Infant of Drug-Abusing Mother]
Clinical Assistant Professor, University of Miami Hospital, Miami, Florida; Attending in Neonatology, Plantation General Hospital, Plantation, Florida, and Hollywood Memorial Hospital, Hollywood, Florida

Veeraiah Chundu, MD
[Extracorporeal Membrane Oxygenation (ECMO), Neural Tube Defects, Thyroid Disorders]
Neonatal/Perinatal Fellow and Clinical Instructor of Pediatrics, Division of Neonatal/Perinatal Medicine, Department of Pediatrics, University of California, Irvine, California College of Medicine

Carol M. Cottrill, MD
[Cardiac Abnormalities]
Professor of Pediatrics and Pediatric Cardiologist, Department of Pediatrics, University of Kentucky College of Medicine, Lexington, Kentucky

M. Douglas Cunningham, MD
[Management of the Extremely Low Birth Weight Infant During the First Week of Life]
Professor of Clinical Pediatrics and Neonatology, University of California, Irvine, California College of Medicine; Director, Infant Special Care Unit, Women's Hospital, Saddleback Memorial Medical Center, Laguna Hills, California

William G. Cvetnic, MD
[Pulmonary Function Testing, Patent Ductus Arteriosus, Persistent Pulmonary Hypertension (Persistent Fetal Circulation)]
Assistant Professor in Residence, Division of Neonatal/Perinatal Medicine, Department of Pediatrics, University of California, Irvine, California College of Medicine

Nirmala S. Desai, MD
[Intrauterine Growth Retardation (Small-for-Gestational-Age Infant)]
Professor of Pediatrics, Division of Neonatology, University of Kentucky College of Medicine, Lexington, Kentucky

Fabian G. Eyal, MD
[Respiratory Management]
Assistant Professor of Pediatrics, The Johns Hopkins University School of Medicine, and Director, Department of Neonatology, Francis Scott Key Medical Center, Baltimore, Maryland

Evan David Frank MD, PhD
[Obstetric Anesthesia and the Neonate]
Assistant Professor, Department of Anesthesiology, Jefferson Medical College of Thomas Jefferson University, Philadelphia, Pennsylvania

Christine A. Gleason, MD
[Resuscitation of the Newborn, Extracorporeal Membrane Oxygenation (ECMO)]
Associate Professor, Department of Pediatrics, The Johns Hopkins University School of Medicine, and Director, Neonatal Intensive Care Unit, The Johns Hopkins Hospital, Baltimore, Maryland

Leonard G. Gomella, MD
[Renal Diseases]
Assistant Professor, Department of Urology, Jefferson Medical College of Thomas Jefferson University, Philadelphia, Pennsylvania

Tricia Lacy Gomella, MD
[Prenatal Testing, Assessment of Gestational Age, Newborn Physical Examination, Temperature Regulation, Nutritional Management, Neonatal Radiology, Procedures, On-Call Problems (Patient Management Problems), Transient Tachypnea of the Newborn]
Part-Time Instructor in Pediatrics, The Johns Hopkins University School of Medicine, and Attending in Neonatology, Francis Scott Key Medical Center, Baltimore, Maryland

Janet E. Graeber, MD
[Retinopathy of Prematurity]
Associate Professor of Pediatrics, Department of Pediatrics, West Virginia University School of Medicine, Morgantown, West Virginia

Bryan D. Hall, MD
[Common Multiple Congenital Anomaly Syndromes]
Professor of Pediatrics and Chief, Division of Genetics and Dysmorphology, University of Kentucky College of Medicine, Lexington, Kentucky

Charles R. Hamm, Jr., MD
[High-Frequency Ventilation]
Instructor, Department of Pediatrics, The Johns Hopkins University School of Medicine, and Assistant Director, Department of Neonatology, Francis

Scott Key Medical Center, Baltimore, Maryland

Mark Damian Harris, MD
[Rickets and Disorders of Calcium and Magnesium Metabolism]
Pediatrician/Neonatologist, Greater Baltimore Medical Center, Baltimore,
Maryland

Dina Herald, RD, CNSD
[Nutritional Management]
Clinical Nutrition Specialist, Women's Hospital, Saddleback Memorial
Medical Center, Laguna Hills, California

C. Kirby Heritage, MD
[Infant of Diabetic Mother]
Assistant Clinical Professor of Pediatrics, Wright State School of Medicine,
and Attending in Neonatology, Miami Valley Hospital, Dayton, Ohio

Marcus C. Hermansen, MD
[Management of the Extremely Low Birth Weight Infant During the First
Week of Life, Thrombocytopenia and Platelet Dysfunction, Hydrocephalus,
Intraventricular Hemorrhage]
Associate Professor of Pediatrics, Medical College of Pennsylvania,
Philadelphia; Director of Neonatology, Allegheny General Hospital,
Pittsburgh, Pennsylvania

Bonnie Boyer Hudak, MD
[Bronchopulmonary Dysplasia]
Assistant Professor of Pediatrics, Divisions of Pediatric Pulmonary and
Neonatology, The Childrens Hospital of Buffalo, Buffalo, New York

Mark L. Hudak, MD
[Surfactant Replacement Therapy, Inborn Errors of Metabolism With Acute
Neonatal Onset]
Associate Professor of Pediatrics, Division of Neonatology, The Childrens
Hospital of Buffalo, Buffalo, New York

William G. Keyes, MD, PhD
[Multiple Gestation]
Attending in Neonatology, Northside Hospital, and Pediatric Intensivist,
Department of Intensive Care Medicine, Scottish Rite Childrens Medical
Center, Atlanta, Georgia

Robert J. Kuhn, PharmD
[Total Parenteral Nutrition, Commonly Used Medications, Commonly Used
Antibiotics, Antivirals, and Antifungals]
Associate Professor, Division of Clinical Practice and Science, University of
Kentucky College of Pharmacy, Lexington, Kentucky

Drew Litzenberger, MD
[Infant Transport]
Co-Director of Neonatology, Memorial Mission Medical Center, Asheville,
North Carolina

Ronald A. Naglie, MD
[Infectious Diseases]
Assistant Clinical Professor, Division of Neonatal/Perinatal Medicine, and
Co-Director of Perinatal Outreach, Department of Pediatrics, University of
California, Irvine, California College of Medicine

Ambadas Pathak, MD
[Neonatal Seizures]
Assistant Professor of Pediatrics, The Johns Hopkins University School of Medicine, and Head, Division of Newborn Medicine, Greater Baltimore Medical Center, Baltimore, Maryland

Thomas H. Pauly, MD
[Air Leak Syndromes, Apnea and Periodic Breathing, High-Frequency Ventilation]
Associate Professor, Department of Pediatrics, Division of Neonatology, University of Kentucky College of Medicine, Lexington, Kentucky

Andrew R. Pulito, MD
[Surgical Diseases of the Newborn]
Professor of Surgery, University of Kentucky College of Medicine, and Chief, Division of Pediatric Surgery, A. B. Chandler Medical Center, Lexington, Kentucky

J. Laurence Ransom, MD
[ABO Incompatibility, Anemia, Polycythemia and Hyperviscosity, Rh Incompatibility]
Director of Neonatal Medicine and Consultant in Pediatric Hematology, The Moses H. Cone Memorial Hospital, Greensboro, North Carolina; Clinical Associate Professor of Pediatrics, University of North Carolina, Chapel Hill, North Carolina

Pamela D. Reiter, PharmD
[Commonly Used Medications]
Pharmacy Resident, Le Bonheur Children's Hospital Medical Center, Memphis, Tennessee

G. Mark Shoptaugh, MD
[Exchange Transfusion, Hyperbilirubinemia]
Neonatal/Perinatal Fellow and Clinical Instructor of Pediatrics, Division of Neonatal/Perinatal Medicine, Department of Pediatrics, University of California, Irvine, California College of Medicine

Melinda Slack, MD
[Meconium Aspiration]
Director of Neonatology, St. John's Regional Health Center, Springfield, Missouri

Michael W. Stelling, MD
[Ambiguous Genitalia]
Associate Professor of Pediatrics, Department of Pediatrics, University of Kentucky College of Medicine, Lexington, Kentucky

Feizal Waffarn, MB, BS
[Necrotizing Enterocolitis]
Associate Professor of Pediatrics in Residence, Division of Neonatal/Perinatal Medicine, Department of Pediatrics, University of California, Irvine, California College of Medicine; Director of Special Care Nurseries and NICU, Fountain Valley Regional Hospital, Fountain Valley, California

Betty Lou Eilers Walfman, MD
[Hyaline Membrane Disease (Respiratory Distress Syndrome)]
Director, Intensive Care Nursery, Humana Women's Hospital, Indianapolis, Indiana

Linda L. Yang, MD
[Perinatal Asphyxia]
Neonatal/Perinatal Fellow and Clinical Instructor of Pediatrics, Division of
Neonatal/Perinatal Medicine, Department of Pediatrics, University of
California, Irvine, California College of Medicine

Karin E. Zenk, PharmD, FASHP
[Effects of Drugs and Substances on Lactation and Breast-Feeding, Effects
of Drugs and Substances Taken During Pregnancy]
Associate Adjunct Professor of Pediatrics, University of California, Irvine,
California College of Medicine; Pharmacist-Specialist in Pediatrics,
University of California, Irvine, Medical Center (Orange); Associate Clinical
Professor of Pharmacy, University of California, San Francisco, School of
Medicine

Preface

The first edition of *Neonatology* proved to be very successful as a practical manual, both here and overseas, providing the opportunity for this second edition.

Many chapters in the second edition of this manual have been extensively updated and revised. However, the format of the manual has remained essentially the same, with one major addition. Section I, Basic Management, includes topics that involve daily care of premature and term infants. Section II, Advanced Management, is new. It addresses newly developed technologies that are typically available only in level III intensive care nurseries and includes Extracorporeal Membrane Oxygenation (ECMO), High-Frequency Ventilation, Surfactant Replacement Therapy, and Management of the Extremely Low Birth Weight Infant During the First Week of Life.

Section III, Procedures, discusses the procedures used in neonatal intensive care units. In this edition, we have added a section on intraosseous infusion.

Section IV, On-Call Problems, proved to be so popular because of its practicality on the "front lines" that it has given rise to a new "On-Call" manual series in other medical specialties, including surgery, obstetrics and gynecology, and internal medicine. Several new neonatal problems (Arrhythmia, Cyanosis) have been added to this edition, and the existing problems have been updated to keep pace with current therapy.

Section V, Diseases and Disorders, has been extensively revised, and drugs have been added to Section VI, Neonatal Pharmacology. In the neonatal pharmacology section, a new chapter, Drugs and Substances Taken During Pregnancy, has also been added and includes the FDA fetal-risk category for specific drugs and substances. Isolation Guidelines is a new appendix in this edition.

The management principles and protocols in the update of this manual are not based on practices at only one institution. Contributors are from all over the United States, and the associate editor and consulting editor are from the West Coast and East Coast, respectively. I feel this has enabled us to produce a manual that is not institution-specific but reflects a cross section of contemporary approaches to neonatal management.

Neonatology is a relatively young and rapidly evolving pediatric subspecialty. If treatment protocols vary from center to center, we have identified them as *controversial*. This clearly indicates to the reader that specific institutions may not treat the same problem in the same way and that different approaches may have been used successfully at other institutions.

The authors and editors have made every effort to assure timely and accurate guidelines in this manual. However, it is impossible to list every clinical situation or institution-specific approach to diagnosis and treatment.

My sincerest thanks to the contributors, the editorial staff at Appleton & Lange, and my family for their continued support, which has been indispensable to the completion of this second edition.

The editor welcomes suggestions and comments about this manual. Letters should be addressed to:

Tricia Lacy Gomella, MD
c/o Appleton & Lange
25 Van Zant Street
East Norwalk, CT 06855
June, 1991

Preface To First Edition

The information offered in this *Manual* represents current recommendations that are applicable in any hospital where sick infants may require immediate treatment and stabilization to prepare them for transfer to an intensive care unit.* It is the editors' and authors' intention that the *Manual* present what has been learned over the past five decades about caring for normal and sick newborns in a readily accessible format for direct, practical application.

Several points about the content and structure of this *Manual* should be emphasized. It is intended for both the novice and the veteran in the neonatal intensive care unit. It is designed to make clinical guidelines quickly available whether the physician is faced with performing a specific procedure, diagnosing a presenting problem, managing a disease, or administering and monitoring drug therapy. For these purposes, the *Manual* is divided into five sections: Basic Procedures, Special Procedures, On-Call Problems, Diseases and Conditions, and Neonatal Pharmacology.

The first two sections—Basic Procedures and Special Procedures—are devoted to general management. Basic Procedures includes chapters not only on prenatal testing and delivery room management but also on the day-to-day management of infants with respect to nutritional, fluid, and respiratory care. A unique chapter in this section is Neonatal Radiology, which contains representative x-rays and radiographic pearls. Section II, Special Procedures, describes the technique for performing each procedure in a step-by-step format, with selected illustrations and practical hints on the proper technical performance of the procedure.

Section III, On-Call Problems, is a unique feature of this *Manual.* It describes the 25 most common problems encountered in a neonatal intensive care unit when "on call," beginning with a statement and definition of the problems and the immediate diagnostic questions that must be dealt with, key differential diagnoses that must be considered, and proceeding then to characterize the data base that must be assembled in order to answer the key questions and make the diagnosis. Immediate management required is also described in each case.

In Section IV, Diseases and Conditions, we have avoided overloading the text with every disorder we could think of and have instead prepared complete but concise discussions intended to convey a clear understanding of the more common diseases encountered in the newborn and their management.

Section V, Neonatal Pharmacology, is intended to provide greater understanding of the medications used to treat infants and not merely to provide

---

*In the last 10 to 15 years neonatology has become a pediatric subspecialty with a highly developed system of regional neonatal centers. Today, regionalization of sick infant care revolves around a system of referrals, beginning with Level 1 hospitals and extending through larger Level II hospitals and ending with Level III medical centers. In general, the Level I nurseries care for normal newborns or those with minor medical problems. Neonatal intensive care at Level II institutions usually serves infants who may require short-term mechanical ventilatory life support. Level III centers are responsible for maternal and infant transport from Level I and Level II facilities and usually provide long-term ventilatory and intensive care support for critically ill infants.

dosage schedules. It includes information on dosages, routes of administration, mechanisms of action, indications, adverse effects, dosage forms, and other relevant data about drugs for newborns.

The first manual used at the University of Kentucky, Medical Center's neonatal intensive care unit was written by one of the first fellows in the program. Beth Wade. It consisted of basic information to help house officers survive rotation in the unit, and it continued to be used for many years. The concept of such a project appealed to me, and I initially prepared handouts and note cards for interns and residents to help them get through the long nights in the unit. These were well received, and this *Manual* represents a natural progression from those early efforts to make practical information available for in-house application. I hope this *Manual* will provide in a readily usable form helpful and practical guidelines on the general care of the normal newborn and on the specific management and specific needs of the sick newborn.

I am indebted to my husband for the enormous amount of work he did on the *Manual* and for the guidance he provided. I also want to thank my family, my in-laws, and my good friend Enda, all of whom helped me care for my sons while I tried to complete my fellowship training program, work on this *Manual,* and maintain some semblance of normal family life.

I wish to acknowledge the support of Dr. Jackie Noonan, Chairman of Pediatrics, during my pediatric residency and the fellowship program at the University of Kentucky. Drs. Cunningham, Desai, and Hermansen provided immense support throughout all aspects of the project and taught me many of their excellent clinical skills during my fellowship in Lexington. The nurses in the neonatal intensive care unit at the University of Kentucky deserve special thanks for showing me the joys of caring for newborns.

Kathleen O'Brien at Appleton & Lange provided outstanding editorial guidance. I am grateful to all the contributors for helping me accomplish this task.

Because of my twin pregnancy, I was able to complete only 18 months of the fellowship program at the University of Kentucky. I want to thank Dr. Doug Jones, Director of Neonatology at The Johns Hopkins University School of Medicine, for allowing me to complete my last six months of training in his program. I extend my thanks also to everyone at the neonatal unit at the Francis Scott Key Medical Center for their support during the last six months of work on this project.

Tricia Lacy Gomella
Silver Spring, Maryland
June, 1988

1 Prenatal Testing

AMNIOCENTESIS

Amniotic fluid can be analyzed for prenatal diagnosis of congenital defects and determination of fetal lung maturity. Testing for congenital abnormalities is usually done at 14–16 weeks' gestation. A sample of amniotic fluid is removed under ultrasound guidance. Fetal cells contained in the fluid can be grown in tissue culture for genetic study. This is indicated (1) in women over 35 years of age, because of the increased incidence of trisomy 21; (2) in those who have already had a child with a chromosomal abnormality; (3) in those in whom X-linked disorders are suspected; and (4) to rule out inborn errors of metabolism.

BIOPHYSICAL PROFILE

The biophysical profile (Table 1–1) is used to assess fetal well-being. A 30-minute ultrasound examination is performed to measure 5 parameters: fetal breathing movements, gross fetal body movements, fetal tone, reactive fetal heart rate, and amniotic fluid volume. A score of 8–10 is considered normal; a score of 4–6 indicates possible poor fetal well-being; and a score of 0–2 is a strong indication of poor fetal well-being.

FETAL HEART RATE MONITORING

Fetal heart rate monitoring may be internal (direct)—electrode attached to fetal scalp—or external (indirect)—electrode attached to maternal abdomen. The baseline heart rate, beat-to-beat variability, and periodic heart rate are measured.

   I. **Baseline fetal heart rate.** The baseline fetal heart rate is the rate that is maintained apart from periodic variations caused by uterine contractions. The **normal fetal heart rate** is 120–160 beats/min. **Fetal tachycardia** is present at 160 beats/min or more. Causes of fetal tachycardia include maternal or fetal infection, fetal hypoxia, thyrotoxicosis, and maternal use of drugs

TABLE 1–1. BIOPHYSICAL PROFILE*

Variable	Normal (2)	Abnormal (0)
Fetal breathing	One episode > 30 seconds in 30 minutes	None or episode < 30 seconds in 30 minutes
Body movement	Three or more movements in 30 minutes	Two or less movements in 30 minutes
Fetal tone	One episode of active limb or trunk extension with flexion	No movement
Nonstress test	Reactive	Nonreactive
Amniotic fluid	One pocket of amniotic fluid 1 cm or more	No fluid pockets or pocket < 1 cm

*Scoring system used to assess fetal well-being, as described in text.
Based on guidelines from Manning F et al: Fetal biophysical profile scoring: A prospective study in 1,184 high-risk patients. *Am J Obstet Gynecol* 1981;**40**:289.

such as parasympathetic blockers or betamimetic agents. **Moderate fetal bradycardia** is defined as a heart rate of 100–120 beats/min with normal variability. **Severe fetal bradycardia** is a heart rate of less than 100 beats/min. The most common cause of bradycardia is hypoxia; other causes include hypothermia, complete heart block, and maternal use of drugs such as beta blockers.

II. **Beat-to-beat variability.** In the normal mature fetus, there are slight rapid fluctuations in the interval between beats (beat-to-beat variability). An **amplitude range** (baseline variability) > **6 beats/min indicates normal beat-to-beat variability** and suggests the absence of fetal asphyxia. Absence of variability may be caused by severe asphyxia, anencephaly, complete heart block, and maternal use of drugs such as magnesium sulfate or morphine.

III. **Periodic fetal heart rate.** The periodic fetal heart rate is the rate that occurs during uterine contractions. There are 3 types of decelerations (Fig 1–1).

   A. **Early decelerations.** Early decelerations (decelerations of head compression) occur secondary to vagal reflex tone, which follows minor, transient fetal hypoxic episodes. These are benign and not associated with fetal compromise.

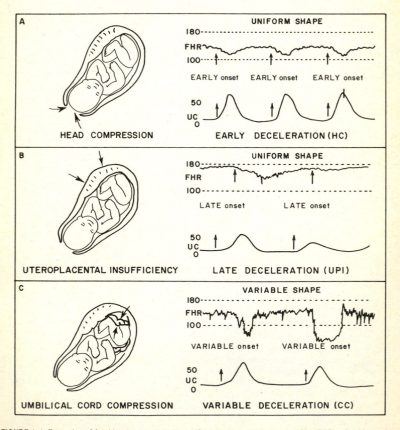

FIGURE 1-1. Examples of fetal heart rate monitoring. UC = uterine contraction (mm Hg); FHR = fetal heart rate in beats per minute (bpm). (Modified and reproduced, with permission, from McCrann JR, Schifrin BS: Fetal monitoring in high-risk pregnancy. *Clin Perinatol* 1974;1:149.)

B. **Late decelerations.** Two types of late decelerations are described.
   1. **Reflex late decelerations.** These are seen in the setting of normal fetal heart rate variability. They are associated with a sudden insult (eg, maternal hypotension) that affects a normally oxygenated fetus and signifies uteroplacental insufficiency. The normal variability of the fetal heart rate signifies that the fetus is physiologically compensated.
   2. **Late decelerations with loss of beat-to-beat variability ("myocardial hypoxia late decelerations").** These are associated with decreased or absent fetal heart rate variability. They result from prolonged asphyxia and signify "fetal decompensation," which may be seen with preeclampsia and intrauterine growth retardation.
C. **Variable decelerations.** These are vagal in origin and are most frequently associated with umbilical cord compression. They are classified as severe when the fetal heart rate is below 60 beats/min, the deceleration is longer than 60 seconds in duration, or the fetal heart rate is 60 beats/min below baseline. If beat-to-beat variability is maintained, the fetus is compensated physiologically and oxygenated normally. If severe variable decelerations are present for more than 30 minutes, the fetus may be decompensated, and maneuvers such as maternal oxygen supplementation and maternal positioning in the left lateral decubitus position may improve placental circulation and should be attempted.

FETAL SCALP BLOOD SAMPLING

Fetal scalp blood sampling is used to determine the fetal acid-base status. This procedure can be performed only after rupture of the membranes. It is contraindicated in cases of known blood dyscrasias, infection due to herpesvirus, or obvious chorioamnionitis. A blood sample is obtained from the fetal presenting part (usually the scalp but sometimes the buttocks), and the fetal blood pH is determined. A pH of 7.25 or greater has been shown to correlate (with 92% accuracy) with a 2-minute Apgar score of 7 or greater. A pH of less than 7.15 correlates with a 2-minute Apgar score of less than 6 (80% accuracy). The following results are usually used as a standard protocol.

pH > 7.25: Normal result; fetus is probably normal.
pH < 7.20: Abnormal result; fetus is acidotic. If this result occurs in the absence of maternal acidosis, and a repeat test done 10 minutes after the first one reveals the same or more acidotic pH, delivery is indicated.
pH between 7.20 and 7.25: The test should be repeated. Decisions regarding delivery depend on the clinical situation.

Complications of this test are scalp infections (< 1% of infants) and soft tissue damage to the scalp.

TESTS OF FETAL LUNG MATURITY

Phospholipids can be measured in amniotic fluid to gauge fetal lung maturity.
I. **Lecithin:sphingomyelin (L:S) ratio.** Lecithin, a saturated phosphatidylcholine (the condensation product of a phosphatidic acid and choline), can be measured specifically in amniotic fluid and is a principal active component of surfactant. It is manufactured by type II alveolar cells. Sphingomyelin is a phospholipid found predominantly in body tissues other than the lungs. The L:S ratio compares levels of lecithin (which increase in late gestation) to levels of sphingomyelin (which remain constant). The L:S ratio is usually 1:1 by 31–32 weeks' gestation and 2:1 by 35 weeks' gestation. The following are guidelines to L:S ratios.
   L:S 2:1 or greater: Lungs are mature (98% accuracy). Only 2% of these infants will develop respiratory distress syndrome.

L:S 1.5–1.9:1: 50% will develop respiratory distress syndrome.

L:S less than 1.5:1: 73% will develop respiratory distress syndrome.

Some disorders are associated with delayed lung maturation, and higher than normal L:S ratios must be present before lung maturity has been reached. The 2 most common are diabetes mellitus (L:S ratio of 3:1 is usually accepted as indicating maturity) and Rh isoimmunization associated with hydrops fetalis.

Acceleration of mature L:S ratios is seen in sickle cell disease, maternal narcotic addiction, prolonged rupture of the membranes, chronic maternal hypertension, intrauterine growth retardation (IUGR), and placental infarction. Differences may also occur in various racial groups.

II. **Phosphatidylglycerol measurement.** Phosphatidylglycerol appears in amniotic fluid at about 35 weeks, and levels increase at 37–40 weeks. This substance is a useful marker for lung maturation. It is reported as either present or absent.

NONSTRESS TEST

The nonstress test (NST) is used to detect fetal hypoxia. Fetal well-being is confirmed if there is an increase in the fetal heart rate in response to fetal activity. The baseline fetal heart rate is measured by external monitoring devices. Fetal movements and heart rate are then recorded for 20 minutes.

Decreased fetal movements can occur with fetal sleep, central nervous system depressants, chronic smoking, and medications such as propranolol.

The following guidelines can be used.

I. **Reactive test.** A normal fetal baseline heart rate is present, and there are at least 4 fetal movements in 20 minutes. The heart rate accelerates by at least 15 beats/min during fetal movement. This result indicates that the fetus is usually normal.

II. **Nonreactive test.** No fetal movements occur during a 20-minute period, or there is no acceleration of the fetal heart rate with fetal movements. This result is associated with a poor outcome and should be followed up with the oxytocin challenge test (see below).

III. **Uncertain reactivity.** Fewer than 4 fetal movements occur within a 20-minute period, or the fetal heart rate accelerates less than 15 beats/min during fetal movement. The nonstress test should be repeated, or the oxytocin challenge test should be performed.

CONTRACTION STRESS TEST

The contraction stress test (CST) is used to assess a fetus at risk for uteroplacental insufficiency. A monitor is placed on the mother's abdomen to continuously record the fetal heart rate and uterine contractions. An adequate test consists of more than 3 contractions, each lasting at least 40–60 seconds, within a period of 10 minutes. If sufficient contractions do not occur, oxytocin is administered by intravenous pump at a rate of 0.5 mU/min until adequate contractions occur. If oxytocin is needed to produce contractions for the contraction stress test, it is called **oxytocin challenge test (OCT).** Normally, the fetal heart rate increases in response to a contraction and no decelerations occur during the contraction. If late decelerations occur during contractions, uteroplacental insufficiency is probably present.

The CST is contraindicated in patients with placenta previa, those who have had a previous cesarean section with a vertical incision, and those who are at high risk for preterm delivery (premature rupture of the membranes, multiple gestation, incompetent cervix).

Test results are interpreted as follows.

I. **Negative (normal) test.** No late decelerations occur during adequate uterine contractions. The baseline fetal heart rate is normal. This result is associated with a good fetal outcome. A repeat test is usually performed in 1 week.

II. **Positive (abnormal) test.** Persistent late decelerations occur during adequate uterine contractions. This result can signify poor fetal outcome, perinatal death, meconium-stained amniotic fluid, or respiratory distress (low 5-minute Apgar score). If the test is positive, delivery is usually recommended.

III. **Equivocal (suspicious) test.** Intermittent late decelerations occur with adequate uterine contractions. The test should be repeated within 24 hours; most repeat tests will be negative.

ULTRASOUND TESTING

Ultrasound examination is used in the following circumstances.

I. **To estimate gestational age and weight.** The following parameters are used:

A. **To determine crown-rump length.** Measurements are most accurate in the first 12 weeks of gestation, with a margin of 3–5 days. Measurements are more difficult to make later in pregnancy as the fetus assumes a more curled-up position.

B. **To determine biparietal diameter.** Measurement of the biparietal diameter is most accurate at 12–18 weeks' gestation. The measurement is made from the outer edge of one side of the skull to the inner edge of the opposite side.

C. **To determine femur length.** The femur is measured from the greater trochanter to the distal metaphyses and plotted against a graph for age assessment.

D. **To determine abdominal circumference.** This measurement is an indication of gestational age and is an accurate indication of intrauterine growth retardation.

II. **To follow fetal intrauterine growth and detect intrauterine growth retardation (IUGR).**

III. **To assess fetal movements and breathing activity.**

IV. **As an adjunct to amniocentesis and intrauterine transfusion.**

V. **To help guide the choice of method of delivery.** Detection of gross anomalies with ultrasonography can be used to decide on the type of delivery and support personnel needed (eg, anencephaly, gastroschisis, multiple gestation).

VI. **To determine amniotic fluid volume**

A. **Oligohydramnios** (lack of amniotic fluid) is associated with a major anomaly 15% of the time. Renal agenesis and prune-belly syndrome are the most common, along with amniotic fluid leak, severe cardiac disease, and chylothorax. The kidneys can be seen with ultrasonography at 15 weeks and the bladder at 16 weeks.

B. **Polyhydramnios (hydramnios)** (excess of amniotic fluid) is associated with major anomalies 15% of the time. It is associated with anencephaly, neural tube defects, bowel obstruction such as duodenal atresia, multiple gestation, nonimmune hydrops fetalis, and exstrophy of the bladder.

VII. **To determine fetal death.** Ultrasound findings of absence of cardiac motion, scalp edema, and overlapping of cranial bones indicate fetal death.

VIII. **To determine fetal sex.**

IX. **To detect fetal heart motion.** Fetal heart activity can be detected at 7–8 weeks.

X. **To assess the placenta for location.**

XI. **To guide fetal surgeons, for example, in surgical intervention for fetal hydronephrosis.**

XII. **To evaluate uterine size and shape.**

XIII. To rule out placenta previa and abruptio placentae in cases of vaginal bleeding.

REFERENCE

Manning FA et al: Fetal biophysical profile scoring: A prospective study in 1184 high-risk patients. *Am J Obstet Gynecol* 1981;**140**:289.

2   Delivery Room Management

OBSTETRIC ANESTHESIA AND THE NEONATE

During birth, the status of the fetus is influenced by many factors. One major factor is obstetric analgesia and anesthesia. Care in choosing analgesic and anesthetic agents can often prevent depression in the newborn, especially in high-risk deliveries.

I. **Placental transfer of drugs.** Drugs administered to the mother may affect the fetus via placental transfer or (less commonly) may cause a maternal disorder that affects the fetus (eg, maternal drug-induced hypotension may cause fetal hypoxia). All anesthetic and analgesic drugs cross the placenta to some degree. Passive diffusion is the usual mechanism, and since most agents are highly permeable, they are also flow-dependent.

Most anesthetic and analgesic drugs have a high degree of lipid solubility, a low molecular weight (< 500), and variable protein-binding and ionization capabilities. These characteristics cause them to be transferred rapidly across the placenta. Local anesthetics and narcotics (which are lipid-soluble and have low ionization) cross the placenta easily, whereas neuromuscular blocking agents (highly ionized) are transferred much more slowly.

II. **Analgesia in labor**

A. **Inhalation analgesia.** Inhalation analgesia is rarely used in the USA. Entonox (50% O_2 and 50% N_2O) is widely used in other countries. Amounts used are generally much lower than those used in general anesthesia.

B. **Pudendal block and paracervical block.** Paracervical block may be associated with severe fetal bradycardia caused by uterine vasoconstriction and is now rarely used. If a paracervical block is performed, fetal heart rate monitoring must be used. Pudendal blocks have little direct effect on the fetus. However, seizures have been reported with several local anesthetic agents used for both pudendal and paracervical blocks. Paracervical blocks are used in the first stage of labor and pudendal in the second stage of labor.

C. **Narcotics.** All narcotics are rapidly transferred to the fetus and cause dose-related respiratory depression and alterations in the Apgar score and neurobehavioral scores.

1. **Meperidine (Demerol)** causes severe neonatal depression (as measured by Apgar scoring) if the drug is administered more than 1 hour before delivery. If meperidine is given within 1 hour of birth, there is no significant difference in the neonate when compared to controls (Shnider, 1964). Depression is manifested as respiratory acidosis, decreased oxygen saturation, decreased minute ventilation, and increased time to sustained respiration. Fetal normeperidine (a meperidine metabolite that may cause significant central nervous system depression) increases with longer intervals between drug administration and delivery. Levels are highest at 4 hours after intravenous administration of the drug to the mother. The half-life of meperidine is 13 hours in neonates, whereas the half-life of normeperidine is 62 hours (Moore, 1973).

2. **Morphine** has a delayed onset of action and perhaps causes more neonatal depression than meperidine (Jouppila, 1982).
3. **Butorphanol (Stadol)** and **nalbuphine (Nubain)** are agonist-antagonist narcotic agents. They are thought to cause less respiratory depression than morphine, particularly when used in high doses.
4. **Pentazocine (Fortral)** is said to have a lower rate of placental transfer than meperidine, but most studies have not shown significant differences in the severity of neonatal depression caused by the 2 drugs.

D. **Narcotic antagonist (naloxone [Narcan]).** The effect of naloxone given intramuscularly may last for 48 hours in the fetus. When the drug is injected into the umbilical vein, effects may last for only 30 minutes. With maternal reversal of narcotic, some researchers have shown temporary improvement in neonatal depression due to narcotic effect.

E. **Sedatives and tranquilizers**
   1. **Barbiturates.** Barbiturates cross the placenta rapidly and can have pronounced neonatal effects lasting for days. These include somnolence, flaccidity, hypoventilation, and failure to feed. Effects are intensified if narcotics are used simultaneously.
   2. **Benzodiazepines (diazepam [Valium], lorazepam [Ativan], midazolam [Versed]).** These agents cross the placenta rapidly and equilibrate within minutes after intravenous administration. Fetal levels are often higher than maternal levels. Diazepam given in low doses (< 10 mg) may cause decreased beat-to-beat variability and tone but has little effect on Apgar scores or blood gas levels. Larger doses of diazepam may persist for days and can cause hypotonia, lethargy, decreased feeding, and impaired thermoregulation, with resulting hypothermia. All benzodiazepines share these features; however, diazepam is the most thoroughly studied of the benzodiazepine series. In addition to the above adverse effects, benzodiazepines are less frequently used because they induce childbirth amnesia in the mother, which can be distressing.
   3. **Phenothiazines.** Phenothiazines are rarely used today, because they may induce hypotension via central alpha blockade. Phenothiazines are sometimes combined with a narcotic ("neuroleptanalgesia"). Innovar, a combination drug containing the narcotic fentanyl and droperidol, may be safe because of the relatively short half-life of the agents.
   4. **Ketamine (Ketaject, many others).** Ketamine may be used for dissociative analgesia or anesthesia. Doses greater than 1 mg/kg may be dangerous, causing neonatal depression and uterine hypotonia. Much smaller doses are normally used in labor (0.1–0.2 mg/kg) and are relatively safe, producing minimal effects in the mother and neonate.

F. **Lumbar epidural analgesia.** Lumbar epidural analgesia is the most frequently used invasive anesthetic technique for childbirth. Lumbar epidural analgesia is safely administered regional anesthesia that may be beneficial to the fetus. Maternal catecholamine levels may be reduced (catecholamines cause prolonged incoordinate labor and decreased uterine blood flow), leading to diminished maternal hyperventilation and improved fetal oxygen delivery. Vasospasm of uterine arteries in pregnancy-induced hypertension may be relieved (Jouppila, 1982; Shnider, 1979).

   Continuous administration of a local anesthetic (eg, bupivicaine, lidocaine) through a catheter placed in the epidural space at the L2 or L3 interspace is usually used. Alternatively, repeated injections through the catheter (so-called topping-off technique) may be used. Epinephrine is sometimes added to prolong the effect and decrease systemic absorption of the agents. Small doses of a narcotic may also be added; these have no effect on the neonate. Maternal hypotension caused by sympathetic blockade is easily treated with fluid administration or small doses of ephedrine given intravenously.

G. **Caudal epidural analgesia.** Caudal epidural analgesia blocks the sacral nerve roots and is excellent for relief of pain in the second stage of labor. There is a high incidence of pelvic floor relaxation with less rotation of the neonate's head. Systemic absorption of anesthetic agents is greater than with lumbar epidural anesthesia. Caudal epidural analgesia is not efficient during the first stage of labor because large doses are needed to block the T11–12 nerve roots. Because of reports of fetal intracranial injections of anesthetic, this technique is becoming less popular.

H. **Saddle block.** Use of saddle block, a form of low spinal block, is decreasing. It is generally safe for the neonate, provided the block stays low to avoid maternal hypotension. In this technique, a spinal anesthetic is given, and the mother sits up so that the hyperbaric agent settles low in the spinal cord around the conus medullaris. Saddle block is best for the second stage of labor.

I. **Local anesthetics.** All of the regional anesthetic/analgesic techniques (eg, epidural, spinal) and local blocks (eg, pudendal) depend on the use of local anesthetic agents. Bupivicaine is the most commonly used agent due to its longer half-life.

1. **Lidocaine (Xylocaine).** Placental transfer of lidocaine is significant, but Apgar scores are usually not affected (Abboud, 1982).

2. **Bupivacaine (Marcaine).** Bupivacaine is theoretically less harmful than lidocaine for the fetus because it has a higher degree of ionization and protein-binding than lidocaine. Reports of maternal toxicity leading to convulsions and cardiac arrest after inadvertent intravascular injection have been reported.

3. **Chloroprocaine (Nesacaine).** After systemic absorption, chloroprocaine is rapidly broken down by pseudocholinesterase, so very little reaches the placenta or fetus. Neurobehavioral studies indicate no difference between controls and neonates whose mothers have been given chloroprocaine. Recent reformulation of this agent may increase its use (the earlier formulation was linked to some cases of neurotoxicity).

4. **Mepivacaine (Carbocaine).** Mepivacaine has been largely abandoned in neonatology because of its adverse effects, in particular, lower neurobehavioral scores and higher fetal serum levels of the agent.

J. **Psychoprophylaxis.** The **Lamaze technique** of prepared childbirth involves instruction in a series of classes for prospective parents. The process of childbirth is explained, and exercises, breathing techniques, and relaxation techniques are taught to relieve labor pain. However, the popular assumption that the neonate benefits if the mother receives no drugs during childbirth is not necessarily justified. Pain and discomfort may cause psychological stress and hyperventilation in the mother and have a profoundly negative impact on the neonate; supplemental anesthesia may be needed. Fifty to 70% of women who have learned the Lamaze method request drugs or an anesthetic block at the time of delivery. **Other psychoprophylaxis techniques** include transcutaneous electric nerve stimulation (TENS), hypnosis, and acupuncture, but these are not currently in widespread use.

III. **Anesthesia for cesarean delivery.** Regional anesthesia is becoming the technique of choice for cesarean deliveries, but in certain circumstances, general anesthesia is used. If *immediate* delivery is needed, general anesthesia is the method of choice because it has the shortest induction time.

However, immediate delivery is usually not mandatory, so regional anesthesia is commonly used.

A. Lumbar epidural anesthesia. Placental transfer of local anesthetics may occur (see above). Maternal hypotension may occur, but preloading the mother with crystalloids usually helps avoid this problem. Use of epidural anesthesia is clearly advantageous to the fetus. There are minimal drug effects, which can be detected only by detailed neurobehavioral testing.

B. Spinal anesthesia. Spinal anesthesia (injection of agent directly into cerebrospinal fluid) uses a lower dose than does epidural anesthesia (infiltration of the epidural space). Maternal and fetal drug levels have been detected but are about one-third those of epidural anesthesia. Hypotension occurs more rapidly and is more difficult to control than with epidural anesthesia. Spinal anesthesia has a shorter induction time than the other regional techniques, so it is preferred for emergency situations. In most studies, the Early Neonatal Neurobehavioral Score (ENNS) (see p 12) is more normal following spinal anesthesia than general anesthesia for cesarean section.

C. General anesthesia. There is a trend away from use of general anesthesia, but it is still used in certain circumstances. These include strong patient preference, emergency delivery (eg, in cases of hemorrhage, cord prolapse, or fetal distress), and contraindications to regional anesthesia (eg, maternal coagulopathy, fetal neurologic problems, sepsis, or infection).

After induction of anesthesia, the mother is usually maintained on a combination of nitrous oxide and oxygen with low doses of other agents such as halothane. Narcotics or benzodiazepines are rarely given until the cord is clamped.

1. Agents used in general obstetric anesthesia

    a. Surgical premedication. Premedications traditionally used in surgery are rarely given. Atropinics (used to decrease oral secretions) are seldom used. Glycopyrrolate (Robinul) crosses the placenta much less readily than atropine or scopolamine. Fetal tachycardia and loss of beat-to-beat variability may occur. Cimetidine (Tagamet) and ranitidine (Zantac) (H_2 receptor antagonists) are used by some to decrease gastric volume and increase the pH of gastric secretions as prophylaxis against aspiration pneumonitis. The neonate is not affected by these agents.

    b. Thiopental (Pentothal). Thiopental, up to 4 mg/kg, is used for induction of general anesthesia. This dosage exposes the fetus to low concentrations, which are usually achieved within 2–3 minutes. Metabolites may affect fetal brain waves (as seen on EEG) for several days and depress the sucking response. Fetal outcome, as measured by Apgar scoring, is not affected by doses of less than 4 mg/kg.

    c. Ketamine. Ketamine is used in doses of less than 1 mg/kg for induction of anesthesia. Neonatal neurobehavioral test scores are slightly better than those of infants of mothers who received thiopental.

    d. Muscle relaxants. Muscle relaxants, which are highly ionized, cross the placenta in small amounts and have little effect on the neonate.

        (1) Succinylcholine (Anectine, many others) crosses the placenta in minimal amounts. In twice-normal doses, it is detectable in the fetus, but no respiratory effects are seen until the dose is 5 times normal.

        (2) Pancuronium (Pavulon) and tubocurarine (Tubarine) do not affect the neonate. These agents are currently rarely used.

(3) Atracurium (Tracrium) and vecuronium (Norcuron) are fairly new agents that are shorter acting. Atracurium may be safer due to its spontaneous degradation, not relying on renal or hepatic clearance.

  e. **Nitrous oxide** has rapid placental transfer. With inhaled concentrations of greater than 50% nitrous oxide, fetal outcome is proportionate to the interval between induction and delivery (the longer the interval, the worse the fetal status). Prolonged administration of high concentrations of nitrous oxide results in low Apgar scores because of central nervous system depression and perfusion hypoxia. Concentrations of up to 50% are safe, but neonates need supplemental oxygen after delivery, especially if the interval between induction and delivery is long.

  f. **Halogenated anesthetic agents (enflurane [Ethrane], halothane [Fluothane])** are used to maintain general anesthesia. Beneficial effects include decreased catecholamines and increased uterine blood flow when compared to nitrous oxide alone. Low concentrations of these agents usually do not cause neonatal depression. If depression is seen, it is usually transient, since these volatile agents are readily excreted. These agents cause much more neonatal respiratory depression in compromised fetuses. Higher doses may halt labor by causing decreased uterine contractility (Crawford, 1984). When used, the lowest effective level is chosen and the agent is promptly discontinued at the point of delivery to help decrease uterine atony and further blood loss.

2. **Neonatal effects of general anesthesia.** Failure of endotracheal intubation or aspiration with associated maternal hypoxia can cause deleterious fetal effects. Maternal hyperventilation ($Paco_2 < 20$ mm Hg) leads to fetal hypoxia and acidosis because of decreased placental blood flow and a shift in the oxyhemoglobin curve. Aortocaval compression may occur during general anesthesia, resulting in decreased placental perfusion (the mother should be positioned with the left side slightly tilted down to help prevent this). Intubation will increase oxygen saturation of maternal blood up to 300 mm Hg; this will increase oxygen tension and saturation of fetal blood.

3. **Interval between incision of the uterus and delivery.** Incision and manipulation of the uterus cause reflex uterine vasoconstriction, resulting in fetal asphyxia. Long intervals between incision and delivery (> 90 seconds) are associated with significant lowering of Apgar scores. If the interval is longer than 180 seconds, lower Apgar scores and fetal acidosis occur in both regional and general anesthesia (Datta, 1981). Epidural blockade may decrease reflex vasoconstriction, so the length of the interval is of less importance. The interval may be prolonged with breech delivery, multiple delivery, or preterm delivery; if there is scarring of the uterus due to a previous delivery or operation; or if the fetus is large.

4. **Regional versus general anesthesia**

  a. **Apgar scores.** Early studies showed that neonates were less depressed on 1- and 5-minute Apgar scores with regional than with general anesthesia (Benson, 1965). Refinements in general anesthetic techniques lower Apgar scores at 1 minute only. This probably represents transient sedation rather than asphyxia. If the interval between induction and delivery is short, there is less difference between the effects of regional and general anesthesia. If a prolonged delivery time is anticipated, regional anesthesia is preferred because it is less harmful to the neonate.

  b. **Acid-base status.** The differences in acid-base status are minimal and probably not significant. Infants of diabetic mothers may be

less acidotic with general than with regional anesthesia, particularly spinal anesthesia, because of the higher incidence of hypotension with regional anesthesia and exacerbation of uteroplacental insufficiency seen in diabetics.
   c. **Neurobehavioral examinations** are used to detect subtle changes in the neonate in the first few hours after birth that may be missed by Apgar scoring or acid-base assessment. After delivery, there is a 1-hour period of alertness, followed by a 3- to 4-hour period of deep sleep and decreased responsiveness. The **Early Neonatal Neurobehavioral Score (ENNS)** was initially developed to detect neurobehavioral changes 2–8 hours after birth (the half-life of most local anesthetics). These changes are usually manifested as decreased tone or decrement in an otherwise alert infant. The **Neonatal Neurologic and Adaptive Capacity Score (NNACS)** uses portions of the ENNS, Brazelton Neonatal Behavioral Assessment Scale, and Amiel-Tison Neurologic Examination. This score is more weighted toward assessment of neonatal tone and is helpful in differentiating abnormalities caused by birth trauma rather than depression. Early neurobehavioral examinations show clear-cut advantages of regional over general anesthesia. Although infants of mothers receiving spinal and epidural anesthesia had similar results at 15 minutes, by 2 hours the epidural group had lower scores. This probably reflects higher local anesthetic uptake. However, there are no significant differences in long-term studies comparing regional and general anesthesia.

RESUSCITATION OF THE NEWBORN

Approximately 3.5 million infants are born in the USA each year in about 5000 hospitals, only 15% of which have neonatal intensive care facilities (Standards and Guidelines for Cardiopulmonary Resuscitation and Emergency Cardiac Care, 1986). Six percent of newborns require some form of resuscitation. This cannot always be anticipated in time to transfer the mother before delivery to a facility with specialized neonatal support. Therefore, every hospital with a delivery suite should have an organized, skilled resuscitation team and appropriate equipment available (Table 2–1) (Ballard, 1984; Bloom, Cropley, 1987).
   I. **Normal physiologic events at birth.** Normal transitional events at birth begin with initial lung expansion, generally requiring large, negative intrathoracic pressures, followed by a cry (expiration against a partially closed glottis). Umbilical cord clamping is accompanied by a rise in blood pressure and massive stimulation of the sympathetic nervous system. With onset of respiration and lung expansion, pulmonary vascular resistance falls, followed by a gradual (over minutes to hours) transition from fetal to adult circulation, with closure of the foramen ovale and ductus arteriosus.
   II. **Abnormal physiologic events at birth.** The asphyxiated newborn infant undergoes an abnormal transition. A rhesus monkey model has been used to study changes in physiologic parameters during asphyxiation and resuscitation (Dawes, 1968). Shortly after acute asphyxiation (the cord is clamped while the head is held in a bag filled with saline), the monkey fetus has **primary apnea,** during which spontaneous respirations can be induced by appropriate sensory stimuli. This lasts for about 1 minute, and the fetus then begins deep gasping for 4–5 minutes, ending with the "last gasp." This is followed by a period of **secondary apnea,** during which spontaneous respirations cannot be induced by sensory stimuli. Death occurs if secondary apnea is not reversed by vigorous ventilatory support within several minutes. Because one can never be certain whether an apneic newborn has primary or secondary apnea, resuscitative efforts should proceed

TABLE 2-1. EQUIPMENT FOR NEONATAL RESUSCITATION

STANDARD EQUIPMENT SETUP
Radiant warmer
Stethoscope
Oxygen source with warmer and humidifier
Suction source, suction catheter, DeLee trap
Nasogastric tubes
Apparatus for bag-and-mask ventilation
Ventilation masks
Laryngoscope (handles, blades, and batteries)
Endotracheal tubes (2.5, 3, 3.5, and 4.0 mm)
Intravenous fluids (10% dextrose, normal saline, Ringer's lactate)
Drugs:
  Epinephrine (1:10,000 solution)
  Naloxone hydrochloride (0.4 mg/mL or 1.0 mg/mL)
  Sodium bicarbonate (0.5 meq/mL)
  Volume expanders (5% albumin, O-negative whole blood [cross-matched against the mother's blood])
Clock
Syringes, hypodermic needles, and tubes for collection of blood samples
Equipment for umbilical vessel catheterization
Micro blood gas analysis availability
Warm blankets
ADDITIONAL EQUIPMENT SETUP
All of the above plus the following:
  Pressure manometer for use during ventilation
  Oxygen blender
  Heart rate and blood gas monitoring equipment
  Umbilical vessel catheter setup (ready to insert)
  Transcutaneous oxygen tension or saturation monitor
  Blood gas laboratory immediately available
  Apgar timer
  Camera

as though secondary apnea were present. This experimental model of acute total asphyxia is comparable to asphyxia in an infant with umbilical cord prolapse. A more common clinical occurrence is prolonged partial asphyxia (eg, with maternal hemorrhage or severe placental insufficiency). Resuscitative measures are the same for both situations. The outcome is often worse following prolonged partial asphyxia in utero (Brann, 1967).

III. **Preparation for high-risk delivery.** Preparation for high-risk delivery is often the key to a successful outcome. Cooperation between the obstetric staff and the pediatric staff is important. Knowledge of potential high-risk situations and appropriate interventions is essential (Table 2-2). It is useful to have an estimation of weight and gestational age, so that drug dosages can be calculated and the appropriate endotracheal tube and umbilical

TABLE 2-2. SOME HIGH-RISK SITUATIONS FOR WHICH RESUSCITATION MAY BE ANTICIPATED

High-Risk Situation	Primary Intervention
Preterm delivery	Intubation, lung expansion
Thick meconium	Endotracheal suction
Maternal hemorrhage	Volume expansion
Use of narcotics in labor	Administration of naloxone
Hydrops fetalis	Intubation, paracentesis, and/or thoracentesis
Polyhydramnios: gastrointestinal obstruction	Nasogastric suction
Oligohydramnios: pulmonary hypoplasia	Intubation, lung expansion
Maternal infection	Administration of antibiotics
Maternal diabetes	Early glucose administration

catheter size chosen (Table 2–3). While waiting for the infant to arrive, it is useful to think through potential problems, steps that may be undertaken to correct them, and which member of the team will handle each step.

IV. **Assessment of need for resuscitation.** The Apgar score (Appendix B) is assigned at 1, 5, and, occasionally, 10–20 minutes after delivery. It gives a fairly objective retrospective idea of how much resuscitation a term infant required at birth and how it responded to resuscitative efforts. It is not particularly useful during resuscitation. During those long, tense moments, assessment of heart rate, skin color, and respiratory activity provides the quickest and most accurate evaluation of the need for continuing resuscitation. For preterm infants, Apgar scores may be particularly misleading, even in assessment of response to resuscitation, because of developmental differences in tone and response to stimulation.

   A. **Heart rate.** The heart rate is ideally monitored by a cardiotachometer via electrodes taped to the chest. Most often, however, evaluation is done by listening to the apical beat or feeling the pulse by lightly grasping the base of the umbilical cord. The evaluator should tap out each beat so that all team members can hear it. If no heart rate can be heard or felt, ventilatory efforts should be halted for a few seconds so that this finding can be verified by another team member.

   B. **Skin color.** Assessment of skin color may be difficult when there is severe bruising, especially in preterm infants. Marked acrocyanosis may also complicate the picture. Looking at the mucous membranes of the mouth may be helpful under these circumstances. Bluish coloring indicates central cyanosis; oxygen supplementation or assisted ventilation is needed. Pinkish membranes indicate normal oxygen levels, and resuscitation may not be needed.

   C. **Respiratory activity.** Assessment of respiratory activity is made by observing chest movement or listening for breath sounds. If there is no respiratory effort or the effort is poor, the infant needs respiratory assistance, either by manual stimulation or bag-and-mask ventilation.

V. **Technique of resuscitation**

   A. **Ventilatory resuscitation**

      1. **General measures**

         a. **Suctioning.** First, nasal and oropharyngeal secretions should be partially removed with a brief period of suctioning, either with a bulb syringe, a suction catheter, or a DeLee trap. More prolonged suctioning delays resuscitation and may cause a profound vagal response in the infant (Cordero, 1971).

         b. **Mechanical ventilation.** Most infants can be adequately ventilated with a bag and mask, provided that the mask is the correct size with a close seal around the mouth and nose and provided there is appropriate flow of oxygen to the bag (Fig 2–1). The stom-

TABLE 2–3. EXPECTED BIRTH WEIGHT (50TH PERCENTILE) AT 24–38 WEEKS' GESTATION

Gestational Age (weeks)	Birth Weight (g)
24	700
26	900
28	1100
30	1350
32	1650
34	2100
36	2600
38	3000

Modified and reproduced, with permission, from Battaglia FC, Lubchenco LO: A practical classification of newborn infants by weight and gestational age. *J Pediatr* 1967;**71**:159.

FIGURE 2-1. Bag-and-mask ventilation of the neonate.

ach should be emptied during and after bag-and-mask ventilation.

c. **Endotracheal intubation.** Endotracheal intubation should be performed when indicated. However, multiple unsuccessful attempts at intubation by inexperienced persons may make a bad situation worse, and in such situations, it may be best to continue mask ventilation until experienced help arrives. Absolute indications for aggressive ventilatory support with endotracheal intubation are difficult to list here, since institutional guidelines and clinical situations vary widely. The procedure for endotracheal intubation and some general guidelines are discussed in Chapter 20.

2. **Specific measures**

a. **Term infant with meconium staining.** Infants born through thick meconium may aspirate meconium. These may be the most critically ill infants in the intensive care nursery. Gregory and associates (1974) were among the first to show that endotracheal suctioning could be lifesaving for such infants. Meconium aspiration is discussed in detail in Chapter 69.

   (1) **Hypopharyngeal suctioning should be started as soon as the head is delivered, before the infant has started to cry.**

   (2) **Endotracheal suctioning.** Subsequently, **endotracheal intubation is performed and suction applied directly to the endotracheal tube.** Suctioning can be done directly from the wall unit via a connector to the endotracheal tube, or a suction catheter can be attached to the wall suction unit and inserted down the endotracheal tube. Suction is applied as the endotracheal tube is slowly withdrawn.

   The presence of thin or watery meconium in the amniotic fluid indicates that the fetus may have been in distress at some time. This type of fluid may not cause airway obstruction, and endotracheal intubation may not be routinely required.

(3) If meconium has been suctioned "below the cords," suctioning should be repeated after reintubation.

(4) The procedures described above may continue for up to 2 minutes after delivery if needed, but other resuscitative measures (particularly, ventilation and oxygenation) must then begin.

(5) **Supplemental oxygen.** Infants born through thick meconium may have experienced prolonged partial asphyxia in utero and may have developed pulmonary vascular constriction, leading to pulmonary hypertension after delivery. It is wise, therefore, to provide generous amounts of supplemental oxygen to these infants.

b. **Term infant with perinatal asphyxia**

   (1) **A term infant with a heart rate of less than 100 beats/min and no spontaneous respiratory activity needs immediate lung expansion and supplemental oxygen provided by bag-and-mask ventilation.** Initially, the lungs should be slowly expanded (5–10 breaths) with peak inflating pressures of 25–30 cm water. If this is not successful in stimulating spontaneous respiratory effort or an improved heart rate, the ventilation rate should be increased to 40–60 breaths/min and peak inflating pressures maintained as high as necessary to expand the lungs. If bag-and-mask ventilation is ineffective or if prolonged positive-pressure ventilation is necessary, endotracheal intubation is indicated. If effective spontaneous respiratory effort results, the infant may be extubated and closely observed while breathing supplemental oxygen.

   (2) **A term infant with a heart rate of more than 100 beats/min but with poor skin color and weak respiratory activity requires stimulation (rubbing the back is often effective), supplemental oxygen blown across the face, and, occasionally, bag-and-mask ventilation to expand the lungs.** Most of these infants will respond with improved skin color and good spontaneous respiratory effort by 5 minutes of age.

c. **Preterm infant.** Preterm infants weighing less than 1200 g most often require immediate lung expansion in the delivery room. Ventilatory support measures should proceed as described for the asphyxiated term infant, with several important differences:

   (1) If intubation is required, a smaller endotracheal tube is selected (2.5 or 3 mm internal diameter).

   (2) Although high peak inflating pressures may initially be needed to expand the lungs, as soon as the lungs "open up," the pressure should be quickly decreased to as low as 10–15 cm of water by the end of the resuscitation if the clinical course permits.

   (3) If available, one of several forms of liquid surfactant may be administered intratracheally as prophylaxis for hyaline membrane disease (see Chap 13).

B. **Cardiac resuscitation.** During delivery room resuscitation, efforts should be directed first to assisting ventilation and providing supplemental oxygen. A sluggish heart rate will usually respond to these efforts.

1. **If the heart rate continues to be less than 60 beats/min by 1 minute of age, chest compression should be initiated.** The thumbs are placed on the mid sternum just below a line connecting the nipples, while the palms of the hands encircle the torso and support the back (Fig 2–2). The sternum is compressed ½–¾ inch (1.3–1.9 cm) at a regular rate of 120 compressions/min. The heart rate should be

FIGURE 2-2. Technique of external cardiac massage (chest compression) in the neonate. Note the position of the thumbs on the mid sternum, just below the level of the nipples.

checked periodically and chest compression discontinued when the heart rate is > 80 beats/min.

2. **An infant born with no heart rate who does not respond to ventilation and oxygenation may be considered stillborn. Further resuscitative efforts for these infants are a matter of ethical consideration.**

C. **Drugs used in resuscitation.** (See also Emergency Drugs, Inside Front and Back Covers.) The AAP's *Textbook of Neonatal Resuscitation* recommends giving medications if the heart rate remains less than 80 beats/min despite adequate ventilation and chest compressions for a minimum of 30 seconds.

1. **Route of administration**
   a. **The umbilical vein** is the preferred route for drug administration in the delivery room. A 3.5F or 5F umbilical catheter should be inserted just until blood is easily withdrawn (usually less than 5 cm); this should avoid inadvertent placement in the hepatic or portal vein.
   b. **Alternate routes** of administration include peripheral venous, interosseous, and intratracheal.

2. **Drugs**
   a. **Epinephrine** may be necessary during resuscitation when adequate ventilation, oxygenation, and chest compression have failed and the heart rate is still less than 80 beats/min. This drug causes peripheral vasoconstriction, enhances cardiac contractility, and increases the heart rate. The dose is 0.1–0.3 mL/kg of 1:10,000 solution given intravenously or by endotracheal tube. This may be repeated every 5 minutes. If an endotracheal tube is used, the solution should be diluted 1:1 with normal saline.

    b. Volume expanders. Hypovolemia should be suspected in any infant requiring resuscitation, particularly when there is evidence of acute blood loss with extreme pallor despite adequate oxygenation, poor peripheral pulse rates despite a normal heart rate, long capillary refill times, or poor response to resuscitative efforts. Appropriate volume expanders include O-negative whole blood (cross-matched against the mother's blood), 10 mL/kg; 5% albumin, 10 mL/kg; Ringer's lactate and normal saline, 10 mL/kg. All are given intravenously over a 5- to 10-minute period.

    c. Naloxone hydrochloride. Naloxone (Narcan) is a narcotic antagonist and should be administered to an infant with respiratory depression unresponsive to ventilatory assistance whose mother has received narcotics within 4 hours before delivery. One major exception to this recommendation is the newborn infant of a drug-addicted mother. These infants should never receive Narcan because acute withdrawal symptoms may develop. The AAP has recently issued a change in the dosage of Narcan (*Pediatrics* 1989;**83**:803). The new intravenous or intratracheal dosage for Narcan is 0.1 mg/kg. Two concentrations of naloxone are available: 0.4 mg/mL and 1.0 mg/mL. Neonatal Narcan (0.02 mg/mL) is no longer available. The dose may be repeated every 5 minutes as necessary.

    d. Dextrose. Dextrostix should be checked within 30 minutes after delivery in asphyxiated term infants, infants of diabetic mothers, and preterm infants, especially those whose mothers received tocolysis with ritodrine. Large boluses of dextrose should be avoided, even when the Dextrostix reading is less than 25 mg/dL. It is preferable to avoid wide glucose swings by giving a small bolus of 10% dextrose (2–4 mL/kg intravenously) and then beginning an infusion of 10% dextrose at a rate of 6 mg/kg/min (100 mL/kg/d).

    e. Sodium bicarbonate is usually not useful during the acute phase of neonatal resuscitation. Without adequate ventilation and oxygenation, it will not improve the blood pH. After prolonged resuscitation, however, sodium bicarbonate may be useful in correcting documented metabolic acidosis. Give 1–2 meq/kg intravenously (usually over a period of 20 minutes).

    f. Atropine and calcium. Although previously used during resuscitation of the asphyxiated newborn, atropine and calcium are no longer recommended by the AAP or AHA. Current evidence does not support their effectiveness during delivery room resuscitation.

D. Other supportive measures

  1. Temperature regulation. Although some degree of cooling in a newborn infant is desirable because it provides a normal stimulus to respiratory effort, excessive cooling increases oxygen consumption and exacerbates acidosis. This is a problem especially with preterm infants, who have thin skin, decreased stores of body fat, and an increased body surface area. Heat loss may be prevented by the following measures.

    a. Dry the infant thoroughly immediately after delivery.

    b. Maintain a warm delivery room.

    c. Place the infant under a prewarmed radiant warmer. See also Chapter 5.

  2. Preparation of the parents for resuscitation. Initial resuscitation usually occurs in the delivery room with one or both parents present. It is helpful to prepare the parents in advance, if possible. Describe what will be done, who will be present, who will explain what is happening, where the resuscitation will take place, where the father should stand, and why crying may not be heard.

REFERENCES

Abboud TK et al: Maternal, fetal, and neonatal responses after epidural anesthesia with bupivacaine, 2-chloroprocaine, or lidocaine. *Anesth Analg* 1982;**61**:638.

Ballard RA: Neonatal resuscitation. Pages 689–692 in: *Current Pediatric Therapy*, 11th ed. Gellis SS, Kagan BM (editors). Saunders, 1984.

Benson RC et al: Fetal compromise during elective cesarean section. *Am J Obstet Gynecol* 1965;**91**:645.

Bloom RS, Cropley C: *Textbook of Neonatal Resuscitation*. American Heart Association, American Academy of Pediatrics, 1987. Pages 1–37.

Cordero L Jr, Hon EH: Neonatal bradycardia following nasopharyngeal stimulation. *J Pediatr* 1971;**78**:441.

Crawford JS: Caesarean section. Chapter 5 in: *Principles and Practice of Obstetric Anesthesia*, 5th ed. Blackwell, 1984.

Datta S et al: Neonatal effect of prolonged anesthetic induction for cesarean section. *Obstet Gynecol* 1981;**58**:331.

Dawes GS: *Foetal & Neonatal Physiology*. Year Book, 1968.

Dubowitz LM et al: Clinical assessment of gestational age in the newborn infant. *J Pediatr* 1970;**77**:1.

Gregory GA et al: Meconium aspiration in infants: A prospective study. *J Pediatr* 1974;**85**:848.

Jouppila P et al: Lumbar epidural analgesia to improve intervillous blood flow during labor in severe preeclampsia. *Obstet Gynecol* 1982;**59**:158.

Kuhnert BR et al: Effects of low doses of meperidine on neonatal behavior. *Anesth Analg* 1985;**64**:335.

Lindemann R: Endotracheal administration of epinephrine during cardiopulmonary resuscitation. (Letter.) *Am J Dis Child* 1982;**136**:753.

Moore J, McNabb TG, Glynn JP: The placental transfer of pentazocine and pethidine. *Br J Anaesth* 1973;**45(Suppl)**:798.

Ravlo O et al: A randomized comparison between midazolam and thiopental for elective cesarean section anesthesia: II. Neonates. *Anesth Analg* 1989;**68**:234.

Sepkoski CM: Neonatal neurobehavior: Development and its relation to obstetric anesthesia. *Clin Anaesthesiol* 1986;**4**:209.

Shnider SM, Moya F: Effects of meperidine on the newborn infant. *Am J Obstet Gynecol* 1964;**89**:1009.

Shnider SM et al: Uterine blood flow and plasma norepinephrine changes during maternal stress in the pregnant ewe. *Anesthesiology* 1979;**50**:524.

Standards and guidelines for cardiopulmonary resuscitation and emergency cardiac care. 6. Neonatal advanced life support. *JAMA* 1986;**255**:2969.

Usher R et al: Judgment of fetal age. 2. Clinical significance of gestational age and objective measurement. *Pediatr Clin North Am* 1966;**13**:835.

3 Assessment of Gestational Age

Gestational age can be determined prenatally by means of the techniques discussed in Chapter 1. Techniques for determining gestational age in the immediate postnatal period are discussed in this chapter.

I. **Classification.** Infants are classified as **preterm (< 38 weeks), term (38–42 weeks),** or **postterm (> 42 weeks).** Refinements developed in neonatal assessment have provided additional classifications based on a combination of features.

   A. **Small for gestational age (SGA)** is defined as 2 standard deviations below the mean weight for gestational age or below the 10th percentile (see Appendix G). See Chapter 64, Intrauterine Growth Retardation, for a full discussion. SGA is commonly seen in infants of mothers with hypertension or preeclampsia, and those who smoke. It is also associated with TORCH infections (see p 339), chromosomal abnormalities, and other congenital malformations.

   B. **Appropriate for gestational age (AGA).** See Appendix G.

   C. **Large for gestational age (LGA)** is defined as 2 standard deviations above the mean weight for gestational age or above the 90th percentile (see Appendix G). LGA can be seen in infants of diabetic mothers (see Chap 62), in infants with Beckwith's syndrome, in constitutionally large infants with large parents, or in infants with hydrops fetalis (see p 267).

II. **Methods of determining postnatal gestational age**

   A. **Rapid delivery room assessment.** The clinical signs most useful in differentiating the premature from borderline mature from full-term infants are (in order of usefulness) creases on the sole of the foot, size of the breast nodule, nature of the hair, cartilaginous development of the earlobe, and scrotal rugae and testicular descent in males. These signs and findings are listed in Table 3–1, which enables one to make a rapid assessment at delivery.

   B. **Ballard examination.** The Ballard examination is best performed 30–42 hours after delivery, with the infant in the supine position.

      1. **Accuracy.** The examination is accurate, whether or not the infant is sick or well, to within 2 weeks of gestational age.

      2. **Criteria.** The examination consists of 6 neuromuscular criteria and 6 physical criteria. The neuromuscular criteria are based on the understanding that passive tone is more useful than active tone in indicating gestational age.

      3. **Procedure.** The examination is administered twice by 2 separate examiners to ensure objectivity, and the data is entered on the **Newborn Maturity Rating and Classification Form** (Fig 3–1), available in most nurseries. The "First Exam and Second Exam" designations refer to the 2 independent examiners. The exam consists of 2 parts, **Neuromuscular Maturity** and **Physical Maturity.** The 12 scores are totaled and maturity rating is expressed in weeks of gestation, estimated by using the chart provided on the form. Part 2 of the form (Fig 3–2) is then used to plot gestational assessment against length, height, and head circumference to determine if the baby is SGA, AGA, or LGA. These are the so-called **Lubchenco charts.**

         a. **Neuromuscular maturity**

TABLE 3-1. CRITERIA FOR RAPID GESTATIONAL ASSESSMENT AT DELIVERY

	36 Weeks and Earlier	37–38 Weeks	39 Weeks and Beyond
Creases in soles of feet	One of 2 transverse creases; posterior three-fourths of sole smooth	Multiple creases; anterior two-thirds of heel smooth	Entire sole covered with creases, including heel
Breast nodule*	2 mm	4 mm	7 mm
Scalp hair	Fine and woolly; fuzzy	Fine and woolly; fuzzy	Coarse and silky; each hair single-stranded
Earlobe	No cartilage	Moderate amount of cartilage	Stiff earlobe with thick cartilage
Testes and scrotum	Testes partially descended; scrotum small, with few rugae	?	Testes fully descended; scrotum normal size, with prominent rugae

*The breast nodule is not palpable before 33 weeks. Underweight full-term infants may have retarded breast development.
Modified and reproduced, with permission, from Usher R, McClean F, Scott KB: Judgment of fetal age. *Pediatr Clin North Am* 1986;3:835.

FIGURE 3-1. Newborn maturity rating and classification. (Reproduced, with permission, from Ballard JL et al: A simplified assessment of gestational age. *Pediatr Res* 1977;11:374.)

(1) **Posture.** Score 0 if the arms and legs are extended, 1 beginning flexion of the knees and hips, arms extended; other degrees scored are based on the diagram.

(2) **Square window.** Flex the hand on the forearm between the thumb and index finger of the examiner. Apply sufficient pressure to get as much flexion as possible. Visually measure the angle between the hypothenar eminence and the ventral aspect of the forearm. Determine the score based on the diagram.

(3) **Arm recoil.** Flex the forearms for 5 seconds; then grasp the hand and fully extend the arm and release. If the arm returns to full flexion, a score of 4 is given. For lesser degrees of flexion, score as noted on the diagram.

(4) **Popliteal angle.** The thigh is held in the knee-chest position by the examiner's left index finger and the thumb supporting the knee. The leg is then extended by gentle pressure from the right index finger behind the ankle. Measure the angle at the popliteal space and score accordingly.

FIGURE 3–2. Classification of newborns based on maturity and intrauterine growth. (X = first examination; O = second examination.) (Modified and reproduced, with permission, from Lubchenco LC, Hansman C, Boyd E: *Pediatrics* 1966;**37**:403; and Battaglia FC, Lubchenco LC: *J Pediatr* 1967;**71**:159.)

(5) **Scarf sign.** Take the infant's hand and try to put it around the neck posteriorly as far as possible over the opposite shoulder and score according to the diagram.

(6) **Heel to ear.** Keeping the pelvis flat on the table, take the infant's foot and try to put it as close to the head as possible without forcing it. Grade according to the diagram.

b. **Physical maturity.** These characteristics are scored as shown in Figure 3–1. Lanugo hair is examined on the infant's back, between and over the scapulae.

C. **Direct ophthalmoscopy.** Another method for determination of gestational age uses direct ophthalmoscopy of the lens. Prior to 27 weeks, the cornea is too opaque to allow visualization; after 34 weeks there is atrophy of the vessels of the lens. Therefore, this technique allows for accurate determination of gestational age at 27–34 weeks only. The pupil must be dilated under the supervision of an opthalmologist, and the assessment must be done within 24 hours of birth, before the vessels atrophy. The following grading system is used (Fig 3–3).

Grade 4: 27–28 weeks. Vessels cover the entire anterior surface of the lens or the vessels meet in the center of the lens.

FIGURE 3-3. Grading system for assessment of gestational age by examination of the anterior vascular capsule of the lens. (Reproduced, with permission, from Hittner HM, Hirsch NJ, Rudolph AJ: Assessment of gestational age by examination of the anterior vascular capsule of the lens. *J Pediatr* 1977;**91**:455.)

Grade 3: 29–30 weeks. Vessels do not meet in the center but are close. Central portion of the lens is not covered by vessels.

Grade 2: 31–32 weeks. Vessels go only to the middle-outer part of lens. The central clear portion of the lens is larger.

Grade 1: 33–34 weeks. Vessels are seen only at the periphery of the lens.

REFERENCES

Amiel-Tison C: Neurological evaluation of the maturity of newborn infants. *Arch Dis Child* 1968;**43**:89.

Ballard JL, Novak KK, Driver M: A simplified score for assessment of fetal maturation of newly born infants. *J Pediatr* 1979;**95**:769.

Dubowitz LM et al: Clinical assessment of gestational age in the newborn infant. *J Pediatr* 1970;**77**:1.

Farr V et al: The definition of some external characteristics used in the assessment of gestational age in the newborn infant. *Dev Med Child Neurol* 1966;**8**:657.

Hittner HM, Hirsch NJ, Rudolph AJ: Assessment of gestational age by examination of the anterior vascular capsule of the lens. *J Pediatr* 1977;**91**:455.

Usher R et al: Judgement of fetal age: 2. Clinical significance of gestational age and objective measurement. *Pediatr Clin North Am* 1966;**13**:835.

4 Newborn Physical Examination

The newborn infant should be examined within 24 hours of birth. It is easier to listen to the heart and lungs first while the infant is quiet.

I. **Vital signs**
   A. **Temperature.** Indicate if the temperature is rectal (which is usually 1 degree higher than oral), oral, or axillary (which is usually 1 degree lower than oral).
   B. **Respirations.** The normal respiratory rate in a newborn is 40–50 breaths/min.
   C. **Blood pressure.** See Appendix C for normal blood pressure curves.
   D. **Pulse rate.** The normal rate is 100–180 beats/min (bpm) in the newborn (usually 120–160 bpm awake, 70–80 bpm while sleeping).

II. **Head circumference, length, weight, and gestational age**
   A. **Head circumference and percentile** (see Appendix G, Growth Charts). Place the measuring tape around the front of the head, above the brow (the frontal area), to the occipital area. The tape should be above the ears. It is known as the occipitofrontal circumference. The normal is 32–37 cm at term.
   B. **Length, percentile** (see Growth Charts, Appendix G).
   C. **Weight, percentile** (see Growth Charts, Appendix G).
   D. **Assessment of gestational age** (see Chap 3).

III. **General appearance.** Observe the infant and record the general appearance (eg, activity, skin color, obvious congenital abnormalities).

IV. **Skin**
   A. **Color**
      1. **Plethora (deep, rosy red color).** Plethora is more common in infants with polycythemia but can be seen in an overoxygenated or overheated infant. It is best to obtain a central hematocrit on any plethoric infant.
      2. **Jaundice (yellowish color).** With jaundice, bilirubin levels are usually greater than 5 mg/dL. It is abnormal in infants less than 24 hours old and may signify Rh incompatibility, sepsis, and TORCH infections (see p 339). After 24 hours, it may be due to the above diseases, but the more common cause is either ABO incompatibility or physiologic causes.
      3. **Pallor (washed-out, white appearance).** Pallor may be secondary to anemia, birth asphyxia, shock, or patent ductus arteriosus. **Ductal pallor** is the term sometimes used to denote pallor associated with patent ductus arteriosus.
      4. **Cyanosis**
         a. **Central cyanosis (bluish skin, including the tongue and lips).** Central cyanosis is caused by low oxygen saturation in the blood. It may be associated with congenital heart or lung disease.
         b. **Peripheral cyanosis (bluish skin with pink lips and tongue).** Peripheral cyanosis may be associated with methemoglobinemia. **Methemoglobinemia** occurs when hemoglobin oxidizes from the ferrous to the ferric form, and the blood actually can have a chocolate hue. Methemoglobin is incapable of transporting oxygen or carbon dioxide. This disorder can be caused

by exposure to certain drugs or chemicals (nitrates or nitrites) or may be hereditary (eg, NADH-methemoglobin reductase deficiency, hemoglobin M disease). Treatment is with either ascorbic acid or methylene blue.

   c. **Acrocyanosis (bluish hands and feet only).** Acrocyanosis may be normal for an infant that has just been born (or within the first few hours after birth) or one that is experiencing cold stress. Consider decreased peripheral perfusion secondary to hypovolemia if seen in an older infant with a normal temperature.

5. **Extensive bruising** may be associated with a prolonged and difficult delivery and may result in early jaundice.

6. **"Blue on pink" or "pink on blue."** Some infants are pink and well perfused, and others are clearly cyanotic, but some do not fit either of these categories. These infants may appear bluish with pink undertones or pink with bluish undertones. This may be secondary to poor perfusion, inadequate oxygenation, inadequate ventilation, or polycythemia.

7. **Harlequin coloration (clear line of demarcation between an area of redness and an area of normal coloration).** The cause is usually unknown. The coloration can be benign and transient (usually less than 20 minutes duration), or it can be indicative of shunting of blood (persistent pulmonary hypertension, coarctation of the aorta). There can be varying degrees of redness and perfusion. The demarcating line may run from the head to the belly, dividing the body into right and left halves, or it may develop in the dependent half of the body when the newborn is lying on one side.

8. **Mottling (lacy red pattern)** may be seen in a normal infant or one with cold stress, hypovolemia, or sepsis. Persistent mottling, referred to as **cutis marmorata,** is seen in infants with Down's syndrome, trisomy 13, or trisomy 18.

B. **Rashes**

1. **Milia.** Milia is a rash in which tiny sebaceous retention cysts are seen. They appear as whitish, pinhead-sized concretions and are usually on the chin, nose, forehead, and cheeks. These cysts are benign and disappear within a few weeks.

2. **Erythema toxicum.** In erythema toxicum, numerous small areas of red skin are seen, with a yellowish white papule in the center. Lesions are most noticeable at 48 hours but may appear as late as 7–10 days. Wright's staining of the papule will reveal eosinophils. The rash resolves spontaneously.

3. *Candida albicans. Candida albicans* diaper rash appears as erythematous plaques with sharply demarcated edges. Satellite bodies (pustules on contiguous areas of skin) are also seen. Usually the skin folds are involved. Gram's stain of a smear or 10% potassium hydroxide preparation of the lesion reveals budding yeast spores, which are easily treated with Nystatin ointment or cream applied to the rash 4 times daily for 7–10 days.

4. **Neonatal pustular melanosis** is characterized by 3 different stages of lesions that may appear over the entire body: pustules, ruptured vesicopustules with scaling, and hyperpigmented macules. It is a benign, self-limiting lesion that requires no specific therapy.

5. **Acne neonatorum.** The lesions are typically seen over the cheeks, chin, and forehead and consist of comedones and papules. The condition is usually benign and requires no therapy; however, severe cases may require treatment with mild keratolytic agents, such as 3% sulfur salicylic acid.

C. **Nevi**

1. **Macular hemangioma ("stork bites").** A macular hemangioma is a true vascular nevus normally seen on the occipital area, eyelids, and glabella. The lesions disappear spontaneously within the first year of life.

2. **Port-wine stain (nevus flammeus)** is usually seen at birth, does not blanch with pressure, and does not disappear with time. If the lesion appears over the forehead and upper lip, then **Sturge-Weber syndrome** (port-wine stain over the forehead and upper lip, glaucoma, and contralateral jacksonian seizures) needs to be ruled out.

3. **Mongolian spot.** Mongolian spots are dark blue or purple bruise-like macular spots usually located over the sacrum. They are usually present in 90% of blacks and Asians and 59% of whites. They disappear by 4 years of age.

4. **Cavernous hemangioma.** A cavernous hemangioma usually appears as a large, red, cystic-appearing, firm, and ill-defined mass that may be found anywhere on the body. The majority of these lesions regress with age, but some require corticosteroid therapy. In more severe cases, surgical resection may be needed. If associated with thrombocytopenia, consider **Kasabach-Merritt syndrome.** Transfusions of platelets and clotting factors are usually required in these patients.

5. **Strawberry hemangioma (macular hemangioma).** Strawberry hemangiomas are flat, bright red, sharply demarcated lesions, most commonly found on the face. Spontaneous regression usually occurs (70% by 7 years of age).

V. **Head.** Note the general shape of the head.

A. **Anterior and posterior fontanelles.** The anterior fontanelle usually closes at 9–12 months and the posterior fontanelle at 2–4 months. A large anterior fontanelle is seen with hypothyroidism and may also be seen in small-for-gestational-age infants. A bulging fontanelle may be associated with increased intracranial pressure, meningitis, or hydrocephalus. Depressed (sunken) fontanelles are seen in newborns with dehydration.

B. **Molding.** Molding is a temporary asymmetry of the skull resulting from the birth process. It is most often seen with prolonged labor and vaginal deliveries but can be seen in cesarean deliveries if the mother had a prolonged course of labor prior to delivery. A normal head shape is usually regained within 1 week.

C. **Caput succedaneum.** Caput succedaneum is a diffuse edematous swelling of the soft tissues of the scalp and it may extend across the suture lines. It is secondary to the pressure of the uterus or vaginal wall on areas of the fetal head bordering the caput. Usually it resolves within several days.

D. **Cephalhematoma** is a subperiosteal hemorrhage that *never* extends across the suture line. It can be secondary to a traumatic delivery or forceps delivery. X-ray films or CT scans of the head should be obtained if an underlying skull fracture is suspected (approximately 5% of all cephalhematomas). The hematocrit and bilirubin levels should be followed in these patients. Most cephalhematomas resolve in 6 weeks. Aspiration of the enclosed blood is rarely necessary.

E. **Increased intracranial pressure.** In an infant with increased intracranial pressure, the following can be seen: bulging anterior fontanelle, separated sutures, paralysis of upward gaze (**setting-sun sign**), and prominent veins of the scalp. The increased pressure may be secondary to hydrocephalus, hypoxic-ischemic brain injury, intracranial hemorrhage, or subdural hematoma.

   F. **Craniosynostosis.** Craniosynostosis is the premature closure of one or more sutures of the skull. It should be considered in any infant that has an asymmetric skull. On palpation of the skull, a bony ridge over the suture line may be felt, and inability to freely move the cranial bones may occur. X-ray studies of the head should be done, and surgical consultation may be necessary.

VI. Neck. Eliciting the rooting reflex (see p 32) will cause the infant to turn its head and allow easier examination of the neck. Palpate the sternocleidomastoid for a hematoma and the thyroid for enlargement and check for thyroglossal duct cysts. A short neck is seen in **Turner's** and **Noonan's syndromes.**

VII. Face. Look for obvious abnormalities. Note the general shape of the nose, mouth, and chin. The presence of hypertelorism (eyes widely separated) or low-set ears should be noted. Facial asymmetry with crying may indicate facial nerve paralysis.

VIII. Ears. Look for unusual shape or abnormal position. The normal position is determined by drawing an imaginary horizontal line from the inner and outer canthus of the eye across the face, perpendicular to the vertical axis of the head. If the helix of the ear lies below this horizontal line, the ears are designated as low-set. Preauricular skin tags (papillomas) are often seen and are benign. Hairy ears are seen in infants of diabetic mothers.

IX. Eyes. Check the **red reflex.** If a cataract is present, there is opacification of the lens and loss of the reflex. Congenital cataracts require early evaluation by an ophthalmologist. The sclera is normally white. It can have a bluish tint if the infant is premature because the sclera is thinner in these infants than in term infants. If the sclera is deep blue, **osteogenesis imperfecta** should be ruled out.

   A. **Brushfield's spots** (salt-and-pepper speckling of the iris) are often seen with Down's syndrome.

   B. **Subconjunctival hemorrhage.** Rupture of small conjunctival capillaries can occur normally but is more common after a traumatic delivery. It is seen in 5% of newborn infants.

   C. **Conjunctivitis.** (See Chap 33.)

X. Nose. Verify the patency of the nostrils with a nasogastric tube if unilateral or bilateral choanal atresia is suspected. Nasal flaring is indicative of respiratory distress. Sniffling and discharge are typical of congenital syphilis.

XI. Mouth. Examine the hard and soft palate for evidence of a cleft palate. A short lingual frenulum (tongue-tie) may require surgical treatment.

   A. **Ranula.** A ranula is a cystic swelling in the floor of the mouth. Most disappear spontaneously.

   B. **Epstein's pearls.** These keratin-containing cysts are located on the hard and soft palate, are normal, and resolve spontaneously.

   C. **Mucocele.** This small lesion on the oral mucosa occurs secondary to trauma to the salivary gland ducts. It is usually benign and subsides spontaneously.

   D. **Natal teeth.** Supernumerary teeth are found in 1 in 4000 births. Removal is necessary to avoid aspiration.

   E. **Macroglossia.** Enlargement of the tongue can be congenital or acquired. Localized macroglossia is usually secondary to congenital hemangiomas. Macroglossia can be seen in **Beckwith's syndrome** (macroglossia, giantism, omphalocele, severe hypoglycemia), or **Pompe's disease** (type II glycogen storage disease).

   F. **Frothy or copious saliva** is commonly seen in infants with a tracheoesophageal fistula.

G. **Thrush.** Oral thrush is common in newborns and is a sign of infection due to *Candida albicans.* Whitish patches appear on the tongue, gingiva, and/or buccal mucosa. Thrush is easily treated with nystatin suspension, 0.1–1.0 mL applied to each side of the mouth, often with a cotton-tipped swab, 3–4 times per day for 7 days.

XII. Chest

A. **Observation.** First note if the chest is symmetrical. An asymmetric chest may signify a tension pneumothorax. Tachypnea, sternal and intercostal retractions, and grunting on expiration indicate respiratory distress.

B. **Breath sounds.** Listen for presence and equality of breath sounds. Absent or unequal sounds may indicate pneumothorax or atelectasis.

C. **Pectus excavatum.** Pectus excavatum is a sternum that is altered in shape; usually it is of no clinical concern.

D. **Breasts in a newborn** may be abnormally enlarged secondary to the effects of maternal estrogens. It is of no clinical concern, and the effect lasts less than a week.

XIII. Heart

A. **Listen for any murmurs** that may be associated with the following conditions.

1. **Ventricular septal defect (VSD)** is the most common heart defect and it accounts for approximately 25% of congenital heart disease. Typically a loud, harsh, blowing pansystolic murmur is heard (best heard over the lower left sternal border). Symptoms, such as congestive heart failure, usually do not begin until after 2 weeks of age, typically from 6 weeks to 4 months. The majority of these defects close spontaneously by the end of the first year of life.

2. **Patent ductus arteriosus (PDA)** is a harsh, continuous, machinery-type, or "rolling thunder" murmur localized to the second left intercostal space. It may radiate to the left clavicle or down the left sternal border. It usually presents on the second or third day of life. A hyperactive precordium is also seen. Clinical signs of PDA include wide pulse pressure and bounding pulses.

3. **Coarctation of the aorta** is a systolic ejection murmur that radiates down the sternum to the apex. It also radiates to the interscapular area and is often heard loudest in the back.

4. **Peripheral pulmonic stenosis.** A systolic murmur is heard bilaterally in the anterior chest, in both axillas, and across the back. It is secondary to the turbulence caused by disturbed blood flow because the main pulmonary artery is larger than the peripheral pulmonary arteries. This murmur is usually benign and may persist up to 3 months of age, but it may also be associated with rubella syndrome.

5. **Hypoplastic left heart syndrome.** A short, midsystolic murmur can be heard. It usually presents anywhere from day 1–21. A gallop is usually heard.

6. **Tetralogy of Fallot** typically has a loud and harsh systolic or pansystolic murmur heard best at the left sternal border. The second heart sound is single.

7. **Pulmonary atresia**
   a. **With VSD.** An absent or soft systolic murmur with the first heart sound is followed by an ejection click; the second heart sound is loud and single.
   b. **With intact intraventricular septum.** Most frequently, there is no murmur and a single second heart sound is heard.

8. **Tricuspid atresia.** A pansystolic murmur along the left sternal border with a single second heart sound is typically heard.

9. **Transposition of the great vessels** is more common in males than in females.

    a. **Isolated (simple).** Cardiac examination is often normal, but cyanosis and tachypnea are present along with a normal chest x-ray film and ECG.

    b. **With VSD.** The murmur is loud, pansystolic, and heard best at the lower left sternal border. The infant typically presents with congestive heart failure at 3–6 weeks of life.

10. **Ebstein's disease.** A long systolic murmur is heard over the anterior portion of the left chest. A diastolic murmur and gallop may be present.

11. **Truncus arteriosus.** A systolic ejection murmur, often with a thrill, is heard at the left sternal border. The second heart sound is loud and single.

12. **Single ventricle.** A loud systolic ejection murmur with a loud, single second heart sound is heard.

13. **Atrial septal defects (ASD)**

    a. **Ostium secundum defect** rarely presents with congestive heart failure in infancy. A soft systolic ejection murmur is best heard at the upper left sternal border.

    b. **Ostium primum defect** rarely presents in infancy. A pulmonary ejection murmur and early systolic murmur are heard at the lower left sternal border. A split second heart sound is heard.

    c. **Common atrioventricular canal** presents with congestive heart failure in infancy. A harsh systolic murmur is heard all over the chest. The second heart sound is split if pulmonary flow is increased.

14. **Anomalous pulmonary venous return**

    a. **Partial.** Findings are similar to those for ostium secundum defect (see above).

    b. **Total.** With a severe obstruction, no murmur may be detected on examination. With a moderate degree of obstruction, a systolic murmur is heard along the left sternal border and occasionally a gallop murmur is heard. A continuous murmur along the left upper sternal border over the pulmonary area is also possible.

15. **Congenital aortic stenosis.** A coarse systolic murmur with a thrill is heard at the upper right sternal border and can radiate to the neck and down the left sternal border. If left ventricular failure is severe, the murmur is of low intensity. Symptoms that present only when the stenosis is severe in infancy are pulmonary edema and congestive heart failure.

16. **Pulmonary stenosis (with intact ventricular septum).** If the stenosis is severe, a loud systolic ejection murmur is audible over the pulmonary area and radiates over the entire precordium. Right ventricular failure and cyanosis may be present. If the stenosis is mild, a short pulmonary systolic ejection murmur is audible over the pulmonic area along with a split second heart sound.

B. **Palpate the pulses** (femoral, pedal, radial, and brachial). Bounding pulses can be seen with patent ductus arteriosus. Absent or delayed femoral pulses are associated with coarctation of the aorta.

C. **Check for signs of congestive heart failure.** Signs may include hepatomegaly, gallop, tachypnea, wheezes and rales, tachycardia, and abnormal pulses.

XIV. **Abdomen**

A. Observation. Obvious defects may include an **omphalocele** (the intestines are covered by peritoneum and the umbilicus is centrally located) or a **gastroschisis** (the defect is usually to the right of the umbilicus and the intestines are not covered by peritoneum). A **scaphoid abdomen** may be associated with a diaphragmatic hernia.

B. Auscultation. Listen for bowel sounds.

C. Palpation. The abdomen is most easily palpated when the infant is quiet or during feeding. Check for distention, tenderness, or masses. It is normal to palpate the liver 1–2 cm below the costal margin and the spleen tip at the costal margin. Hepatomegaly can be seen with congestive heart failure (CHF), hepatitis, or sepsis, and splenomegaly with cytomegalovirus (CMV) or rubella infections or sepsis. The kidneys (especially on the right) can often be palpated. Kidney size may be increased with polycystic disease, renal vein thrombosis, or hydronephrosis. Abdominal masses are more commonly related to the urinary tract.

XV. Umbilicus. Normally, the umbilicus has 2 arteries and 1 vein. If only 2 vessels are present (1 artery, 1 vein), it could indicate renal problems or genetic problems (most commonly trisomy 18). If the umbilicus is abnormal, ultrasonography of the abdomen is recommended. Also inspect for any discharge, redness, or edema around the base of the cord, which may indicate a patent urachus or omphalitis. The cord should be translucent; if greenish-yellow, it suggests meconium staining, usually secondary to fetal distress.

XVI. Genitalia. Any infant with ambiguous genitalia should not undergo gender assignment until a formal endocrinology evaluation has been performed (see Chap 55). Any male infant with hypospadius should not undergo circumcision.

A. Male. Check for dorsal hood, hypospadias, epispadias, or chordee. Normal penile length is greater than 2 cm at birth. Newborn males always have a marked phimosis. Determine the site of the meatus. Hydroceles are common and usually disappear by age 1. Palpate the testicles and examine for groin hernias.

B. Female. Examine the labia and clitoris. A mucosal tag is commonly attached to the wall of the vagina. Discharge from the vagina is common and is often blood-tinged secondary to maternal estrogen withdrawal. If the labia are fused and the clitoris is enlarged, suspect adrenal hyperplasia. A large clitoris can be associated with maternal drug ingestion.

XVII. Anus and rectum. Check for patency of the anus to rule out imperforate anus. Check the position of the anus. Meconium should pass within 48 hours of birth.

XVIII. Extremities. Examine the arms and legs, with close attention to the digits and palmar creases.

A. Syndactyly is abnormal fusion of the digits.

B. Polydactyly is supernumerary digits on hands and/or feet. An x-ray film of the extremity is usually obtained to verify if there are bony structures in the digit. If there are no bony structures, a suture can be tied around the digit until it falls off. If bony structures are present, surgical removal is necessary. Axial extra digits are associated with heart anomalies.

C. Simian crease. A single transverse palmar crease most commonly seen in Down's syndrome but occasionally a normal variant.

D. Talipes equinovarus (club foot) is more common in males. The foot is turned downward and inward, and the sole is directed medially. If it can be corrected with gentle force, it will resolve spontaneously. If not, orthopedic treatment and follow-up is necessary.

    E. Metatarsus varus is adduction of the forefoot. It usually corrects spontaneously.

XIX. **Trunk and spine.** Check for any gross defects of the spine. Any abnormal pigmentation or hairy patches over the lower back should increase the suspicion that an underlying vertebral abnormality might exist. A sacral or pilonidal dimple may indicate a small meningocele or other anomaly.

XX. **Hips.** Evaluate for congenital hip dislocation by using the **Ortolani and Barlow maneuver.** It is done by placing the infant in the frog leg position. Then, the hips are either abducted (Ortolani's sign) or adducted (Barlow's sign). (Some clinicians suggest omitting the Barlow maneuver, because this may contribute to hip instability by stretching the capsule unnecessarily.) A click of reduction and a click of dislocation is elicited in infants with hip dislocation. If this disorder is suspected, radiographic studies and orthopedic consultation should be obtained.

XXI. **Nervous system.** First, observe the infant for any abnormal movement (eg, seizure activity) or excessive irritability. Then, evaluate the following parameters.

    A. Muscle tone

        1. **Hypotonia.** Floppiness and head lag will be seen.

        2. **Hypertonia.** Increased resistance is seen when the arms and legs are extended. Hyperextension of the back and tightly clenched fists are often seen.

    B. Reflexes. The following reflexes are normal for a newborn infant:

        1. **Rooting reflex.** Stroke the lip and corner of cheek with a finger and the infant will turn in that direction and open his mouth.

        2. **Glabellar reflex (blink reflex).** Tap gently over the forehead and the eyes will blink.

        3. **Grasp reflex.** Place your finger in the palm of the infant's hand and he will grasp your finger.

        4. **Neck-righting reflex.** Turn the infant's head to the right or left and movement of the contralateral shoulder should be obtained in the same direction.

        5. **Moro reflex.** Allow the baby to fall back 1–2 cm before catching with both hands. This should cause abduction of both arms and extension of the fingers.

    C. Cranial nerves. Note the presence of gross nystagmus, the reaction of the pupils, and the ability of the infant to follow moving objects with its eyes.

    D. Movement. Check for spontaneous movement of limbs, trunk, face, and neck. A fine tremor is usually normal. Clonic movements are not normal and may be seen with seizures.

    E. Peripheral nerves

        1. **Erb-Duchenne paralysis** involves injury to the fifth and sixth cervical nerves. The shoulder is rotated with the forearm supinated and elbow extended ("waiter's tip" position). The grasping function of the hand is preserved. It can be associated with diaphragm paralysis.

        2. **Klumpke's paralysis** involves the seventh and eighth cervical nerves and the first thoracic nerve. The hand is flaccid with little or no control. If the sympathetic fibers of the first thoracic root are injured, ipsilateral ptosis and miosis can occur.

    F. General signs of neurologic disorders

        1. Symptoms of increased intracranial pressure (bulging anterior fontanelle, dilated scalp veins, setting-sun sign) (see p 27).

        2. Hypotonia, hypertonia.

        3. Irritability/hyperexcitability.

        4. Poor sucking and swallowing reflexes.

5. Shallow, irregular respirations.
6. Apnea.
7. Apathy.
8. Staring.
9. Seizure activity (sucking or chewing of the tongue, blinking of eyelids, eye rolling, hiccups).
10. Absent, depressed, or exaggerated reflexes.
11. Asymmetrical reflexes.

5 Temperature Regulation

The newborn infant must be kept warm and dry to prevent heat loss and its consequences. For this reason, a **neutral thermal environment** should be maintained. At this temperature the least amount of oxygen consumption and metabolic expenditure is needed for the infant to maintain a normal body temperature (Table 5–1). The **normal skin temperature** in the neonate is 36.0–36.5 °C (96.8–97.7 °F). The **normal core temperature** is 36.5–37.5 °C (97.7–99.5 °F).

I. **Hypothermia.** Preterm infants are especially likely to experience heat loss because they have less subcutaneous fat, an increased surface area–to–body weight ratio, and reduced glycogen and brown fat stores. They also have hypotonia and are therefore not able to curl up to keep warm, as a normal infant would.

A. **Mechanisms of heat loss** in the newborn include:
1. **Radiation.** Radiation is heat loss from the infant (warm object) to a colder object in the room.
2. **Conduction.** Conduction is direct heat loss from the infant to the surface with which it is in contact.
3. **Convection.** Convection is heat loss from the infant to the air.
4. **Evaporation.** Heat may be lost by water evaporation from the skin of the infant (especially likely immediately after delivery).

B. **Consequences of hypothermia**
1. **Hypoglycemia.**
2. **Metabolic acidosis,** caused by peripheral vasoconstriction with anaerobic metabolism and acidosis.
3. **Increased oxygen demands.**
4. **Decreased growth with increased metabolic rate.**
5. **Clotting disorders.** Pulmonary hemorrhage can accompany severe hypothermia.
6. **Shock.**
7. **Apnea.**
8. **Intraventricular hemorrhage.**

C. **Prevention and treatment of hypothermia.** There is some controversy about whether rewarming should be done rapidly or slowly; however, rapid rewarming may lead to apnea, and most clinicians recommend slow rewarming at a rate of 0.5–1.0 °C/h (infant < 1000 g: rate should not exceed > 0.6 °C/h).

1. **Equipment**
a. **Closed incubator.** Incubators are usually used for infants less than 1800 g. One disadvantage is that it is difficult to observe a sick infant closely or perform any type of procedure. Temperature changes due to sepsis may be masked by the automatic temperature control. The infant can be weaned from the incubator when the body temperature can be maintained at an environmental temperature of less than 30 °C (usually when the body weight reaches about 1800 g). The enclosed incubator maintains a constant body temperature by one of the following devices.
(1) **Servocontrolled skin probe,** which is attached to the abdomen of the infant. If the temperature falls, additional heat is delivered. Once the desired skin temperature is reached, the heat-

TABLE 5-1. APPROXIMATE NEUTRAL THERMAL ENVIRONMENTAL TEMPERATURES (IN DEGREES CELSIUS)*

	Weight (g)			
Age	1200 or Less	1201–1500	1501–2500	More Than 2500 or More Than 36 Weeks
0–24 hours	34–35.4	33.3–34.4	31.8–33.8	31–33.8
24–48 hours	34–35	33–34.2	31.4–33.6	30.5–33.5
48–72 hours	34–35	33–34	31.2–33.4	30.1–33.2
72–96 hours	34–35	33–34	31.1–33.2	29.8–32.8
4–14 days	*	32.6–34	31–33.2	29–32.6
2–3 weeks	*	32.2–34	30.5–33	*
3–4 weeks	*	31.6–33.6	30–32.7	*
4–5 weeks	*	31.2–33	29.5–32.2	*
5–6 weeks	*	30.6–32.3	29–31.8	*

*Data not established. In general, the smaller the infant, the higher the temperature required.
Data from Scopes J, Ahmed I: Range of initial temperatures in sick and premature newborn babies. *Arch Dis Child* 1966;41:417.

ing unit turns off automatically. Disadvantages include over-heating, which may occur if the skin sensor is loose.

(2) **Air temperature control device.** With the use of this device, the temperature of the air in the incubator is controlled. It is increased or decreased depending on the temperature of the infant. Use of this mode requires constant attention from a nurse. It is usually used in older infants.

(3) **Air temperature probe** is a probe that hangs in the incubator near the infant and maintains a constant air temperature around the baby. There is less temperature fluctuation with this use.

b. **Radiant warmer.** The radiant warmer is usually used for very un-stable infants or during the performance of medical procedures. The temperature can be maintained in the "servo mode" (ie, by means of a skin probe) or the "nonservo mode," which is also called *manual mode* (a certain temperature is maintained regard-less of the infant's temperature).

2. **Normal term infant (> 2500 g)**
   a. Place the infant under a preheated radiant warmer immediately after delivery.
   b. Dry the infant completely to prevent evaporative heat loss.
   c. Cover the head with a cap.
   d. Place the infant in a crib, wrapped in blankets.
   Note: It has been shown that normal term infants can be wrapped in warm blankets and go directly into their mother's arms without any significant heat loss.

3. **Sick term infant.** Follow the same procedure as for the term infant, except place the infant under a radiant warmer with temperature servoregulation.

4. **Premature infant (1000–2500 g)**
   a. For an infant weighing 1800–2500 g who has no medical prob-lems, use of a crib, cap, and blankets is usually sufficient.
   b. For an infant 1000–1800 g:
      (1) **Well infant.** Closed incubator with servocontrol.
      (2) **Sick infant.** Radiant warmer with servocontrol.

5. **Very low birth weight infant (< 1000 g).** Either the radiant warmer or the incubator can be used, depending on the individual situation.
   a. **Radiant warmer**
      (1) Use servocontrol, with the temperature for abdominal skin set at 36.5 °C.

    (2) Cover the infant's head with a cap.

    (3) Use an inner heat shield. The humidity level under the heat shield should be 40–50%.

    (4) Place plastic wrap (eg, Saran Wrap) loosely over the infant.

    (5) Use a black mattress cover to absorb heat.

    (6) Maintain an inspired air temperature of the hood or ventilator of at least 32–35 °C.

    (7) Place a K-pad (heating pad) under the infant and set at 37 °C (*controversial*).

    (8) If the temperature cannot be stabilized, move the infant to a closed incubator.

  b. Closed incubator

    (1) Use servocontrol, with the temperature for abdominal skin set at 36.5 °C.

    (2) Use a double-walled incubator if possible.

    (3) Cover the infant's head with a cap.

    (4) Keep the humidity level at 40–50% or higher. (**Note:** Excessive humidity and dampness of the clothing and incubator can lead to excessive heat loss or accumulation of fluid and possible infections.)

    (5) Keep the temperature of the ventilator at 32–35 °C or higher.

    (6) Line the ends of the incubator with aluminum foil if needed.

    (7) Place a K-pad under the infant and set the temperature at 35 °C.

    (8) Place plastic wrap loosely over the infant.

    (9) If the temperature is difficult to maintain, try increasing the humidity level.

II. Hyperthermia. Hyperthermia is defined as a temperature that is greater than the normal core temperature of 37.5 °C.

  A. Differential diagnosis

    1. **Environmental causes.** Excessive temperature, overheating, overbundling the infant.

    2. **Infection.** Bacterial or viral infections (eg, herpes).

    3. **Dehydration.**

    4. **Drug withdrawal.**

    5. **Unusual causes**

      a. Hyperthyroid crisis or storm.

      b. Drug effect (eg, prostaglandin E_1).

      c. Riley-Day syndrome (periodic high fevers secondary to defective temperature regulation).

  B. Consequences of hyperthermia. Hyperthermia can cause several problems in the neonate, including tachycardia, tachypnea, irritability, apnea, and periodic breathing.

  C. Treatment

    1. **Turn down any heat source.**

    2. **Remove excess clothing from the infant.**

    3. **Treat underlying cause.**

    4. **Additional measures for older infants** with significant temperature elevation.

      a. Tepid water sponge bath.

      b. Tylenol, 5–10 mg/kg/dose orally or rectally every 4 hours.

REFERENCE

Scopes J, Ahmed I: Range of initial temperatures in sick and premature newborn babies. *Arch Dis Child* 1966;**41**:417.

6 Respiratory Management

See Glossary at the end of the chapter for abbreviations and definitions of terms.

INVASIVE RESPIRATORY MONITORING: BLOOD GAS DETERMINATIONS

I. **Arterial blood gases.** Arterial blood gases are the best indicators of pH, $Paco_2$ and Pao_2. Normal values: pH 7.35-7.45, $Paco_2$ 35-45 mm Hg (higher values may be accepted if the blood pH remains normal), Pao_2 55-65 mm Hg on room air.

II. **Capillary blood gases.** Capillary blood gases will give a lower pH value and a higher Pco_2. Normal values: pH 7.30-7.35, Pco_2 40-45 mm Hg, and Po_2 40-60 mm Hg.

III. **Venous blood gases.** Venous blood gases provide information about pH and Pco_2 but not oxygenation. This is *controversial* (some believe venous Po_2 is an excellent indicator of the adequacy of tissue perfusion/oxygenation). Normal values: pH 7.25-7.30, Pco_2 45-50 mm Hg, and Po_2 30-45 mm Hg.

NONINVASIVE OXYGEN MONITORING SYSTEMS

There are 2 types of noninvasive oxygen monitoring systems: pulse oximetry and transcutaneous oxygen monitoring.

I. **Pulse oximetry.** The pulse oximeter utilizes a photo sensor on the skin to measure the percentage of oxygen saturation of hemoglobin available for oxygen transport. It is affected by the oxyhemoglobin dissociation curve. A higher saturation for a given oxygen tension (curve shifted to the left) occurs with alkalosis, hypothermia, fetal hemoglobin, high altitude, and hypometabolism. A lower saturation for a given oxygen tension (curve shifted to the right) occurs with acidosis, hyperthermia, hypermetabolism, and hypercapnia. Table 6-1 shows oxygen saturation of arterial blood (Sao_2) as a function of Pao_2 and pH and is useful in the interpretation of pulse oximeter readings. Figure 6-1 shows saturation in adult and fetal hemoglobin.

   A. **Advantages**
   1. Unlike transcutaneous oxygen monitoring (see **B,** below), pulse oximetry is not dependent on skin perfusion (however, when there is poor perfusion with weak pulsatile activity, the monitor may not provide an accurate reading).
   2. No regular calibration is needed.
   3. It is more accurate in infants with bronchopulmonary dysplasia (BPD) than transcutaneous oximetry.
   4. There is no trauma to the skin.

   B. **Disadvantages**
   1. Pulse oximetry does not provide accurate readings in patients with abnormal hemoglobin, such as methemoglobinemia.
   2. Any strong light source, such as phototherapy, may skew the readings.
   3. Increased motion may cause inaccurate readings.

TABLE 6–1. SaO₂ AS A FUNCTION OF PO₂ and pH[a,b]

PO₂	pH				
	7.30	7.35	7.40	7.45	7.50
			SaO₂		
120	98	98	98	98	99
100	97	97	97	98	98
90	96	96	97	97	97
80	95	95	96	96	97
70	92	93	94	95	95
65	91	92	93	94	94
60	88	90	91	92	93
55	85	87	89	90	91
50	81	83	85	87	88
45	76	78	80	83	85
40	69	71	74	77	79
35	61	63	66	69	72
30	51	54	57	60	62
20	29	32	34	36	39
10	7	8	9	10	11

[a] Assuming a temperature of 37° C, normal levels of 2,3-DPG, a PaCO₂ of 40 mm Hg, and adult hemoglobin.
[b] This graph is merely a reference tool and is not to be used for deriving precise values of PO₂ or pH from the Ohmeda Biox saturation readings.
Reproduced, with permission, from the Ohmeda Company, Boulder, Colorado.

FIGURE 6–1. Comparison between normal mean oxyhemoglobin dissociation curves of (**A**) term infants at birth and (**B**) adults. The pH is 7.40. (Modified and reproduced, with permission, from Sherwood WC, Cohen A (editors): *Transfusion Therapy: The Fetus, Infant, and Child.* Masson, 1980.)

4. Accuracy decreases when the saturation drops below 60%.
5. It does not discriminate for the high end of the oxygenation scale, ie, it gives a reading of 99–100% whether the Pao_2 is 100 or 300 mm Hg.

II. **Transcutaneous oxygen monitoring** measures the oxygen partial pressure from the skin surface by means of an electrochemical oxygen skin sensor that heats the skin. It is important to draw an arterial blood gas sample and confirm the accuracy of the reading. It is usually done every 6 to 24 hours, depending on the accuracy of the monitor.

A. **Advantages**
   1. Transcutaneous monitoring measures tissue Pao_2, not saturation. It discriminates for the high end of the oxygenation scale and is also more accurate at the low end of the scale.
   2. It allows simultaneous readings of pre- and postductal oxygenation to diagnose conditions such as persistent pulmonary hypertension.

B. **Disadvantages**
   1. Certain conditions can decrease the reliability of the readings.
      a. Temperature variation of the sensor (44 °C is best for a term infant; a premature infant needs to be evaluated to access which temperature is the best).
      b. Placement of the sensor on bony or hairy areas.
      c. Use on infants with edema or poor perfusion.
   2. The site must be changed every 4–6 hours to prevent burning.
   3. The instrument must be recalibrated with each site change.
   4. Transcutaneous oxygen monitoring can be used on babies weighing less than 1000 g, but the site should be changed more frequently (usually every 2 hours) because of skin breakdown or burns.

END-TIDAL CARBON DIOXIDE MONITORING

An end-tidal CO_2-monitoring unit measures the CO_2 concentration as a partial pressure of CO_2 ($Petco_2$) from the exhaled ventilator air. The majority of units measure both inspired and expired gases. A waveform is included in the read-out, and the peak of this waveform is the end-tidal CO_2 ($ETCO_2$). This number, the $ETCO_2$, correlates with the alveolar and arterial Pco_2. It can provide early warning and detection of changes in lung pathology, shunting, changes in dead space ventilation, and hyper- or hypocapnia. Correlation with arterial blood gases needs to be done periodically. Two types of $ETCO_2$ monitoring are available.

I. **Main stream.** In this unit the measuring device (called *infrared bench*) that reads the CO_2 is placed proximal to the endotracheal tube. Although it gives the best breath-to-breath data and clearest waveform, the extra dead space added and the weight of the device pulling on the endotracheal tube are factors that need to be considered in evaluations for use in the neonatal intensive care unit (NICU).

II. **Side stream.** This unit pumps air samples from a port in the proximal airway through a small lumen tube into the unit where the infrared bench is located. Although weight and dead space are not an issue, this method is plagued with problems associated with condensation and mucus in the tubing and delayed or dampened waveforms.

VENTILATORY SUPPORT

The need for ventilatory support in the neonate falls broadly into 2 categories, which often coexist in the same patient: **(1) inability to oxygenate,** which occurs when the Pao_2 is under 50 mm Hg and **(2) inability to ventilate,** which can occur with severe apnea or respiratory acidosis ($Paco_2 > 60$ mm Hg).

I. **Oxygen supplementation.** Improvement in oxygenation can be provided by the following methods: oxygen hood, nasal cannula, nasal or endotracheal continuous positive airway pressure (CPAP), and mechanical ventilation. Initially, the infant is placed under an oxygen hood. If this does not improve oxygenation, a trial of nasal CPAP is used. Mechanical ventilation is used next. The nasal cannula is usually reserved for "older" infants (> 1 week old) who have problems with oxygenation.

A. **Oxygen hood ("cake box").** Air and oxygen are blended to form oxygen concentrations that range from 0.21 to 1.0. The oxygen-air mixture is heated and humidified before it is delivered to the baby.

1. **Advantages.** Oxygen hoods work well with all types of infants. Precise oxygen concentrations can be maintained by using an oxygen analyzer to sample the fraction of inspired oxygen (F_{IO_2}) inside the hood.

2. **Disadvantages.** Oxygen hoods are cumbersome to work with and can interfere with interactions between the infant and parents and the hospital personnel. Active infants may be uncomfortable as they come in contact with the plastic hood.

B. **Nasal cannula.** The nasal cannula is an alternative method for delivering oxygen. A graduated pediatric flowmeter (eg, Timeter Instrument Corporation) can deliver oxygen flows from 0.025 L/min to 3.0 L/min. Nasal cannulas are well suited for infants with chronic lung diseases such as BPD or those requiring low oxygen concentrations for prolonged periods. Flow rates greater than 1 L/min should be avoided because of the drying effect as well as the discomfort caused by the turbulent flow. Table 6-2 shows an estimation of the percentage of administered oxygen based on the flow rate (from 0.25 to 1.0 L/min) and blender F_{IO_2} settings.

1. **Advantages.** Nasal cannulas allow a greater opportunity for contact and interaction with the infant. The infant can also be more mobile and feed while cannulas are in place.

2. **Disadvantages.** Nasal cannulas do not deliver precise oxygen concentrations. When changing from an oxygen hood to a nasal cannula, a transcutaneous P_{O_2} monitor or pulse oximeter is needed to establish a baseline reading on a known percentage of oxygen. After the infant is placed on the cannula, the oxygen flow is adjusted until the baseline reading is the same as the preexisting reading while under the oxygen hood.

C. **Continuous positive airway pressure (CPAP).** Nasal or endotracheal CPAP can be used to improve oxygenation in an infant. It is provided through nasal prongs or an endotracheal tube. In nasal CPAP, a supportive device such as a Zee Frame is generally used to hold the prongs against the infant's face.

1. **Advantages**

a. Nasal CPAP allows some infants to be spared endotracheal intubation and mechanical ventilation.

b. It is also useful after extubation to prevent areas of atelectasis.

TABLE 6-2. NASAL CANNULA CONVERSION TABLE*

Flow Rate (L/min)	F_{IO_2}			
	100%	80%	60%	40%
0.25	34%	31%	26%	22%
0.5	44%	37%	31%	24%
0.75	60%	42%	35%	25%
1	66%	49%	38%	27%

*General guidelines; numbers are not exact.

     c. It is beneficial in some cases of apnea of prematurity.
   2. Disadvantages
     a. An infant on nasal CPAP usually cannot be fed orally and must have a gastric tube in place to prevent gastric distention. (*Controversial*. Many institutions feed infants on nasal CPAP without any problems.)
     b. Nasal CPAP should not be used in the following types of patients.
       (1) Infants with gastrointestinal disorders.
       (2) Infants who are easily agitated or who are in frank respiratory failure.
       (3) Infants not capable of spontaneous breathing efforts, such as those with central nervous system disorders.
 D. Mechanical ventilation. If the above measures fail to improve oxygenation, mechanical ventilation is usually indicated (see next section).

II. Mechanical ventilation
 A. Indications
   1. Inability to ventilate occurs with the following disorders.
     a. Apnea. Apnea is initially treated with pharmacologic agents or nasal CPAP, and if apnea still occurs, mechanical ventilation is indicated.
     b. CO_2 retention. CO_2 retention greater than 60 mm Hg with an acidotic pH is usually treated with mechanical ventilation if no other correctable cause (eg, pneumothorax) is found. Some infants have a chronically high CO_2 but with a pH compensation (such as infants with chronic lung disease); these infants are usually not intubated.
   2. Inability to oxygenate. Mechanical ventilation is indicated when the oxygen hood or nasal CPAP fails to improve oxygenation.
 B. Types of positive-pressure ventilators. Conventional ventilators are classified by the mechanism for initiating inspiration (cycle) and for terminating inspiration (limit). They are further classified by the drive mechanism and the controlled parameter. There are 2 types: pressure control and volume control.
   1. Pressure control. The following ventilators are those most commonly found in a neonatal unit. They are all time-cycled and time-limited. Tidal volume (V_T) exchanged is dependent on peak inspiratory pressure (PIP) delivered and will vary relative to the compliance and resistance of the pulmonary system. The pressure-control ventilators are described below.
     a. Bear-medical BP-200, Bear-medical BP-2001 (Bear Cub), Healthdyne 105, Babybird 2A, Infrasonic Infant Star
       (1) User-controlled parameters: Rates up to 150 breaths/min, PIP, inspiratory time (IT), positive end-expiratory pressure (PEEP)/CPAP, flow, F_{IO_2}.
       (2) Flow is continuous, constant, and adjustable.
       (3) All are pneumatically driven and electrically controlled.
       (4) Expiratory time (ET) and the ratio of inspiratory time to expiratory time (I:E ratio) are a factor of IT and rate.
       (5) Distinctive qualities
         (a) Bear-medical BP-200. This ventilator has an I:E ratio limiter and must be used with an adjunct monitor. It will deliver inadvertent PEEP at high flows; therefore an inadvertent PEEP reducer must be used.
         (b) Bear-medical BP-2001 (Bear Cub). There are digital displays of IT, ET, I:E ratio, rate, and mean airway pressure (MAP). Total airway pressure (PAP) and PEEP/CPAP are read off the manometer. This ventilator can give a negative end-expiratory pressure of −2 cm water.

    (c) Healthdyne 105. The only digital display is I:E ratio. It must be used with an adjunct monitor.

    (d) Babybird 2A. This ventilator does not display values and must be used with an adjunct monitor.

    (e) Infrasonic Infant Star

        (i) Has digital displays of I:E ratio, ET, measured PEEP/CPAP, measured PAP, and MAP as well as all the controlled parameters.

        (ii) Has the option of demand intermittent mandatory ventilation (IMV) and demand CPAP. Regardless of the flow selected, baseline flow (during exhalation) is 4 L/min. Flow is increased as needed to maintain PEEP/CPAP. Initial flow on a mandatory breath is as set, then tapers to 4 L/min to maintain desired PIP during inspiratory time limit.

        (iii) Has numerous alarms and safety features.

        (iv) Can be obtained with a high-frequency flow interrupter.

  b. Babybird, Sechrist Model IV-100 and IV-100B

    (1) User-controlled parameters: IT, ET, PIP, PEEP/CPAP, flow, F_{IO_2}.

    (2) Rate is a factor of IT and ET.

    (3) Flow is continuous, constant, and adjustable.

    (4) Pneumatically driven and electrically controlled.

    (5) Distinctive qualities

        (a) Babybird is one of the earliest infant ventilators. It needs an adjunct monitor and alarm system.

        (b) Sechrist Model IV-100 and IV-100B. IT and ET are controlled by an oscillating quartz crystal that is highly accurate. It has a digital display of IT, ET, I:E ratio, and rate. MAP is not monitored.

  c. Siemens Servo 900-C

    (1) User-defined parameters. Rate (5–150), PIP, PEEP/CPAP, IT% (20%, 25%, 33%, 50%, 67%, and 80%). IT is expressed as a percentage of a breath cycle (based on control rate). **Note:** The servo defines PIP as pressure above PEEP. If you have a PEEP of 4 cm water and set the PIP for 12 cm water, total peak airway pressure (PAP) will be 16 cm water. When writing orders for the Servo 900-C, always specify whether your order is for a change in PIP or PAP.

    (2) Flow is delivered only on inspiration and is not user controlled. Each breath is delivered at a constant pressure. Flow is high at the initiation of a breath and then tapers as needed during the inspiratory phase to maintain the requested pressure.

    (3) Is a time/patient-cycled (assist-cycled) system (not IMV). A patient's inspiratory effort sufficient to trigger the ventilator (sensitivity is adjustable) results in a pressure-controlled breath regardless of the rate set on the ventilator.

    (4) IT is not infinitely variable and is set as a percentage of a breath cycle. As the control rate is changed, the inspiratory percentage may need to be adjusted to maintain an appropriate inspiratory time.

    (5) Measured data are displayed digitally and include rate (total), exhaled tidal volume, delivered tidal volume, exhaled minute volume, PIP, pause pressure, and MAP.

    (6) This ventilator is best used for large neonates (> 1500 g) with strong inspiratory efforts.

2. Volume control. The volume-control ventilator is used infrequently in the NICU. It is generally considered appropriate only for term infants. The 2 models discussed are very different from one another.

   a. Bourns LS-104-150. This ventilator is a time/patient-cycled (assist-cycled), volume-limit and volume-control unit. It is a piston-driven (volume is a function of stroke length) system with a high pressure limit that can be set for safety.

      (1) User-defined parameters. Rate (5–80), flow, V_T (5–150 mL), PEEP, and pressure limit.

      (2) IT is a function of V_T and flow. I:E ratio is a function of IT and rate.

      (3) Rates are in increments of 5 up to 40 breaths/min and in increments of 10 from 40 to 80 breaths/min.

   b. Siemens Servo 900-C (in synchronous intermittent mandatory ventilation [SIMV] and volume-control mode). This unit is a time/patient-cycled (assist-cycled), time-limit, volume-control system. It is pneumatically driven and electrically controlled. In SIMV, the infant may breathe unassisted between mandatory breaths. In volume control, every breath, regardless of how it is initiated (by patient or ventilator), is volume controlled.

      (1) User-defined parameters. Rate (5–40 breaths/min in SIMV, 5–120 breaths/min in volume control), minute volume, inspiratory percentage time, PEEP/CPAP, pressure limit, and trigger sensitivity.

      (2) Tidal volume (V_T) is calculated from set minute volume (V) and control rate (f) ($V/f = V_T$). When in the volume-control mode, the set minute volume must be adjusted each time the rate is changed in order to maintain the same V_T.

      (3) IT is a function of inspiratory percentage time and control rate.

      (4) Flow is a function of inspiratory percentage time, rate, and set minute volume.

  3. Pressure support is a relatively new modality available on the Siemens Servo 900-C and other adult ventilators. Its use in the neonatal intensive care unit is essentially limited to infants > 1500 g. It is strictly a spontaneous mode. Every breath is initiated by the patient. It is a patient-cycled, flow-limit pressure-control system. Only the PEEP and PIP are set. Its use is still *controversial* but may have application for the larger infant when one wants to avoid pharmacologic paralyzation, such as in meconium aspiration or persistent pulmonary hypertension.

C. Methods of ventilation. Two methods of ventilation most commonly used in the neonate are **conventional ventilation** and **high-frequency positive-pressure ventilation (HFPPV),** which is available on conventional ventilators. Conventional ventilation involves a rate less than 60 breaths/min, whereas HFPPV involves a rate between 60 and 150 breaths/min. Conventional ventilation is used most of the time. Table 6–3 compares the 2 different ventilatory methods and indicates the ranges of parameters used for each method. Initially, most patients are started on conventional ventilation unless there are specific reasons

TABLE 6–3. COMPARISON OF CONVENTIONAL VENTILATION AND HFPPV

	Rate (breaths/min)	IT (seconds)	PIP (cm water)	PEEP (cm water)	MAP (cm water)
Conventional ventilation	Less than 60	0.4–1	15–45	2–6	10–20
HFPPV	60–150	Less than 0.4	15–20	Less than 3	Less than 10

to use HFPPV, such as in infants with specific pulmonary problems (persistent pulmonary hypertension, diaphragmatic hernia, or pulmonary interstitial emphysema), or in any other situation in which pressures generated by the ventilator must be reduced. Three other types of high-frequency ventilation are available—**high-frequency "jet," oscillatory, and flow-interrupter ventilation.** These are discussed in Chapter 14.

D. **Ordering routine initial ventilator settings.** The following must be specified: PIP, PEEP, F_{IO_2}, rate, and I:E ratio (or IT). MAP is not directly set but is a factor that needs to be considered when ordering ventilator settings.

   1. **PIP (peak inspiratory pressure).** Use the lowest peak pressure necessary to adequately move the chest. Prior to beginning mechanical ventilation, bag-and-mask ventilation can be done to see what pressure is necessary, or the following weight guidelines can be used: < 1000 g, PIP = 12–14 cm water; 1000–2000 g, PIP = 15–20 cm water; > 2000 g, PIP = 20–25 cm water.

   2. **PEEP.** A "physiologic PEEP" of 2 cm water is most often used, except that in pulmonary interstitial emphysema (PIE) no PEEP is used and in hyaline membrane disease (HMD) 4 cm water or more is used.

   3. **F_{IO_2}.** Use the concentration necessary to maintain adequate oxygenation. The range is from 0.21 to 1.0 (21–100%).

   4. **Rate.** Rates between 40 and 60 breaths/min are often used.

   5. **IT or I:E ratio.** One value or the other can be set, and the remaining one calculated. The IT should always be less than or equal to ET. Make sure that whatever I:E ratio is selected, the IT is not above 1 second. An IT of 0.35–0.45 is generally recommended. At higher rates (> 60 breaths/min), care should be taken that ET does not exceed IT. If it is necessary to increase the ventilator rate, adjust the IT to maintain appropriate I:E ratios. Normal I:E ratios range from 1:1 to 1:2.

      a. **Calculation of I:E ratio or inspiratory time (IT)**
         (1) First, determine the Tc (total cycle time) based on the rate ordered: Tc = 60 seconds divided by rate in breaths/min. **Example:** Desired rate = 60 breaths/min, Tc = 60/60, Tc = 1 second/breath.
         (2) Next, decide on the ratio you wish to use (most commonly 1:1 or 1:2). To establish the I:E or IT use the following formula: Tc/(I + E) = IT; and Tc = IT + ET. Therefore with an I:E ratio of 1:1 at a rate of 60 breaths/min, IT = 0.50 second and ET = 0.50 second.

   6. **Mean airway pressure (MAP).** Although not directly controlled, MAP is a function of any variable that affects the amount of positive pressure or the amount of time that pressure is delivered (eg, rate, flow, PIP, PEEP, and IT). Use the lowest MAP possible to achieve adequate oxygenation. High MAP has been associated with the development of pulmonary interstitial emphysema.

E. **Usual ventilator treatment plans in specific diseases**
   1. **Hyaline membrane disease (HMD)**
      a. **PEEP.** PEEP of 4 cm water or greater (range, 4–6 cm water).
      b. **PIP.** Minimal pressures to move the chest adequately (range, 18–30 cm water).
      c. **IT.** Lowest possible with the designated rate to maintain adequate oxygenation (range, 0.4–0.75 seconds).
      d. **Rate.** Usually 30–60 breaths/min.
      e. **Oxygen.** Use whatever percentage is necessary to maintain adequate oxygenation (range 0.21–1.0). Adequate oxygenation is defined as Pa_{O_2} of 50–70 mm Hg.

2. Persistent pulmonary hypertension (PPH)
   a. PEEP. Generally a low PEEP (usually 2 cm water) is used. Higher PEEP may be harmful in a patient with no parenchymal damage.
   b. PIP. Set as needed to maintain oxygenation. The usual range is 20–40 cm water.
   c. Rate. High rates, usually over 60 breaths/min, are used. If oxygenation is a problem, low rates with longer inspiratory times can sometimes be tried. Remember, changes in FiO_2 and PIP should be made slowly. Changes in FiO_2 are usually made by 2% and changes in PIP by 1 cm water pressure. Lower $PaCO_2$ values are often acceptable and desirable.
   d. Oxygen. Keep the infant well oxygenated (usually PaO_2 > 80 mm Hg).
3. Pulmonary interstitial emphysema (PIE) (use a conventional ventilator for high-frequency positive-pressure ventilation)
   a. PEEP. PEEP of 0 or 1 cm water is most often used.
   b. PIP. Low peak inspiratory pressures are used.
   c. IT. IT is usually low (range, 0.1–0.2 second).
   d. Rate. Higher rates are used (range, 60–150 breaths/min).
   e. Oxygen. Use whatever percentage is necessary to maintain an adequate PaO_2.
   f. See Chapter 14, High-Frequency Ventilation.
4. Apnea
   a. PEEP. PEEP of 2 cm water (physiologic).
   b. PIP. Low peak inspiratory pressures are used (range, 10–15 cm water).
   c. IT. IT is usually 0.5 second.
   d. Rate. Range is usually 10–30 breaths/min.
   e. Oxygen. Oxygen requirement is usually low.
5. Meconium aspiration. Ventilatory techniques are not well established in meconium aspiration.
   a. PEEP. PEEP of 2–5 cm water.
   b. PIP. Use whatever pressure adequately moves the chest.
   c. Rate. Range, > 60 breaths/min.
   d. Oxygen. Use as high an oxygen concentration as necessary to keep the infant well oxygenated (usually PaO_2 > 80 mm Hg).
F. Changing ventilator settings. The effects of changes in ventilator parameters on arterial blood gas levels are shown in Table 6-4. These parameters are provided as general rules. As clinical expertise increases, other factors come to play important roles in interpreting arterial blood gas levels. Ventilator changes should be based on blood gas values. In general, the following guidelines can be used.
1. $PaCO_2$. $PaCO_2$ is inversely proportionate to minute ventilation (tidal volume [proportional to the PIP] × rate).
   a. An increase in minute ventilation will decrease the $PaCO_2$.
   b. Minute ventilation can be increased by increasing the PIP and/or

TABLE 6-4. CHANGES IN BLOOD GAS LEVELS CAUSED BY CHANGES IN VENTILATOR SETTINGS[a]

	Rate	PIP	PEEP	IT	FiO_2
To increase $PaCO_2$	Decrease	Decrease	NA	NA	NA
To decrease $PaCO_2$	Increase	Increase	NA[b]	NA[c]	NA
To increase PaO_2	NA	Increase	Increase	Increase	Increase
To decrease PaO_2	NA	Decrease	Decrease	NA	Decrease

[a] NA, not applicable.
[b] In severe pulmonary edema and pulmonary hemorrhage, increased PEEP can decrease $PaCO_2$.
[c] Not applicable unless the I:E ratio is excessive.

the rate. Minute ventilation can be decreased by a decrease in the rate or PIP. For example, if the $Paco_2$ is high and you want to lower it, the PIP or the rate (or both) can be increased. This will increase the minute ventilation, thereby decreasing the $Paco_2$.

2. **Pao_2.** Pao_2 is proportionate to the Fio_2 and MAP.
   a. An increase in Fio_2 or MAP will increase oxygenation, whereas a decrease in Fio_2 will decrease oxygenation.
   b. MAP is proportionate to PIP, PEEP, IT, and the I:E ratio. An increase in these parameters will increase the MAP and result in an increased Pao_2. The choice of which parameter to change depends on whether a change in $Paco_2$ is necessary. For example, if oxygenation is needed, the following can be done.
      (1) If $Paco_2$ is normal, increase Fio_2, increase PEEP, increase IT (done less frequently now and should be done with caution).
      (2) If $Paco_2$ is high, increase PIP (to increase oxygenation and decrease $Paco_2$); increase Fio_2; increase PEEP (will increase Pao_2 and may have no effect or may increase or decrease the $Paco_2$).
      (3) If $Paco_2$ is low, increase Fio_2; increase PEEP; increase IT.

G. **Weaning from ventilatory support**
   1. **General approach.** Weaning can start when the Pao_2 is greater than 70 mm Hg and the $Paco_2$ is less than 45–50 mm Hg. Many believe that parameters that cause an increase in the mean airway pressure should be weaned first. As the oxygen concentration is reduced to or equals 50% and the PIP is 20–25 cm H_2O for an infant weighing over 2000 g, 15–20 cm water for an infant 1000–2000 g, or 12–15 cm water for an infant under 1000 g, further weaning should be done by decreasing the respiratory rate. Weaning can be done usually by decrements of 5 breaths/min, depending on how the $Paco_2$ is responding and what disease process the infant has. In an infant with persistent pulmonary hypertension, the weaning is done *slowly;* an infant who was intubated only for surgery can be weaned quickly, eg, in decrements of 10 breaths/min.
   2. **Methods.** Weaning can be achieved by several methods.
      a. Wean the rate down to 5–10 breaths/min and then extubate.
      b. Wean the rate down to 5–10 breaths/min and if this is tolerated for 1 hour, use endotracheal CPAP set at 3–4 cm water for 2–4 hours. Increase the oxygen concentration by 5% when the infant is placed on CPAP. If the infant tolerates this (acceptable blood gas levels, no respiratory distress), extubation can be attempted. If CPAP is not tolerated, perform either of the following:
         (1) **Slow weaning of rate.** Lower the rate by 2–4 breaths/min every 12 hours or every day until a rate of 5 breaths/min is reached, and then extubate.
         (2) **Start endotracheal CPAP weaning.** Start the infant on 5 minutes of CPAP and then give 55 minutes of full ventilatory support. Increase the interval on CPAP by 5 minutes per hour. Once 60 minutes of CPAP is tolerated, continuous CPAP can be attempted. Perform extubation if 2–4 hours of CPAP is tolerated.
   3. **After extubation, the infant should be placed on hood oxygen or nasal CPAP.**
      a. **Hood oxygen.** Infants placed on hood oxygen usually weigh more than 1500 g, were not considered clinically unstable, and are not expected to have problems with apnea or atelectasis.
         (1) Give supplemental oxygen. Increase the oxygen concentration in the hood by at least 5% over the last oxygen level obtained while the infant was on the ventilator.

      (2) Perform frequent percussion and postural drainage.
      (3) Observe the infant closely for signs of tachypnea or increasing oxygen requirement.
      (4) If the infant has had an increasing oxygen requirement or has clinically deteriorated, obtain an anteroposterior chest x-ray film at 6 hours postextubation to monitor for atelectasis.
   b. Place on nasal CPAP. Many institutions routinely place infants on nasal CPAP after extubation. It helps to prevent areas of atelectasis and to decrease the risk of apnea associated with weaning. Nasal CPAP is commonly used for infants less than 1500 g or for any infant believed to have problems with extubation.
      (1) Place on nasal CPAP 4–6 cm water, with an increase in the oxygen concentration of approximately 5% over the previous level.
      (2) Follow guidelines given in **a.(2)–(4),** above.
  4. Precautions during weaning
   a. When decreasing the rate, do not increase the IT. An IT of 0.5 second should be adequate at rates of 5–15 breaths/min.
   b. If an extubated infant on hood oxygen becomes apneic or requires more oxygen, consider nasal CPAP before reintubation. Nasal CPAP improves oxygenation, but its effect on $Paco_2$ varies.
H. Nebulized medications. In the process of extubation, the following medications are sometimes used. They are also used in patients with BPD and bronchospasm.
  1. Racemic epinephrine (Vaponefrin, others)
   a. Indications. To treat postextubation inspiratory stridor, laryngeal edema, and bronchospasm.
   b. Actions. Alpha-adrenergic action results in decongestion of inflamed mucosa.
   c. Dosage (nebulized treatment). 0.1–0.3 mL in 2–3 mL normal saline every 30 minutes to 2 hours as needed. Observe for tachycardia, hypertension, and tremor. Always reassess the patient after 4 treatments.
  2. Beta-2 agonists. The following are beta-2 agonists: terbutaline (Brethine), isoetharine (Bronkosol), metaproterenol (Alupent), and albuterol (Proventil).
   a. Terbutaline sulfate (Brethine, others)
      (1) **Indications.** Treatment of bronchospasm in patients with BPD or wheezing in a patient with an already increased heart rate.
      (2) **Action.** A potent beta-2 agonist, causing prolonged bronchodilation and peripheral vasodilation.
      (3) **Dosage (nebulized treatment).** 0.1–0.3 mg/kg in 2–3 mL normal saline every 2–8 hours.
      (4) **Adverse reactions.** At high doses, decreased blood pressure may occur.
   b. Isoetharine (Bronkosol, others)
      (1) **Indications.** Treatment of bronchospasm and wheezing, usually in patients with BPD.
      (2) **Action.** This sympathomimetic amide has more beta-2 activity than beta-1 activity. It causes bronchodilation (beta-2) and increased contractility and heart rate (beta-1).
      (3) **Dosage (nebulized treatment).** 0.1–0.2 mg/kg in 2–3 mL normal saline every 2–8 hours.
      (4) **Adverse reactions.** May cause tachycardia, arrhythmias, blood pressure changes.
   c. Metaproterenol sulfate (Alupent)
      (1) **Indications.** Treatment of bronchospasm in infants with BPD.
      (2) **Action.** Same as **b(2),** above.

      (3) Dosage (nebulized treatment). 0.25–0.5 mg/kg in 2–3 mL normal saline every 2–8 hours.

      (4) Adverse reactions. Same as **b(4),** above.

   d. Albuterol (Ventolin)

      (1) Indications. Treatment of bronchospasm.

      (2) Action. Same as **b(2),** above.

      (3) Dosage (nebulized treatment). 0.05–0.15 mg/kg in 2–3 mL normal saline every 2–8 hours.

      (4) Adverse reactions. Same as **b(4),** above.

  3. Other topical respiratory agents

   a. Atropine sulfate

      (1) Indications. To reduce bronchospasm mediated by vagal reflexes and decrease secretions. May improve ventilatory function in infants with BPD.

      (2) Action. Anticholinergic; blocks neurotransmission of acetylcholine to the smooth muscle, thus inhibiting bronchoconstriction.

      (3) Dosage (nebulized treatment). 0.025–0.08 mg/kg in 2–3 mL normal saline every 6–8 hours.

      (4) Adverse reactions. Flushing, tachycardia, decreased gastrointestinal activity, CNS stimulation.

   b. Intal (cromolyn sodium)

      (1) Indications. To prevent bronchospasm.

      (2) Action. Stabilizes mast cells, which prevents subsequent release of mediators of inflammation.

      (3) Dosage (nebulized treatment). 20 mg/2 mL normal saline, every 6–8 hours.

      (4) Adverse reactions. Anaphylaxis, bronchospasm.

PULMONARY FUNCTION TESTING

Individualizing mechanical ventilatory care to match the alterations in lung mechanics of sick newborns has become important during the last several years. Instruments have been developed to measure pulmonary function in the newborn that are minimally invasive, are performed at the bedside, and afford continuous breath-to-breath recording with on-line computer-assisted calculations.

Pulmonary mechanics refers to the actual outputs from the infant, ie, esophageal pressure (reflecting intrathoracic pressure), airway pressure, airflow, and volume. Pulmonary function refers to the specific parameters that are calculated from these outputs, eg, compliance and resistance.

  I. Indications. In the following instances, pulmonary function testing (PFT) may be helpful.

   A. To assist with ventilatory care in an infant with any form of acute lung disease.

   B. To follow improvement or deterioration in infants with BPD.

   C. Prior to extubation, airway resistance in particular can be evaluated, and again 12 hours after extubation.

   D. To determine the effectiveness of bronchodilator therapy.

   E. To determine the optimal level of PEEP.

   F. In infants with apnea.

   G. To evaluate pulmonary mechanics in infants with surgical conditions or abdominal distention.

   H. In infants with stridor or wheezing.

   I. In infants with neuromuscular disease.

  II. Equipment. The essential items necessary to make measurements are:

   A. An endotracheal tube or a face mask (for nonintubated infants).

   B. An esophageal catheter or balloon for intrathoracic pressure monitoring.

   C. A pneumotachograph inserted between the endotracheal tube and ventilator circuit or attached to the face mask for measurement of flow and pressure gradients.

   D. A differential pressure transducer to which the esophageal catheter and the pneumotachograph are connected. It transmits the signals of airflow, airway pressure, and esophageal pressure to the recording device.

   E. A multichannel recorder interfaced with a microcomputer. The recorder displays the tracings of changes in airway pressure, esophageal pressure, airflow, and tidal volume for each breath. During continuous monitoring, the computer is necessary to calculate the actual pulmonary function values.

      1. Currently available PFT systems differ in the following respects.

         a. Computer software. There are differences in graphic capabilities, tabulation of data, and the ability to perform statistical procedures.

         b. The use of an esophageal balloon vs the occlusion method. Airway occlusion at the end of inspiration is accomplished by the use of a shutter-valve mechanism. Through the Hering-Breuer inflation reflex, it results in a period of apnea during which the respiratory muscles are relaxed. This occlusion method may be used to determine the passive compliance of the total respiratory system. This method is also noninvasive, as it avoids the use of an air-filled balloon or water-filled catheter.

         c. The ability to perform functional residual capacity (FRC) measurements. FRC is a measurement of the volume of air in the lungs after a normal expiration.

         d. The ability to distinguish between spontaneous and mechanical breaths. Some systems will automatically mark breaths as spontaneous or mechanical, while others need to be reviewed and individually marked by the operator.

III. Procedure (for use with esophageal balloon method)

   A. The infant should be supine and in a quiet state. Older infants require sedation (chloral hydrate, 50–70 mg/kg orally).

   B. The esophageal balloon is gently passed through the mouth and positioned in the lower third of the esophagus. An estimation is made as follows: The distal tip of the catheter is aligned with the tip of the xiphoid. Measure from this point to the ear lobe and then to the corner of the mouth.

      1. Allow at least 20 minutes after feeding before placement.

      2. Attach the syringe to the balloon catheter and inject approximately 0.1–0.5 mL air. The proper signals on the recorder showing the pressure tracing will confirm the correct placement of the balloon and the correct amount of air.

   C. The system must be calibrated and the transducer zeroed.

   D. The pneumotachograph is placed in line with the ventilator or with the face mask, and along with the esophageal catheter, it is connected to the differential pressure transducer.

   E. Breaths are then sampled for 1–2 minutes. Real-time scalar analyses of each breath may be followed with reference to pressure, flow, and volume signals. Volume is integrated in the computer from the flow signal across the pneumotachograph.

   F. By accessing the computer, the desired parameters are then calculated and may be visualized on the screen as well as printed.

IV. Interpretation. Following are definitions of the pulmonary function values and graphic representations obtained.

A. **Tidal volume (V_T).** The volume (in mL or mL/kg) of air that is delivered during each spontaneous or mechanical breath. It can be represented graphically as a continuum for each breath.

B. **Transpulmonary pressure (P_{tp}).** This is the approximate difference between the proximal airway pressure taken at any point minus the esophageal pressure at the corresponding point. It may be represented graphically for each breath.

Since esophageal pressure is therefore essential in measuring transpulmonary pressure, **placement of the balloon** is important. **Chest wall distortion** may lead to inaccurate results.

C. **Airflow.** Flow (L/min) measured with the pneumotachograph; the change in inspiratory and expiratory flow pattern can be shown graphically.

D. **Compliance.** The change in lung volume per unit of pressure generated (mL/cm water).

   1. **Static compliance.** The elastic properties of the lungs. It is calculated from the change in pressure in the respiratory system when flow is momentarily obstructed at peak inspiration and volume held constant for several breaths (occlusion method).

   2. **Dynamic compliance.** Dynamic compliance during spontaneous or mechanical breathing as influenced by airway resistance and respiratory rate. It is measured at points of no flow during peak inspiration and expiration. Knowing the change in V_T and transpulmonary pressure, dynamic compliance (C_{dyn}) is:

$$C_{dyn} = \Delta V_T / \Delta P_{tp}$$

   3. Changes in compliance may be seen graphically by plotting the pressure along the abscissa and the volume along the ordinate (pressure-volume loop). The loop traces the change in volume that occurs as pressure changes on inspiration and then expiration. The diagonal of this loop represents the compliance (Fig 6-2).

E. **Resistance.** Airway resistance is calculated from the changes in trans-

FIGURE 6-2. Pressure-volume loop demonstrating changes in pulmonary compliance.

pulmonary pressure and flow with inspiration and expiration as follows.

$$R = \Delta P_{tp}/\Delta V \ (\Delta V = Flow)$$

1. The pneumotachograph allows for measurement of total respiratory system resistance. It includes the difference between total pulmonary resistance and total airway resistance.
2. Similar to the pressure-volume loop, a flow-volume loop may also be plotted with volume on the abscissa and flow on the ordinate. Relative changes in resistance may be determined by observing the characteristics of these loops (Fig 6–3).

F. **Time constants (sec).** The time constant of the respiratory system, a measure of how long it takes for alveolar and proximal airway pressures to equilibrate, is equal to the product of the compliance and resistance. At the end of 3 time constants, 95% of the tidal volume is expired from the alveoli. To avoid gas trapping, the measured expiratory time should be greater than this value.

G. **Work of breathing (g·cm/min).** During inspiration and expiration, elastic and frictional resistance (airway resistance and tissue viscous resistance) must be overcome. The work of breathing is an estimate of the work expenditure required to sustain the respiratory effort.

V. **Normal PFT values.** It is very difficult to discuss a normal set of pulmonary function tests. Values will be different, depending on the presence or absence of pulmonary disease, the chronologic age of the infant, and whether or not spontaneous or mechanical breaths are measured. The following are **average values** measured by a number of different investigators for infants less than 3 kg and less than 1 month of age: tidal volume, 5–8 mL/kg; dynamic compliance (total), 1.5–2.5 mL/cm water/kg; resistance (total), 25–50 cm water/L/sec; work of breathing, 1–3 g·cm/min; respiratory time constant (total), 0.15–0.33 second; functional residual capacity, 20–30 mL/kg.

VI. **Complications.** To date, no complications of significance have been reported.

FIGURE 6-3. Flow-volume loop demonstrating relative changes in pulmonary resistance.

GLOSSARY OF TERMS USED IN RESPIRATORY SUPPORT

Assist. A setting at which the infant initiates the mechanical breath, triggering the ventilator to deliver a preset tidal volume or pressure.

Assist/control. The same as assist, except that if the infant becomes apneic, the ventilator will deliver the number of mechanical breaths per minute set on the rate control.

Continuous positive airway pressure (CPAP). A spontaneous mode in which an increase in ambient intrapulmonary pressure is maintained throughout the respiratory cycle.

Control. A setting at which a certain number of mechanical breaths per minute is delivered. The infant is unable to breathe spontaneously between mechanical breaths.

End-tidal carbon dioxide (ETCO$_2$). A measure of the Pco_2 of end expiration.

Expiratory time (ET). The amount of time set for the expiratory phase of each mechanical breath.

Flow rate. The amount of gas per minute passing through the ventilator. It must be sufficient to prevent rebreathing (ie, 3 times the minute volume) and to achieve the peak inspiratory pressure during inspiratory time. Changes in the flow rate may be necessary if changes in the airway waveform are desired. The normal range is 6–10 L/min, with 8 L/min normally being used.

Fraction of inspired oxygen (F$_{IO_2}$). The percentage of oxygen concentration of inspired gas expressed as decimals (room air = 0.21).

I:E ratio. Ratio of inspiratory time to expiratory time. The normal values are 1:1, 1:1.5, or 1:2.

Inspiratory time (IT). The amount of time set for the inspiratory phase of each mechanical breath.

Intermittent mandatory ventilation (IMV). Mechanical breaths are delivered at intervals. The infant breathes spontaneously between mechanical breaths.

FIGURE 6-4. Graphic representation of ventilator airway pressure waveforms and other ventilator terminology. See Glossary, p 52, for explanations.

Mean airway pressure (MAP). Mean airway pressure is the average proximal pressure applied to the airway throughout the entire respiratory cycle. It can be calculated by the following formula.

$$\frac{(R)\,(IT)\,(PIP) + [60 - (R)\,(IT)] \times PEEP}{60}$$

Minute ventilation. Tidal volume (proportional to PIP) multiplied by rate.

Oxyhemoglobin dissociation curve. A curve showing the amount of oxygen that combines with hemoglobin as a function of Pao_2 and $Paco_2$. The curve will shift to the right when oxygen take-up by the blood is less than normal at a given Po_2, and it will shift to the left when oxygen take-up is greater than normal.

$Petco_2$. Measured concentration of carbon dioxide from exhaled ventilator gases.

$Paco_2$. Partial pressure of arterial carbon dioxide.

Pao_2. Partial pressure of arterial oxygen.

PAP. The total airway pressure. In the Siemens Servo 900-C, it is the PIP + PEEP.

Pco_2. Carbon dioxide partial pressure.

Peak inspiratory pressure (PIP). The highest pressure reached within the proximal airway with each mechanical breath. *Note:* In the Siemens Servo 900-C, the PIP is defined as the inspiratory pressure above the PEEP.

Po_2. Oxygen partial pressure.

Positive end-expiratory pressure (PEEP). The pressure in the airway above ambient pressure during the expiratory phase of mechanical ventilation.

Rate. Number of mechanical breaths per minute delivered by the ventilator.

Sao_2. Oxygen saturation of arterial blood.

Tidal volume (V_T). The volume of gas inspired or expired during each respiratory cycle.

Total cycle time (Tc). Inspiratory time plus expiratory time.

Transpulmonary pressure (P_{tp}). Approximate difference between proximal airway pressure at any point minus esophageal pressure at the corresponding point.

Waveform. A pattern of change in airway pressure during the entire respiratory cycle. The 3 types of waveforms are square, sine, and triangular. The sine and square forms are the most common. The square wave indicates that the volume is being delivered at a constant rate; the sine wave, at a variable rate (see Fig 6–4).

REFERENCES

Anday EK, Godart-Wlodavar A, Delivoria-Papadopoulos M: Sequential pulmonary function measurements in very low birth weight infants during the first week of life. *Pediatr Pulmonol* 1987;**3**:392.

Beardsmore CS et al: Improved esophageal balloon technique for use in infants. *Appl Physiol* 1980;**49**:735.

Cunningham MD: Intensive care monitoring of pulmonary mechanics for preterm infants undergoing mechanical ventilation. *J Perinatol* 1989;**9**:56.

Cunningham MD, Desai NS: Methods of assessment and findings regarding pulmonary function in infants less than 1000 grams. *Clin Perinatol* 1986;**13**:299.

Goldsmith JP, Karotkin EH (editors): *Assisted Ventilation of the Neonate,* 2nd ed. Saunders, 1988.

Masters IB et al: Longitudinal study of lung mechanics in normal infants. *Pediatr Pulmonol* 1987;**3**:3.

Uhl RR, Lewis FJ: Digital computer calculation of human pulmonary mechanics using a least squares fit technique. *Comput Biomed Res* 1974;**7**:489.

Vyas H et al: Determinants of the first inspiratory volume and functional residual capacity at birth. *Pediatr Pulmonol* 1986;**2**:189.

Wald A et al: A computers system for respiratory parameters. *Comput Biomed Res* 1969;**2**:411.

Wilkie RA, Bryan MH: Effect of bronchodilators on airway resistance in ventilator-dependent neonates with chronic lung disease. *J Pediatr* 1987;**111**:278.

7   Fluids and Electrolytes

The management of fluid and electrolyte therapy is at the center of many management issues of disease in the newborn infant. Therefore, fluid and electrolyte therapy for neonates must be undertaken with careful planning. The needs of small infants must be met without placing stress on organ systems that are immature or have not yet adapted to extrauterine function. Physiologic principles of fluid and electrolyte balance in newborn infants must be thoroughly understood (Costarino, 1986).

Historically, fluid management in the newborn has oscillated from early feeding to fluid restriction. In the 1940s and 1950s an association between aspiration and edematous, preterm infants in respiratory distress suggested fluid restriction might be beneficial. In 1966, Cornblath described significantly reduced mortality rates in very low birth weight infants following early parenteral administration of fluids (glucose [dextrose] in water). In the 1970s the general shift in fluid therapy goals toward supplementation for growth, combined with the findings of increased insensible water loss and immature renal function, led to widespread acceptance of routine administration of large volumes of intravenous fluids. In the 1980s, excessive fluid administration was associated with bronchopulmonary dysplasia, patent ductus arteriosus, necrotizing enterocolitis, and intraventricular hemorrhage. Today, as the physiology of the newborn is further understood, it is critical that immediate fluid and electrolyte management, with close monitoring, be established to ensure the best outcome for each newborn.

MECHANISMS OF FLUID AND ELECTROLYTE BALANCE

I. **Renal function.** Water in the body is either **intracellular fluid (ICF)** or **extracellular fluid (ECF)**. With increasing gestational age, total body water and ECF volume both decrease, whereas ICF increases. However, in late gestation and the first few weeks of life, renal function undergoes changes that influence the balance of salt and water. At birth (of term as well as preterm infants) the ECF is acutely expanded by shifts of fluids from the ICF to the ECF compartments. Extrauterine renal adaptation differs for term versus preterm infants.

  A. **Infants greater than 34 weeks' gestation** have a low glomerular filtration rate (GFR) at birth and an increased renal tubular reabsorption, resulting in a positive sodium and a negative fluid balance. Secondarily, a low GFR leaves term infants with a delayed response to fluid loads.

  B. **Preterm infants** have an even lower GFR than term infants at birth, along with high basal excretion rates of sodium (driven by a negative fluid balance) and limited renal concentrating abilities (to 50% of adult function). Additionally, preterm infants have a paradoxical inability to rapidly increase sodium excretion in the face of a sodium load; thus they are susceptible to sodium loss, as well as to sodium and water overload.

II. **Insensible water loss.** Insensible water loss (IWL) is evaporization of water through the skin and mucous membranes.

  A. **Term infants.** In term infants, maintenance fluid requirements can be expressed as a function of metabolism, as shown in Table 7–1.

TABLE 7–1. THE RELATIONSHIP BETWEEN METABOLISM AND MAINTENANCE FLUIDS

Route	Loss/Gain	Fluid Replacement (mL/100 kcal Metabolized Energy)
Insensible loss		
Skin	Loss	25
Respiration	Loss	15
Urine	Loss	60
Stool	Loss	10
Water of oxidation	Gain	10
Total for maintenance		100

Modified and reproduced, with permission, from Winters RW: Maintenance fluid therapy. Pages 113–133 in: *The Body Fluids in Pediatrics.* Little, Brown, 1973.

B. **Preterm infants.** The relationship between metabolism and maintenance fluid requirements does not hold true for infants of less than 800
g birth weight or 27 weeks' gestation, because their immaturity and
thinness of skin allows for passive evaporation of large quantities of
body water. Maturation of the skin occurs rapidly with exposure to air,
and transepidermal water loss diminishes three- to fourfold during the
first week of life. Average IWL in preterm infants, according to birth
weight, is listed in Table 7–2. Overall, IWL is greatest for infants less
than 800 g. However, insensible water loss is influenced not only by
the birth weight of the infant, but also by the respiratory status and
environmental factors, such as type of radiant warmer, mode of phototherapy, and room humidity. Table 7–3 summarizes the percent change
10 factors have on IWL. In general, for well premature infants nursed
in closed incubators and weighing 800–2000 g, IWL increases linearly
as body weight decreases. However, for sick infants of similar weight,
nursed on an open radiant warmer and undergoing assisted ventilation,
IWL increases exponentially as body weight decreases. When assess-

TABLE 7–2. INSENSIBLE WATER LOSS (IWL) IN PRETERM INFANTS

Birth Weight (g)	Average IWL (mL/kg/d)
> 750–1000	64
1001–1250	56
1251–1500	38
1501–1750	23
1751–2000	20
2001–3250	20

Modified and reproduced, with permission, from Nash M: Nutrition, body fluids, and acid-base homeostasis. Pages 445–472 in: *Neonatal-Perinatal Medicine,* 4th ed. Mosby, 1987.

TABLE 7–3. FACTORS IN THE NURSERY ENVIRONMENT THAT AFFECT INSENSIBLE WATER LOSS (IWL)

Increases IWL*	Decreases IWL*
1. Severe prematurity, 100–300%	1. Humidification in incubator, 50–100%
2. Open warmer bed, 50–100%	2. Plastic heat shield in incubator, 30–50%
3. Forced convection, 30–50%	3. Plastic blanket under radiant warmer, 30–50%
4. Phototherapy, 30–50%	4. Tracheal intubation with humidification, 20–30%
5. Hyperthermia, 30–50%	
6. Tachypnea, 20–30%	

*Estimates of percent change represent empirical data.
Modified and reproduced, with permission, from Costarino A, Baumgart S: Modern fluid and electrolyte management of the critically ill premature infant. *Pediatr Clin North Am* 1986;**33**:153.

ing the appropriate fluid management for an individual case, birth weight, phototherapy, ambient humidity (ideally 40-50%), type of warmer, and respiratory status must be carefully considered.

III. **Electrolytes.** The principle electrolytes in body fluids are sodium (Na^+), chloride (Cl^-), potassium (K^+), and calcium (Ca^+). Na^+ and Cl^- are present in the ECF and K^+ in the ICF. Na^+ is of greatest concern in neonates. Imbalances of Cl^- are seldom a major problem. Imbalance of K^+ is a frequent problem in extreme prematurity; it is also seen in renal dysfunction and sometimes with potassium-containing medications (ie, tromethamine [THAM], amphotericin B). Increased serum K^+ levels in the face of acidosis is indicative of shifts of K^+ from the intracellular to the extracellular compartments and not necessarily an increase in whole body K^+. Ca^+ imbalances are usually seen with endocrine disturbances and extended diuretic use. Care needs to be taken in interpreting hypocalcemic levels in the face of hypoalbuminemia; in these cases, ionized calcium values give a truer picture of body calcium status.

FLUID AND ELECTROLYTE REPLACEMENT THERAPY

Fluid replacement in neonates must be carefully calculated to allow for normal loss of ECF and weight while preventing dehydration from insensible water loss, which may lead to hypotension, acidosis, and hypernatremia. It is important to avoid excessive fluid therapy, which has been associated with an increased incidence of patent ductus arteriosus, bronchopulmonary dysplasia, intraventricular hemorrhage, and necrotizing enterocolitis in premature infants. Fluid recommendations given below are based on historically averaged values for well infants managed in a single-walled incubator (Baumgart, 1982; Bell, 1979; Costarino, 1986; Nash, 1987). For estimated adjustments for environmental variables, see Table 7-3.

I. **Protocol**
  A. **First day**
    1. **Term infants.** Give 10% dextrose in water (D10W) at a rate of 60-80 mL/kg/d. This amount will provide approximately 6-7 mg/kg/min of glucose. Although there are no accepted guidelines for Ca^+ supplementation in this time frame, it is our practice to supplement 2 mg calcium gluconate per milliliter of maintenance intravenous fluid at birth (*controversial*).
    2. **Preterm infants.** Preterm infants, particularly those weighing less than 1000 g, require more fluids and are less tolerant of glucose. For infants between 800-1000 g, begin fluids at a rate of 80-100 mL/kg/d, adding the appropriate amount of glucose to provide 5-6 mg/kg/min (approximately D7.5W) and 2 mg calcium gluconate per milliliter. Infants less than 700 g usually require fluids in excess of 120-140 mL/kg/d to compensate for transdermal insensible losses and to avoid hyperkalemia, hypovolemia, and hypotension.
  B. **Second and third days.** Once tolerance of fluid therapy has been established and urine output is satisfactory (1-2 mL/kg/h), the rate and composition of the solution can be modified.
    1. **Fluid volume.** Increase by 10-20 mL/kg/d on either the second or the third day, depending on tolerance of previous fluid therapy, estimation of IWL, and clinical status of infant (ie, patent ductus arteriosus, congestive heart failure, pulmonary edema).
    2. **Sodium.** Na^+ requirements range from 2-4 meq/kg/d. However, in some infants, especially the more premature infants (with immature kidneys), a larger Na^+ supplementation may be necessary to compensate for sodium diuresis. These infants are susceptible to both hypo- and hypernatremia, both of which have been associated with permanent brain injury.

3. **Potassium.** K^+ requirements range from 1-2 meq/kg/d. K^+ supplementation is usually not required on the first day of life and sometimes is not necessary until the third day of life. Extreme care should be taken to document renal function prior to adding K^+ (determination of urine output is usually adequate).

4. **Laboratory monitoring.** Continue to monitor serum and urine electrolyte values as in day 1 of life. Laboratory data, estimations of IWL, and clinical assessment are all factors used in readjusting fluid and electrolyte requirements.

C. **Fourth day**

1. **Fluid volume.** Again, fluids may be increased by 20 mL/kg/d. Glucose intake can be gradually increased over these first few days to 12-15 mg/kg/min, depending on tolerance (serum and urine glucose).

2. **Sodium and potassium.** Basic requirements remain unchanged from days 2 and 3. Individual adjustments will need to be made in response to serum levels and clinical status. K^+ requirements increase with diuretic (especially furosemide) use. Keep in mind that renal function will slowly improve as the kidneys mature and IWL will decrease as the skin matures; thus infants may begin showing improved ability to conserve Na^+ and water by the fourth day of life.

3. **Enteral feedings.** By the third or fourth day, the neonate may be ready for enteral feeds. If not, parenteral nutrition may be required. If enteral feeding is begun, intravenous fluids are progressively decreased as enteral fluid intake is slowly increased, maintaining a combined fluid intake of approximately 150 mL/kg/d. Enteral feeds will supply adequate electrolytes, vitamins, trace elements, and the basic proteins, fats, and carbohydrates when appropriate volumes are given.

II. **Monitoring of fluid and electrolyte status.** Fluid and electrolyte replacement therapy should be monitored by daily weights, vital signs, and specific urine and serum laboratory studies.

A. **Body weight.** The body weight should be recorded daily. A loss of more than 20% of birth weight during the first week of life is excessive and suggests uncompensated insensible water loss. If the weight loss is less than 2%/d for the first 4-5 days, fluid administration is probably excessive. A useful tool, especially for sick neonates, is an in-bed scale for measuring body weight 2 or 3 times per day.

B. **Serum levels.** Test for serum hematocrit, sodium, potassium, BUN, creatinine, osmolality, acidosis, and base deficit. Increases in any of these parameters may indicate inadequate fluid therapy. Na^+ supplementation of 2-4 meq/kg/d becomes necessary usually no sooner than the second 12 hours of life. Because K^+ is mainly an intracellular ion, the total K^+ balance cannot be effectively measured in the serum; however, hyperkalemia may become a life-threatening problem in infants less than 800 g and thus electrolytes should be followed frequently (every 4-6 hours) in these infants.

C. **Fluid intake and output.** Fluid status should be measured by accurate fluid intake and output. Urine output measuring < 1.0 mL/kg/h may indicate a need for increased fluid intake, whereas urine output > 3.0 mL/kg/h may indicate overhydration and the need for restriction. Urine specific gravity, electrolytes, and osmolality may be useful in further assessing fluid status.

D. **General appearance and vital signs.** Hypotension, poor perfusion, tachycardia, and poor pulses may all be signs of inadequate fluid intake.

FLUID CALCULATIONS

I. **Environmental factors.** Sick infants under radiant warmers or receiving phototherapy will have dramatically increased IWL and additional fluids must be given to compensate (Table 7–3).

II. **Glucose.** The normal glucose requirement is 6–8 mg/kg/min; however, intake can be slowly increased to 12–15 mg/kg/min, as tolerated, to allow for growth (Table 7–4).

$$\frac{\text{Percentage of glucose} \times \text{Rate (cc/h)} \times 0.167}{\text{Weight (kg)}} = \text{mg/kg/min}$$

Alternate method:

$$\left(\frac{\text{Amount of glucose/mL [from Table 7–4]} \times \text{Total fluids}}{\text{Weight (kg)}}\right) \div 60 \text{ min}$$

$$= \text{mg glucose/kg/min}$$

III. **Sodium. The normal sodium requirement in infants is 2–3 meq/kg/d.** It may be higher in premature infants. The following calculations can be used to determine the amount of sodium the infant is receiving.

Amount of Na^+/mL (from Table 7–5) × Total fluids/day = Amount of Na^+/day

Amount of Na^+/day ÷ Infant's weight (kg) = Amount of Na^+/kg/day

IV. **Potassium. The normal requirement for potassium in infants is 1–2 meq/ kg/d.** It can be easily calculated and added to the intravenous fluids as potassium chloride.

MODIFIERS OF FLUID AND ELECTROLYTE REQUIREMENTS

I. **Insensible water loss.** As previously mentioned (see p 55, II), physiologic and environmental factors influence IWL and thus total fluid requirements.

II. **Diabetes insipidus.** Either secondary to a central (decreased production) or a nephrogenic (unable to be used by the kidneys) etiology, there is decreased activity of antidiuretic hormone (ADH), and thus an increased urine output. Hydration is best maintained by replacement of urine volume and Na^+ loss in addition to IWL. Frequent measurements of body weight (every 12 hours) and Na^+ (every 6–8 hours) are necessary to gauge efficacy of therapy. With diabetes insipidus of central nervous system origin, 1-deamino-8-D-arginine vasopressin (DDAVP) therapy may be helpful.

TABLE 7–4. GLUCOSE CONCENTRATIONS IN COMMONLY USED INTRAVENOUS FLUIDS

Solution (%)	Glucose Concentration (mg/mL)
D5W	50
D7.5W	75
D10W	100
D12.5W	125
D15W	150

TABLE 7–5. SODIUM CONTENT OF COMMONLY USED INTRAVENOUS FLUIDS

Solution	Sodium Concentration (meq/mL)
3% normal saline	0.500
Normal saline	0.154
$\frac{1}{2}$ normal saline	0.075
$\frac{1}{4}$ normal saline	0.037
$\frac{1}{8}$ normal saline	0.019

III. **Syndrome of inappropriate secretion of antidiuretic hormone (SIADH).** An inappropriate increase in the secretion of ADH results in a decreased urine output with urine osmolality > 100 mosm/L, decreased serum osmolality, and hyponatremia (usually on the basis of volume expansion). SIADH is treated by restriction of fluid to approximately 50–60 mL/kg/d or less.

IV. **Renal failure.** If renal failure occurs in the neonate, it is usually secondary to hypoxia or shock. Fluids should be adjusted to compensate only for IWL and replacement of urine volume, if any. K^+ supplementation should be avoided.

REFERENCES

Al-Dahhan J et al: Sodium homeostasis in term and preterm neonates. 1. Renal aspects. *Arch Dis Child* 1983;**58**:335.

Aperia A, Herin P, Zetterstrom R: Sodium chloride and potassium needs in very low birth weight infants. In: *Vitamin and Mineral Requirements in Preterm Infants*. Tsang RC (editor). Marcel Dekker, 1985.

Baumgart S et al: Fluid, electrolyte, and glucose maintenance in the very low birth weight infant. *Clin Pediatr* 1982;**4**:199.

Bell EF et al: Effect of fluid administration on the development of symptomatic patent ductus arteriosus and congestive heart failure in premature infants. *N Engl J Med* 1980;**320**:598.

Bell E, Oh W: Fluid and electrolyte balance in very low birth weight infants. *Clin Perinatol* 1979;**6**:139.

Cornblath M et al: A controlled study of early fluid administration on survival of low birth weight infants. *Pediatrics* 1966;**38**:547.

Costarino A, Baumgart S: Modern fluid and electrolyte management of the critically ill premature infant. *Pediatr Clin North Am* 1986;**33**:153.

Day GM et al: Electrolyte abnormalities in very low birth weight infants. *Pediatr Res* 1976;**10**:522.

Fanaroff A, Klaus M (editors): The gastrointestinal tract: Feeding and selected disorders. In: *Care of the High-Risk Neonate*. Saunders, 1986.

Lorenz J et al: Water balance in very low birth weight infants: Relationship to water and sodium intake and effect on outcome. *J Pediatr* 1982;**101**:423.

Nash M: Nutrition, body fluids, and acid-base homeostasis. In: *Neonatal-Perinatal Medicine,* 4th ed. Mosby, 1987.

Rees L et al: Hyponatremia in the first week of life in preterm infants. *Arch Dis Child* 1984;**59**:423.

Schrier RW, Gabow P: Hyponatremia and hypernatremia. In: *Textbook of Nephrology*. Massry SG, Glassock RJ (editors). Williams & Wilkins, 1983.

Zenk K: Calculating dextrose infusion in mg/kg/min. *PeriScope* Aug (1984):5.

8 Nutritional Management

NUTRITIONAL REQUIREMENTS IN THE NEONATE

I. **Calories**
   A. **To maintain weight,** give 50–60 kcal/kg/d to a term infant; give 60–75 kcal/kg/d to a premature infant.
   B. **To gain weight,** give 100–120 kcal/kg/d to a term infant; give 110–150 kcal/kg/d to a premature infant (to gain 15–30 g/d).
II. **Carbohydrates.** 11–15 g/kg/d is needed (40–50% of total calories).
III. **Proteins.** Adequate protein intake has been estimated at between 2.25 and 4.0 g/kg/d (7–15% of total calories). To achieve fetal accretion rate, 3.5–4.0 g/kg/d is recommended. (**Note:** protein intakes greater than 4.0 g/kg/d may be excessive in some premature infants.)
IV. **Fats.** Fat requirements are 4–6 g/kg/d (limit to < 50% of total calories, or ketosis may result). One to 5% of total calories should be in the form of linoleic acid to meet the essential fatty acid requirements.
V. **Vitamins.** Vitamin requirements are not clearly established. Guidelines are provided in Table 8–1 for low birth weight infants. Vitamin supplementation is dependent on the type of formula used (Table 8–2).
VI. **Fluids.** See Chapter 7 for fluid requirements.

TABLE 8–1. DAILY VITAMIN AND MINERAL REQUIREMENTS FOR THE LOW BIRTH WEIGHT INFANT

Nutrient	Amount
Vitamins	
Choline	5–9 mg/kg
Folate	15 µg/kg
Niacin	4 mg/100 kcal
Pantothenic acid	1.0–1.4 mg/kg
A	1400 IU
B_1 (Thiamine)	250 µg/100 kcal
B_2 (Riboflavin)	335 µg/100 kcal
B_6 (Pyridoxine)	250 µg/100 kcal
B_{12}	0.15 µg/100 kcal
C	30 mg/100 kcal
D	400 IU
E	25 IU (1st 2–4 wk)
	5 IU (after 2–4 wk)
K	5 µg/kg/d
Minerals	
Calcium	200–250 mg/kg
Copper	100–200 µg/kg
Iron	2–3 mg/kg (after wgt > 1500 g)
Magnesium	5–6 mg/kg
Manganese	10–20 µg/kg
Phosphorus	up to 113 mg/kg
Potassium	1–3 meq/kg
Sodium	3–8 meq/kg to 3 wk
	1–3 meq/kg after 3 wk
Zinc	800–1200 µg/kg

PRINCIPLES OF INFANT FEEDING

I. **Criteria for initiating infant feeding.** Most normal term infants are fed within the first 4 hours. The following criteria should usually be met before initiating infant feedings.

  A. **An abdominal examination should have been performed.** If the abdomen is normal (including normal bowel sounds and a nondistended, soft abdomen), feeding can usually be started, provided the baby is otherwise clinically stable. If the examination is abnormal, an abdominal x-ray film should be obtained.

  B. **The infant should have passed meconium;** however, term infants may not pass meconium for up to 24 hours. In a sick or premature infant, passage of meconium may be delayed (see Chap 45).

  C. **The infant should be clinically stable.** The infant can be intubated but should be clinically stable. Feeding should not be started in an infant receiving pancuronium or dopamine (*controversial*). Some institutions feel that if an infant is on dopamine his gut is probably not well perfused, so they do not initiate feeds.

  D. **If the infant has recently been extubated, at least 6 hours should be allowed to pass after extubation** before attempting feeding. The infant should be tolerating extubation well.

  E. **The respiratory rate should be < 60 breaths/min for oral feeding and < 60-80 breaths/min for gavage feeding.** If the respiratory rate is > 80 breaths/min, the infant should not be fed orally because of increased risk of aspiration.

  F. **Umbilical vein or arterial catheters should be removed 24 hours before initiation of feeding.** (This view is *controversial;* some centers feed infants with these catheters in place.)

  G. **If the infant was birth asphyxiated** (Apgar score < 5 at 1 and 5 minutes and initial blood gas levels revealed acidosis), **feeding should be delayed until the infant is 3-5 days of age** to allow the gut to recover (*controversial*).

II. **Feeding guidelines and choice of formula.** Although most normal newborns can be easily started on formula or breast milk, preterm infants and those weighing < 2000 g require more careful consideration. Many different, highly specialized formulas are available. Table 8-2 outlines indications for various formulas. The composition of commonly used infant formulas and breast milk can be found in Table 8-3.

  A. **Formulas**

   1. **Isoosmolar formulas (270-300 mosm/kg water).** The majority of infant formulas are isoosmolar (Similac 20, Enfamil 20, and SMA 20 with and without iron). These are the formulas used most often and tolerated by most healthy infants. Premature formulas containing 24 cal/oz (Similac 24, Enfamil 24, "preemie" SMA 24) are also isoosmolar and are indicated for rapidly growing premature infants.

   2. **Hypoosmolar formulas (< 270 mosm/kg water)** have a lower osmolality, which can improve feeding tolerance. Similac 13 has an osmolality of 200 mosm/kg water. This formula was specifically designed for a conservative initial feeding for infants who have not been fed enterally for several days or weeks. It is not for long-term feeding because it does not meet the nutrient needs for most infants. Other hypoosmolar formulas include most of the premature formulas containing 20 cal/oz (Similac Special Care 20, Enfamil Premature Formula 20, "preemie" SMA 20), which are designed to be better tolerated by premature infants and meet the nutritional requirements.

   3. **Hyperosmolar formulas (> 300 mosm/kg water)** are formulas that are 24 and 27 cal/oz with the exception of the 24 cal/oz premature formulas that are isoosmolar. These formulas (Similac 24, Enfamil

TABLE 8–2. INFANT FORMULA INDICATIONS AND USES

Formula	Indications	Vitamin and Mineral Supplements[a]
HUMAN MILK		
Donor	Preterm infant < 1200 g.	Multivitamins; iron if > 1500 g; fluoride at 40 weeks' gestation; folic
Maternal	All infants.	acid until 7000 g.
Breast milk fortifiers (see p 73)		
STANDARD FORMULAS		
Isoosmolar		
Enfamil 20	Full-term infants: as supplement to breast milk.	Multivitamins if taking < 32 oz/d.
Similac 20	Preterm infants: > 1800–2000 g.	
SMA 20[b]		
Higher Osmolality		
Enfamil 24	Term infants: for infants on fluid restriction or who cannot handle required volumes of 20-cal formula	
Similac 24 & 27	to grow.	
SMA 24 & 27		
Low Osmolality		
Similac 13	Preterm and term infants: for conservative initial feeding in infants who have not been fed orally for	
	several days or weeks. *Not for long-term use.*	
SOY FORMULAS		
ProSobee (lactose and sucrose free)	Term infants: milk sensitivity, galactosemia, carbohydrate intolerance. *Do not use in preterm in-*	Multivitamins if taking < 32 oz/d.
Isomil (lactose free)	*fants. Phytates can bind calcium and cause rickets.*	
Nursoy (lactose free)		
PROTEIN HYDROSYLATE FORMULAS		
Nutramigen	Term infants: Gut sensitivity to proteins, multiple food allergies, persistent diarrhea, galactosemia.	Multivitamins if taking < 32 oz/d.
Pregestimil	Preterm and term infants: disaccharidase deficiency, diarrhea, GI defects, cystic fibrosis, food al-	
	lergy, celiac disease, transition from TPN to oral feeding.	
Alimentum	Term infants: protein sensitivity, pancreatic insufficiency, diarrhea allergies, colic carbohydrate	
	and fat malabsorption.	
SPECIAL FORMULAS		
Portagen	Preterm and term infants: pancreatic or bile acid insufficiency, intestinal resection.	Multivitamins if taking < 32 oz/d; calcium needed.
Similac PM 60/40	Preterm and term infants: problem feeders on standard formula; infants with renal, cardiovascular,	Multivitamins and iron if weight > 1500 g.
	digestive diseases that require decreased protein and mineral levels, breast-feeding supple-	
	men; initial feeding.	
PREMATURE FORMULAS		
Low Osmolality		
Similac Special Care 20	Premature infants (< 1800–2000 g) who are growing rapidly. These formulas promote growth at	Routine vitamin supplementation not required (*controversial*).
Enfamil Premature 20	intrauterine rates. Vitamin and mineral concentrations are higher to meet the needs of growth.	
Preemie SMA 20	Usually started on 20 cal/oz and advanced to 24 cal/oz as tolerated.	
Isoosmolar		
Similac Special Care 24	Same as for low-osmolality premature formulas.	Same as for low-osmolality premature formulas.
Enfamil Special Care 24		
Preemie SMA 24		

[a] Such as Polyvisol (Mead Johnson) ½ mL/d.
[b] SMA has decreased sodium content and can be used in patients with congestive heart failure, bronchopulmonary dysplasia, and cardiac disease.

TABLE 8-3. COMPOSITION OF INFANT FORMULAS

Characteristics	Mature Human Breast Milk	Similac 20, Similac with Iron 20	Enfamil 20, Enfamil with Iron 20	SMA, SMA with Iron 20
Calories per liter	680	676	670	676
Osmolality (mosm/kg water)	290	300	300	300
Osmolarity (mosm/liter)	255	270	270	271
Protein				
Grams per liter	10.5	15	15	15
Percent total calories	6	9	9	8.9
Source		Cow's milk	Reduced minerals; whey, nonfat milk	Nonfat milk, demineralized whey
Fat				
Grams per liter	39	36.3	38	36
Percent total calories	52	48	50	48.2
Source		Oils: soy and coconut	Oils: soy and coconut	Oils[a]
Carbohydrate				
Grams per liter	72	72.3	69	72
Percent total calories	42	43	41	42.9
Source	Lactose	Lactose	Lactose	Lactose
Minerals	mg/L (meq/L)	mg/L (meq/L)	mg/L (meq/L)	mg/L (meq/L)
Calcium	280 (14)	510 (25.4)	460 (23)	420 (20.9)
Chloride	420 (11.9)	450 (12.7)	420 (12)	375 (11)
Iodine	0.11	0.1	0.068	0.06
Iron	0.03	12[b]	12.7[c]	12.0[d]
Magnesium	35	41	52	45
Phosphorus	140	390	310	280
Potassium	525 (13.4)	730 (18.7)	720 (18)	560 (14.3)
Sodium	180 (7.8)	230 (8.3)	181 (8)	150 (6.5)
Zinc	1.2	5.1	5.2	5.0
Vitamins per liter				
Vitamin A (IU)	2230	2030	2100	2000
Vitamin B_1 (mg)	0.21	0.68	0.52	0.67
Vitamin B_2 (mg)	0.35	1.01	1.05	1.0
Vitamin B_6 (mg)	0.20	0.41	0.42	0.42
Vitamin B_{12} (μg)	0.50	1.7	1.5	1.3
Vitamin C (mg)	40	60	54	55
Vitamin D (IU)	20	410	420	400
Vitamin E (IU)	2.3 (mg)	20	21	9.5
Vitamin K (μg)	2.1	54	58	55
Folic acid (μg)	50	100	105	55
Niacin (mg)	1.5	7.1	8.4	5.0
Pantothenic acid (mg)	1.8	3.04	3.1	2.1

[a] Oleo, coconut, oleic, and soy oils.
[b] Similac 20 Low Iron contains 1.5 mg iron/liter.
[c] Enfamil 20 Low Iron contains 1.1 mg iron/liter.
[d] SMA LO-IRON contains 1.5 mg iron/liter.
[e] MCT = medium-chain triglycerides.
[f] Special Care 24 Low-Iron 3.0 mg iron/liter.
[g] Low iron formula.

(continued)

Characteristics	Similac Special Care 20	Enfamil Premature Formula 20	Similac Special Care 24 and with Iron 24	Enfamil Premature Formula 24
Calories per liter	676	670	812	810
Osmolality (mosm/kg water)	250	240	300	300
Osmolarity (mosm/liter)	230	220	260	260
Protein				
Grams per liter	18.3	20	22	24
Percent total calories	11	12	11	12
Source	Cow's milk and whey	Nonfat milk, whey protein concentrate	Cow's milk and whey	Nonfat milk, whey protein concentrate
Fat				
Grams per liter	36.7	34	44.1	41
Percent total calories	47	44	47	44
Source	Oils: MCT,* soy, and coconut	Oils: MCT, soy and coconut	Oils: MCT, soy and coconut	Oils: MCT, soy and coconut
Carbohydrate				
Grams per liter	71.7	74	86.1	89
Percent total calories	42	44	42	44
Source	Lactose and polycose glucose polymers	Lactose and corn syrup solids	Lactose and polycose glucose polymers	Lactose and corn syrup solids

Minerals (mg/L, and meq/L where shown)

Characteristics	Similac Special Care 20 mg/L	meq/L	Enfamil Premature Formula 20 mg/L	meq/L	Similac Special Care 24 and with Iron 24 mg/L	meq/L	Enfamil Premature Formula 24 mg/L	meq/L
Calcium	1220	60.8	790	40	1460	73	950	47
Chloride	640	15.5	570	16	660	18.6	690	20
Iodine	0.04		0.05		0.15		0.06	
Iron	2.5		1.7		15^f		2	
Magnesium	81		68		100		81	
Phosphorus	610		400		730		480	
Potassium	870	22.3	750	19	1050	25.9	900	23
Sodium	290	12.6	260	11	350	15.2	320	14
Zinc	10.1		6.8		12.2		8.1	

Vitamins per liter

Characteristics	Similac Special Care 20	Enfamil Premature Formula 20	Similac Special Care 24 and with Iron 24	Enfamil Premature Formula 24
Vitamin A (IU)	4600	8100	5520	9700
Vitamin B$_1$ (mg)	1.69	1.69	2.03	2.00
Vitamin B$_2$ (mg)	4.19	2.3	5.03	2.9
Vitamin B$_6$ (mg)	1.69	1.69	2.03	2.0
Vitamin B$_{12}$ (µg)	3.7	2.0	4.5	2.4
Vitamin C (mg)	250	230	300	290
Vitamin D (IU)	1010	2200	1220	2600
Vitamin E (IU)	27	31	32	37
Vitamin K (µg)	81	88	100	106
Folic acid (µg)	250	230	300	290
Niacin (mg)	33.8	27.2	40.6	33.0
Pantothenic acid (mg)	12.8	8.1	15.4	9.7

[a] Oleo, coconut, oleic, and soy oils.
[b] Similac 20 Low Iron contains 1.5 mg iron/liter.
[c] Enfamil 20 Low Iron contains 1.1 mg iron/liter.
[d] SMA LO-IRON contains 1.5 mg iron/liter.
* MCT = medium-chain triglycerides.
[f] Special Care 24 Low-Iron 3.0 mg iron/liter.
[g] Low iron formula.

(continued)

TABLE 8-3. COMPOSITION OF INFANT FORMULAS (continued)

Characteristics	Similac PM 60/40		Similac 27	
Calories per liter	676		913	
Osmolality (mosm/kg water)	280		430	
Osmolarity (mosm/liter)	250		370	
Protein				
Grams per liter	15.8		24.7	
Percent total calories	9		11	
Source	Whey and caseinate		Cow's milk	
Fat				
Grams per liter	37.6		48.1	
Percent total calories	50		47	
Source	Oils: soy and coconut		Oils: soy and coconut	
Carbohydrate				
Grams per liter	69		95.9	
Percent total calories	41		42	
Source	Lactose		Lactose	
Minerals	mg/L	meq/L	mg/L	meq/L
Calcium	380	19	820	41
Chloride	400	11	740	21
Iodine	0.041		0.14	
Iron	1.5		2.0	
Magnesium	41		64	
Phosphorus	190		640	
Potassium	580	14.8	1210	31
Sodium	160	7	310	13.5
Zinc	5.1		6.9	
Vitamins per liter				
Vitamin A (IU)	2030		2740	
Vitamin B$_1$ (mg)	0.68		0.91	
Vitamin B$_2$ (mg)	1.01		1.37	
Vitamin B$_6$ (mg)	0.41		0.55	
Vitamin B$_{12}$ (µg)	1.7		2.3	
Vitamin C (mg)	60		80	
Vitamin D (IU)	410		550	
Vitamin E (IU)	20		27	
Vitamin K (µg)	54		73	
Folic acid (µg)	100		140	
Niacin (mg)	7.1		9.59	
Pantothenic acid (mg)	3.04		4.11	

a Oleo, coconut, oleic, and soy oils.
b Similac 20 Low Iron contains 1.5 mg iron/liter.
c Enfamil 20 Low Iron contains 1.1 mg iron/liter.
d SMA LO-IRON contains 1.5 mg iron/liter.
e MCT = medium-chain triglycerides.
f Special Care 24 Low-Iron 3.0 mg iron/liter.
g Low iron formula.

(continued)

Characteristics	Isomil 20		ProSobee 20		Nutramigen 20		Pregestimil 20	
Calories per liter	676		670		670		670	
Osmolality (mosm/kg water)	240		200		320		320	
Osmolarity (mosm/liter)	220		170		290		290	
Protein								
Grams per liter	18		20		19		19	
Percent total calories	11		12		11		11	
Source	Soy protein isolate		Soy protein isolate		Casein, hydrolysate, cystine, tyrosine, tryptophan		Casein, hydrolysate, cystine, tyrosine, tryptophan	
Fat								
Grams per liter	36.9		36		26		38	
Percent total calories	49		48		35		48	
Source	Oils: soy and coconut		Oils: soy and coconut		Corn oil		Oils: corn and MCT and high oleic safflower	
Carbohydrate								
Grams per liter	68.3		68		91		69	
Percent total calories	40		40		54		41	
Source	Corn syrup and sucrose		Corn syrup solids		Corn syrup and modified corn starch		Corn syrup and modified corn starch	
Minerals	mg/L	meq/L	mg/L	meq/L	mg/L	meq/L	mg/L	meq/L
Calcium	710	35.4	630	31	630	32	630	31
Chloride	420	11.9	560	16	580	16.4	580	16
Iodine	0.1		0.07		0.48		0.48	
Iron	12		12.7		12.7		12.7	
Magnesium	51		74		74		74	
Phosphorus	510		500		420		420	
Potassium	730	18.7	820	20	740	19	740	19
Sodium	300	13.0	240	10	320	14	320	14
Zinc	5.1		5.3		5.3		5.3	
Vitamins per liter								
Vitamin A (IU)	2030		2100		2100		2100	
Vitamin B1 (mg)	0.41		0.52		0.52		0.53	
Vitamin B2 (mg)	0.61		0.63		0.63		0.63	
Vitamin B6 (mg)	0.41		0.42		0.42		0.42	
Vitamin B12 (µg)	3.0		2.1		2.1		2.1	
Vitamin C (mg)	60		55		55		55	
Vitamin D (IU)	410		420		420		420	
Vitamin E (IU)	20		21		21		15.9	
Vitamin K (µg)	100		106		106		106	
Folic acid (µg)	100		106		106		106	
Niacin (mg)	9.13		8.5		85		85	
Pantothenic acid	5.07		3.2		3.2		3.2	

a Oleic, coconut, oleic, and soy oils.
b Similac 20 Low Iron contains 1.5 mg iron/liter.
c Enfamil 20 Low Iron contains 1.1 mg iron/liter.
d SMA LO-IRON contains 1.5 mg iron/liter.
e MCT = medium-chain triglycerides.
f Special Care 24 Low-Iron 3.0 mg iron/liter.
g Low iron formula.

(continued)

TABLE 8–3. COMPOSITION OF INFANT FORMULAS (continued)

Characteristics	Similac, Similac with Iron 24		SMA, SMA with Iron 24		Enfamil, Enfamil with Iron 24		Similac 13	
Calories per liter	812		811		810		440	
Osmolality (mosm/kg water)	380		364		360		200	
Osmolarity (mosm/liter)	340		322		320		190	
Protein								
Grams per liter	22		18		17.8		11.9	
Percent total calories	11		8.9		9		11	
Source	Cow's milk		Nonfat milk, demineralized whey		Nonfat milk, reduced mineral whey		Cow's milk	
Fat								
Grams per liter	42.8		43.2		45		23.2	
Percent total calories	47		48.2		50		47	
Source	Oils: soy and coconut		Oils: soy, coconut, oleo, and oleic		Oils: soy and coconut		Oils: soy and coconut	
Carbohydrate								
Grams per liter	85.3		86.4		83		46.2	
Percent total calories	42		42.9		41		42	
Source	Lactose		Lactose		Lactose		Lactose	
Minerals	mg/L	meq/L	mg/L	meq/L	mg/L	meq/L	mg/L	meq/L
Calcium	730	36.4	504	25.1	560	28	400	20
Chloride	660	18.6	450	12.7	500	14	360	10.2
Iodine	0.12		0.072		0.081		0.066	
Iron	15(1.8)[g]		14.4(1.8)[g]		15.2(1.3)[g]		1.0	
Magnesium	57		54		63		31	
Phosphorus	570		336		380		310	
Potassium	1070	27.4	672	17.2	870	22	580	14.8
Sodium	280	12.2	180	7.8	220	10	150	6.5
Zinc	6.1		6		6.3		3.3	
Vitamins per liter								
Vitamin A (IU)	2240		2400		2500		1320	
Vitamin B₁ (mg)	0.81		0.804		0.65		0.440	
Vitamin B₂ (mg)	1.22		1.20		1.3		0.66	
Vitamin B₆ (mg)	0.42		0.504		0.49		0.26	
Vitamin B₁₂ (µg)	2.0		1.6		1.9		1.1	
Vitamin C (mg)	70		66		66		40	
Vitamin D (IU)	490		480		510		260	
Vitamin E (IU)	24		11.4		25		13	
Vitamin K (µg)	65		66		70		35	
Folic acid (µg)	120		60		126		66	
Niacin (mg)	8.53		6.00		10.1		4.62	
Pantothenic acid (mg)	3.65		2.52		3.8		1.98	

a Oleo, coconut, oleic, and soy oils.
b Similac 20 Low Iron contains 1.5 mg iron/liter.
c Enfamil 20 Low Iron contains 1.1 mg iron/liter.
d SMA LO-IRON contains 1.5 mg iron/liter.
e MCT = medium-chain triglycerides.
f Special Care 24 Low-Iron 3.0 mg iron/liter.
g Low iron formula.

Characteristics	"Preemie" SMA 20	"Preemie" SMA 24	Nursoy 20	Alimentum
Calories per liter	676	676	676	676
Osmolality (mosm/kg water)	268	280	296	370
Osmolarity (mosm/liter)	242	246	266	330
Protein				
Grams per liter	20	20	21	18.6
Percent total calories	11.9	9.6	12.3	11
Source	Nonfat milk, demineralized whey	Nonfat milk, demineralized whey	Soy protein isolate	Casein hydrolysate, cystine, tyrosine, tryptophan
Fat				
Grams per liter	35	44	36	37.5
Percent total calories	46.7	48.5	47.4	48
Source	Oils: soy, coconut, oleic, oleo and MCT	Oils: soy, coconut, oleic, oleo and MCT	Oils: soy, coconut, oleo and oleic	Oils: soy, safflower, MCT
Carbohydrate				
Grams per liter	70	86	69	46.2
Percent total calories	41.5	41.9	40.3	42
Source	Lactose and glucose polymers	Lactose and glucose polymers	Sucrose	Sucrose and modified tapioca starch
Minerals	mg/L — meq/L	mg/L — meq/L	mg/L — meq/L	mg/L — meq/L
Calcium	750 — 37.4	750 — 37.4	600 — 29.9	710 — 35.4
Chloride	530 — 14.9	530 — 14.9	375 — 10.6	540 — 15.3
Iodine	0.083	0.083	0.060	0.100
Iron	3	3	11.5	12
Magnesium	70	70	67	51
Phosphorus	380	380	420	510
Potassium	750 — 19.2	750 — 19.2	700 — 17.9	800 — 20.5
Sodium	320 — 13.9	320 — 13.9	200 — 8.7	300 — 13
Zinc	8	8	5	5.1
Vitamins per liter				
Vitamin A (IU)	3200	2400	2000	2030
Vitamin B_1 (mg)	0.80	0.800	0.67	0.41
Vitamin B_2 (mg)	1.30	1.30	1.0	0.61
Vitamin B_6 (mg)	0.50	0.410	0.42	0.41
Vitamin B_{12} (µg)	2.0	2.0	2.0	3.0
Vitamin C (mg)	70	70	55	60
Vitamin D (IU)	510	480	400	260
Vitamin E (IU)	15	15	9.5	20
Vitamin K (µg)	70	70	100	100
Folic acid (µg)	100	100	50	100
Niacin (mg)	6.3	6.3	5.0	9.13
Pantothenic acid (mg)	3.60	3.60	3.0	5.07

[a] Oleic, coconut, oleic, and soy oils.
[b] Similac 20 Low Iron contains 1.5 mg iron/liter.
[c] Enfamil 20 Low Iron contains 1.1 mg iron/liter.
[d] SMA LO-IRON contains 1.5 mg iron/liter.
[e] MCT = medium-chain triglycerides.
[f] Special Care 24 Low-Iron 3.0 mg iron/liter.
[g] Low iron formula.

24, and SMA 24; and Similac 27 and SMA 27) are hypercaloric formulas designed to provide a greater percentage of the calories as protein and provide increased mineral concentrations. They are appropriate for an infant on fluid restriction so they can meet nutritional requirements.

B. **General guidelines**
   1. **For the initial feeding** for all infants, use sterile water or D5W if the infant is not being breast-fed. Formula is not recommended for the initial feeding so that if aspiration occurs, severe pneumonitis will not result. D10W is also not a good choice because it is hypertonic and not well tolerated.
   2. **Subsequent feedings.** Controversy surrounds dilution of infant formulas for the next several feedings if the infant tolerates the initial feeding. Some clinicians advocate diluting formulas with sterile water and advance as tolerated (eg, $\frac{1}{4}$ strength, increase to $\frac{1}{2}$ and then $\frac{3}{4}$ strength). Others feel this is unnecessary and that full-strength formula can be used if infants tolerate the initial feeding without difficulty. Breast milk is never diluted.
C. **Specific guidelines** are based on birth weight.
   1. **Weight $<$ 1200 g.** Gavage feed through a nasogastric tube.
      a. **Type of formula**
         (1) Initial feeding: Similac 13, diluted premature formulas.
         (2) Maintainence feeding: Premature formulas (20 or 24 cal/oz).
      b. **Procedure for initial feeding.** Give sterile water 0.5–1 mL/h. If tolerated, use initial formula stated in **a,** above.
      c. **Procedure for subsequent feedings**
         (1) **Volume.** Give 0.5–1.0 mL/h continuously; increase by 0.5–1.0 mL every other shift. When 10 mL/h is tolerated, change feedings to every 2 hours and advance as tolerated.
         (2) **Strength.** Use Similac 13 or diluted premature formula for 24–48 hours; then advance to premature formula. Once full feedings of 20 cal/oz are tolerated, consider advancing to 24 cal/oz feedings.
   2. **Weight 1200–1500 g.** Gavage feed through a nasogastric tube.
      a. **Type of formula.** See **1.a,** above.
      b. **Initial feeding.** Give sterile water 2 mL/kg every 2 hours; if tolerated for 4 hours, begin formula.
      c. **Subsequent feedings**
         (1) **Volume.** Give 2 mL/kg every 2 hours; increase by 1 mL every shift up to 20 mL every 2 hours. Then change to feedings every 3 hours.
         (2) **Strength.** Use Similac 13 or diluted premature formulas for 24 hours, then advance to premature formulas. Once full feedings of 20 cal/oz are tolerated, advance to 24 cal/oz if desired.
   3. **Weight 1500–2000 g.** Gavage feed through a nasogastric tube. A bottle can be attempted if the infant is $>$ 1600 g, $>$ 34 weeks' gestation, and neurologically intact.
      a. **Type of formula.** Use premature formulas (usually diluted the first 24 hours). For infants $>$ 1800 g, may consider regular formula (*controversial*).
      b. **Initial feeding.** Give sterile water, 2.5 mL/kg. If tolerated, begin regular formula.
      c. **Subsequent feedings.** Give 2.5 mL/kg every 3 hours; advance as tolerated.
   4. **Weight 2000–2500 g.** Use bottle if infant neurologically intact.
      a. **Type of formula.** Use standard formula.
      b. **Initial feeding.** Give sterile water, 2.5 mL/kg. If tolerated, begin formula or breast milk.

      c. **Subsequent feedings.** Give 5 mL/kg every 3–4 hours. Advance as tolerated.
   5. Weight > 2500 g. Use bottle if neurologically intact.
      a. **Type of formula.** Use standard formula.
      b. **Initial feeding.** See **4.b,** above.
      c. **Subsequent feedings.** Feed every 3–4 hours and advance as tolerated. Use 5 mL/kg; advance 2–5 mL per feeding.

III. Management of feeding intolerance. If feeding is initiated but not tolerated, the following should be done.

   A. Perform a complete abdominal examination; consider abdominal x-ray studies if physical findings are suspicious.

   B. If the abdominal evaluation is normal:
      1. Attempt continuous feedings with a nasogastric or orogastric tube. Check the **gastric aspirate** and follow the recommendations noted in Chapter 34.
      2. A different formula (eg, PM 60/40, Pregestimil) or breast milk may be better tolerated. Occasionally, diluting a formula with sterile water will be successful (start at $\frac{1}{4}$ strength, advance slowly to $\frac{1}{2}$ strength, $\frac{3}{4}$ strength, and full strength).

IV. Nutritional supplements. Supplements are sometimes added to feedings, primarily to increase caloric intake (Table 8–4). They increase energy needs without a concomitant increase in nutrients. Some clinicians feel strongly that if caloric supplementation is needed, it should be given in the form of a high-calorie formula (ie, 24 kcal/oz) instead of in the form of a supplement, because all nutrients in a high-calorie formula are in proportion to one another and allow maximum absorption. The nutritional supplements are often used in patients with bronchopulmonary dysplasia (BPD) who are not gaining weight and need an increase in calories without an increase in protein or fat.

BREAST-FEEDING

I. Advantages
   A. Protein quality. The whey predominance and mixture of amino acids is compatible with the metabolic needs of low birth weight infants.
   B. Digestion and absorption are improved with breast milk.
   C. Immunologic benefits. Breast-feeding provides immunologic protection against bacterial and viral infection (particularly upper respiratory tract and gastrointestinal infection). Studies of infants breast-fed more than 6 months show that they have a decreased incidence of cancer.
   D. Bonding between the mother and infant is promoted.
   E. Lower renal solute load, which facilitates better tolerance.

II. Contraindications
   A. A mother with active tuberculosis should not breast-feed.
   B. A mother with certain viral and bacterial infections should not breast-feed. See Appendix H, Isolation Guidelines, for specific recommendations.
   C. A mother who is taking medications that are passed in the breast milk and may harm the infant. See Chapter 77 for the effects of medications and substances on lactation and breast-feeding.

III. Possible contraindications
   A. A preterm infant may have a poorly developed sucking reflex and may not be able to nurse.
   B. A weak or ill infant or one with a cleft lip or palate may also have difficulty. In some cases, the mother can express her milk with a breast pump, and it can be bottle-fed to the infant.
   C. Protein, sodium, calcium, and phosphorus in breast milk may be inadequate for the premature infant. Supplementation may be needed.

TABLE 8–4. NUTRITIONAL SUPPLEMENTS USED IN INFANTS

Supplement	Nutrient Content	Calories	Indications and Contraindications	Amount to Use
CARBOHYDRATE				
Polycose	Glucose polymers	3.8 kcal/g powder; 2 kcal/mL liquid	Calorie supplementation[a]	**Powder** 0.5 g/oz of 20-cal formula = 22 cal/oz; 1 g/oz of 20-cal formula = 24 cal/oz **Liquid** 1 mL to 1 oz of 20 cal formula = 22 cal/oz
Infant rice cereal	Rice	15 cal/tbs	Thickens feedings	1 tsp/4 oz formula
FAT				
Medium-chain triglyceride (MCT) oil	Lipid fraction of coconut oil	8.3 kcal/g, 7.7 cal/mL	Limit to 50% calories from fat to prevent ketosis; may cause diarrhea; do not use if infant has BPD due to risk of aspiration pneumonia[b]	0.5 mL/4 oz formula = 21 cal/oz; 1 mL/4 oz formula = 22 cal/oz
Vegetable oil	Soy, corn oil	9.0 cal/g (120 cal/tbs)	To increase calories if fat absorption normal[c]	See MCT above
PROTEIN				
Casec	Calcium caseinate	3.4 cal/g (4 g protein/tbs)	Useful in chronic fluid restriction and as breast milk supplement; do not use in premature infants due to high solute load	

[a] Limiting formula intake while increasing calories may compromise protein, vitamin, and mineral intake, which may also lead to hyperglycemia and diarrhea.
[b] Always mix with formula to avoid possibility of lipid aspiration and/or pneumonia.
[c] Vitamin E may need to be increased to at least 1 IU per gram linoleic acid.

Note: Temporary problems (eg, sore or cracked nipples, mastitis) will resolve with treatment (eg, antibiotics for mastitis) and do not preclude nursing.

IV. **Donor breast milk.** The use of donor breast milk is both regional and *controversial.* If the mother is unable to provide breast milk for an infant who needs it, breast milk from a donor can be obtained from a human milk bank and bottle-fed to the infant. (The mother's milk is always preferable to donor milk unless contraindicated for one of the reasons given above.) Donor milk is almost always mature breast milk and should be used only until the infant can tolerate formula with adequate vitamin and mineral content.

  A. **Storage.** Breast milk can be stored frozen at $-20\ °C$ for up to 6 months and refrigerated at $4\ °C$ for up to 24 hours.

  B. **Screening of breast milk donors.** Potential donors are screened for chronic disease. The blood is tested (and must be negative) for hepatitis core antibody and surface antigen and HTLV-III antibody. The tuberculin skin test must be negative. A history of sexually transmitted disease or infection due to herpesvirus makes the donor unacceptable. Donors must not be taking any medication, must be nonsmokers, and must limit alcohol intake to 60 mL/d. Once donors are accepted, they are taught sterile techniques for milk collection.

  C. **Acceptable bacteria levels in donor breast milk.** Samples are tested from each donor for colony-forming units and specific pathogenic organisms. Acceptable standards for raw milk are less than 10,000 colony-forming units per milliliter and absence of *Staphylococcus aureus* and gram-negative rods. Pasteurization is required for more than 10,000 colony-forming units per milliliter or if *S aureus* or gram-negative organisms are present. Breast milk is not checked for viruses. Cytomegalovirus is destroyed by freezing for more than 7 days.

V. **Breast milk fortifiers (supplements).** The breast milk fortifiers (Table 8–5) are designed as a supplement to be added to mother's milk in rapidly growing premature infants. Preterm human milk beyond the second and third week may contain insufficient amounts of protein, calcium phosphorus, and possibly copper, zinc, and sodium. Currently, 2 fortifiers are available.

  A. **Enfamil Human Milk Fortifier**

    1. **Indications.** This is indicated for those premature infants who tolerate unfortified human milk at full feedings, usually at 2–4 weeks of age up to time of discharge or birth weight 2500–3000 g.

    2. **Composition.** The protein is 60% whey protein and 40% casein, similar to breast milk. The carbohydrate is 75% glucose polymers and 25% lactose. The fat amount is negligible. It comes in a powder form.

    3. **Calories**

      a. One packet of fortifier added to 50 mL of human milk provides an additional 2 cal/fl oz.

      b. One packet of fortifier added to 25 mL of human milk provides an additional 4 cal/fl oz.

    4. Once the powder is added to human milk, the container should be capped and mixed well. It can be covered and stored under refrigeration but should be used within 8 hours of preparation.

    5. Clinical experience has shown that Enfamil Human Milk Fortifier added to preterm mother's milk:

      a. Decreases the time needed to grow from 1500–1800 g by 25%.

      b. Achieves better alkaline phosphatase levels.

      c. Does not dilute anti-infective factors in breast milk.

      d. Enables the premature infant to tolerate it well.

  B. **Similac Natural Care**

    1. **Indications.** This is indicated for those premature infants who toler-

TABLE 8–5. A COMPARISON OF 2 COMMERCIALLY AVAILABLE BREAST MILK SUPPLEMENTS

	Similac Natural Care (Ross)	Enfamil Human Milk Fortifier (Mead Johnson)
Volume	100 mL (50 mL breast milk plus 50 mL forti- fier)	100 mL (4 packets fortifier plus 100 mL breast milk)
Total calories	73 (24 cal/oz)	81 (24 cal/oz)
Osmolality (mosm/kg water)	300	365
	These supplements add the following to the breast milk	
Calories	9	14
Protein	0.1 g	0.7 g
Fat	0.4 g	0.04 g
Carbohydrate	1.3 g	2.7 g
Minerals		
Calcium	71 mg	60 mg
Chloride	9 mg	17.7
Copper	62 μg	40 μg
Iron	0.1 mg	—
Magnesium	3.4 mg	4 mg
Phosphorus	36 mg	33 mg
Potassium	28 mg	15.6 mg
Sodium	8 mg	7 mg
Vitamins per liter		
Vitamin A (IU)	150	780
Vitamin B$_1$ (μg)	96	187
Vitamin B$_2$ (μg)	233	250
Vitamin B$_6$ (μg)	99	193
Vitamin B$_{12}$ (μg)	0.2	0.21
Vitamin C (mg)	12.8	24
Vitamin D (IU)	58.8	210
Vitamin E (IU)	1.3	3.4
Vitamin K (μg)	4.0	9.1
Folic Acid (μg)	12.8	23
Niacin (μg)	1920	3100
Pantothenic acid (μg)	640	790

ate unfortified breast milk at full feedings, usually at 2–4 weeks of age up until time of discharge or weight > 2500–3000 g.
2. **Composition.** The protein is whey predominant. The carbohydrate is lactose in equal proportion to glucose polymers. The fat is a mixture of 50% medium chain triglyceride, 30% soy oil, and 20% coconut oil. It is a ready-to-use liquid formula that can be mixed with human milk.
3. **Calories.** 24 cal/fl oz. It is most commonly made as a 50–50% dilution with human milk.
4. **Storage.** Same as **A.4,** above.
5. **Clinical experience.** Increased bone mineralization has been observed in infants given the fortifier compared to those who were not.

TOTAL PARENTERAL NUTRITION

Total parenteral nutrition (TPN) is **intravenous administration of all nutrients** (fats, carbohydrates, proteins, vitamins, and minerals) necessary for metabolic requirements and growth. Parenteral nutrition (PN) is supplemental intravenous administration of nutrients. Enteral nutrition (EN) is oral or gavage feedings.
  I. **Intravenous routes used in PN**
    A. **Central parenteral nutrition.** Central parenteral nutrition is **usually re-**

served for patients requiring long-term administration of most calories. The advantage of this route is that hypertonic solutions (15–25% dextrose) can be administered through the central catheter. Disadvantages include increased risk of infection and complications due to catheterization placement. There are 2 methods commonly used for placement.

1. A **percutaneous catheter,** placed in the **antecubital or external jugular vein,** is usually advanced into the superior vena cava. This technique avoids surgical placement, and fewer complications are seen. See Chapter 27, p 160, for details of the procedure.
2. A **central vein, usually the subclavian vein,** is used. The **indwelling catheter** is surgically placed, either by a percutaneous route or by cutdown. The disadvantages are that anesthesia and surgery are needed for placement of the catheter.

B. **Peripheral parenteral nutrition.** A peripheral vein is used. This route is **more commonly used in the neonatal intensive care unit (NICU)** than central parenteral nutrition and is usually associated with fewer complications. The maximum concentration of dextrose that can be given is 12.5%.

Note: Parenteral nutrition can be given through an umbilical artery catheter, and this route has been used in some centers. However, the umbilical artery is not a preferred site and should be used with caution.

II. **Indications.** PN is used as a supplement to enteral feedings or as a complete substitution (TPN) for it when adequate nourishment cannot be achieved by the enteral route. Common indications in neonates include congenital malformation of the gastrointestinal tract, gastroschisis, meconium ileus, short bowel syndrome, necrotizing enterocolitis, paralytic ileus, respiratory distress syndrome, extreme prematurity, sepsis, and malabsorption. PN is usually started on day 3 or 4 of life, depending on how ill the patient is.

III. **Caloric concentration.** Caloric densities of various energy sources are as follows:

Dextrose (anhydrous)	3.4 kcal/g
Protein	4 kcal/g
Fat	9 kcal/g
10% fat emulsion	1.1 kcal/mL
20% fat emulsion	2 kcal/mL

IV. **Composition of PN solutions**

A. **Carbohydrates.** The only commercially available carbohydrate source is **dextrose (glucose).** A solution of 5.0–12.5% g/dL is used in peripheral PN and up to 25% g/dL in central PN. Dextrose concentrations should be calculated as milligrams per kilograms per minute. To allow for an appropriate response of endogenous insulin and to prevent the development of osmotic diuresis secondary to glucosuria, neonates should not routinely be started on more than 6–8 mg/kg/min of dextrose. Frequent testing of urine for the presence of glucose is required. Infusion rates can be increased by 0.5–1 mg/kg/min each day as tolerated to achieve adequate caloric intake. See p 59, II, for the formula used in calculating the amount of glucose in milligrams per kilogram per minute that an infant is receiving.

B. **Proteins. Inadequate protein** intake may result in failure to thrive, hypoalbuminemia, and edema. **Excessive protein** can cause hyperammonemia, serum amino acid imbalance, metabolic acidosis, and cholestatic jaundice. The formulations of amino acids specifically designed for use in neonates and pediatric patients has resulted in fewer metabolic complications. Products such as TrophAmine and Aminosyn are designed to decrease the production of organic acids and provide additional taurine and histidine, which are essential during the neonatal period. Use of TrophAmine has resulted in far fewer complications of

hyperammonemia, cholestasis, and elevation of BUN levels. These solutions also have a lower pH to allow for the addition of sufficient quantities of calcium (2 meq/dL) and phosphorus (1–2 mm/dL), in order to
meet daily requirements. *Note:* It is no longer necessary, except in very
low birth weight infants, to gradually increase the protein concentration of PN over several days (Kerner, 1983). It is best not to begin amino
acids unless a minimum of 40 cal/kg/d are given as glucose, because
the amino acids will be poorly utilized and acidosis and hyperammonemia will develop. Amino acids can be started at a rate of 0.5 g/kg/d
in infants weighing less than 1500 g and can be increased by increments of 0.5 g/kg/d. In term infants, the starting rate can be 1.5 g, with
increases of 1 g/kg/d; to avoid hyperammonemia and acidosis, the final
concentration should not exceed 3 g/kg/d.

At most institutions, amino acid solutions are prepared in 1%, 2%,
and 3% concentrations. This works out to the following equivalents.

100 mL/d of 1% solution = 1 g/kg/d protein
100 mL/d of 2% solution = 2 g/kg/d protein
100 mL/d of 3% solution = 3 g/kg/d protein

C. **Fats.** Because of their high caloric density, intravenous fat solutions
(eg, Intralipid) are an excellent source of calories and will provide a
significant portion of the daily caloric needs. Most intravenous fat solutions are isotonic (270–300 mosm/L) and are therefore not likely to
cause infiltration of peripheral lines. Caution should be used when administering fat solution to neonates with unconjugated hyperbilirubinemia because of the competitive binding of bilirubin and nonesterified
fatty acids on albumin, which may increase significantly during infusion. Fat solution should not be administered to infants with bilirubin
levels above 8 mg/dL (> 5 mg/dL for very low birth weight infants).

1. **Concentrations.** A common regimen is 0.5 g/kg/d on the first day, 1
g/kg/d on the second day, and 2 g/kg/d (maintenance dose) on the
third day. The **infusion rate** should not exceed 0.24 g/kg/h. The infusion is given continuously over 24 hours. For example, in an infant
weighing 2 kg who is to start at an amount of 0.5 g/kg/d:

   a. 2 kg × 0.5 g/kg/d = 1 g/d
   b. 1 mL of Intralipid = 0.1 g
   c. $\frac{1\,mL}{0.1\,g} = \frac{x\,mL}{1\,g}$
   d. 0.1 x = 1
   e. x = 10 mL. This infant should receive a total of 10 mL of Intralipid in a 24-hour period to equal 0.5 g/kg/d.
   f. The volume (eg, 10 mL) is divided by 24 hours. It should run at 0.4
   mL/h × 24 hours.

2. **Complications.** Fat intolerance may be seen. Blood triglyceride levels should be monitored weekly. If they are greater than 150 mg/dL,
infusion of fats should be stopped. "Lipidcrits" (checks of the serum
for cloudiness caused by excessive fats) are no longer considered
reliable.

D. **Vitamins.** Vitamins are added to intravenous solutions in the form of a
pediatric multivitamin suspension, based on recommendations by the
Nutritional Advisory Committee. Neonates, regardless of weight, receive two-thirds the dose of pediatric patients. Except for vitamin D,
patients receive daily requirements for all vitamins. As soon as possible, vitamin D drops should be added to enteral feedings.

E. **Trace elements.** Trace elements are added to the solution based on
weight and total volume (0.5 mL/kg/wk) for patients on short-term TPN
and 0.5 mL/kg/d for long-term TPN. Additional amounts of zinc (1–2 mg/
d) are often added for patients requiring gastrointestinal surgery to

TABLE 8-6. RECOMMENDATIONS FOR TRACE ELEMENT SUPPLEMENTATION IN TPN SOLUTIONS FOR NEONATES

Element	Full term	Premature
Zinc (μg)	100–200	400–600
Copper (μg)	10–20	20
Chromium (μg)	0.14–0.2	0.14–0.2
Manganese (μg)	2–10	2–10
Fluoride (μg)	1	1*
Iodine (μg)	3–5	3–5*

* Not well defined in the premature infant.

help promote healing. At many institutions, a prepared solution is available. See Table 8-6 for recommended doses of trace elements.

F. **Electrolytes.** Electrolytes can be added according to specific needs, but for low birth weight infants, requirements are usually satisfied by standard amino-acid solution formulations, containing electrolytes (Table 8-7).

V. **Monitoring of PN.** Hyperalimentation can cause many alterations in biochemical function, and compulsive anthropometric and laboratory monitoring is essential for all patients. Recommendations for monitoring are shown in Table 8-8.

VI. **Complications of PN.** Most complications of TPN are associated with use of central hyperalimentation and primarily involve infections and problems associated with catheterization. However, metabolic problems can occur with both central and peripheral TPN. The major complication of peripheral hyperalimentation is accidental infiltration of the solution, causing sloughing of the skin.

A. **Infection.** Sepsis can occur in infants receiving central hyperalimentation. The most common organisms include coagulase-positive and -negative *Staphylococcus, Streptococcus viridans, Escherichia coli, Pseudomonas* species, *Klebsiella* species, and *Candida albicans*. Contamination of the central line can occur as a result of contamination at the insertion site or use of the line for blood sampling or administration of blood. It is best not to open the line.

B. **Complications of catheterization.** Complications associated with placement of central catheters (specifically in the subclavian vein) occur in approximately 4–9% of patients. Complications include pneumothorax, pneumomediastinum, hemorrhage, and chylothorax (caused by

TABLE 8-7. COMPOSITION OF AMINO ACID SOLUTIONS FOR LOW BIRTH WEIGHT INFANTS—STANDARD FORMULATIONS

Electrolytes (meq/L)	Amino Acid Concentration					
	1.0%		2.0%		3.0%	
	A[a]	T[b]	A	T	A	T
Na$^+$	20	20	20	20	20	20
C1$^-$	20	20	20	20	20	20
K$^+$	15	15	15	15	15	15
Mg^{++}	11	11	11	11	11	11
Ca^{++}	15	15	15	15	15	15
Acetate	7.6	9.3	15.3	18.6	22.8	27.9
Phosphorus (mmol/L)	10	10	10	10	10	10

[a] A = Aminosyn PF.
[b] T = TrophAmine.

TABLE 8-8. MONITORING SCHEDULE FOR NEONATES RECEIVING PARENTERAL NUTRITION

Measurement	Baseline Study	Frequency of Measurement
Anthropometric		
Weight	Yes	Daily
Length	Yes	Weekly
Head circumference	Yes	Daily
Metabolic		
Glucose	Yes	Daily
(Dextrostix when changing detrose concentrations)		
Calcium and phosphorus	Yes	Twice per week initially, then weekly
Electrolytes (Na, Cl, K, CO$_2$)	Yes	Once a day for 3 days, then twice a week
Magnesium	Yes	Weekly
Hematocrit	Yes	Every other day for 1 week, then weekly
BUN and creatinine	Yes	Twice a week, then weekly
Bilirubin	Yes	Weekly
Ammonia	Yes	Weekly if using high protein
Total protein and albumin	Yes	Weekly
SGOT or SGPT	Yes	Weekly
Triglycerides	Yes	Weekly for patients on intravenous fat
Urine		
Specific gravity and glucose	Yes	For first week, test each urine sample; then once/shift

injury to the thoracic duct). Thrombosis of the vein adjacent to the catheter tip may occur, resulting in "superior vena caval syndrome" (edema of the face, neck, and eyes). Once collateral circulation is established, the syndrome resolves. Pulmonary embolism can also occur secondary to thrombosis. Malpositioned catheters may result in collection of fluid in the pleural cavity, causing hydrothorax, or in the pericardial space, causing tamponade.

C. **Metabolic complications**
   1. **Hyperammonemia** occurs secondary to metabolic immaturity and substrate deficiency in ammonia metabolism.
   2. **Hyperchloremic metabolic alkalosis** is secondary to increased amounts of chloride.
   3. **Serum amino-acid imbalance.**
   4. **Elevated blood urea nitrogen levels** occurs secondary to excessive protein administration.
   5. **Cholestatic liver disease.** With prolonged administration of intravenous dextrose and protein and absence of enteral feeding, cholestasis usually occurs. The incidence ranges from as high as 80% in very low birth weight infants receiving TPN for longer than 30 days (with no enteral feeding) to as low as 15% (or lower) in neonates weighing more than 1500 g receiving TPN for 14 days or less. Monitoring for abnormalities in liver function and the development of direct hyperbilirubinemia is important in long-term TPN. Some authors suggest that enteral feedings be started in small amounts as soon as possible to help alleviate this problem.
   6. **Hypoglycemia or hyperglycemia** may occur with administration of dextrose. (See also Chaps 38 and 41.)
   7. **Complications of fat administration.** Infusion of fat emulsion has been associated with several metabolic disturbances, hyperlipidemia, platelet dysfunction, acute allergic reactions, deposition of pigment in the liver, and lipid deposition in the blood vessels of the lung. Most metabolic problems seem to be associated with rapid rates of infusion and exceeding the recommended dose. Contro-

versy over administering Intralipid in severe lung disease arose when an excessive dose was given and the lipids did not clear but were deposited in blood vessels in the lung. This sequence of events resulted in carbon dioxide retention and oxygenation problems; therefore lipids were being avoided in infants with severe lung disease. Because the dose of lipids and the rate at which to give it are now well defined, this problem no longer occurs.

8. **Essential fatty acid deficiency.** If PN is administered without adding fat emulsion, deficiency of essential fatty acids may occur. Essential fatty acid deficiency is associated with decreased platelet aggregation (thromboxane A_2 deficiency), poor weight gain, scaly rash, sparse hair growth, and thrombocytopenia. These problems usually occur after 10 days in full-term infants and after 2 days in preterm infants.

9. **Mineral deficiency.** Most minerals are transferred to the fetus during the last trimester of pregnancy. The following problems may be seen.

   a. **Osteopenia, rickets, and pathologic fractures** (see Chap 72).

   b. **Zinc deficiency** occurs if zinc is not added to TPN after 4 weeks. Zinc deficiency can present as poor growth, diarrhea, alopecia increased susceptibility to infection, and skin desquamation surrounding the mouth and anus (**acrodermatitis enteropathica**). Zinc losses are increased in patients with an ileostomy or colostomy.

   c. **Copper deficiency** presents as osteoporosis, hemolytic anemia, neutropenia, and depigmentation of the skin.

CALORIC CALCULATIONS

An infant should receive 100–120 kcal/kg/d for growth and for maintenance of a positive nitrogen balance, at least 60–80 kcal/kg/d for oral intake. (Infants require fewer calories [80–90 cal/kg/d] for growth if receiving TPN only.) Some hypermetabolic infants may require more than 120 kcal/kg/d for growth. Equations for calculation of caloric intake for oral formula and TPN are as follows.

I. **Infant formulas. Most standard infant formulas contain 0.67 kcal/mL.** Specific caloric concentrations of formulas are given in Table 8–3. To calculate total daily calories, use the following equation.

$$\text{kcal/kg/d} = \frac{\text{kcal/mL} \times \text{Total mL (of formula)}}{\text{Weight of patient (kg)}}$$

TABLE 8-9. CALORIC CONCENTRATIONS OF VARIOUS PARENTERAL SOLUTIONS

Dextrose Solutions (Anhydrous) in kcal/mL	
D5 = 0.17	D15 = 0.51
D7.5 = 0.255	D20 = 0.68
D10 = 0.34	D25 = 0.85
D12.5 = 0.425	

Protein Solutions (g/d)	Percent Concentration	Caloric Concentration (kcal/mL)
0.5 g	0.5%	0.02
1.0 g	1%	0.04
1.5 g	1.5%	0.06
2.0 g	2.0%	0.08
2.5 g	2.5%	0.10
3.0 g	3.0%	0.12
(0.5% solution, if given 100 mL/d = 0.5 g protein/d)		

II. Carbohydrates. If only dextrose infusion is given, the total daily caloric intake is calculated as follows. (See Table 8–9 for caloric concentrations of common solutions.)

$$\text{kcal/kg/d} = \frac{\text{mL (solution)/h} \times 24 \text{ h} \times \text{kcal in solution}}{\text{Weight of patient (kg)}}$$

III. Proteins. Use the same formula given for carbohydrates (see above). Use the caloric concentrations given in Table 8–9.

IV. Fat emulsions. A 10% fat emulsion (Intralipid) contains 1.1 kcal/mL; 20%, 2 kcal/mL. Use the following formula to calculate daily caloric intake supplied by Intralipid 10%.

$$\text{kcal/kg/d} = \frac{\text{Total mL/d (solution)} \times 1.1 \text{ kcal/mL}}{\text{Weight of patient (kg)}}$$

REFERENCES

Baker SS, Dwyer E, Queen P: Metabolic derangements in children requiring parenteral nutrition. *JPEN* 1986;**10**:279.

Cox MA: Nutrition. Pages 448–456 in: *Manual of Neonatal Care,* 2nd ed. Cloherty JP, Stark AR (editors). Little, Brown, 1985.

Fitzgerald KA, MacKay MW: Calcium and phosphate solubility in neonatal parenteral nutrient solutions containing TrophAmine. *Am J Hosp Pharm* 1986;**43**:88.

Kerner JA Jr (editor): *Manual of Pediatric Parenteral Nutrition.* Wiley, 1983.

Kushner RF: Total parenteral nutrition-associated metabolic acidosis. *JPEN* 1986;**10**:306.

Merritt RJ: Cholestasis associated with total parenteral nutrition. *J Pediatr Gastroenterol Nutr* 1986;**5**:9.

Moore MC et al: Evaluation of pediatric multiple vitamin preparation for total parenteral nutrition in infants and children. 1. Blood levels of water-soluble vitamins. *Pediatrics* 1986;**77**:530.

9 Neonatal Radiology

COMMON RADIOLOGIC TECHNIQUES

I. **X-ray.** The need for x-ray studies must always be weighed against the risks of neonatal exposure to radiation (3–5 mrem per x-ray). No studies have been done on infants' exposure to radiation in neonatal intensive care units (NICUs). It is known that 1000 rem delivered to the mother causes abortion of the fetus. The infant's gonads should be shielded as much as possible. Anyone holding an infant during the x-ray procedure should also wear a protective shield. Persons standing 6–10 feet from the x-ray machine will receive negligible radiation, as 10 feet is the maximum area of "scatter" for this type of radiation.

A. **Chest x-ray studies**

1. **Anteroposterior (AP) view** is the single best view for identification of heart or lung disease or verification of endotracheal tube placement. It also is the best view to obtain in an emergency if an air leak is suspected.

2. **Cross-table lateral view** can be used to diagnose pneumothorax in conjunction with an AP view. The cross-table lateral view will not show which side the pneumothorax is on.

3. **Lateral decubitus view** is the best view for ruling out a small pneumothorax or one that is difficult to assess on the AP view. In a newborn infant there is a tendency for the denser tissue of the lung to collapse posteriorly. For example, if a pneumothorax is suspected to be on the left side, a right lateral decubitus view of the chest should be obtained (infant is placed on its right side, with the left side up). An air pocket will be visible on the side on which the pneumothorax is present. The only disadvantage of this view is that it is sometimes difficult to do in an unstable infant and it takes more time than a regular AP view.

4. **Upright view** is not used as much in the NICU as in other areas. It can identify abdominal perforation by showing free air under the diaphragm.

B. **Abdominal x-ray studies**

1. **Anteroposterior (AP) view** is the single best view for diagnosis of abdominal disorders and to check placement of umbilical artery and vein catheters.

2. **Cross-table lateral view** will help diagnose abdominal perforation, but the left lateral decubitus view is better for this purpose. Abdominal perforations may be missed on cross-table lateral views.

3. **Left lateral decubitus view** (infant placed on its left side, with the right side up) is the best view for diagnosis of perforation, which will be seen as an air pocket above the liver.

C. **Barium contrast studies (barium swallow, barium enema).** Barium is inert and is not absorbed from the gastrointestinal tract. It does not cause fluid shifts, except in infants in whom there is a high possibility of barium retention in the colon, where water may be absorbed.

1. **Indications.** The use of barium as a contrast agent is recommended for:

    a. Imaging the GI tract. Barium enema is used to rule out lower abdominal obstruction.

    b. Suspected tracheoesophageal fistula. Barium swallow is sometimes used. However, most tracheoesophageal fistulas can be diagnosed by inserting a radiopaque nasogastric tube; the tube will be seen curled up in the blind esophageal pouch.

    c. Suspected esophageal perforation. Barium swallow is used if previous studies with water-soluble agents have been negative.

    d. Suspected gastroesophageal reflux. Barium swallow is used as the first-line study.

  2. Contraindications. Barium-contrast studies are not recommended in infants with **suspected abdominal perforation,** because barium is toxic to the peritoneum.

D. High-osmolality water-soluble contrast studies (Hypaque or Gastrografin enema)

  1. Advantages of these agents

    a. They are not toxic to the peritoneum if they leak from the GI tract, and they are absorbed and cleared from the body.

    b. They draw water into the lumen of the bowel, so they may be used therapeutically to relieve some cases of bowel obstruction or treat meconium ileus.

  2. Disadvantages

    a. Severe shifts of fluid may occur; therefore, if used, fluid and electrolyte status must be followed closely.

    b. Extremely toxic if aspirated into the lungs.

    c. Bowel necrosis has occurred following the use of these agents for meconium ileus.

    d. NEC resulting in death has been reported.

  3. Indications

    a. Evaluation of the bowel if perforation is suspected.

    b. Differentiation of ileus from obstruction.

    c. Treatment of meconium obstruction syndromes.

E. Low-osmolality water-soluble contrast agents. These agents (metrizamide, iohexol, iopamidol, and ioxaglate) are being studied now because of their benefits over barium and the high-osmolality contrast agents.

  1. Advantages

    a. They do not cause fluid shifts.

    b. If perforation is suspected, they are nontoxic.

    c. They do not damage the bowel mucosa.

    d. They do not cause severe problems if aspiration occurs.

  2. Disadvantages

    a. High cost.

    b. Lower quality images as compared to barium.

  3. Indications

    a. Suspected tracheoesophageal fistula.

    b. Suspected gastroesophageal reflux.

    c. Suspected esophageal obstruction.

    d. Evaluation of the bowel if perforation is suspected.

    e. Unexplained pneumoperitoneum.

    f. Suspected intussusception or distal small bowel or colon obstruction.

II. Ultrasonography

A. Ultrasonography of the head is performed to rule out intraventricular hemorrhage and to grade the size of ventricles. It can be performed in most NICUs with a portable machine. No special preparation is needed; however, an open anterior fontanelle must be present, and there should be no intravenous lines placed in the scalp. The classification of intra-

FIGURE 9-1. Ultrasonogram of the head (right sagittal view) showing a small germinal matrix hemorrhage (grade I intraventricular hemorrhage).

ventricular hemorrhage based on ultrasonographic findings (developed by Papile) is given below. Examples are shown in Figures 9-1 to 9-4.

Grade I. Subependymal, germinal matrix hemorrhage.

Grade II. Intraventricular extension without ventricular dilatation.

Grade III. Intraventricular extension with ventricular dilatation.

Grade IV. Intraventricular and intraparenchymal hemorrhage.

   B. **Abdominal ultrasonography** is useful in the evaluation of abdominal masses and renal failure.

III. **Computed tomographic (CT) scanning.** CT scanning of the head is more complicated than ultrasonography, because the patient must be moved to the CT unit and be adequately sedated. CT scanning does provide more information than ultrasonography of the head. It can be used to diagnose intraventricular, subdural, or subarachnoid bleeding and cerebral edema or infarction. Infusion of contrast medium is needed to diagnose cerebral infarction. If infusion is used, blood urea nitrogen and creatinine determinations must be obtained before the test to rule out renal impairment, which may be a contraindication to the use of contrast media. An intravenous line must be placed, preferably not in the head.

IV. **Magnetic resonance imaging (MRI).** Use of MRI in the neonate is now an acceptable mode of imaging and its use in neonates is expanding. It is superior to CT for imaging the brain stem, spinal cord, soft tissues, and areas of high CT bony artifact. Advantages are that there is no ionizing radiation, and visualization of vascular anatomy can be obtained without contrast dye. The major disadvantages are (1) that it cannot be done on critically ill infants requiring ventilator support, (2) the scanning time is longer, and (3) the infants must be heavily sedated.

NORMAL RADIOGRAPHIC EXAMPLES

Caution is necessary when identifying ribs in the newborn and correlating ver-

FIGURE 9-2. Ultrasonogram of the head (left sagittal view) showing germinal matrix and intraventricular hemorrhage but minimal ventricular enlargement. Same patient as in Fig 9-3.

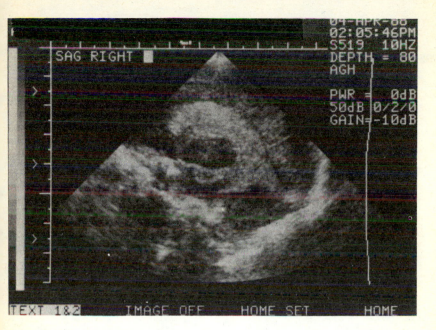

FIGURE 9-3. Ultrasonogram for same patient as in Fig 9-2, right sagittal view, demonstrating a large intraventricular hemorrhage with enlarged ventricle (grade III).

tebrae. Occasional errors are made because it is assumed that there are 12 ribs in infants as in older children and adults. In fact, it is not at all uncommon for infants to have a noncalcified 12th rib, and thus the 11th rib is mistaken for the 12th rib and an incorrect count of the lumbar vertebrae follows.

I. **Endotracheal intubation.** The endotracheal tube should be approximately at the level of T2. Correct tube placement is shown in Figure 9-5. If the tube has been placed in the right main-stem bronchus, a chest x-ray film will show atelectasis of the left lung and hyperinflation of the right lung. If the tube has been placed in the esophagus, x-ray studies may show gaseous distention of the esophagus below the carina. If the tube is directed toward the left main-stem bronchus, suspect esophageal intubation first and not left main-stem bronchus intubation. If the tube is too high, the tip will lie above the clavicle and the x-ray film may show diffuse atelectasis. If correct placement cannot be verified by the x-ray film, direct laryngoscopy should be performed.

II. **Umbilical vein catheterization (UVC).** The catheter should be in the inferior vena cava, just above the diaphragm. The catheter will appear to the right of the vertebrae on an x-ray film and will follow the ductus venosus. Figure 9-6 demonstrates correct placement.

III. **Umbilical artery catheterization (UAC).** The use of high versus low umbilical artery catheterization depends on institutional preference. Some clinicians feel that high catheters are associated with a higher risk of hypertension and that low catheters are associated with a higher risk of vasospasms, but this has not been proved. If **high placement** is desired, the tip should be between thoracic vertebrae 6 and 9 (above the origin of the celiac axis) (Fig 9-7). For **low placement,** the tip should be below the lumbar vertebrae (L3) and optimally between L3 and L4 (Fig 9-8). A catheter placed

FIGURE 9-4. Ultrasonogram of the head (left sagittal view) showing intraventricular hemorrhage and localized intraparenchymal hemorrhage (grade IV).

FIGURE 9-5. Chest x-ray film showing proper placement of endotracheal tube.

below L5 usually does not function well and carries a risk of severe vaso-spasm in small arteries. Note that the catheter turns downward and then upward on an abdominal x-ray film. The upward turn is the point at which the catheter passes through the internal iliac artery (hypogastric artery).
Note: If both a UAC and UVC are placed and an x-ray study is obtained, it will be necessary to differentiate the two so proper line placement can be ob-tained. Remember, the UAC will turn downward and then upward on the x-ray film. The UVC will appear to the right of the vertebrae and not make a turn downward.

RADIOGRAPHIC PEARLS

I. **Lung disease**
   A. **Hyaline membrane disease.** A fine, diffuse reticulogranular pattern is seen secondary to microatelectasis of the alveoli. An x-ray film of the bronchi will reveal radiolucent areas (known as air bronchograms) caused by air in the major airways.
   B. **Meconium aspiration.** Bilateral patchy, coarse infiltrates and hyperin-flation of the airways are seen.
   C. **Pneumonia.** Diffuse alveolar or interstitial disease is usually asymmet-ric and localized. Group B streptococcal pneumonia can appear much the same as hyaline membrane disease. Pneumatoceles can be seen with staphyloccal pneumonia. Pleural effusions and empyema can be seen with any bacterial pneumonia.
   D. **Transient tachypnea of the newborn.** Hyperaeration with symmetrical perihilar infiltrates is seen. Pleural fluid may be seen as prominence of the minor fissure.
   E. **Bronchopulmonary dysplasia.** Many centers no longer rely on the fol-lowing grading system, but it is included for historical purposes.

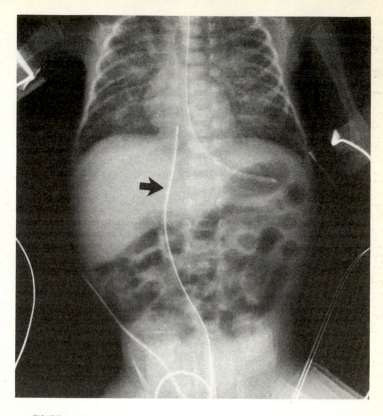

FIGURE 9-6. Abdominal x-ray film showing correct placement of umbilical venous catheter.

Grade I: X-ray findings are similar to those of severe hyaline membrane disease.

Grade II: Dense parenchymal opacification is seen.

Grade III: A bubbly fibrocytic pattern is seen.

Grade IV: Hyperinflation is present, with multiple fine, lacy densities extending to the periphery and with areas of lucency extending to the bullae.

F. **Wilson-Mikity syndrome.** Hyperaeration and a bubblelike appearance of the lung are seen (cystic lesions with thickening of interstitial structures).

G. **Air leak syndromes**

  1. **Pneumopericardium.** Air completely surrounds the heart, including the inferior border (Fig 9–9).

  2. **Pneumomediastinum**

    a. **AP view.** A hyperlucent rim of air is present lateral to the cardiac border and thymus. This rim may displace the thymus superiorly away from the cardiac silhouette **(angel wing sign)** (Fig 9–10, right).

    b. **Lateral view.** An air collection is seen either substernally (anterior pneumomediastinum) or in the retrocardiac area (posterior pneumomediastinum) (Fig 9–10, left).

  3. **Pneumothorax.** The lung is displaced away from the chest wall by a

FIGURE 9-7. X-ray film showing correct positioning of high umbilical artery catheter.

radiolucent band of air. The affected lung is collapsed (Fig 9–11). In many cases, the pneumothorax is not that obvious. In some cases, it is very difficult to see (only a subtle rim of air) and requires careful inspection of the x-ray films.

4. **Tension pneumothorax.** The diaphragm on the affected side is depressed, the mediastinum is shifted to the contralateral hemithorax, and collapse of the ipsilateral lobes is seen.

5. **Pulmonary interstitial emphysema.** Single or multiple circular radiolucencies with well-demarcated walls are seen in a localized or diffuse pattern. There is a marked increase in volume of the involved portion of the lung (Fig 9–12).

FIGURE 9-8. Abdominal x-ray film showing correct positioning of low umbilical artery catheter.

H. Atelectasis. A decrease in lung volume or collapse of part or all of a lung is seen. The mediastinum is shifted toward the affected side of collapse. Compensatory hyperinflation of the involved lung is seen. The area that is affected appears whited-out.

1. **Microatelectasis.** See p 87, **A.**

2. **Generalized atelectasis.** An area of "white-out" is seen on the x-ray film. It may be seen in severe respiratory distress syndrome or airway obstruction, or it may occur if the endotracheal tube is not in the trachea. It may also be seen in hypoventilation.

3. **Lobar atelectasis.** Lobar atelectasis is atelectasis of one lobe. The most common site is the right upper lobe, which will appear as an

FIGURE 9-9. Chest x-ray film showing pneumopericardium in a 2-day-old infant.

FIGURE 9-10. Pneumomediastinum. **Right:** Cross-table lateral chest x-ray film. **Left:** Anteroposterior chest x-ray film.

FIGURE 9-11. Left pneumothorax as shown on an anteroposterior chest x-ray film in a ventilated infant on day 2 of life.

area of "white-out" on the x-ray film. Also, the right minor fissure may be elevated. It commonly occurs after extubation.

I. Pulmonary hypoplasia. Small lungs and thorax are seen. The lungs appear radiolucent. The thorax is bell-shaped.

J. Pulmonary edema. There is a diffuse, hazy appearance of the lungs, with the area of greatest density around the hilum of each lung. The heart size is usually increased.

II. Cardiac disease. The normal cardiac/thoracic index should be < 0.6. The cardiac/thoracic index is the ratio of the length of the base of the heart divided by the length of the thorax. If the index is > 0.6, it suggests cardiomegaly. The pulmonary vascularity is increased if there are more than 2 or 3 end-on vessels and if the diameter of the descending branch of the right pulmonary artery is greater than that of the trachea.

A. Cardiac dextroversion. The cardiac apex is on the right and the aortic arch and stomach bubble on the left. There is a high incidence of congenital heart disease associated with this finding.

B. Congestive heart failure. The following are seen: cardiomegaly; pulmo-

FIGURE 9-12. Chest x-ray film showing bilateral pulmonary interstitial emphysema (PIE) in a 7-day-old ventilated infant.

nary venous congestion (engorgement and increased diameter of the pulmonary veins); diffuse opacification in the perihilar regions; and pleural effusions (sometimes).

C. **Patent ductus arteriosus.** Cardiomegaly, pulmonary edema, ductal haze (pulmonary edema seen with a patent ductus arteriosus), and increased pulmonary vascular markings are seen.

D. **Ventricular septal defect.** Findings include cardiomegaly, increase in pulmonary vessels, enlargement of the left ventricle and left atrium, and enlargement of the main pulmonary artery.

E. **Coarctation of the aorta**
   1. **Preductal coarctation.** Generalized cardiomegaly, with normal pulmonary vascularity, is seen.
   2. **Postductal coarctation.** An enlarged left ventricle and left atrium and a dilated ascending aorta are seen.

F. **Tetralogy of Fallot.** The heart is boot-shaped. There is enlargement of the right atrium, right ventricle, and small pulmonary artery and a normal left atrium and left ventricle. There is decreased pulmonary vascularity.

G. **Transposition of the great arteries.** The x-ray film may show cardiomegaly, with an enlarged right atrium and right ventricle, narrow mediastinum, and increased pulmonary vascular markings, but in most cases it is normal.

H. **Total anomalous pulmonary venous return.** Pulmonary venous markings are increased. Cardiomegaly is minimal or absent. Congestive heart failure and pulmonary edema may be present.

I. **Hypoplastic left heart syndrome.** Can be normal at first but then may show cardiomegaly, pulmonary vascular congestion, and an enlarged right atrium and ventricle.

J. **Tricuspid atresia.** Cardiac enlargement, enlargement of the left ventricle, small pulmonary arteries, and decreased pulmonary vascularity are seen.

FIGURE 9-13. Abdominal x-ray film showing pneumoperitoneum in a 3-day-old infant.

K. Truncus arteriosus. Biventricular cardiomegaly, increased pulmonary vascularity, and straightening of the left cardiac border are seen.

L. Atrial septal defect. Varying degrees of enlargement of the right atrium and ventricle are seen. The aorta and left ventricle are small, and the pulmonary artery is large. Increased pulmonary vascularity is also seen.

M. Ebstein's anomaly. Gross cardiomegaly and decreased pulmonary vascularity, are seen.

N. Pulmonary stenosis. Cardiomegaly and decreased pulmonary markings are seen.

III. Abdominal disorders

    A. Alteration in the following normal patterns should raise suspicion of gastrointestinal tract disease.

        1. Air in the stomach should occur within 30 minutes after delivery.

        2. Air in the small bowel should be seen by 3–4 hours of age.

        3. Air in the colon and rectum should be seen by 6–8 hours of age.

    B. Intestinal obstruction. Air-fluid levels are seen proximal to the obstruction. There is gaseous intestinal distention. Distal to the obstruction, gas may be decreased or absent.

FIGURE 9-14. Abdominal x-ray film showing pneumatosis intestinalis in a 4-day-old infant.

C. **Ascites.** Gas-filled loops of bowel, if present, are located in the center of the abdomen. The abdomen may be distended, with relatively small amounts of gas (**"ground glass" appearance**). A uniform increase in the density of the abdomen, particularly in the flank areas, may be seen.

D. **Calcification in the abdomen** is most often seen secondary to meconium peritonitis, which may also cause calcifications within the scrotum in male infants. Calcifications in the abdomen may also be seen in infants with neuroblastoma or teratoma or may signify calcification of the adrenals following adrenal hemorrhage.

E. Pneumoperitoneum
   1. **Supine view.** Free air is seen as a central lucency (Fig 9–13).
   2. **Upright view.** Free air is present in a subdiaphragmatic location.
   3. **Left lateral decubitus view.** Air collects over the lateral border of the liver, separating it from the abdominal wall.
F. Pneumatosis intestinalis. Intraluminal gas in the bowel wall (produced by bacteria that have invaded the bowel wall) appears as a string of submucosal bubbles. It is most frequently seen in infants with necrotizing enterocolitis (Fig 9–14).
G. Situs inversus. The stomach, aortic arch, and cardiac apex are on the right. This finding is not associated with an increased incidence of intrinsic heart disease.
H. Ileus. Distended loops of bowel are present. Air-fluid levels may be seen on the upright or cross-table lateral x-ray film.
I. Absence of gas in the abdomen. Absence of gas in the abdomen may be seen in patients taking muscle-paralyzing medications (eg, pancuronium) because they do not swallow air. It may also be seen in infants with esophageal atresia without tracheoesophageal fistula.
J. Intraportal air. Air is seen in the portal veins (often seen best on a lateral view). This finding may indicate bowel necrosis, such as that which occurs in advanced stages of necrotizing enterocolitis. It may also be seen in patients with intestinal infarction secondary to mesenteric vessel occlusion. Another possible cause of this finding is iatrogenically introduced gas into the portal vein, which can occur during umbilical vein catheterization or exchange transfusion.

10 Infant Transport

As regionalization and specialization of care for newborn infants have developed, a new type of team has been created especially for transport of these infants from a referring hospital to a level III center (neonatal intensive care unit [NICU]). A great deal of planning must take place in order for these teams to function effectively, and clear guidelines must be set up regarding personnel, procedures, and equipment needed (Guidelines for Perinatal Care, 1988). Policies and procedures will reflect the unique characteristics of each region (eg, size, geography, economics, sophistication of medical services). Lines of communication must always be open between the referring hospital and the NICU at all levels (administrators, physicians, nurses) and with ambulance or air services. Ideally, the mother would be transferred to the level III center before delivery of a high-risk infant, but this is not always possible.

I. **Transport team.** The team may include physicians, nurses, respiratory therapists, and/or emergency medical technicians (Bose, 1984). Special training must be provided in the care of sick infants. A specific medical protocol is set up. The team should be able to contact the attending neonatologist at any time during transport. Appropriate insurance coverage is necessary for team members, and questions of liability must be worked out with legal consultation between hospitals, ambulance services, and aircraft services.

At the referring hospital, team members should conduct themselves as professional representatives of the NICU, avoiding conflict with or criticism of the referring hospital staff. Questions about transport protocol should be worked out directly between the referring physician and the attending neonatologist.

II. **Equipment.** Each transport team should be self-sufficient. Medications and equipment can be chosen according to published lists (Ferrara, 1980). Special emphasis is placed on maintaining thermal neutrality (eg, plastic swaddling; heated, humidified inspired air mixtures). Noise and vibration often compromise auditory and visual monitoring, and well-calibrated indwelling blood pressure and oxygen tension monitors (or transcutaneous oximetry) may be useful. An instant camera is a "must" because pictures of the infant may be the mother's only psychological support for days.

III. **Protocol for stabilization and transfer.** The goal of stabilization is to make the transfer uneventful.

   A. **General procedures.** *Attention to the details of stabilization is important!* Unless active resuscitation is under way, the team's first task at the referring hospital is to *listen* to the history and assessment of the infant's status. The vital signs are then obtained. At this point, a precise diagnosis of all the infant's problems may be less important than predicting what the infant will need during transport. It is prudent to initiate anticipated interventions before leaving the referring hospital. For example, an infant with increasing work of breathing and increasing needs for inspired oxygen who faces a 2-hour journey probably should be placed on mechanical ventilation and have an intravenous line in place before transfer begins. In most cases, an infant is not ready for transport until basic neonatal needs are met: **thermoneutrality, acceptable cardiac and respiratory function, and blood glucose levels in the normal range.** Vital signs must be stable and catheters and tubes appropriately placed. Problems that may occur during transport should be anticipated. The NICU should be given an expected arrival time. The parents should be allowed to see and touch the infant before transport. During transport, vigilant monitoring should continue for unexpected changes in the infant's status. The respiratory rate, heart rate, blood pressure, and oxygen saturation levels should be followed. Transcutaneous oximetry should be used if available. After transfer is completed, the team should talk with the parents and, if possible, with the referring physician.

B. **Prophylactic antibiotic therapy.** Infants at risk for sepsis and those with indwelling catheters should probably receive antibiotic therapy. Culture of blood samples may be performed at the referring hospital or at the NICU. Antibiotic dosages are given in Chapter 76.

C. **Gastric intubation.** If the infant has a gastrointestinal disorder (including ileus accompanying critical illness) or diaphragmatic hernia or if continuous positive airway pressure is administered through the nose or a mask, venting of the stomach with a nasogastric or orogastric tube is indicated, especially if airplane or helicopter transport will be used. Venting should be done prior to transport, because the air trapped in the gastrointestinal tract will expand in volume as atmospheric pressure decreases (see below, **V.B, Dysbarism**).

D. **Temperature control and fluid balance.** Special attention to temperature and fluid balance is required for infants with open lesions (eg, myelomeningocele, omphalocele). A dry or moist protective dressing over the lesion can be covered by thin plastic wrap to reduce radiant heat loss.

IV. **Evaluation of transport.** Each transport should have a scoring system that reflects the "before" and "after" status of the infant (Hermansen, 1988). For example, vital signs and Dextrostix measurements taken when the team first arrives at the referring hospital should be compared to the same measurements taken on admission to the NICU. This system provides quality control of transports and is useful in outreach education to convey constructive criticism to referring hospitals.

V. **Special considerations in air transport.** Each region should develop protocols for choosing ground or air transport, based on distance, nature of terrain, location of landing sites, and availability of aircraft and ambulances (American Academy of Pediatrics, 1986).

A. **Safety guidelines.** Clear guidelines should be established regarding air transport. Decisions regarding flight safety should be made according to weather and other flight conditions (ie, the pilot should not be given information on the age of the patient or the severity of the illness before making decisions on flight safety). Controlled landing sites familiar to the pilot should be used. Loading and unloading of the aircraft should not take place while engines are running; an idling helicopter is dangerous.

B. **Dysbarism.** In helicopters and unpressurized aircraft, dysbarism (imbalance between air pressure in the atmosphere and the pressure of gases within the body) causes predictable problems. Partial pressures of inspired gases decrease as altitude increases, so infants will require an increased concentration of inspired oxygen (Ferrara, 1980). Trapped free air in the thorax or intestines will expand in volume and may cause significant pulmonary embarrassment. A cuffed tube or catheter should be evacuated before takeoff. **Note:** Because blood pressure varies with changing gravitational force, fluctuations noted during climbing or descent should not be cause for alarm.

REFERENCES

American Academy of Pediatrics Committee on Hospital Care: Guidelines for air and ground transportation of pediatric patients. *Pediatrics* 1986;**78**:943.

Bose CL, Jung AL, Thornton JW: Neonatal transport. *Perinatol Neonatal* 1984;**8**:61.

Ferrara A, Harin A: *Emergency Transfer of the High-Risk Neonate.* Mosby, 1980.

Hermansen MC et al: A validation of a scoring system to evaluate the condition of transported very low birth weight neonates. *Am J Perinatol* 1988;**5**:74.

Interhospital care of the perinatal patient. Chapter 8 in: *Guidelines for Perinatal Care,* 2nd ed. American Academy of Pediatrics, 1988.

11 Follow-Up of High-Risk Infants

As neonatal intensive care continues to develop as a medical specialty, concern has grown regarding the quality of life of high-risk infants. Follow-up clinics are a valuable, and even necessary, adjunct to neonatal intensive care in that they provide both service to infants and families and feedback to neonatologists and obstetricians.

I. **Goals of neonatal follow-up clinic**
   A. **Early identification of developmental disability.** Some infants will be referred for further diagnostic evaluation and/or community services.
   B. **Parent counseling.** Parents of children who do well can be reassured by positive feedback. Parents of children with disabilities will need help in coping with their child's problems. Physical and occupational therapists can provide valuable suggestions regarding positioning, handling, and feeding infants.
   C. **Identification and treatment of medical complications.** Some disorders may not be anticipated at the time of discharge from the neonatal intensive care unit (NICU).
   D. **Feedback for neonatologists, pediatricians, obstetricians, and pediatric surgeons** regarding developmental progress, medical status, and unusual or unforeseen complications in these infants is essential.

II. **Staff of neonatal follow-up clinic.** Pediatricians, developmental pediatricians, and neonatologists make up the regular staff of the clinic. Special consultation may be needed from audiologists, ophthalmologists, psychologists, physical therapists, occupational therapists, speech and language specialists, social workers, nutritionists, respiratory therapists, pediatric surgeons, and orthopedic surgeons.

III. **Risk factors for developmental disability.** It is virtually impossible to diagnose developmental disability with certainty in the neonatal period, but a number of perinatal risk factors have been identified.
   A. **Prematurity.** Although the majority of preterm infants are not significantly handicapped, they do have a higher incidence of cerebral palsy and mental retardation than the general population (5–10% of preterm infants with birth weight below 1500 g, higher in those with birth weight below 750 g). Preterm infants also have a higher risk of minimal cerebral dysfunction, including language disorders, visual perception problems, attention deficits, and learning disabilities. Preterm infants with slow head growth (especially in the postnatal period), asphyxia, sepsis (especially meningitis), chronic lung disease, abnormal neonatal neurodevelopmental examinations, and abnormalities on cranial ultrasonography or CT scanning have an increased risk of developmental disability. Cranial abnormalities, including intraventricular hemorrhage (especially grades III and IV), ventricular dilatation (with or without hemorrhage), cortical atrophy and periventricular echodensities (periventricular leukomalacia), are all associated with a poor prognosis. The incidence of handicaps is very high with periventricular echodensities, especially if they are bilateral and large.
   B. **Intrauterine growth retardation (IUGR).** Although full-term infants who are small for gestational age (SGA) appear to have no (or only slightly higher) risk of cerebral palsy and mental retardation, they have a high incidence of minimal cerebral dysfunction, especially learning disabil-

ity. Preterm SGA infants have a high incidence of cerebral palsy and mental retardation (Pena, 1988). The risk of developmental disability in SGA infants is usually determined by the cause of IUGR, timing of the insult, and subsequent perinatal complications (eg, asphyxia, hypoglycemia, polycythemia) (Allen, 1984).

C. **Asphyxia.** Perinatal asphyxia is associated with later developmental disability but is frequently difficult to define. Apgar scores are useful in predicting the outcome only when they are very low (score of 0–3) for extended periods of time (> 10 minutes) in full-term newborns (Nelson, 1981). Most outcome studies have focused on severely asphyxiated infants who required prolonged resuscitation or who were symptomatic as newborns. The mortality rate for this group is high (50%); however, 75% of the survivors are free of major handicap. Those with handicaps usually have multiple handicaps, including severe mental retardation, spastic quadriplegia, microcephaly, seizures, and sensory impairment. The number and type of neonatal symptoms correlate with the degree of later disability, as do abnormalities on EEG and CT scan (Brown, 1974; Samat, 1976; Fenichal, 1983; Fitzhardinge, 1982).

D. **Other risk factors.** Other perinatal factors are less common but are associated with a high risk of handicap.

1. **TORCH infections.** Infants with congenital cytomegalovirus infection, toxoplasmosis, or rubella who are symptomatic at birth have a high incidence (60–90%) of developmental disability. Even if asymptomatic as neonates, they are at risk for sensory impairment and learning disability.

2. **Infection,** especially meningitis, carries a risk of later developmental disability.

3. **Hypoglycemia and polycythemia.** The presence of symptomatic hypoglycemia or polycythemia (hyperviscosity) at birth is associated with handicap.

IV. **Parameters requiring follow-up**

A. **Growth.** Growth parameters and trends should be carefully monitored at each follow-up visit. These include **length, weight, and head circumference** (see also Appendix G). Although most preterm infants "catch up" in growth during the first year, some SGA infants, extremely immature infants, and infants with severe chronic lung disease may always remain small. Slow head growth may be an early indication of developmental disability.

B. **Blood pressure.** A silent sequela of neonatal intensive care that may have serious long-term consequences is high blood pressure. Blood pressure measurements should be performed for all infants on a periodic basis.

C. **Breathing disorders**

1. **Apnea.** Infants requiring home apnea monitors and/or those receiving theophylline for apnea require close follow-up, with special attention paid to whether or not resuscitation has been required. When to discontinue monitoring is a matter of debate and is usually decided by the physician and the family. Most clinicians recommend that monitoring be continued for at least 6–12 months or for several months after the last episode of apnea or bradycardia. (See also Apnea and Periodic Breathing, p 173.)

2. **Chronic lung disease.** Infants with chronic lung disease require specialized medical and developmental follow-up. The decision to discontinue administration of supplemental oxygen or to taper the amount should be based on pulse oximeter studies during periods of sleep, wakefulness, and feeding and on clinical criteria (ie, growth, exercise intolerance). Poor growth, sleeping or feeding difficulties, rising hematocrit, increasing abnormalities on ECG and echocardio-

gram, and plateauing or loss of developmental progress after discontinuing oxygen all suggest intermittent hypoxia; oxygen administration should be resumed, and the infant should be restudied. Some infants with chronic lung disease who have done well breathing room air for some time may have problems if they develop upper or lower respiratory tract infections.

D. Hearing. Infants with a family history of childhood hearing impairment, congenital perinatal hearing (eg, TORCH) infection, congenital malformations of the head or neck, birth weight less than 1500 g, hyperbilirubinemia requiring exchange transfusion, bacterial meningitis, or severe perinatal asphyxia or who were exposed to ototoxic drugs (eg, furosemide, gentamicin, vancomycin) are at risk for hearing impairment and should be referred for evaluation. Because hearing is essential for the acquisition of language, it is important to diagnose hearing impairment as early as possible. Some NICUs screen for hearing loss with **brain-stem auditory evoked potentials.** This test can identify infants with a high risk of hearing impairment who need careful audiologic follow-up. However, because of the high false-positive results, it is usually difficult to diagnose hearing loss with certainty in the neonatal period by the use of this or any other technique.

E. Vision. Preterm infants who were given oxygen in the neonatal period are at risk for developing **retinopathy of prematurity.** An indirect ophthalmoscopic examination should be performed at 4–6 weeks by a pediatric ophthalmologist. Until the retina is fully vascularized, follow-up ophthalmologic examinations should be performed every 2 weeks (or every week if active disease is progressing). Infants with congenital infection and asphyxia should also have ophthalmologic examinations and follow-up. All high-risk infants should have an assessment of visual acuity at 1–5 years.

F. Language and motor skills. For each infant, a history of language and motor milestones should be obtained and compared to norms for the age (Capute, 1980). Infants with persistent delay, dissociation, or deviance should be carefully assessed for disability by a developmental pediatrician or multidisciplinary team.

1. **Delay** is late acquisition of milestones.
2. **Dissociation** is delay in one area of development compared to other areas and can help diagnose disability (eg, delay in gross and fine motor development with normal language development suggests cerebral palsy, whereas delay in language acquisition with normal motor development suggests mental retardation, language disorder, or hearing impairment).
3. **Deviance** is acquisition of milestones out of normal sequence (eg, the child is able to stand but does not sit well).

G. Neurologic development is a dynamic process, and what is normal at a certain age may be abnormal at another. The examiner must know what is normal at each age and must decide if deviations from normal are significant. Preterm infants are often hypotonic at birth but develop flexor tone in a caudocephalad direction. Preterm infants at term and full-term newborns have flexor hypertonia and lose this flexor tone in a caudocephalad direction (ie, at 1–2 months from term there is more flexor tone in the arms than the legs). By 4 months from term, muscle tone should be the same (normal) in the upper and lower extremities.

1. **Neurodevelopmental examination** of high-risk infants should include assessment of:
   a. Posture.
   b. Muscle tone in the extremities.
   c. Axial (neck and trunk) muscle tone.
   d. Deep tendon reflexes.

      e. Pathologic reflexes (eg, Babinski reflex).

      f. Primitive reflexes (eg, Moro reflex, asymmetric tonic neck reflex).

      g. Postural reactions (eg, righting or equilibrium response).

  2. Abnormalities in high-risk infants. Many high-risk infants have some abnormalities during the first year of life that may resolve by age 1 year. However, the presence of multiple persistent abnormalities in conjunction with motor delay suggests cerebral palsy. These infants should be referred for multidisciplinary evaluation. Because damage to the central nervous system is seldom focal, infants with motor impairment are likely to have associated deficits (eg, mental retardation, learning disability, sensory impairment) that eventually may be more debilitating. The following developmental abnormalities are commonly seen in high-risk infants during the first year of life.

    a. Hypotonia (generalized or axial) is especially common in preterm infants and infants with chronic lung disease.

    b. Hypertonia is seen most often in the lower extremities (hips and ankles) in preterm infants.

    c. Asymmetry of function, tone, posture, or reflexes may be seen.

    d. Neck extensor hypertonia and shoulder retraction is common in infants with chronic lung disease, tracheostomy, or prolonged intubation.

    e. Involuntary movements, grimacing, and poor coordination are indicative of extrapyramidal involvement.

    f. Feeding problems may occur.

H. Cognitive development. Language development is one of the most reliable predictors of intelligence and can help identify children with cognitive impairment. Cognitive evaluation may be difficult in infants. High-risk children should have a psychological evaluation at age 1–3 years and before starting school because of the risk of learning disability. An audiologic evaluation should be performed at an early age to rule out hearing impairment.

V. Correction for prematurity. Correcting for prematurity when assessing physical or psychological development continues to be *controversial*. Recent data suggest that motor milestone development proceeds according to age from conception and that one should correct for the degree of prematurity. Recommendations regarding correction for cognitive abilities varies widely: some correct completely throughout childhood; some correct only to age 1 or 2; some use partial correction. We recommend calculating both the child's chronologic age and age corrected for degree of prematurity (term age equivalent, or adjusted age). A child's language and problem-solving abilities should fall between these 2 ages. The older a child becomes the less important this issue is: By the time a child is 5, arithmetically 3 months' difference (eg, 60 vs 57 months) matters little.

VI. Multidisciplinary evaluation. The presence of one disability is an indication for careful evaluation in other areas. Brain damage is seldom focal and often diffuse. These infants should be referred for complete multidisciplinary evaluation to identify areas of strength and weakness and to formulate an appropriate rehabilitation program. A comprehensive overview allows for a more realistic determination of prognosis. Appropriate counseling can then be given the parents.

REFERENCES

Allen MC: Developmental outcome and follow-up of the small for gestational age infant. *Semin Perinantol* 1984;8:123.

Allen MC, Alexander GR: Gross motor milestones in preterm infants: Correction for degree of prematurity. *J Pediatr* 1990;**116**:955.

Allen MC, Jones MD: Medical complications of prematurity. *Obstet Gynecol* 1986;**67**:427.

Barrera ME, Rosenbaum P, Cunningham CE: Corrected and uncorrected Bayley scores:

Longitudinal developmental patterns in low and high birthweight preterm infants. *Infant Behav Dev* 1987;**10**:337.

Brown JK et al: Neurological aspects of perinatal asphyxia. *Dev Med Child Neurol* 1974;**16**:567.

Capute AJ, Palmer FB: A pediatric overview of the spectrum of developmental disabilities. *J Dev Behav Pediatr* 1980;**1**:66.

Capute AJ et al: Normal gross motor development: The influence of race, sex and socioeconomic status. *Dev Med Child Neurol* 1985;**27**:635.

Capute AJ et al: Clinical linguistic and audiotory milestone scale: Prediction of cognition in infancy. *Dev Med Child Neurol* 1986;**28**:762.

Fitzhardinge PM, Flodmark D, Ashby S: The prognostic value of computed tomography of the brain in asphyxiated premature infants. *J Pediatr* 1982;**100**:476.

Hack M, Fanaroff AA: Outcomes of extremely low birth weight infants between 1982 and 1988. *N Engl J Med* 1989;**24**:1262.

Miller G, Dubowitz LMS, Palmer P: Follow-up of preterm infants: Is correction of the developmental quotient for prematurity helpful? *Early Hum Dev* 1984;**9**:137.

Nelson KB, Ellenberg JH: Apgar scores as predictors of chronic neurologic disability. *Pediatrics* 1981;**68**:36.

Palisano RJ: Use of chronologic and adjusted ages to compare motor development of healthy preterm and full term infants. *Dev Med Child Neurol* 1984;**28**:180.

Pena IC, Teberg AJ, Finello KM: The premature small for gestational age infant during the first year of life: Comparison by birthweight and gestational age. *J Pediatr* 1988;**113**:1066.

Samat HB, Samat MS: Neonatal encephalopathy following fetal distress: A clinical and electroencephalographic study. *Arch Neurol* 1976;**33**:696.

Siegal LS: Correction for prematurity and its consequences for the assessment of the very low birth weight infant. *Child Dev* 1983;**54**:1176.

12 Management of the Extremely Low Birth Weight Infant During the First Week of Life

This chapter addresses the initial care of premature infants of less than 1000 g birth weight, also known as "extremely low birth weight infants." Many aspects of this care are *controversial,* and each institution has developed its own philosophy, style, and techniques for managing these infants, especially those weighing less than 750 g at birth. Therefore, it is of utmost importance to learn and follow the practices of your own institution. This chapter presents guidelines we have found useful for stabilizing and caring for extremely small infants.

I. **Temperature and humidity control.** Because the tiny baby has little subcutaneous tissue, relatively large skin surface area and minimal energy reserves, a **neutral thermal environment** is essential for its survival. A neutral thermal environment is defined as the environmental temperature that minimizes heat loss so that oxygen consumption is not increased and metabolic stress is not incurred. Also, to maintain minimal evaporative heat loss, it is best if the environmental humidity is at least 50%.

A. **Incubators or radiant warmers.** Extremely low birth weight infants may initially be managed either in **double-walled incubators or under radiant heaters with protective plastic sheeting or covers.** Hypothermia must be avoided, although the definition of hypothermia is not readily agreed upon. Some centers strive for core temperatures of 37.0 °C, whereas others allow the infants to be maintained at temperatures as low as 35.5 °C. Guidelines for Perinatal Care, of the American College of Obstetrics and Gynecology and the American Academy of Pediatrics, recommend maintaining either a skin temperature of 36.0–36.5 °C or a core body temperature of 36.0–37.5 °C.

B. **Humidification.** Tiny infants have increased insensible water loss due largely to evaporation. In particular, the ratio of their body surface area to body weight is greatly increased. They also have a greater proportion of body water relative to body mass. Furthermore, transcutaneous water loss is enhanced by their thin epidermis and underdeveloped stratum corneum. These evaporative losses are minimized by increased environmental humidity. **Humidification within the incubator or the area beneath the plastic protective cover of a radiant warmer is recommended.**

1. Use a **respiratory care humidification unit,** the same as that used with oxygen hoods. (If the manufactured humidity reservoirs of the incubators are used, special attention to infection control is needed, especially to prevent skin infections.)

2. Maintain a surrounding **humidity of at least 40–50%.** Use of a hand-held humidistat or hygrometer will allow hourly checking of ambient humidity.

C. **Monitoring and maintenance of body temperature and ambient humidity**

1. Maintain skin temperature of 36–36.5 °C. Rectal temperatures in tiny babies are discouraged.
2. Using a servocontrol skin probe, record skin temperature and environmental temperature every hour until skin temperature is stable (36–36.5 °C) and follow thereafter with recordings at 2-hour intervals.
3. Check axillary temperature only if skin temperature is outside the range of 36–36.5 °C. Periodically check axillary temperature. You may need to change from servo- to non-servocontrol (manual) to warm the smallest infants.
4. Record incubator humidity every hour until it is stable (40–50%), then every 2 hours for maintenance.
5. If minor surgical procedures are required, convert the overhead radiant warmer to servocontrol set at 37–38 °C. Use prewarmed sterile drapes.
6. Low birth weight infants must be weighed at least once daily for management of fluids and electrolytes. The incubator should have an **in-bed scale for continuous weighing of infant to minimize handling and removal from a controlled environment,** thus maximizing temperature control. The **scale should be preheated** with the incubator prior to admission and should be calibrated after optimal air temperature and humidity have been established.
7. **Accessory items for infant care must be prewarmed.** These items include all new linens, blood pressure cuffs, x-ray cassettes, air mattresses, sterile towels, intravenous fluids, stethoscope, and saline lavages.

D. **Rewarming hypothermic infants.** Rewarming of infants who become hypothermic must be gradual. Overhead radiant warming units added to the double-walled incubators provide the best sources of heat. Both units should be operated on manual controls to achieve rewarming of the infant. In general, the rewarming rate should not exceed 0.6 °C per hour. When skin temperature of 36.5 °C is achieved, rewarming efforts should be discontinued and temperature maintenance by servocontrol should be followed. Excessive warming of these infants must be avoided, as core body temperatures greater than 37.5 °C will cause an increase of insensible water losses and increased oxygen consumption.

E. **Infants on mechanical ventilation**
1. For all infants receiving mechanical ventilation, especially those weighing less than 1000 g, **humidification and warming of administered respiratory gases** is important to minimize insensible fluid losses.
2. **In-line warming of respiratory gas circuits** minimizes "rain out" of the humidified air and oxygen and maintains airway temperature, which should be 32–35 °C.

II. **Fluids and electrolytes.** Because of increased insensible water loss and immature renal function, these infants have increased fluid requirements, necessitating **intravenous fluid therapy** or, in some cases, infusion of fluids through the umbilical artery.
A. **Intravenous fluid therapy (fluid volume and type of fluid)**
1. **First day of life.** Guidelines for the type of fluid and volume per kilogram of body weight are given in Table 12–1 for the first day of life. The table gives suggested volumes (including line flushes and medications) for infants in double-walled incubators with a constant humidity of 40–50% and stable skin temperatures of 36–36.5 °C. For babies of the same weight, small-for-gestational-age infants require lesser amounts of fluid.
a. **Additional fluid will be required if phototherapy is used** (see

TABLE 12-1. GUIDELINES FOR INTRAVENOUS FLUIDS IN THE VERY LOW BIRTH WEIGHT INFANT THE FIRST DAY OF LIFE

Weight (g)	Type of Fluid	SGA*	AGA*
500–599	D5W	140 . . . . . . 200 mL/kg/d	
600–699	D5W	120 . . . . . . 180 mL/kg/d	
700–799	D5W	100 . . . . . . 160 mL/kg/d	
800–899	D5W	80 . . . . . . 120 mL/kg/d	
900–999	D10W	70 . . . . . . 100 mL/kg/d	

* SGA = small for gestational age; AGA = appropriate for gestational age.

p 112, **C.2**); the fluid volume should be increased by 10–20 mL/kg/d.

    b. **Additional fluid will be required if the infant is exposed to direct overhead radiant heat.** Extreme insensible body fluid losses occur in tiny babies under direct radiant heat if not shielded by protective plastic barrier sheeting or enclosed in protective plastic hoods or other types of enclosures. However, be aware that excessive fluid intake may contribute to the development of a hemodynamically significant patent ductus arteriosus and should be avoided.

  2. **Second and subsequent days of life.** Fluid management on the second and subsequent days depends on changes in body weight, renal function (BUN, creatinine and urine output), and serum electrolyte concentrations (see Chap 7).

B. Infusion of fluids through umbilical catheters. Add **heparin,** 1 unit/mL, to fluids infused through umbilical catheters. For the fluid volume and type, see Table 12–1.

C. For line flushes, use the same fluids as those being infused as intravenous fluids. Avoid normal saline flushes because of excessive sodium. Also, avoid hypotonic solutions (less than 0.45 normal saline or less than 5% dextrose); these solutions cause red cell hemolysis.

D. Monitoring of fluid therapy. The infant's fluid status should be evaluated at least twice daily and the fluid intake should be adjusted accordingly. Monitoring of fluid status is done by measurements of body weight, urine output, urine specific gravity, serum sodium, and other less reliable parameters such as hematocrit and physical examination.

  1. **Body weight.** The most important way of monitoring fluid therapy is by measurement of body weight. If an in-bed scale is used, weigh the baby every 12 hours. If an in-bed scale is not available, weighing may have to be delayed to every 24 to 48 hours, depending on the stability of the tiny infant, to prevent excessive handling and cold stress. A weight loss of up to 15% of birth weight may be experienced by the end of the first week of life. Greater weight loss is considered excessive, and environmental controls for insensible fluid losses and fluid management must be carefully reviewed.

  2. **Urine output and specific gravity.** Monitoring urine output is the second most important method of monitoring fluid therapy. In addition to urine volume, urine specific gravity should be determined to check renal function and the state of hydration.

    a. **First 12 hours:** Any amount of urine output is acceptable.

    b. **Twelve to 24 hours:** The minimum acceptable urine output is 0.5 mL/kg/h, with urine specific gravity of 1.008–1.015.

    c. **Second day and after:** Normal urine output for the second day is 1–2 mL/kg/h. After the second day of life, urine output may increase to 3.0–3.5 mL/kg/h; 4–5 mL/kg/h is excessive and indicates early fluid overload, which may lead to electrolyte loss. Urine specific gravity should fluctuate between 1.008 and 1.015. Values outside this range warrant reevaluation of fluid management or environmental humidity control.

3. **Electrolyte values.** Serum electrolyte levels should be monitored at least twice daily, or every 4–8 hours for the most immature infants.

   a. **Sodium.** Initially, tiny infants have a sufficient sodium level (132–138 meq/L) and require no sodium intake. However, when the serum sodium level begins to decrease (usually on the third or fourth day of life), sodium should be added to the intravenous fluids (3–8 meq/kg/d of sodium). In subsequent monitoring of the serum sodium levels:

      (1) If sodium is greater than 142 meq/L, consider that the sodium intake is too high or the infant is dehydrated.

      (2) If sodium is less than 133 meq/L, more sodium may be needed, or the infant may have fluid overload. If the decrease in the serum sodium level is believed to be due to fluid overload, the total daily fluids should be reduced.

      Note: Hypernatremia in the first few days of life may be due to dehydration or to inadvertent sodium administration from normal saline catheter flushes. Flush catheters only with the intravenous fluids being used for maintenance fluid therapy. If infusion is being done through an umbilical artery catheter, heparinized intravenous fluid must be used for flushing.

   b. **Potassium**

      (1) **During the first 48 hours after birth,** tiny babies are prone to the development of increased serum potassium levels of 5 meq/L or more (range 4.0–8.0 meq/L). The increase is due mostly to immature renal tubular function. Most clinicians recommend that no potassium be given during this time. Electrocardiographic changes are not usually seen until the serum potassium level is greater than 9.0 meq/L. The following clinical guidelines are offered.

         (a) **Serum potassium 7–8 meq/L.** Accept the value as the upper limit and observe the infant and the ECG. Repeat serum studies every 4–6 hours.

         (b) **Serum potassium 8–9 meq/L.** Check urine output. The minimal acceptable output is 1–2 mL/kg/h (2–3 mL/kg/h is preferred) with urine specific gravity of 1.006 to 1.012). Observe for elevated or peaked T wave changes on the bedside heart rate monitor. Monitor BUN and creatinine.

         (c) **Serum potassium levels greater than 9 meq/L** are usually pathologic and are associated with decreasing renal function, cardiac irregularities, or both. Consider administration of sodium bicarbonate, calcium solutions, or glucose/insulin infusions (consultation required) (see Chap 39 for details on the management of hyperkalemia). Kayexalate enemas and exchange transfusion have had little effect and may further complicate the infant's condition.

      (2) **Third to sixth day after birth.** Usually by the third to the sixth day, the initially elevated serum potassium level begins to decrease. As potassium levels approach 4 meq/L, add supplemental potassium to IV fluids. Begin with 1–2 meq/kg/d. Measure serum potassium every 6–12 hours until the level is stabilized at 4.1–4.8 meq/L.

III. **Blood glucose.** As with larger high-risk infants, extremely low birth weight infants should be supported with 4–6 mg/kg/min glucose infusion. This support can usually be achieved by starting with a 5% dextrose solution. (Use of a 10% dextrose solution may result in hyperglycemia.) Reagent strip testing of blood glucose should be of performed every 2 hours until a stable blood glucose level (50–60 mg/dL) has been established. All urine samples should be checked for glucosuria. Trace glucosuria is acceptable and may occur with a blood glucose level as low as 120 mg/dL, but higher levels of serum glucose and glycosuria require recalculation of glucose administration and total fluid administration.

IV. **Calcium.** Serum calcium should be monitored once or twice daily. When the serum calcium decreases below 7.5 mg/dL, we institute treatment with calcium gluconate (for dosage, see p 460). This decrease usually happens on the second day of life. Although a few infants may not require calcium therapy, some centers routinely institute daily maintenance calcium supplementation in their intravenous solutions (eg, 2 mg calcium gluconate per milliliter of intravenous solution).

V. **Hyperalimentation.** Hyperalimentation should be started as soon as the infant's fluid and electrolyte (sodium and potassium) and glucose have stabilized, usually late in the first week of life.

VI. **Respiratory support.** Virtually all of these infants will initially require **mechanical ventilation.** Although some centers prefer a trial of nasal continuous positive airway pressure (CPAP) prior to intubation, we have found that it is often prudent to electively intubate these infants in the delivery room.

   A. **Endotracheal intubation**

      1. **Type of endotracheal tube.** When possible, use an endotracheal tube with 1-cm markings on the side. The internal diameter (ID) of the tube should routinely be 2.5 cm or 3.0 cm, according to body weight:

         (a) 500–1000 g: 2.5 cm ID

         (b) 1000–1250 g: 3.0 cm ID

      2. **Endotracheal tube placement.** (The procedure for endotracheal tube placement is described in detail in Chapter 20.) Proper placement should be confirmed by a chest x-ray study, performed with the infant's head in the midline position. After correct placement has been confirmed, the numbers (or letters) on the tube that are at the infant's gum line should be noted. As a means of subsequently checking proper tube position, every shift the nurse responsible for the infant should check and record the numbers or letters at the gum line. Any adjustment of the endotracheal tube requires a subsequent chest x-ray study to confirm the tube position.

   B. **Mechanical ventilation.** Initial ventilator settings vary from institution to institution. Tiny infants respond to a wide range of ventilator settings. Some do relatively well on 20–30 cycles/min; others require 50–60 cycles/min, with inspiratory times ranging from 0.28 to 0.50 second. The minimum airway pressure possible should be used. Seek to maintain mechanical breath tidal volumes of 3–5 mL/kg; often this may be achieved with as little as 8–12 cm inspiratory pressure and 2–3 cm positive end-expiratory pressure. Higher pressures increase the risk of barotrauma and the development of chronic lung disease and must be avoided. We have found that pressures can be kept to a minimum by allowing a mild to moderate respiratory acidosis (pH 7.25–7.32 and pco_2 45–55 torr). The following ventilatory support guidelines are offered for the initiation of respiratory care. Each tiny infant will require frequent reassessment and revision of settings and parameters. **Recommended initial settings for pressure-limited time-cycled ventilators are:**

      1. **Rate:** 20–60 breaths/min (usually 30).

      2. **Inspiratory time (IT):** 0.3–0.5 second (usually 0.33).

3. **Peak inspiratory pressure:** 12–20 cm water (select oxygen concentration on the basis of tidal volume if it can be measured; usually 3.5–5.0 mL/kg).
4. **Mean airway pressure (MAP):** Less than 8 cm water.
5. **Fio_2:** As required per initial Po_2 values.
6. **Flow rate:** 6–8 L/min.

C. **Monitoring of ventilatory status**
   1. **Oxygenation**
      a. **Blood gas sampling.** Arterial catheterization (see pp 132–137 for details) should be performed for frequent blood gas sampling. Routinely, these infants require blood gas sampling every 2–4 hours. Sampling may need to be done more frequently, possibly as often as every 20 minutes, but less frequent sampling is desirable as soon as possible to minimize stress and blood loss and the need for blood replacement.
         (1) **Desirable arterial blood gas values**
             (a) **Pao_2:** 45–60 torr.
             (b) **$Paco_2$:** 45–55 torr. A slightly higher $Paco_2$ is acceptable if the pH remains acceptable.
             (c) **pH:** 7.25–7.32 is acceptable.
         (2) **Abnormal blood gas values** indicate the need for immediate chest x-ray (see **3**, below), chest wall transillumination (see p 230, **IV.C.1**), and repeat blood gas determinations.
      b. **Continuous oxygen monitoring** should also be performed, preferably by pulse oximetry. Transcutaneous electrode monitoring of oxygen and carbon dioxide is discouraged because of possible skin damage in tiny babies. The air/oxygen mixture should be adjusted to maintain the pulse oximeter reading between 88 and 92% hemoglobin oxygen saturation.
   2. **Infant's appearance.** Abrupt changes in the infant's color or the appearance of cyanosis indicate the need for immediate assessment by chest x-ray study and blood gas sampling.
   3. **Chest x-ray study**
      a. **Indications**
         (1) Abnormal or sudden change in blood gas values.
         (2) Adjustment of the endotracheal tube (to confirm proper positioning).
         (3) Sudden change in infant's color.
      b. **Technique.** Chest x-ray should be performed with the infant's head in the midline position to check for endotracheal tube placement.
      c. **X-ray evaluation.** Check chest x-ray film for expansion of the lung, chest wall, and diaphragm. Overexpansion (hyperlucent lungs and diaphragms below 9th rib) must be avoided. If overexpansion is present, consider decreasing the peak airway pressure. Some tiny babies do very well with peak inspiratory pressures as low as 8 cm water.

D. **Suctioning.** Suctioning should be done only as needed and not more frequently than every 4 hours.
   1. **Assessment of the need for suctioning.** To assess need for suction, the nurse and/or physician should consider:
      a. **Breath sounds.** Wet or diminished breath sounds may indicate secretions obstructing the airways and the need for suctioning.
      b. **Blood gas values.** If the $Paco_2$ is increasing above 50 mm Hg, suctioning should be considered to clean the airways and avoid the "ball-valve" effect of thick secretions.
   2. **Technique**
      a. Suctioning should be done only to the depth of the endotracheal

tube. Use suctioning guide or marked (1-cm increments) suction catheter.

  b. Lavage fluid for suctioning should be sterile normal saline. Use 1–2 drops for each suctioning procedure. Lavage solution should be warmed to 36–37 °C.

E. Extubation
  1. Indications. Occasionally extremely low birth weight infants may be extubated by the end of the first week of life. Many require maintenance mechanical ventilation beyond the first month of life. Indications for extubation include:
  a. Ventilator rate less than 10 breaths/min.
  b. Oxygen requirements less than 30% F_{IO_2}.
  c. Regular spontaneous respiratory rate.
  d. Adequate spontaneous tidal volume (3.8–5.0 mL/kg).
  e. Pulmonary function tests (if available) revealing a compliance of 1 mL/cm water.
  f. Stable blood gas values (within normal ranges).
  g. Stable chest x-ray findings on serial examinations.
  2. Technique. Apnea is usually not a problem for tiny babies in the first few days of life, perhaps because of the use of mechanical ventilation. To prevent apnea, we start treatment with **theophylline prior to extubation** (see p 483). The procedure for tube removal is the same as for larger infants.

VII. Surfactant. (See Chap 13.) Most centers administer surfactant to these infants. Surfactant may be given either prophylactically or as rescue therapy. It should be administered according to the protocol provided with the specific surfactant product.

VIII. Patent ductus arteriosus. (See p 281.) Efforts should be made to minimize the risk of patent ductus arteriosus (PDA). Overhydration must be avoided. If the infant shows any sign of a hemodynamically significant PDA, medical treatment should commence. Some centers institute prophylactic indomethacin therapy, although this is somewhat *controversial.*

IX. Transfusion. These infants are usually born anemic, with hematocrits less than 40, and they will require numerous transfusions. We try to keep the hematocrit between 35 and 45%.

X. Skin care. Meticulous skin care is advised. Maintenance of intact skin provides care to the tiny baby's most effective barrier against infection, insensible fluid loss, and protein and blood loss and provides for more effective body temperature control. Additionally, the very thin skin of the tiny baby allows absorption of many substances. Skin care must focus on maintaining skin integrity and minimizing exposure to topical agents.
  A. **Cut servocontrol skin probe covers to the smallest size possible** (try a 2-cm diameter circle) to diminish skin damage due to the adhesive.
  B. **Monitoring of oxygen therapy is best accomplished by use of a pulse oximeter** for hemoglobin oxygen saturations. Alternative means of oxygen monitoring include umbilical catheter blood sampling. The use of transcutaneous oxygen and carbon dioxide gel electrodes is discouraged. Heated gel electrodes have caused serious skin burns in extremely low birth weight infants.
  C. **Urine bags and blood pressure cuffs should not routinely be used** because of adhesives and sharp plastic edge cuts. For urine collection, turn diaper plastic side up. Bladder aspirations are discouraged.
  D. **Prophylactic eye ointment should be applied** per routine admission plan. If the eyelids are fused, apply along the lash line.
  E. **When the physician prepares the skin for a procedure (eg, placement of UAC, UVC, chest tube) 1 mL of warm full-strength Betadine solution should be measured out.** (One milliliter is sufficient to effectively dis-

infect 50–60 sq cm of skin.) After the procedure is completed, the solution should be washed off immediately with warm sterile water.

F. **Attach ECG electrodes using as little adhesive as possible.** Options are:

1. Consider using electrode jacket.
2. Consider stretch gauze to strap the ECG leads to the extremities if limit leads are used.
3. Trim the adhesive electrode patch to minimize adhesive on the skin.

G. **Bathing is not appropriate for the tiny baby.** Soiled areas can be gently cleansed with cotton balls and warm water.

H. **Avoid the use of anything that dries out the skin,** such as soaps and alcohol.

I. **Medium-chain triglyceride (MCT) oil is useful for helping remove adhesive tape, probe covers, and electrode patches.**
Note: When skin appears dry, thickened, and no longer shiny or translucent (usually 10–14 days), these skin care recommendations and procedures may be modified or discontinued.

XI. **Other special considerations for the extremely low birth weight infant**

A. **Infection**

1. **Cultures.** Many of these infants are born infected or from an infected environment. Blood and urine cultures should be obtained. Unless there is a strong suspicion of meningitis, lumbar puncture should not be performed.
2. **Antibiotics.** After obtaining cultures, these infants should be started on **ampicillin** and an **aminoglycoside.** The aminoglycoside is usually started at a dosing interval of once a day. The peak and trough serum levels of the aminoglycoside must be monitored and the dosage should be adjusted appropriately. (See Chap 76.)
3. **Intravenous gamma globulin therapy.** Preliminary studies suggest that prophylactic treatment with intravenous gamma globulin may prevent infections in these small infants. This therapy will depend on the practice of your individual institution (see p 467).

B. **Central nervous system hemorrhage**

1. **Pharmacologic prevention.** Although many prophylactic therapies have been proposed—phenobarbital, indomethacin, ethamsylate, pancuronium, vitamin K, and vitamin E—none has received widespread acceptance and none can be recommended at this time. As much as possible, these infants should be maintained with normal blood pressures, blood volumes, acid-base status, and oxygenation. Transfusions should be given slowly (over at least 30 minutes, preferably slower). The use of sodium bicarbonate should be kept to a minimum.
2. **Monitoring.** Initial **cranial ultrasonography** is usually performed as soon after birth as practical. It should always be performed within the first 4 to 7 days of life.

C. **Hyperbilirubinemia**

1. **Risk.** There appears to be little risk from mild or moderate hyperbilirubinemia in these infants. Still, efforts should be made to keep the serum bilirubin below 10 mg/dL. Serum bilirubin should be monitored at least twice daily, and an exchange transfusion should be considered when the bilirubin exceeds 12 mg/dL.
2. **Phototherapy.** Phototherapy to reduce the serum bilirubin level appears to have little or no risk in these infants and can be used to prevent the need for exchange transfusion. Many centers start phototherapy immediately after birth. If the infant is treated with phototherapy, the fluid intake should be increased by 10–20 mL/kg/d.

D. **Social problems.** Many of these families have unexpected problems develop at the time of the birth. Nearly all will have numerous social problems prior to the infant's discharge. A social service consultation is mandatory for all of these families.

13 Surfactant Replacement Therapy

I. **Historical background.** In 1959, Avery and Mead reported that the lung lavage extract of infants who died from respiratory distress syndrome (RDS) had surface-active properties that were markedly decreased compared to the lavage of term infants who died from nonrespiratory illnesses. This seminal observation presaged the use of exogenous surfactant replacement in the treatment of RDS. By 1961, the phospholipid dipalmitoylphosphatidylcholine (DPPC, also termed *lecithin*) had been identified as the major component of surfactant. Early clinical trials failed to demonstrate that treatment with DPPC alone improved pulmonary function in infants with RDS, delaying the development of an effective exogenous surfactant. One study even suggested that pulmonary ischemia, and not surfactant deficiency, was the fundamental cause of RDS. These negative results might have been predicted prospectively if the biophysical properties necessary for surfactant function in vivo had been better understood. Over the next decade, investigators described the composition and biophysical properties of natural surfactants and studied the clinical effects of surfactant replacement in different animal models of RDS. In 1980, Fujiwara et al galvanized the perinatal community when they reported that a surfactant preparation derived from calf lung significantly improved pulmonary function in infants with severe RDS. This report precipitated an explosion of further basic and clinical research with a variety of surfactant preparations. By mid-1990, large randomized controlled trials of 2 different surfactant preparations for the prophylaxis and treatment of RDS were complete. On the basis of these trials, Exosurf Pediatric (a synthetic surfactant marketed by the Burroughs Wellcome Company) had received new drug approval (NDA) from the Food and Drug Administration. At this writing, similar approval of Survanta (a calf-lung derived surfactant marketed by Abbott Laboratories) is expected to follow shortly.

II. **Surfactant: basic science essentials**
   A. **Composition.** As determined from analysis of lung lavage fluid, surfactant is a complex mixture of phospholipids (85% by weight), neutral lipids (7%), and surfactant-associated proteins (8%). The phospholipid composition of surfactant is detailed in Table 13–1. This phospholipid profile is identical to that of the lamellar bodies of type II pneumocytes.
   B. **Life cycle.** Type II pneumocytes synthesize all surfactant components. These components are packaged in the smooth endoplasmic reticulum and Golgi apparatus. After posttranscriptional modification of surfactant proteins and dehydration of prelamellar bodies, mature lamellar bodies are ready to be released into the alveoli by exocytosis. Surfactant reuptake occurs by endocytosis and is regulated in part by interactions of surfactant proteins with specific cell membrane receptors. After reuptake, surfactant components are catabolized and recycled.
   C. **Biophysical properties**
      1. **Reduction in surface tension.** Surface forces at an air-liquid interface normally exert a surface pressure that tends to reduce the area of the interface. Critical to the biophysical activity of surfactant (**surface-active agent**) is its ability to lower surface-active forces, thus promoting stability of the air-liquid interface (Figure 13–1[D]). Lung alveoli that lack a functional surfactant lining become atelec-

TABLE 13-1. COMPOSITION OF PULMONARY SURFACTANT (% BY WEIGHT)

Phospholipids		85%
PC	80%	
PG	7%	
PI + PS	5%	
PE	4%	
Sph	2%	
Other	2%	
	100%	
Neutral lipids		7%
(cholesterol, free fatty acids)		
Surfactant-associated proteins		8%
(SP-A, SP-B, SP-C)		
		100%

Note: PC, phosphatidylcholine; PG, phosphatidylglycerol; PI, phosphatidylinositol; PS, phosphatidylserine; PE, phosphatidyl-ethanolamine; Sph, sphingomyelin; SP-A, B, and C, surfactant proteins A, B, and C.

tactic at end-expiration (when transpulmonary pressure = 0). An effective pulmonary surfactant must be able to lower surface tension during dynamic compression-expansion to < 10 dynes/cm (dynes/cm = mN/m). Natural surfactant and calf-lung surfactant extract lower minimum surface tension to < 1 dyne/cm on dynamic cycling; Surfactant-TA lowers surface tension to a minimum of 2–3 dynes/cm.

2. **Rapid and effective adsorption to the air-liquid interface.** For endogenous surfactant to be effective, it must adsorb rapidly to the air-liquid interface of the alveolus after lamellar body exocytosis. Similarly, an effective exogenous surfactant must be able to spread throughout the tracheobronchial tree and adsorb to the alveolar epithelial lining.

3. **Variation of surface tension during dynamic cycling and hysteresis.** These properties are well demonstrated in Figure 13–1. Failure to modulate surface tension as a function of the area of the air-liquid interface (or the volume of the alveolus) would create an unstable population of alveoli. Because the surface pressure (P) promoting alveolar collapse is proportional to the surface tension (T) and inversely proportional to the alveolar "radius" (r) [$P = 2T/r$]; (law of Young and LaPlace), a surfactant that lowered T to the same value independent of alveolar size would create higher P in small than in large alveoli. In effect, small alveoli would empty into large alveoli, resulting in inhomogeneity of alveolar inflation characterized by atelectasis and emphysema.

4. **Respreadability after compression of surfactant lining beyond monolayer collapse.** Certain components of surfactant may become "squeezed out" of the lining during compression (expiration). These components must be able to reenter the surface film with reexpansion; otherwise, the surfactant would soon become biophysically effete. The inability of pure DPPC to respread accounts in part for the loss of hysteresis in Figure 13–1.

D. **Surfactant proteins.** Although surfactant phospholipids can lower surface tension when spread in a surface film, phospholipids have poor adsorption and dynamic respreadability. It has become clear that surfactant proteins are essential for normal biophysical function of surfactant and play important roles in surfactant recycling and possibly in host defense.

1. **SP-A** is the largest (molecular weight 35K daltons) and most common surfactant protein. Its chief biophysical function is to facilitate

NOTE:
Numbers refer to the order of the cycles, eg (1 = first cycle).

FIGURE 13-1. A-D. Surface tension-area diagrams of synthetic (**A-C**) and artificial (Surfactant-TA) (**D**) surfactants (mN/m = dynes/cm). Surfactants were spread onto a clean saline surface. The area of surfactant-coated air-liquid interface was cyclically compressed and reexpanded by means of a modified Wilhelmy balance technique. The synthetic surfactants have inferior biophysical properties compared to those of artificial surfactants, as demonstrated by (1) requirement for much greater compression of area of surface film (50% vs 75%) to achieve minimal surface tension and (2) loss of loop hysteresis with repeated cycles of compression and rexpansion. (Modified and reproduced, with permission, from Fujiuara T, Adams FH: Surfactant for hyaline membrane disease. *Pediatrics* 1980;**66**:795.)

the formation of tubular myelin, the microstructure of surfactant phospholipids and proteins from which adsorption of endogenous surfactant occurs. SP-A, a hydrophilic protein, is lost during the extraction process and is not present in current preparations of surfactant derived from calf lungs.

2. **SP-B and SP-C** are smaller, less prevalent, hydrophobic proteins. Their primary function is to confer adsorptive properties to surfactant. Addition of SP-B,C to the phospholipid moiety of surfactant results in a mixture that both quantitatively and qualitatively repro-

duces all biophysical properties of natural surfactant. SP-B,C probably are important in regulating the secretion and reuptake of surfactant by the type II alveolar pneumocyte. SP-B,C are present in current calf-lung derived surfactants.

E. **Clinical properties.** The following clinical properties of surfactant are consequences of its biophysical effects.
   1. Increased lung compliance.
   2. Decreased work of breathing.
   3. Improved alveolar stability.
   4. Decreased tendency for pulmonary edema formation (by means of influencing Starling forces operative at alveolar surface).

F. **Types of surfactant**
   1. **Natural.** All surfactant phospholipids and proteins are present. *Example:* human amniotic fluid surfactant.
   2. **Artificial.** A subset of surfactant components is present; additional components not present in surfactant may be added. *Examples:* Survanta (Abbott Laboratories), calf lung surfactant extract (CLSE), Curosurf. Survanta is the descendent of Surfactant-TA used by Fujiwara in the first modern study that demonstrated the efficacy of surfactant in the treatment of RDS. It is made by adding certain lipid ingredients to an extraction of calf lung mince. Survanta lacks SP-A. CLSE is extracted from calf lung lavage and also lacks SP-A, but no exogenous components are added after extraction. Curosurf, surfactant used in Europe, is derived from porcine lung mince, from which components are removed by chromatographic methods.
   3. **Synthetic.** Exosurf Pediatric (Burroughs-Wellcome Company) is composed of dipalmitoylphosphatidylcholine (DPPC), hexadecanol, tyloxapol, and sodium chloride. No surfactant proteins are present. Hexadecanol helps DPPC spread on the air-fluid interface of the tracheobronchial tree (including the alveoli), and tyloxapol aids dispersion of both DPPC and hexadecanol.

III. **Clinical trials of surfactant.** Numerous clinical trials using several surfactants, each administered under different protocols, have been published in the past decade. These trials are well reviewed in some of the references. Briefly, all modern surfactants (with the exception of artificial lung expanding compound [ALEC] used in the UK) have decreased the severity of acute RDS. Most have significantly decreased the incidence of pulmonary air leak as well. Surfactants as a group have not consistently decreased mortality or the incidence of chronic lung disease. In general, significant improvement has occurred only when the control population has sustained above-average rates of mortality and chronic lung disease. Surfactant therapy has not had a significant effect on the incidence or severity of other morbidities related to prematurity (IVH, NEC, PDA, sepsis), nor on short- or long-term immunologic function. The few published studies that have examined the effect of surfactant therapy on neurodevelopmental outcome allow no definitive conclusions.

IV. **Surfactant treatment IND protocols.** In the summer of 1989, the FDA approved treatment IND (investigational new drug) protocols for 2 surfactant preparations, Exosurf Pediatric and Survanta. Each surfactant had undergone extensive prospective, controlled double-masked trials and had been shown to be effective in reducing the acute severity of RDS. In addition, under certain circumstances, each of these surfactants was shown to reduce mortality and the incidence of BPD. In August 1990, the FDA granted new drug approval (NDA) to Exosurf Pediatric, thus making Exosurf the first surfactant generally available for the prophylaxis and treatment of neonatal RDS. At this writing, it appears likely that the FDA will soon grant similar NDA status to Survanta.

A. **Exosurf Pediatric**

1. **Composition** (Table 13-2)
2. **Protocol for administration**
   a. **Indications**
      (1) **Prophylaxis**
          (a) Birth weight 500–1350 g; larger infants with evidence of pulmonary immaturity.
          (b) No serious congenital anomalies.
          (c) Intubation required for stabilization.
          (d) Treatment must be given within the first 30 minutes after birth.
      (2) **Rescue**
          (a) Birth weight $\geq$ 700 g.
          (b) No serious congenital anomalies.
          (c) Clinical diagnosis of RDS with an a:A ratio < 0.22, which is calculated as follows:

$$\text{Pao}_2/\text{Pao}_2 = \frac{\text{Pao}_2}{[\text{Fio}_2 (\text{Barometric pressure} - \text{H}_2\text{O vapor pressure}) - \text{Paco}_2]}$$

          (d) Only treatments administered at more than 2 hours but less than 24 hours after birth have been studied.
   b. **Dose.** The dose is 5 mL/kg (67.5 mg DPPC/kg).
   c. **Frequency of dosing**
      (1) **Prophylaxis.** Three doses (at birth and at 12 and 24 hours of life) reduce mortality at 28 days and at 1 year compared to single-dose prophylaxis at birth.
      (2) **Rescue.** Two doses are given. The second dose is given 12 hours after first if infant is still intubated and on IMV.
   d. **Recommended method of administration**
      (1) Connect side-port adapter to endotracheal tube.
      (2) Intubate infant and verify tube is in proper tracheal position. Verification of tube placement is done by auscultation of the chest (with bag-and-mask ventilation) for bilateral breath sounds, inspection of the chest for movement with bag-and-mask ventilation, and clinical response.
      (3) Reconstitute Exosurf Pediatric by injecting 8 mL of preservative free sterile water into vacuum-sealed vial.
      (4) Draw back full 8 mL/solution into syringe and reinject into vacuum-sealed vial to solubilize Exosurf powder; repeat 3–4 times.
      (5) Administer Exosurf Pediatric in 2 doses (2.5 mL/kg each) via side-port adapter.
          (a) Instill each dose slowly over 1–2 minutes (30–50 manual breaths) with infant's head and torso in midline.
          (b) After the first dose, turn infant's head and torso to the right; after the second dose, turn the head and torso to the left. After each dose, continue ventilation for 30 seconds.

Note: Check current protocol recommended by manufacturer. The above recommendations may be modified by the outcome of ongoing clinical trials.

TABLE 13-2. COMPOSITION OF EXOSURF PEDIATRIC*

DPPC	108 mg
Hexadecanol	12 mg
Tyloxapol	8 mg
Sodium chloride	47 mg

*Supplied as powder. Powder reconstituted in 8 mL preservative-free sterile water to achieve a DPPC concentration of 13.5 mg DPPC/mL.

3. **Potential side effects**
   a. **Pulmonary air leak.** Changes in compliance after surfactant administration demand careful clinical assessment of lung compliance. Failure to decrease ventilator pressures as compliance improves could result in barotrauma.
   b. **Pulmonary hemorrhage.** The risk of pulmonary hemorrhage has been significantly increased compared to control (10% vs 2%) only for prophylactically treated infants with birth weights between 500 and 700 g.
   c. **Apnea** (see Chap 29 and Chap 69, p 405).
4. **Results of clinical trials.** Selected results of clinical trials summarized in the Exosurf brochure are listed in Table 13–3. In infants with birth weights between 700 and 1100 g, Exosurf prophylaxis followed by additional treatments at 12 and 24 hours of life significantly decreased mortality compared to single-dose prophylaxis alone.
B. **Survanta (beractant; surfactant-TA)**
   1. **Composition.** The approximate composition of Survanta by weight is 88% phospholipids, 7% other lipids (free fatty acids, triglycerides, and cholesterol), and 1% protein (including SP-B,C but not SP-A). Survanta is extracted from calf lung mince. Certain components are added to the extract following purification (eg, palmitic acid, tripalmitic acid) to achieve a phospholipid profile more analogous to natural surfactant.
   2. **Protocol for administration**
      a. **Indications**
         (1) **Prophylaxis**
             (a) Gestational age 23–29 weeks, inclusive.
             (b) Birth weight 600–1250 g.
             (c) Intubation required for stabilization.
             (d) Only treatments given in the first 15 minutes after birth have been studied.

TABLE 13–3. RESULTS OF CLINICAL TRIALS OF EXOSURF PEDIATRIC IN THE PROPHYLACTIC AND RESCUE TREATMENTS OF RDS

Treatment	P	P	P	P	R	R
Number of doses	1	3 vs 1	1	1	2	2
Birth weight	700–1100	700–1100	700–1350	500–700	700–1350	> 1250
Number of patients analyzed	446	716	361	215	419	1237
Outcome Variable						
RDS						
Incidence	NS	NS	NS	NS	NA	NA
Severity	D	D	D	D	D	D
Air leaks						
Pneumothorax	D	NS	NS	D	D	D
PIE	NS	NS	D	NS	D	D
Total air leaks	NS	NS	NS	NS	D	D
Deaths						
RDS	NS	NS	NS	D	D	D
< 28 days	NS	D	NS	NS	D	D
Total deaths	D	D	NS	NS	D	NS
Complications						
BPD	NS	NS	NS	NS	NS	D
PDA	NS	NS	NS	NS	NS	D
IVH	NS	NS	NS	NS	NS	D
ICPS	NS	NS	I	NS	I	I

Note: P, prophylactic treatment; R, rescue treatment; PIE, pulmonary interstitial emphysema; ICPS, intact cardiopulmonary survival (alive without BPD on day 28); NS, not significant, NA, not applicable; D, significantly decreased; I, significantly increased.

    (2) Rescue
       (a) Weight 600–1750 g on admission to NICU.
       (b) Clinical diagnosis of RDS.
       (c) Requirement for assisted ventilation and $Pao_2 \leq 80$ mm Hg on $Fio_2 \geq 0.40$ between 1 and 6 hours of age.
       (d) Only treatments given before 8 hours of age have been studied.
       (e) No previous treatment with another surfactant.
  b. Dose. The dose is 4 mL/kg (100 mg phospholipid/kg).
  c. Frequency of dosing
    (1) Prophylaxis. After the initial dose, up to 3 re-treatments are permitted within the first 48 hours of life. A minimum of 6 hours must elapse between doses. Criteria include confirmation of RDS on chest radiograph, continued intubation, and $Pao_2 \leq 80$ mm Hg on $Fio_2 \geq 0.30$.
    (2) Rescue. Same as for prophylaxis (see **(1),** above).
  d. Recommended method of administration
    (1) A vial of Survanta is warmed to room temperature.
    (2) Survanta is administered in 4 aliquots of 1 mL/kg via 5F feeding tube positioned at the distal end of the endotracheal tube. After each dose, the infant's head and torso are turned to the right and to left, respectively, as described on p 118, **d.5.(b).**
    (3) Manual ventilation (for prophylaxis) or mechanical ventilation (for rescue) is performed for 30 seconds between aliquots. Ventilator settings are adjusted before dosing.
      (a) Prophylaxis: Manual ventilation with bag and mask as deemed clinically appropriate.
      First rescue: $Fio_2 = 1.00$; IMV set at pretreatment rate or at 60, whichever is greater; pretreatment pressures; IT = 0.5 second.
      Subsequent rescues: Fio_2 set at 0.2 > baseline: IMV set at pretreatment rate or at 30, whichever is greater; pretreatment pressures; IT ≤ 1.0 second.
  Note: Check current protocol recommended by manufacturer. The above recommendations may be modified by the outcomes of ongoing clinical trials.
  3. Potential side effects. Pulmonary air leak may occur (see p 118, **A.3.a).**
  4. Results of clinical trials. Results of many clinical trials using Survanta are not yet published; preliminary results are contained in the Survanta treatment IND drug brochure. In summary, both single- and multiple-dose prophylaxis regimens decreased the incidence and severity of RDS and the percentage of RDS-related deaths. Only the multiple-dose protocol decreased air leak. Single-dose rescue trials decreased the severity of RDS but not total deaths or deaths related to RDS. Preliminary results of the multiple-dose rescue trials are not available at this time.
V. Clinical controversies
  A. Optimal surfactant. At least 4 surfactants are in use in the United States: human amniotic fluid surfactant; Exosurf Pediatric; Survanta; and calf-lung surfactant extract (CLSE). In addition, development and limited clinical testing of a surfactant composed of phospholipids and genetically cloned human surfactant apoprotein is in progress. However, it may be years before large-scale clinical trials of the latter genetically engineered surfactant can be started. Significant differences exist among these surfactants with respect to in vitro tests of biophysical properties and also with respect to functional stability in the presence of a variety of surfactant inhibitors. However, it is as yet unknown

whether these in vitro differences will translate into significant differences in clinical efficacy or side effects or both.

B. Optimal treatment strategies

  a. Prophylaxis vs rescue. Debate continues about whether or not prophylaxis or early treatment of established RDS is optimal. In the largest study to date, CLSE prophylaxis in infants less than 26 weeks resulted in significant improvement in the survival rate, compared to early treatment. Other studies have found no difference in the survival rate but an increased incidence of BPD in infants less than 30 weeks who were randomly assigned to prophylaxis, compared to infants randomly assigned to early treatment. Further studies are needed to define the optimal approach to treatment.

  b. Time of initial rescue treatment. Available evidence supports the use of surfactant therapy earlier rather than later in the course of RDS. In addition, rescue treatment of infants with preexisting pulmonary barotrauma is less effective than of infants with otherwise uncomplicated RDS.

  c. Indications for re-treatment. Available evidence suggests that multiple surfactant treatments are more effective than single-dose therapy; however, comparison of different indications for re-treatment have not been investigated.

C. Method of administration of prophylactic surfactant. Timing of surfactant prophylaxis varies from before the first breath to as late as 30 minutes after birth. Animal studies suggest that even a short period of lung aeration before surfactant administration decreases clinical efficacy as assessed by blood gases (a:A ratio) and lung compliance. However, administration before the first breath requires a high level of technical skill, and an attempt to administer prophylaxis before resuscitation and stabilization of the infant may prolong hypoxia and bradycardia. Clinical trials that compare the timing of prophylaxis in the very premature infants are needed.

D. Surfactant therapy for other diseases. Basic research and anecdotal clinical reports suggest that surfactant deficiency may contribute to the pathophysiology of other respiratory diseases common in newborns (meconium aspiration syndrome, pneumonia, shock lung). Outcome results of trials of surfactant replacement therapy for these conditions are eagerly anticipated. Finally, surfactant may be the first drug developed specifically for the newborn that may have clinical utility in a serious adult disease: ARDS. Clinical trials using Exosurf in the treatment of ARDS are already under way.

REFERENCES

Fujiwara T et al: Artificial surfactant therapy in hyaline membrane disease. *Lancet* 1980;**1**:55.

Jobe A, Ikegami M: Surfactant for the treatment of respiratory distress syndrome. *Am Rev Respir Dis* 1987;**136**:1256.

Shapiro DL, Notter RH: Surfactant replacement therapy. Alan R. Liss, 1989.

Vidyasagar D et al: Surfactant replacement therapy: Clinical and experimental studies. *Clin Perinatol* 1987;**14**:713.

14 High-Frequency Ventilation

High-frequency ventilation refers to a variety of ventilatory strategies and devices designed to provide ventilation at rapid rates and very low tidal volumes, thus reducing the risk of barotrauma. Three types of high-frequency ventilators are being used in increasing numbers in intensive care nurseries: **high-frequency jet ventilators (HFJV), high-frequency flow interrupters (HFFI),** and **high-frequency oscillatory ventilators (HFOV).**

High-frequency positive-pressure ventilation (HFPPV) is available on all current conventional infant ventilators. It is defined as rates between 60 and 150 breaths/min (see p 44, **C**). This chapter will discuss the 3 types of high-frequency ventilators.

I. **High-frequency jet ventilators (HFJV).** The HFJV injects a high-velocity stream of gas into the endotracheal tube, usually at lower frequencies (240–600 breaths/min) and higher tidal volumes (equal to or slightly greater than dead space). During HFJV, expiration is passive. The only FDA approved HFJV is the Bunnell Life Pulse ventilator, which will be discussed here.

A. **Definite indications**
   1. **Pulmonary interstitial emphysema (PIE).** A multicenter trial has demonstrated HFJV to be superior to conventional ventilation in early PIE as well as in neonates failing conventional ventilation.
   2. **Severe bronchopleural fistula.** In severe bronchopleural fistula not responsive to thoracostomy tube evacuation and conventional ventilation, HFJV may provide adequate ventilation and decrease fistula flow.

B. **Possible indications.** HFJV has been used with moderate success in infants with other disease processes; it is usually implemented at the point of severe respiratory failure with maximal conventional ventilation. Further study is needed to develop clear indications and appropriate ventilatory strategies before HFJV can be recommended for routine use in infants with these diseases.
   1. **Patients qualifying for ECMO.**
   2. **Hyaline membrane disease.**
   3. **Meconium aspiration syndrome.**
   4. **Diaphragmatic hernia with pulmonary hypoplasia.**
   5. **Postoperative Fontan procedures.**

C. **Contraindications.** The only contraindication is an infant too small for intubation with a triple-lumen endotracheal tube. The smallest triple-lumen endotracheal tube (2.5 mm inside diameter) has an outside diameter equal to a standard 3.0 mm endotracheal tube.

D. **Equipment**
   1. **Bunnell Life Pulse ventilator.** HFJV is provided by the Bunnell Life Pulse ventilator. The inspiratory pressure (PIP), jet valve "on time" and respiratory frequency are entered into a digital control panel on the jet. Inspiratory pressures are servocontrolled by the Life Pulse from the distal pressure port. The Life Pulse has an elaborate alarm system to ensure safety and to help detect changes in pulmonary function. It also has a special humidification system.
   2. **Triple-lumen endotracheal tube.** Intubation with a special triple-lumen endotracheal tube (ETT) is required. This ETT has a distal port

for measuring airway pressure, a side port for jet injection, and a standard connection for a conventional ventilator circuit.

3. **Conventional ventilator.** A conventional ventilator is needed to generate positive end-expiratory pressure (PEEP) and sigh breaths. Therefore, PEEP and background ventilation are controlled with the conventional ventilator.

E. **Procedure**
   1. **Initiation of HFJV**
      a. **Reintubation with a triple-lumen tube.**
      b. **Settings on the jet ventilator** (pressure measurements are obtained through the distal pressure port on the conventional ventilator to help determine the initial jet settings):
         (1) **Default jet valve "on time":** 0.02 seconds.
         (2) **Frequency of jet:** 420/min.
         (3) **PIP on the jet:** Set 2–3 cm water below what was on the conventional ventilator. Occasionally patients require considerably less PIP during HFJV.
      c. **Settings on the conventional ventilator**
         (1) **PEEP:** Maintained at 3–5 cm water. Once the jet ventilator is up to pressure, PEEP valve is adjusted to maintain PEEP.
         (2) **Rate:** As jet ventilator comes up to pressure, rate decreased to 5–10 breaths/min.
         (3) **PIP:** Once at pressure, PIP is adjusted to a level 3–4 cm water below that on jet.
      d. **Close observation** is required at all times, especially during initiation.
      e. Rarely, an infant will develop worse air trapping on HFJV and require prompt return to the CMV.
   2. **Management on HFJV.** Management of HFJV is based on clinical course and radiographic findings.
      a. **Elimination of carbon dioxide.** Alveolar ventilation is much more sensitive to changes in tidal volume than in respiratory frequency at very low tidal volume ventilation. As a result, the **delta pressure (PIP minus PEEP)** is adjusted to attain adequate elimination of carbon dioxide, while jet valve "on time" and respiratory frequency are usually not adjusted during HFJV.
      b. **Oxygenation.** Oxygenation is often better during HFJV than during conventional mechanical ventilation in these neonates. However, if oxygenation is inadequate and if the infant is already on 100% oxygen, an increase in mean airway pressure will usually result in improved oxygenation. It can be accomplished by:
         (1) Increasing PEEP.
         (2) Increasing PIP.
         (3) Increasing background conventional ventilator, either rates or pressure.
      c. **Positioning of infants.** Positioning infants with the affected side down may speed resolution of PIE. In bilateral air leak, alternating dependent sides may be effective, but diligent observation and frequent radiographs are necessary to avoid hyperinflation of the nondependent side.
   3. **Weaning from the HFJV.** When weaning, the following guidelines are used.
      a. **Reduce PIP** as soon as possible ($PaCO_2$ < 45–50 mm Hg). Because elimination of carbon dioxide is very sensitive to changes in tidal volume, PIP is weaned 1 cm water at a time.
      b. **Wean oxygen concentration** if oxygenation remains good (PaO_2 > 50–60 mm Hg).
      c. Jet valve "on time" and frequency are usually kept constant.

    d. Constant attention is paid to **clinical course** and radiographs to detect early atelectasis or hyperinflation.

    e. Resolution of air leak. Continuation of HFJV occurs until the air leak has been resolved for 12–24 hours, which often corresponds to a dramatic drop in ventilator pressures and oxygen requirement.

    f. No improvement. If there is no improvement in the patient, a trial of conventional ventilation is used after 6–24 hours on jet ventilation.

  4. Special considerations

    a. Airway obstruction. Because of the stiffness of the triple-lumen endotracheal tube, the bevel of the tube may become lodged against the tracheal wall, resulting in airway obstruction. This problem can usually be recognized quickly. Chest wall movement is decreased, although breath sounds may be adequate. The servopressure (driving pressure) is usually very low in this case. (An obstruction in the endotracheal tube proximal to the distal pressure port will result in a high servopressure alarm). Positioning the tube with the jet port facing anteriorly usually will maintain good tube position.

    b. Inadvertent PEEP. In larger patients, the flow of jet gases may result in inadvertent PEEP. Decreasing the background flow on the conventional ventilator may correct the problem, or it may be necessary to decrease the respiratory frequency to allow more time for expiration.

F. Complications

  1. Tracheitis. Necrotizing tracheitis was a frequent complication in the early days of jet ventilation. This problem is much less frequent with the recognition of the critical importance of proper humidification of the jet gases. If tracheitis occurs, emergent bronchoscopy may be indicated. The clinical signs are:

    a. Increased airway secretions.

    b. Evidence of airway obstruction (including air trapping).

    c. Acute respiratory acidosis.

  2. Intraventricular hemorrhage (IVH). There has been no increase in the incidence or severity of IVH with the use of HFJV.

  3. Bronchopulmonary dysplasia. The incidence of PIE appears to be equal in neonates ventilated with HFJV and those ventilated with CMV.

II. High-frequency flow interrupter (HFFI). The HFFI shares some qualities with HFOV and HFJV. It operates at frequencies as high as HFOV but does not have active exhalation. Bursts of gas approximate those of HFJV, but a standard endotracheal tube can be used. The only FDA-approved HFFI is the Infrasonic Infant Star ventilator, which will be discussed here.

A. Indications. The indications are the same as those for HFJV. Pulmonary interstitial emphysema. The Infrasonic Infant Star ventilator may not be effective in infants whose birth weight is greater than 1800 g. If an infant of this size qualifies for high-frequency ventilation, high-frequency jet ventilation may prove to be more effective.

B. Equipment

  1. The Infrasonic Infant Star ventilator. Infrasonics prefers to call its ventilator a *flow oscillator* because of the ventilation technique used and its flow characteristics.

    a. The bursts of gas are 18 msec in duration, which is factory preset. The sudden expansion of gas after the burst creates a rebound negative pressure deflection that closely approximates the active exhalation of oscillatory ventilation.

    b. It can be termed *hybrid oscillator,* with characteristics of a flow interrupter and an oscillator.

    c. The user-defined parameters are frequency (10–20 Hz), mean airway pressure (MAP), and amplitude, which is a function of volume of gas per burst.

  2. Conventional ventilator. The high-frequency mode on the Infant Star must be used in combination with the conventional ventilator. Rate, PEEP, and PAP are set on the conventional ventilator.

  3. Endotracheal tube. A regular endotracheal tube is used.

C. Procedure

  1. Initiation of Infant Star ventilation

    a. Conventional ventilator settings

      (1) Rate is set at 5 breaths/min. It is extremely important to have a conventional rate set during high frequency so that atelectasis does not develop, as tidal volumes will be very small during high frequency.

      (2) PAP and PEEP are not changed from the original settings.

    b. Settings

      (1) Frequency is always maintained at 15 Hz (900 breaths/min). It is not adjusted during high-frequency ventilation.

      (2) MAP is determined by the PEEP level and initially should be set to match the MAP prior to the initiation of high frequency, ie, if MAP was 15 on conventional ventilatory support, it should be set on the high-frequency ventilator by means of setting the PEEP at 15.

      (3) Amplitude. After the frequency and the MAP are set, the amplitude should be adjusted. It should be increased until the chest wall of the infant begins to vibrate visually. This setting is the most difficult and arbitrary to determine. The range is 10–30 mL.

    c. After the high-frequency device is initially set, arterial blood gas values and chest x-ray studies are used to determine adjustment of settings. Chest x-ray studies are usually done every 6 hours until stabilization of the infant.

  2. Management on the Infant Star. It is important to note that the MAP controls oxygenation and the amplitude controls elimination of carbon dioxide.

    a. If Pao_2 is low

      (1) MAP should be increased on the Infant Star. PEEP is the main determinant of MAP and lung volume; therefore PEEP levels should be increased until adequate oxygenation.

      (2) Increase conventional rate, but this is a less effective means of increasing oxygenation.

    b. If $Paco_2$ is high

      (1) If poor oxygenation also exists, it is an indication of poor lung volume (a chest x-ray study at this time will often reveal a hypoventilated lung with atelectasis) and PEEP should be increased.

      (2) If adequate oxygenation exists, amplitude should be increased until adequate removal of carbon dioxide is achieved.

      (3) If hyperoxygenation exists, it may be an indication of air trapping and PEEP should be decreased. A chest x-ray film would reveal lung hyperinflation.

  3. Weaning. Once adequate gas exchange has been achieved and oxygenation is adequate, careful weaning should begin. In general, weaning should follow the pattern described below.

    a. If Pao_2 is acceptable and a chest x-ray film does not show hyperexpansion, wean the FiO_2. (If hyperexpansion is present, PEEP is weaned, followed by **c, d,** and **e** below.)

    b. When the FiO_2 has been weaned to 60%, wean the PEEP.

    c. If $Paco_2$ elimination is good ($Paco_2 < 40$ mm Hg), wean the amplitude.

    d. When the amplitude has reached low levels (around 10 mL), conventional breaths may be added to ventilatory strategy.

    e. Frequency does not need to be decreased during weaning.

    Note: It is necessary to perform serial chest x-ray studies to rule out atelectasis and underinflation while weaning is in progress. The x-ray films may indicate that PEEP has been dropped too low or that amplitude needs to be increased.

  D. Complications. The main complication is gas trapping resulting in hyperexpansion, which can be prevented by meticulously monitoring serial chest x-ray studies and arterial blood gas values and by appropriate weaning procedures, as outlined above.

  E. Prognosis for HFFI (and HFJV). The great promise of high-frequency ventilation has been largely unfulfilled. In pulmonary air leak, there is a definite advantage. The use of high-frequency ventilation in other diseases, especially severe respiratory failure, is becoming more widespread, with some encouraging results. However, the routine application of high-frequency ventilation early in other disease processes awaits the rigorous evaluation of different ventilatory strategies in controlled clinical trials.

III. High-frequency oscillatory ventilation (HFOV). This technique produces tidal volumes generally smaller than the anatomic dead space at frequencies between 600 and 900 breaths/min. The tidal volume is generated by a piston causing both inspiration and expiration to be active. There are no FDA-approved HFOVs commercially available at the time of this publication.

REFERENCES

Hamilton LH et al (editors): *High Frequency Ventilation.* CRC Press, 1986.

Keszler MA et al: Controlled multicenter trial of high frequency jet ventilation vs. conventional ventilation in newborns with interstitial emphysema. *Pediatr Res* 1990;**27(4):**309A.

Lunkenheimer PP et al (editors): High frequency ventilation, 20 years of endeavour reviewed: Final stress or departure to achievement. *Acta Anaesthiol Scand* 1989;**33 (Supp 90).**

Spitzer AR et al: Ventilatory response to combined high frequency jet ventilation and conventional mechanical ventilation for the rescue treatment of severe neonatal lung disease. *Pediatr Pulmonol* 1989;**7:**244.

15 Extracorporeal Membrane Oxygenation (ECMO)

I. **Introduction.** Extracorporeal membrane oxygenation (ECMO) is a technique in which an infant's venous blood is pumped through a membrane oxygenator (artificial lung) whereby oxygen is added and carbon dioxide is removed. The blood is then pumped back into the patient's venous (venovenous ECMO) or arterial circulation (venoarterial ECMO). The procedure allows the lungs to rest and averts continuous high-pressure mechanical ventilation in severe respiratory failure (Zwischenberger, 1986). During ECMO, the lungs continue to function at a low volume and low pressure to prevent atelectasis and to maintain minimal alveolar ventilation. The patient is entirely dependent on the membrane for oxygenation and removal of carbon dioxide.

II. **Indications.** ECMO is currently used primarily for critically ill term newborns with reversible respiratory failure who have failed maximal medical management. Each ECMO center must establish its own specific criteria for both reversible respiratory failure *and* maximal medical management. These criteria should identify infants who would have at least an 80% mortality and significant morbidity without ECMO. Infants should be identified in time to institute ECMO before it's too late.

Diseases that have been treated by ECMO include meconium aspiration syndrome, congenital diaphragmatic hernia, sepsis, persistent pulmonary hypertension (usually secondary to meconium aspiration or severe asphyxia), cardiac failure following open heart surgery, and respiratory distress syndrome in the older infant with pneumonia and sepsis.

A. **ECMO entry criteria.** The following criteria should be applied only after failure of maximal medical therapy (100% FIO_2, induction and maintenance of alkalosis, tolazoline).

1. Weight greater than 2 kg.
2. No more than 7–10 days of assisted ventilation.
3. Reversible lung disease.
4. No major bleeding disorder or major intracranial hemorrhage.
5. The patient must have been screened with echocardiography to rule out cyanotic congenital heart disease.
6. **PLUS** one of the following:

   a. Alveolar-to-arterial oxygen gradient ($A\text{-}aDO_2$) is greater than 610 for 8 hours (80% mortality). (Normal $A\text{-}aDO_2$ is less than 20 mm Hg.)

   $$A\text{-}aDO_2 = \left[(FIO_2)\,(Pb - 47) - \frac{(Paco_2)}{R} \right] - Pao_2$$

   Pb = barometric pressure (760 mm Hg); 47 = water vapor pressure; $Paco_2$ = alveolar CO_2 (approximately equivalent to the $Paco_2$); R = respiratory quotient (0.8).

   b. PIP is greater than or equal to 38 and $A\text{-}aDO_2$ is equal to or less than 605 for 4 hours (84% mortality).

   Note: Some centers use oxygen index (OI) rather than $A\text{-}aDO_2$.

   $$OI = \frac{FIO_2 \times MAP \times 100}{Pao_2}$$

      a. OI is greater than 40 in 3 ABGs (80% mortality).
      b. OI is greater than 25 (50% mortality).
III. Contraindications. See Table 15–1.
IV. Procedure. Uniform guidelines should be established to describe essential equipment, procedures, personnel, and training required for neonatal ECMO. A multidisciplinary team approach is necessary because of the variety of diseases treated by ECMO as well as the variety of resulting complications. The currently accepted ECMO procedure is **venoarterial (VA) bypass.** Venoarterial ECMO is usually preferred for neonatal patients because it provides both cardiac and respiratory support and because it is easier to oxygenate the blood.

  A. Catheters are placed in the right internal jugular vein and right common carotid artery, with the venous catheter advanced so that it rests in the right atrium. The arterial catheter is advanced to the entrance of the aortic arch.

  B. During an ECMO "run," the infant's blood must be heparinized to avoid clotting the circuit. Usually a loading dose of 100–150 units heparin/kg is required during the cannulation procedure, with a heparin drip of 20–70 units/kg/h.

  C. As bypass is achieved, ventilator settings are reduced to final settings: FIO_2, 0.21; ventilator rate, 10–15 breaths/min; pressure limit, 15 cm water and positive end-expiratory pressure (PEEP), 5 cm water. An average ECMO "run" is 5 days but may be as long as 14 days.

  D. Some ECMO centers are successfully re-anastomosing the carotid artery after the procedure, but long-term evaluation of these infants is just beginning.

V. Complications
  A. Infant
    1. Intracranial hemorrhage (incidence varies between 7 and 42%).
    2. Pulmonary hemorrhage.
    3. Nasal bleeding.
    4. Hypertension.
    5. GI hemorrhage.
    6. Cardiac arrhythmias.
    7. Electrolyte abnormalities.
    8. Hemolysis.
    9. Thrombocytopenia.
    10. Acute renal failure.
    11. Seizures.
  B. Mechanical
    1. Oxygenator failure.

TABLE 15–1. CONTRAINDICATIONS TO EXTRACORPOREAL MEMBRANE OXYGENATION (ECMO)

Contraindications	Reason
Gestational age < 35 weeks	Risk of intracranial hemorrhage
Birth weight < 2000 g	Surgical difficulties with vessel cannulation
Mechanical ventilation > 7–10 days	Irreversible lung disease likely
Intracranial hemorrhage > grade I	High risk of progression of hemorrhage
Coagulopathy	Higher risk of bleeding
Severe perinatal asphyxia with evidence of severe brain damage	Poor neurologic outcome
Severe congenital anomalies	Poor outcome despite ECMO
Cyanotic congenital heart disease without cardiopulmonary failure	Other interventions are indicated

2. Tubing rupture.
3. Pump failure.
4. Heat exchanger failure.
5. Air embolization.
6. Membrane lung failure.
7. Cannulation difficulties.

VI. Prognosis. The National Registry of Neonatal ECMO patients was established in 1985 and currently has over 2500 patients, the first of whom was treated in 1975. As of this writing (1990), overall survival is 82.7%. The registry also keeps track of survival rates for specific diseases, and these data are as follows. For meconium aspiration syndrome, the survival rate is 92%; for pulmonary hypertension, 86%; for hyaline membrane disease, 82%; for sepsis/pneumonia, 76%; and for congenital diaphragmatic hernia, 64%.

ECMO centers generally follow their surviving patients closely. Glass et al have published data on neurodevelopmental outcome to age 1 year for neonatal ECMO survivors at Children's Hospital and Medical Center, Washington, DC. So far, these children have done extraordinarily well, especially considering how sick they were prior to ECMO. Currently, the majority are normal, a few are borderline, and only 1 patient is seriously handicapped. Of course, more patients and longer follow-up are necessary before anyone can be reassured about this high-technology procedure.

REFERENCES

Glass P, Miller MK, Short B: Morbidity for survivors of extracorporeal membrane oxygenation: Neurodevelopmental outcome at 1 year of age. *Pediatrics* 1989;**83**:72.
Klein MD: Neonatal ECMO. *ASAIO Trans* 1988;**34(1)**:39.
Marsh TD, Wilkerson SA, Cook LN: Extracorporeal membrane oxygenation selection criteria: Partial pressure of arterial oxygen versus alveolar-arterial oxygen gradient. *Pediatrics* 1988;**82(2)**:162.
Neonatal ECMO Registry Report. October 1989.
Short BL, Miller MK, Anderson KD: Extracorporeal membrane oxygenation in the management of respiratory failure in the newborn. *Clin Perinatol* 1987;**14**:737.
Stolar CJ, Dillow PW: Extracorporeal membrane oxygenation for neonatal respiratory failure. *Surg Ann* 1987;**19**:111.
Toomasian JM et al: National experience with extracorporeal membrane oxygenation for newborn respiratory failure. Data from 715 cases. *ASAIO Trans* 1988;**34**:140.

16 Arterial Access

All procedures involving blood or secretions should be performed with gloves.

ARTERIAL PUNCTURE (RADIAL ARTERY PUNCTURE)

I. **Indications.** Arterial puncture is performed (1) to obtain blood for blood gas measurements or (2) when blood is needed and venous or capillary blood samples cannot be obtained.

II. **Equipment.** A 23- or 25-gauge scalp vein needle, a 1- or 3-mL syringe, povidone-iodine and alcohol swabs, a 4 × 4 gauze pad, gloves, and 1:1000 heparin solution are needed.

III. **Procedure**

A. Draw a small amount of heparin (concentration, 1:1000) into the syringe to be used for submitting the blood gas sample to the laboratory, and then discard the heparin. The small amount of heparin coating the syringe is sufficient to prevent coagulation of the sample. Excessive amounts of heparin may interfere with laboratory results, causing a falsely low pH and Pa_{CO_2}. If a routine chemistry is to be performed, do not use heparin.

B. The radial artery is the most frequently used puncture site and will be described here. An alternative site is the posterior tibial artery. Use of femoral arteries should be reserved for emergency situations. Brachial arteries should not be used, because there is minimal collateral circulation. There is also a risk of median nerve damage.

C. Check for collateral circulation and patency of the ulnar artery by means of the **Allen test.** First elevate the arm and simultaneously occlude the radial and ulnar arteries at the wrist, and then rub the palm to cause blanching. Release pressure on the ulnar artery. If normal color returns in the palm in less than 10 seconds, adequate collateral circulation from the ulnar artery is present. If normal color does not return for 15 seconds or longer or does not return at all, the collateral circulation is poor and it is best not to use the radial artery in this arm. The radial and ulnar arteries in the other arm should then be tested for collateral circulation.

D. To obtain the blood sample, take the patient's hand in your left hand (for a right-handed operator) and extend the wrist. Palpate the radial artery with the index finger of your left hand (Fig 16–1). Marking the puncture site with a fingernail imprint may be helpful.

E. Clean the puncture site first with a povidone-iodine swab and then with an alcohol swab.

F. Puncture the skin at about a 30-degree angle, and slowly advance the needle with the bevel up until blood appears in the tubing (Fig 16–1). With arterial blood samples, little aspiration is needed to fill the syringe.

G. Collect the amount of blood needed (the least amount necessary). The volume of blood taken should not exceed 3–5% of the total blood volume (the total blood volume in a neonate is approximately 80 mL/kg). Therefore, if 4 mL of blood is drawn from an infant weighing 1 kg, this represents 5% of the total blood volume.

FIGURE 16-1. Technique of arterial puncture in the neonate.

   H. Withdraw the needle and apply firm, but not occlusive, pressure to the site for at least 5 minutes with a 4 × 4 gauze pad to ensure adequate hemostasis.

   I. Before submitting an arterial blood gas sample, **expel air bubbles** from the sample and tightly cap the syringe. Failure to do this can lead to errors in testing. (See **IV.D,** below.)

   J. Place the syringe in ice and take it to the laboratory immediately. Note the collection time, the patient's temperature, and hemoglobin on the laboratory slip.

IV. Complications

   A. Hematoma. To minimize the risk of hematoma, use the smallest-gauge needle possible, and immediately after withdrawing the needle, apply pressure for approximately 5 minutes. Hematomas will usually resolve spontaneously.

   B. Arteriospasm, thrombosis, and embolism. These complications can be minimized by using the smallest-gauge needle possible. With thrombosis, the vessel will usually recanalize over a period of time. Arteriospasm will usually resolve spontaneously.

   C. Infection. The risk of infection is rare and can be minimized by using strict sterile technique. Infection is commonly caused by gram-positive organisms such as *Staphylococcus epidermis,* which should be treated with nafcillin or vancomycin and gentamicin (see Chap 76). Drug sensitivities at the specific hospital should be checked.

   D. Inaccuracy of blood gas results. Too much heparin in the syringe may result in a falsely low pH and $Paco_2$. Remove excess heparin before obtaining the blood sample. Air bubbles caused by failure to cap the syringe may falsely elevate the Pao_2 and falsely lower the $Paco_2$.

PERCUTANEOUS ARTERIAL CATHETERIZATION

  I. Indications

   A. When frequent arterial blood samples are required and an umbilical arterial catheter cannot be placed or has been removed because of complications, percutaneous arterial catheterization is required.

   B. This procedure is also indicated when intra-arterial blood pressure monitoring is required.

II. **Equipment.** Use a 22- or 24-gauge needle with a 1-inch catheter encasement (Jelco or Angiocath). A 24-gauge needle is recommended for infants weighing less than 1500 g. Also needed are an armboard (or 2 tongue blades taped together), adhesive tape, sterile drapes, povidone-iodine and alcohol swabs, gloves, antiseptic ointment, a needle holder, suture scissors, 4–0 or 5–0 silk sutures, normal saline or $\frac{1}{2}$ normal saline solution (latter preferred in premature infants to decrease incidence of hypernatremia) in a 1-mL or 3-mL syringe, heparinized saline solution (1 unit of heparin per milliliter of saline) in a pressure bag, and connecting tubing.

III. **Procedure.** Two methods are described here, both using the radial artery (the most commonly used site). An alternative site is the posterior tibial artery. Transillumination may be helpful in locating the artery in premature infants. Arterial catheterization requires a great deal of patience.

A. **Method 1**

1. Check for collateral circulation using the Allen test described previously (see p 131, **III.C**).
2. Place the infant's wrist on an armboard (some prefer to use an intravenous bag), and hyperextend the wrist by placing gauze underneath it. Tape the arm and hand securely to the board (Fig 16–2). Put on gloves, and place sterile drapes around the puncture site. Cleanse the site, first with povidone-iodine swabs and then with alcohol swabs.
3. Puncture both the anterior and posterior walls of the artery at a 30- to 45-degree angle. Remove the stylet. There should be little or no backflow of blood.
4. Pull the catheter back slowly until blood is seen; this signifies that the arterial lumen has been entered.
5. Advance the catheter after attaching the syringe and flush the catheter. Never use hypertonic solutions to flush an arterial line.
6. Secure the catheter with 4–0 or 5–0 silk sutures in 2 or 3 places. Occasionally, it is not possible to suture the catheter, and it should be securely taped instead.
7. Connect the tubing from the heparinized saline pressure bag to the catheter.
8. Place povidone-iodine ointment on the area where the catheter enters the skin, and cover the area with gauze taped securely in place.

FIGURE 16-2. When placing an indwelling arterial catheter, the wrist should be secured as shown. The catheter assembly is introduced at a 30- to 45-degree angle.

B. **Method 2 (alternative method)**
1. Perform steps 1 and 2 from method 1.
2. Puncture the anterior wall of the artery until blood return is seen. At this point, the catheter should be in the lumen of the artery.
3. Advance the catheter into the artery while simultaneously withdrawing the needle. The blood should be flowing freely from the catheter if the catheter is properly positioned.
4. Attach the syringe and flush the catheter.
5. Secure the line as in method 1.

IV. **Complications**
A. **Arteriospasms.** The risk of arteriospasm can be minimized by using the smallest-gauge catheter possible and performing as few punctures as possible. If arteriospasm occurs, the catheter must be removed until the spasm resolves.
B. **Embolism or thrombosis.** To prevent these complications, make certain that air is not introduced into the catheter and that the catheter is flushed with heparinized saline.
C. **Skin ischemia or gangrene.** Adequate collateral circulation decreases the risk of this complication. Always perform the Allen test to verify collateral flow (see p 131, **III.C**).
D. **Hematoma.** See p 132, **IV.A.**
E. **Blood loss.** Accidental loss of catheter position, resulting in hemorrhage, can occur.

UMBILICAL ARTERY CATHETERIZATION

I. **Indications**
A. Umbilical artery catheterization is indicated when frequent measurements of arterial blood gases are required.
B. This procedure is also used for continuous arterial blood pressure monitoring.
C. A third indication is to provide exchange transfusion.

II. **Equipment.** An umbilical artery catheterization tray usually includes sterile drapes, a tape measure, a needle holder, suture scissors, a hemostat, a forceps, and a blunt needle. Also needed are a 3-way stopcock, an umbilical artery catheter (3.5F for an infant weighing < 1.2 kg, 5F for an infant weighing > 1.2 kg), umbilical tape, silk tape (Dermicel), 000 silk sutures, a 4 × 4 gauze pad, antiseptic solution, gloves, mask and hat, a 10-mL syringe, normal saline, or $\frac{1}{2}$ normal saline solution, and a 22-gauge needle.

III. **Procedure**
A. Place the patient supine. Wrap a diaper around both legs and tape the diaper to the bed. This stabilizes the patient for the procedure and allows observation of the feet for vasospasm.
B. Put on sterile gloves, mask, hat, and a sterile gown.
C. Prepare the umbilical catheter tray by attaching the stopcock to the blunt needle and then attaching the catheter to the blunt needle. Fill the 10-mL syringe with flush solution, and inject through the catheter.
D. Clean the umbilical cord area with antiseptic solution. Place sterile drapes around the umbilicus, leaving the feet and head exposed. Observe the infant for vasospasm in the extremities or signs of distress during the procedure.
E. Tie a piece of umbilical tape around the base of the umbilical cord tightly enough to minimize blood loss but loosely enough so that the catheter can be passed easily through the vessel (snug but not tight). Cut off the excess umbilical cord with scissors or a scalpel, leaving a 1-cm stump. A scalpel usually makes a cleaner cut, so that the vessels are more easily seen. There are *usually* 2 umbilical arteries and one

umbilical vein. The arteries are smaller and are usually located at 4 and 7 o'clock. The vein usually has a floppy wall (Fig 16–3A and B).

F. Take the curved hemostat, and grasp the end of the umbilicus to hold it upright and steady.

G. Use the forceps to open and dilate the umbilical artery. First, place one arm of the forceps in the artery, and then use both arms to gently dilate the vessel (Fig 16–3C and D).

H. Once the artery is sufficiently dilated, insert the catheter.

I. Be certain you know the correct length of catheter to be inserted. The catheter is positioned in one of 2 ways. In so-called low catheterization, the tip of the catheter lies below the level of L3 or L4. In so-called high catheterization, the tip lies above the diaphragm at the level of T6 to T9. Positioning is usually determined by the routine at a given institution. The length of catheter needed can be obtained from the Umbilical Catheter Measurements graph in Appendix K. Another method for determining the length needed for low catheterization is to measure two-thirds of the distance from the umbilicus to the midportion of the clavicle.

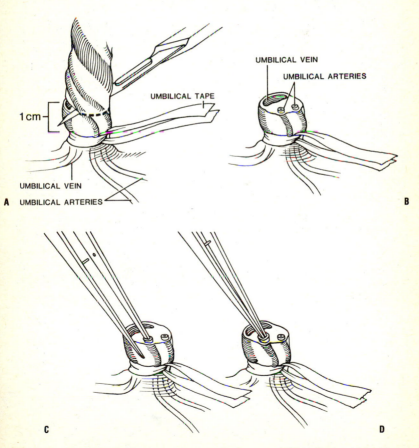

FIGURE 16–3. A: The umbilical cord should be amputated, leaving a 1-cm stump. **B:** Identification of the umbilical vessels. **C and D:** A forceps is used to gently dilate the umbilical artery.

FIGURE 16–4. The umbilical artery catheter is secured with silk tape, which is attached to the base of the umbilicus with 000 silk sutures.

FIGURE 16–5. Important landmarks, related vessels, and path of the umbilical artery. The internal iliac artery is also called the *hypogastric artery.*

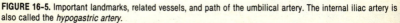

J. Once the catheter is in position, perform aspiration to verify blood return.

K. Secure the catheter as shown in Fig 16-4. The silk tape is folded over part way, the catheter is placed, and the remaining portion of the tape is folded over. Suture the silk tape to the skin at the base of the umbilicus as shown, using 000 silk sutures. Connect the tubing to the monitor and flush it. No special dressing is needed. The umbilical stump with the catheter in place is left open to the air.

L. Obtain an abdominal x-ray film to verify the position of a low catheter. To check the position of a high catheter, obtain a chest x-ray film. Fig 16-5 shows landmarks and the relationship of umbilical arteries to the other major abdominal arteries. X-ray films showing positioning can be found in Chapter 9 (Figs 9-7, 9-8).

IV. Complications

A. **Infection.** Infection can be prevented by using strict sterile technique. No attempt should be made to advance a catheter once it has been placed and sutured into position; instead, the catheter should be replaced.

B. **Vascular accidents.** Thrombosis or infarction may occur. Vasospasm may lead to loss of an extremity. Hypertension is a long-term complication caused by stenosis of the renal artery as a result of improper catheter placement near the renal arteries.

C. **Hemorrhage.** Hemorrhage may occur if the catheter becomes disconnected at one of the stopcocks. The stopcocks must be securely fastened. If hemorrhage occurs, blood volume replacement may be necessary.

D. **Vessel perforation.** The catheter should *never* be forced. If the catheter cannot be easily advanced, use of another vessel should be attempted. If perforation occurs, surgical intervention may be necessary.

17 Bladder Aspiration (Suprapubic Urine Collection)

I. **Indications.** Bladder aspiration is performed to obtain sterile urine for culture.

II. **Equipment.** Necessary equipment includes sterile gloves, povidone-iodine solution, a 23- or 25-gauge 1-inch needle with a 3-mL syringe attached, 4 × 4 gauze pads, gloves, and a sterile container.

III. **Procedure**

    A. Be certain that voiding has not occurred within the previous hour so that there will be enough urine in the bladder to make collection worthwhile.

    B. An assistant should hold the infant's legs in the frog-leg position.

    C. Locate the site of bladder puncture, which should be approximately 0.5 cm above the pubic symphysis, in the midline of the lower abdomen.

    D. Put on sterile gloves, and clean the skin at the puncture site with antiseptic solution.

PUBIC SYMPHYSIS

BLADDER

UTERUS

RECTUM

FIGURE 17-1. Technique of suprapubic bladder aspiration.

E. Palpate the pubic symphysis. Insert the needle approximately 0.5 cm above the pubic symphysis at a 90-degree angle (Fig 17–1).
F. Advance the needle, and perform aspiration while doing so. Do not advance the needle once urine is seen in the syringe. This precaution helps prevent perforation of the posterior wall of the bladder.
G. Withdraw the needle, and maintain pressure over the site of puncture.
H. Place a sterile cap on the syringe or transfer the specimen to a sterile urine cup, and submit the specimen to the laboratory.

IV. **Complications**
A. **Bleeding.** Microscopic hematuria may occur after bladder aspiration but is usually transient and rarely causes concern. Hemorrhage may occur if there is a bleeding disorder. The platelet count should be checked before aspiration is performed. If it is low, the procedure should not be performed.
B. **Infection.** Infection is not likely to occur if strict sterile technique is used.
C. **Perforation of bowel.** With careful identification of the landmarks described above, this complication is rare. If the bowel is perforated, close observation is recommended, and intravenous administration of antibiotics should be considered.

18 Bladder Catheterization

I. **Indications**
   A. Bladder catheterization is performed when a urine specimen is needed and a clean-catch specimen cannot be obtained or suprapubic aspiration cannot be performed.
   B. The procedure is performed to monitor urinary output, to relieve urinary retention, or to obtain a cystogram or voiding cystourethrogram.

II. **Equipment.** The procedure requires sterile gloves, cotton balls, povidone-iodine solution, sterile drapes, lubricant, a sterile collection bottle, and urethral catheters (3.5F umbilical artery catheter for infants weighing < 1000 g; 5F feeding catheter for infants weighing 1000–1800 g; 8F feeding tube for infants weighing > 1800 g).

III. **Procedure**
   A. **Males**
      1. Place the infant supine, with the thighs abducted (frog-leg position).
      2. Cleanse the penis with povidone-iodine solution, starting with the meatus and moving in a proximal direction.
      3. Put on sterile gloves, and drape the area with sterile towels.
      4. Place the tip of the catheter in sterile lubricant.
      5. Hold the penis approximately perpendicular to the body to straighten the penile urethra and help prevent false passage. Advance the catheter until urine appears. A slight resistance may be felt as the catheter passes the external sphincter, and steady, gentle pressure is usually needed to advance past this area. *Never force the catheter* (Fig 18–1).
      6. Collect the urine specimen. If the catheter is to remain in place, some feel it should be taped to the lower abdomen rather than to

FIGURE 18-1. Bladder catheterization in the male.

CLITORIS
URETHRA
VAGINA

ANUS

FIGURE 18-2. Landmarks used in catheterization of the bladder in females.

the leg in males to help decrease stricture formation caused by pressure on the posterior urethra.

B. Females
1. Place the infant supine, with the thighs abducted (frog-leg position).
2. Separate the labia, and cleanse the area around the meatus with povidone-iodine solution. Use anterior-to-posterior strokes to prevent fecal contamination (Fig 18–2).
3. Put on sterile gloves, and drape sterile towels around the labia.
4. Spread the labia with 2 fingers. Lubricate the catheter, and advance it until urine appears. Tape the catheter to the leg if it is to remain in position.

IV. Complications
A. **Infection.** Strict sterile technique is necessary to prevent infection. "In-and-out" catheterization carries a small risk of urinary tract infection. The longer a catheter is left in place, the greater the chance of infection.
B. **Trauma to the urethra ("false passage") or bladder.** Trauma to the urethra or bladder is more common in males. It can be prevented by adequately lubricating the catheter and stretching the penis to straighten the urethra. The catheter should never be forced if resistance is felt.
C. **Hematuria.** Hematuria is usually transient but may require irrigation with normal saline solution.
D. **Stricture.** Stricture is more common in males. It is usually caused by using a catheter that is too large or by prolonged or traumatic catheterization. In males, taping the catheter to the anterior abdominal wall will help decrease the pressure on the posterior urethra.

19 Chest Tube Placement

I. **Indications**

A. A chest tube may be inserted to treat tension pneumothorax causing respiratory compromise and decreased venous return to the heart, resulting in decreased cardiac output and hypotension.

B. A chest tube may be used to treat pneumothorax compromising ventilation and causing increased work of breathing, hypoxia, and increased $Paco_2$.

C. Use chest tubes in pleural effusion to obtain fluid for diagnosis or to drain fluid.

II. **Equipment.** A chest tube tray should consist of sterile towels, 4 × 4 sterile gauze pads, 000 silk suture thread, curved hemostats, a No. 15 or 11 scalpel, scissors, needle holder, antiseptic solution, antibiotic ointment, 1% lidocaine, 3-mL syringe, and 25-gauge needle. The chest tube should be a 10F catheter for infants weighing less than 2000 g and a 12F catheter for infants weighing more than 2000 g. Sterile gloves, mask, hat and gown, and a suction-drainage system (eg, Pleur-evac system) are also needed.

III. **Procedure**

A. The site of chest tube insertion is determined by examining the AP and cross-table lateral or lateral decubitus chest films. Air collects in the uppermost areas of the chest and fluid in the most dependent areas. For air collections, place the tube anteriorly. For fluid collections, place the tube posteriorly and laterally. **Transillumination** of the chest may help detect pneumothorax. With the lights in the room turned down, a strong light source is placed on the anterior chest wall above the nipple and in the axilla. The affected side will usually appear hyperlucent and will "light up" when compared to the unaffected side. Transillumination may not reveal a small pneumothorax. Unless the infant's status is rapidly deteriorating, a chest x-ray film should be obtained to confirm pneumothorax before the chest tube is inserted.

B. Position the patient so that the site of insertion is accessible. The most common position is supine, with the arm at a 90-degree angle on the affected side.

C. Select the appropriate site (Fig 19–1). For anterior placement, the site should be the second or third intercostal space at the midclavicular line. For posterior placement, use the fourth, fifth, or sixth intercostal space at the anterior axillary line. The nipple is a landmark for the fourth intercostal space.

D. Put on a sterile gown, mask, hat, and gloves. Cleanse the area of insertion with povidone-iodine solution, and then drape the area.

E. Infiltrate the area superficially with 0.5–1.0% lidocaine and then down to the rib. Infiltrate into the intercostal muscles and along the parietal pleura. Make a small incision (about 1.5 cm, or approximately the width of the tube) in the skin over the rib just below the intercostal space where the tube is to be inserted (Fig 19–2A).

F. Insert a closed, curved hemostat into the incision, and spread the tissues down to the rib. Using the tip of the hemostat, puncture the pleura just above the rib and spread gently. Remember that the intercostal nerves, arteries, and veins lie below the ribs (Fig 19–2A). This maneuver

FIGURE 19-1. Recommended sites for chest tube insertion in the neonate.

FIGURE 19-2. Procedures of chest tube insertion. A: Level of skin incision and thoracic wall entry site in relation to the rib and neurovascular bundle. B: Opened hemostat through which chest tube is inserted. C: Chest tube secured to skin with silk sutures.

helps create a subcutaneous tunnel that aids in closing the tract when the tube is removed.

G. When the pleura has been penetrated, a rush of air will often be heard.

H. Insert the chest tube through the opened hemostat (Fig 19–2B). Be certain that the side holes of the tube are within the pleural cavity. The presence of moisture in the tube usually confirms proper placement in the intrapleural cavity. Use of a trocar guide is usually unnecessary and may increase the risk of complications. The chest tube should be inserted 2–3 cm for a small preterm infant and 3–4 cm for a term infant. (These are guidelines only; the length of tube to be inserted will vary.) An alternative approach to tube insertion is to measure the length from the insertion site to the apex of the lung and tie a silk suture around the tube the same distance from the tip. Position the tube until the silk suture is just outside the skin.

I. Hold the tube steady first and then allow an assistant to connect the tube to a water-seal vacuum drainage system (eg, Pleur-evac system). Five to 10 cm of suction pressure is usually used. Start at the lower level of suction and increase as needed if the pneumothorax or effusion does not resolve. Systems such as the Pleur-evac provide continuous suction and water seal. Water seal prevents air from being drawn back into the pleural space.

J. Secure the chest tube with 000 silk sutures and silk tape (Fig 19–2C). Close the skin opening with sutures if necessary. Obtain a chest x-ray to verify placement and check for residual fluid or pneumothorax. Positioning of the tube must always be verified by a chest x-ray film.

IV. **Complications**

A. **Infection.** Strict sterile technique must be used to prevent infection. Many institutions recommend beginning prophylactic antibiotics (usually nafcillin, see p 500) when a chest tube is inserted. The use of antibiotics and duration of treatment remains *controversial.*

B. **Bleeding.** Bleeding may occur if one of the major vessels (intercostal, axillary, pulmonary, or mammary) is perforated during the procedure. This complication can be avoided if landmarks are properly identified. Bleeding is less likely to occur if a trocar is *not* used. Bleeding may stop during suctioning. If it continues, immediate surgical consultation is usually necessary.

C. **Nerve damage.** Passing the tube over the top of the rib will help avoid injury to the intercostal nerve running under the rib.

D. **Lung trauma.** Never force the tube into the pleural cavity.

20 Endotracheal Intubation

I. **Indications.** Endotracheal intubation is performed to provide mechanical respiratory support, to obtain aspirates for culture, to provide pulmonary toilet, to alleviate subglottic stenosis, or to clear the trachea of meconium.

II. **Equipment.** Choose the correct tube, using the guidelines in Table 20-1. Also needed are a pediatric laryngoscope handle with blade (No. 0 blade for infants weighing < 3000 g. No. 1 Miller blade for infants weighing > 3000 g), a bag-and-mask apparatus, an adapter, an oxygen source with tubing, a suction apparatus, tape, scissors, a stylet (*optional*), gloves, and tincture of benzoin.

III. **Procedure**
   A. The endotracheal tube should be precut to eliminate some dead space. Some newer tubes are marked "oral" or "nasal" and should be cut appropriately.
   B. Be certain that the light source on the laryngoscope is working before beginning the procedure. A bag-and-mask apparatus with 100% oxygen should be available at the bedside. Place the stylet (if used) in the endotracheal tube. (Flexible stylets are optional but may help guide the tube into position more efficiently.)
   C. Place the infant in the "sniffing position" (the neck is slightly extended). Hyperextension of the neck in infants may cause the trachea to collapse.
   D. Suction the trachea as needed to clear the oropharynx and make the landmarks clearly visible.
   E. Monitor the infant's heart rate and color.
   F. Hold the laryngoscope with the left hand. Insert the scope into the right side of the mouth, and sweep the tongue to the left side.
   G. Advance the blade a few millimeters, passing it beneath the epiglottis.
   H. Lift the blade vertically to elevate the epiglottis and visualize the glottis (Fig 20-1). Remember, the purpose of the laryngoscope is to vertically lift the epiglottis, not to pry it open.
   I. To better visualize the vocal cords, gentle external pressure can be placed on the thyroid cartilage by an assistant.
   J. Pass the endotracheal tube along the right side of the mouth and down past the vocal cords during inspiration. It is best to advance the tube *only* 2-2.5 cm into the trachea to avoid placement in the right main-

TABLE 20-1. RECOMMENDED SIZE OF ENDOTRACHEAL TUBE BASED ON INFANT'S WEIGHT OR GESTATIONAL AGE*

Tube Size (ID mm)	Weight	Gestational Age
2.5	Below 1000 g	Below 28 weeks
3.0	1000–2000 g	28–34 weeks
3.5	2000–3000 g	34–38 weeks
4.0	Above 3000 g	Above 38 weeks

*Based on recommendations by the American Heart Association and American Academy of Pediatrics.
Reproduced, with permission, from *Textbook of Neonatal Resuscitation*, 1987. Copyright American Heart Association.

FIGURE 20-1. Endotracheal intubation in the neonate.

stem bronchus. It may be helpful to tape the tube at the lip when the tube has been advanced 7 cm in a 1-kg infant, 8 cm in a 2-kg infant, or 9 cm in a 3-kg infant. The stylet should be gently removed while the tube is held in position.

K. Confirm the positioning of the tube. The resuscitation bag is attached to the tube, and an assistant provides mechanical breaths while the physician listens for equal breath sounds on both sides of the chest. Auscultate the stomach to be certain that the esophagus was not inadvertently entered.

L. Paint the skin with tincture of benzoin. Tape the tube securely in place.

M. Obtain a chest x-ray film to confirm proper placement of the tube.

IV. Complications

A. Tracheal perforation. Tracheal perforation is a rare complication requiring surgical intervention. It can be prevented by careful use of the laryngoscope and endotracheal tube.

B. Esophageal perforation. Esophageal perforation is usually caused by traumatic intubation. Treatment depends on the degree of perforation. Most injuries can be managed by use of parenteral nutrition until the leak seals, use of broad-spectrum antibiotics, and observation for signs of infection. A barium swallow contrast study may be necessary after several weeks to evaluate healing or rule out stricture formation.

C. Laryngeal edema. Laryngeal edema is usually seen after extubation and may cause respiratory distress. To prevent this, a short course of steroids (eg, dexamethasone) can be given intravenously before and just after extubation.

D. Palatal grooves. Palatal grooves are usually seen in cases of long-term intubation and will resolve with time.

E. Subglottic stenosis. Subglottic stenosis is most often associated with long-term endotracheal intubation (> 3–4 weeks). Surgical correction is usually necessary.

21 Exchange Transfusion

Four types of exchange transfusion are used: (1) simple volumetric 2-volume exchange, (2) isovolumetric 2-volume exchange, (3) partial simple exchange (< 2 volumes) with packed red blood cells or fresh frozen plasma, and (4) isovolumetric partial exchange. These procedures are used primarily in sick newborn infants but may also be used for intrauterine exchanges in fetuses at high risk for central nervous system toxicity (eg, erythroblastosis fetalis) by percutaneous umbilical blood sampling (PUBS) and umbilical vein catheterization under ultrasound guidance.

I. **Indications**

A. **Hyperbilirubinemia.** Exchange transfusions are used in infants with hyperbilirubinemia of any origin when the serum bilirubin level may reach or reaches a level that puts the infant at risk for central nervous system toxicity (eg, kernicterus) if left untreated (see Appendix F). Two-volume exchanges are recommended. A simple volumetric 2-volume exchange may be used if vascular access is difficult, but it tends to take longer to complete in these at-risk infants. Efficiency of bilirubin removal is increased in slower exchanges because of extravascular and intravascular bilirubin equilibration.

B. **Hemolytic disease of the newborn** results from destruction of fetal red blood cells (RBCs) by passively acquired maternal antibodies. Exchange transfusion aids in removing antibody-coated RBCs, thereby prolonging intravascular RBC survival. It also removes potentially toxic bilirubin from an increased bilirubin load resulting from RBC breakdown, and provides plasma volume and albumin for bilirubin binding. Two-volume exchanges are recommended when RBC destruction is rapid.

C. **Sepsis.** Neonatal sepsis may be associated with shock caused by bacterial endotoxins. A 2-volume exchange may help remove bacteria, toxins, abnormal fibrin split products, and acids. It may provide immunoglobulins, complement and coagulating factors, endotoxin inhibitors, and adult white blood cells.

D. **Disseminated intravascular coagulation (DIC)** from multiple causes. A 2-volume exchange transfusion is preferred, but depending on the sick infant's condition, any one of the exchange methods may help provide necessary coagulation factors and may help reduce the underlying etiology for the abnormal coagulation. Repletion of clotting factors by transfusion of fresh frozen plasma (10–15 mL/kg) may be all that is necessary in less severe cases of DIC.

E. **Metabolic disorders causing severe acidosis** (eg, aminoaciduria with associated hyperammonemia). Simple partial exchanges are usually acceptable. Peritoneal dialysis may also be useful for treating some progressive metabolic disorders.

F. **Severe fluid or electrolyte imbalance** (eg, hyperkalemia, hypernatremia, fluid overload). Isovolumetric partial exchanges are recommended to prevent large electrolyte fluctuations with each aliquot of volume. Exchanges with blood products may bind calcium; therefore, calcium gluconate should be handy. Fresh blood products should be used to prevent contribution of the by-products of older blood.

G. **Polycythemia.** It is usually best to give a partial exchange transfusion using a plasma protein fraction (eg, Plasmanate). Isotonic normal saline may also be used.

H. Severe anemia (normovolemic or hypervolemic) causing cardiac failure, as in hydrops fetalis, is best treated with a partial exchange transfusion using packed red blood cells.

I. Any disorder requiring complement, opsonins, or gamma globulin. These infants may require frequent exchanges, and their fluid status must be carefully managed. Partial exchanges are recommended.

II. Equipment

A. Radiant warmer.

B. Equipment for respiratory support and resuscitation (eg, oxygen, suctioning device). This equipment and medications used in resuscitation should be immediately available.

C. Equipment for monitoring the heart rate, blood pressure, respiratory rate, temperature, Pao_2, $Paco_2$, and Sao_2.

D. Equipment for umbilical artery and umbilical vein catheterization (see Chaps 16 and 27).

E. Disposable exchange transfusion tray.

F. Nasogastric tube for evacuating the stomach before beginning the transfusion.

G. A controlled water bath for warming the blood. The bath should have an internal disposable coil and connectors to the donor blood bag and the exchange transfusion circuit. The blood should be warmed to a temperature of 37 °C. Use of makeshift water baths or heaters is not advised, because blood that is too warm may cause hemolysis.

H. An assistant to help maintain a sterile field, monitor and assess the infant, and record the procedure and exchanged volumes.

III. Blood transfusion

A. Blood collection

1. **Homologous blood.** Blood donated by an anonymous donor with a compatible blood type is most commonly used. Donor-directed blood (blood donated by a selected blood type compatible person) is another option.

2. **CMV-negative blood** is recommended, and blood should be freshly washed to remove accumulated metabolites and acids.

B. Blood typing and cross-matching

1. **Infants with Rh incompatibility.** The blood must be type O, Rh negative, low titer anti-A, anti-B blood. It must be cross-matched with the mother's plasma and red blood cells.

2. **Infants with ABO incompatibility.** The blood must be type O, Rh compatible (with the mother and the infant) or Rh negative, low titer anti-A, anti-B blood. It must be cross-matched with the infant's and with the mother's blood.

3. **Other blood group incompatibilities.** In other hemolytic diseases (eg, anti-Rh-c, anti-Kell, anti-Duffy), the blood should be cross-matched to the mother's blood, and the offending antigen should be excluded.

4. **Hyperbilirubinemia, metabolic imbalance, or hemolysis not caused by isoimmune disorders.** The blood must be cross-matched against the infant's plasma and red blood cells.

C. Freshness and preservation of blood.
In newborn infants, it is preferable to use blood or plasma that has been collected in citrate-phosphate-dextrose (CPD). The blood should be less than 72 hours old. These 2 factors will ensure that the blood pH is above 7.0. For disorders associated with hydrops fetalis or fetal asphyxia, it is best to use blood that is less than 24 hours old. In hydrops fetalis, the pH of the donor blood should be determined; if it is less than 7.25, consider buffering

the blood with tromethamine (THAM), 10 mL of molar solution per 500 mL of blood.

D. **Hematocrit.** Most blood banks can reconstitute a unit of blood to a desired hematocrit (Hct) of 50–70%. The blood should be agitated periodically during the transfusion to maintain an even hematocrit.

E. **Potassium levels in donor blood.** Potassium levels in the donor blood should be determined if the infant is asphyxiated or in shock and renal impairment is suspected. If potassium levels are higher than 7 meq/L, consider using a unit of blood that has been collected more recently or a unit of washed red blood cells.

F. **Temperature of the blood.** Warming of blood is especially important in low birth weight and sick newborn infants.

IV. **Plasma transfusions.** Plasma is used in partial exchange transfusions. It should be typed and cross-matched with the infant's plasma. Plasma should be fresh-frozen. A plasma protein fraction (such as Plasmanate) is recommended because it will not carry the HIV virus. Normal saline may also be used successfully.

V. **Procedure**

A. **Simple 2-volume exchange transfusion is used for uncomplicated hyperbilirubinemia**

1. The normal blood volume in a full-term newborn infant is 80 mL/kg. In an infant weighing 2 kg, the volume would be 160 mL. Twice this volume of blood is exchanged in a 2-volume transfusion. Therefore, the amount of blood needed for a 2-kg infant would be 320 mL. Low birth weight and the blood volume of extremely premature newborns (may be up to 95 mL/kg) should be taken into account when calculating exchange volumes.

2. Allow adequate time for **blood typing** and **cross-matching** at the blood bank. The infant's bilirubin level will increase during this time, and this increase must be taken into account when ordering the blood.

3. Perform the transfusion in an **intensive care setting.** Place the infant in the supine position. Restraints must be snug but not tight. A nasogastric tube should be passed to **evacuate the stomach** and should be left in place to maintain gastric decompression and prevent regurgitation and aspiration of gastric juices.

4. Scrub and put on a sterile gown and gloves.

5. Perform **umbilical vein catheterization.**

6. Have the unit of blood prepared.
   a. Check the **blood types** of the donor and the infant.
   b. Check the **temperature** of the blood and warming procedures.
   c. Check the **hematocrit.** The blood should be agitated regularly to maintain a constant hematocrit.

7. Attach the bag of blood to the tubing and stopcocks according to the directions on the transfusion tray. The orientation of the stopcocks for infusion and withdrawal must be double-checked by the assistant.

8. Establish the volume of each aliquot (Table 21–1).

TABLE 21–1. ALIQUOTS USUALLY USED IN NEONATAL EXCHANGE TRANSFUSION

Infant Weight	Aliquot (mL)
More than 3 kg	20
2–3 kg	15
1–2 kg	10
850 g–1 kg	5
Less than 850 g	1–3

B. Isovolumetric 2-volume exchange transfusion. Isovolumetric 2-volume exchange transfusion is performed using a double setup, with infusion via the umbilical vein and withdrawal via the umbilical artery. This method is preferred when volume shifts during simple exchange might cause or aggravate myocardial insufficiency (eg, hydrops fetalis). Two operators are usually needed—one to perform the infusion and one the withdrawal.

1. Perform **steps 1–6** as in simple 2-volume exchange transfusion. In addition, perform umbilical artery catheterization.
2. Attach the unit of blood to the tubing and stopcocks attached to the umbilical vein catheter. If the catheter is to be left in place after the exchange transfusion (usually, to monitor central venous pressure), it should be placed above the diaphragm, with placement confirmed by chest x-ray film.
3. The tubing and the stopcocks of the second setup are attached to the umbilical artery catheter and to a sterile plastic bag for discarding the exchanged blood.
4. If isovolumetric exchange is being performed because of cardiac failure, the central venous pressure can be determined via the umbilical vein catheter; it should be placed above the diaphragm, in the inferior vena cava.

C. Simple partial exchange transfusion. Simple partial exchange transfusion is performed in the same manner as simple 2-volume exchange transfusion. It is used for polycythemia.

$$\text{Volume of exchange (mL)} = \frac{\text{Estimated blood volume (mL)} \times \text{Weight (kg)} \times (\text{Observed Hct} - \text{Desired Hct})}{\text{Observed Hct}}$$

D. Isovolumetric partial exchange transfusion with packed red blood cells is the best procedure in cases of severe hydrops fetalis.

E. Ancillary procedures

1. **Laboratory studies.** Blood should be obtained for laboratory studies before and after exchange transfusion.
   a. **Blood chemistry studies** include total calcium, sodium, potassium, chloride, pH, $Paco_2$, acid-base status, bicarbonate, and serum glucose.
   b. **Hematologic studies** include hemoglobin, hematocrit, platelet count, white blood cell count, and differential count. Blood for retyping and cross-matching following exchange is often requested by the blood bank to verify typing and re-cross-matching, and for study of transfusion reaction, if needed.
   c. **Blood culture** is recommended following exchange transfusion (*controversial*).
2. **Administration of calcium gluconate.** The citrate buffer binds calcium and transiently lowers ionized calcium levels. Treatment of suspected hypocalcemia in patients receiving transfusions is controversial. Some physicians routinely administer 1–2 mL of calcium gluconate 10% by slow infusion after each 100 mL of exchanged blood donor blood. Others maintain that this treatment has no therapeutic effect unless hypocalcemia is documented by ECG showing a change in the QT interval.
3. **Phototherapy.** Begin or resume phototherapy following exchange transfusion for disorders involving a high bilirubin level.
4. **Monitoring of serum bilirubin levels.** Continue to monitor serum bilirubin levels following transfusion at 2, 4, and 6 hours and then at 6-hour intervals. A rebound of bilirubin levels is to be expected 2–4 hours after the transfusion.

5. **Remedication.** Patients receiving antibiotics or anticonvulsants will need to be remedicated. Unless the cardiac status is deteriorating or serum digoxin levels are too low, patients receiving digoxin should *not* be remedicated.

6. **Antibiotic prophylaxis** following the transfusion should be considered on an individual basis. Infection is uncommon but is the most frequent complication.

VI. Complications

A. **Infection.** Bacteremia (usually due to a *Staphylococcus* organism), hepatitis, cytomegalovirus infection, malaria, and acquired immune deficiency syndrome (AIDS) have been reported.

B. **Vascular complications.** Clot or air embolism, arteriospasm of the lower limbs, thrombosis, and infarction of major organs may occur.

C. **Coagulopathies.** Coagulopathies may be due to thrombocytopenia or diminished coagulation factors. Platelets may decrease by more than 50% after a double-volume exchange transfusion.

D. **Electrolyte abnormalities.** Hyperkalemia and hypocalcemia can occur.

E. **Hypoglycemia.** Hypoglycemia is especially likely in infants of diabetic mothers and those with erythroblastosis fetalis.

F. **Metabolic acidosis.** Metabolic acidosis from stored donor blood (due to the acid load) occurs less often in citrate-phosphate-dextrose (CPD) blood.

G. **Metabolic alkalosis.** Metabolic alkalosis may occur because of delayed clearing of citrate preservative from the donated blood by the liver.

H. **Necrotizing enterocolitis.** An increased incidence of necrotizing enterocolitis following exchange transfusion has been suggested. For this reason, the umbilical vein catheter should be removed immediately if central venous pressure monitoring is not required. Also, feedings should be delayed for at least 24 hours to observe the infant for ileus.

22 Gastric Intubation

I. **Indications**
   A. **Enteric feeding.** Gastric intubation is needed for enteric feeding in the following situations.
      1. **High respiratory rate.** At some institutions, the infant is given enteric feedings if the respiratory rate is greater than 60 breaths/min in order to decrease the risk of aspiration pneumonia.
      2. **Neurologic disease.** If neurologic disease impairs the sucking reflex or ability to feed, enteric feeding is needed.
      3. **Premature infants.** Many premature infants tire before they can take in enough calories with normal feeding to maintain growth.
   B. **Gastric decompression.** Gastric decompression may be required in infants with necrotizing enterocolitis, bowel obstruction, or ileus.
II. **Equipment.** Necessary equipment includes a 5F or 8F infant feeding tube, a stethoscope, sterile water (to lubricate the tube), a syringe (5–10 mL), $\frac{1}{2}$-inch adhesive tape, gloves, and suctioning equipment.
III. **Procedure**
   A. Monitor the patient's heart rate and respiratory function throughout this procedure.
   B. Place the infant in the supine position, with the head of the bed elevated.
   C. The length of tubing needed is determined by measuring the distance from the nose to the xiphoid process. Mark the length on the tube.
   D. Moisten the end of the tube with sterile water.
   E. **Insertion**
      1. **Nasal insertion.** Flex the neck, push the nose up, and insert the tube, directing it straight back. Advance the tube the desired distance.
      2. **Oral insertion.** Push the tongue down with a tongue depressor and pass the tube into the oropharynx. Advance the tube slowly the desired distance.
   F. Continue to observe the infant for respiratory distress or bradycardia.
   G. Determine the location of the tube. One method is to inject air into the tube with a syringe and listen for a rush of air in the stomach. If the location is uncertain, obtain an x-ray film.
   H. Aspirate the gastric contents.
   I. Secure the tube to the face with $\frac{1}{2}$-inch tape.
IV. **Complications**
   A. **Apnea and bradycardia.** Apnea and bradycardia are usually mediated by a vagal response and will usually resolve without specific treatment.
   B. **Perforation of the esophagus, posterior pharynx, stomach, or duodenum.** The tube should never be forced during insertion.
   C. **Hypoxia.** Always have bag-and-mask ventilation with 100% oxygen available to treat this problem.
   D. **Aspiration.** Aspiration can occur if feeding has been initiated in a tube that is accidentally inserted into the lung.

23 Heelstick (Capillary Blood Sampling)

I. Indications
A. Heelstick is performed to collect blood samples when only a small amount of blood is needed or when there is difficulty in obtaining samples by venipuncture.

B. Heelstick may be performed to obtain a capillary blood gas sample.

II. Equipment.
A lancet is used to perform the procedure. A 2-mm lancet can be used if the infant weighs less than 1500 g or if only a small amount of blood is needed. A 4-mm lancet is used if the infant is larger or if more blood is required. Also needed are alcohol swabs, 4 × 4 sterile gauze pads, a capillary tube (for hematocrit and bilirubin tests) or a caraway tube (if more blood is needed [eg, for blood chemistry determinations]), clay to seal the end of the tube, a warm washcloth, gloves, and a diaper.

III. Procedure
A. Wrap the foot in a warm washcloth and then a diaper for 5–10 minutes. Although this is not mandatory, it will produce hyperemia, which increases vascularity, making blood collection easier.

B. Choose the area of puncture (Fig 23–1). Do not use the center of the heel, because there is an increased incidence of osteomyelitis if this area is used.

C. Wipe the area with an alcohol swab, and let it dry. If the area is wet with alcohol, hemolysis may occur, altering the results of blood testing.

D. Encircle the heel with the palm of the hand and the index finger (Fig 23–1).

E. Make a quick, deep puncture with a lancet. Wipe off the first drop of blood. Gently squeeze the heel, and place the collection tube at the site of the puncture. The tube should automatically fill by capillary action. It may be necessary to gently "pump" the heel to continue the blood

FIGURE 23–1. Use the shaded area when performing a heelstick in an infant.

flow. Allow enough time for capillary refill of the heel. Seal the end of the tube with clay.

F. Maintain pressure on the puncture site with a dry sterile gauze pad until the bleeding stops. A 4 × 4 gauze pad can be wrapped around the heel and left on to provide hemostasis.

IV. **Complications**

A. **Cellulitis.** Cellulitis may occur if sterile technique is not properly followed. A culture of tissue from the affected area should be obtained, and use of broad-spectrum antibiotics should be considered.

B. **Osteomyelitis.** This complication usually occurs in the calcaneus bone. Avoid the center area of the heel and do not make the puncture opening too deep. If osteomyelitis occurs, tissue should be obtained for culture and broad-spectrum antibiotics started until a specific organism is identified. Consultation with specialists in infectious disease and orthopedics is usually obtained.

C. **Scarring of the heel.** Scarring occurs when there have been multiple punctures in the same area. It is best to avoid another heelstick in this situation and use another technique of blood collection such as central venous sampling.

D. **Pain.** Pain caused by routine heelsticks in premature infants can cause marked declines in hemoglobin oxygen saturation as measured by pulse oximetry. Some institutions advocate topical lidocaine (0.5–1.0%) prior to the procedure.

24 Lumbar Puncture (Spinal Tap)

I. Indications
  A. To obtain cerebrospinal fluid (CSF) for the diagnosis of central nervous system disorders such as meningitis or subarachnoid hemorrhage.
  B. To drain cerebrospinal fluid in communicating hydrocephalus.
  C. To give intrathecal medications.
II. Materials required. Lumbar puncture kit (usually contains 3 sterile specimen tubes, sterile drapes, sterile gauze, 22-gauge 1-inch spinal needle with stylet, 1% lidocaine), gloves, povidone-iodine solution, 1-mL syringe.
III. Procedure. (Normal CSF values are listed in Appendix D.)
  A. An assistant restrains the infant in a sitting or lateral decubitus position. The position to use depends on personal preference. Obviously an intubated, critically ill infant must be treated in the lateral decubitus position. Some clinicians feel that if CSF cannot be obtained in the lateral decubitis position, the sitting position should be used. In the lateral decubitus position, the head and legs must be flexed (knee-chest position). Make sure airway patency is maintained.
  B. Once the infant is in position, check for landmarks (Fig 24–1). Palpate the iliac crest and slide your finger down to the L4 vertebral body. Then use the L4–L5 interspace as the site of the lumbar puncture. It is sometimes easier to make a nail imprint at the exact location to mark the site.
  C. Prepare the materials (open sterile containers, pour antiseptic [Betadine solution] solution into the well located in the plastic lumbar puncture kit).
  D. Put gloves on.
  E. Clean the lumbar area with antiseptic solution, starting at the interspace selected. Prep in a widening circle from that interspace up and over the iliac crest.
  F. Drape the area with one towel under the infant and one towel covering everything but the selected interspace.
  G. Palpate again to find the selected interspace. At this time, 0.1–0.2 mL of 1% lidocaine can be injected subcutaneously for pain relief (*optional*).
  H. Insert the needle in the midline with steady force aimed toward the umbilicus.
  I. Advance the needle slowly and then remove the stylet to check for appearance of fluid. One usually does not feel a "pop" as the ligamentum flavum and dura are penetrated, as is the case with older children and adults. It is therefore necessary to remove the stylet frequently to keep from going too far and getting a bloody specimen.
  J. Collect about 1 mL of CSF in each of the 3 sterile specimen tubes by allowing the fluid to drip into the tubes.
  K. Replace the stylet and withdraw the needle.
  L. Maintain pressure on the area, and clean off the antiseptic solution.
  M. For routine CSF examination, send 3 tubes of CSF to the laboratory.

  Tube 1: For Gram stain, culture, and sensitivity testing.
  Tube 2: For glucose and protein levels.
  Tube 3: For cell count and differential.

FIGURE 24-1. Positioning and landmarks used for lumbar puncture. The iliac crest (dotted line) marks the approximate level of L4.

    N. If a bloody specimen is obtained in the first tube, observe for clearing in the second and third tubes.
      1. If bleeding clears, the tap was traumatic.
      2. If blood does not clear but forms clots, a blood vessel has probably been punctured. Since CSF has not been obtained, a repeat tap must be done.
      3. If blood does not clear and does not clot, the infant probably has had intraventricular bleeding.
IV. Complications
    A. Infection. If sterile technique is not used, bacteria may be introduced into the CSF and cause infection. Bacteremia may result if a blood vessel is punctured after the needle has passed through contaminated CSF.
    B. Intraspinal epidermoid tumor. This tumor occurs as a result of performing a lumbar puncture with a needle that does not have a stylet.
    C. Herniation of cerebral tissue through the foramen magnum. This is not a common problem in neonatal intensive care units because of the open fontanelle in infants.
    D. Spinal cord and nerve damage. To avoid this complication, it is best to use only interspaces below L4.
    E. Apnea and bradycardia sometimes occur from respiratory compromise caused by the infant being held too tightly during the procedure.

25 Abdominal Paracentesis

I. Indications
A. To obtain peritoneal fluid for diagnostic tests to determine the cause of ascites.

B. For therapeutic reasons such as removal of peritoneal fluid to aid in ventilation.

II. Materials required.
Sterile drapes, sterile gloves, povidone-iodine solution, sterile gauze pads, sterile tubes for fluid, 10-mL syringe, 22- or 24-gauge catheter-over-needle assembly. The smaller (24-gauge) needle is for infants less than 2000 g, the larger for infants weighing more than 2000 g.

III. Procedure
A. The infant should be supine with both legs restrained. To restrict all movements of the legs, a diaper can be wrapped around the legs and secured in place.

B. Choose the site for paracentesis. The area between the umbilicus and the pubic bone is not generally used in neonates because of the danger of perforating the bladder or bowel wall. The sites most frequently used are the right and left flanks. A good rule is to draw a horizontal line passing through the umbilicus and select a site between this line and the inguinal ligament (Fig 25–1).

C. Prepare the area with povidone-iodine in a circular fashion, starting at the puncture site.

D. Put on sterile gloves, and drape the area.

E. Insert the needle at the selected site. A "Z-track" technique is usually used to prevent persistent leakage of fluid after the tap. Insert the needle perpendicular to the skin. When the needle is just under the skin, move it 0.5 cm before puncturing the abdominal wall.

F. Advance the needle, aspirating until fluid appears in the barrel of the syringe. Then remove the needle, and aspirate the contents *slowly* with the catheter. It may be necessary to reposition the catheter to obtain an adequate amount of fluid. Once the necessary amount of fluid is taken (usually 3–5 mL for specific tests, or enough to aid ventilation), remove the catheter.

G. Cover with a sterile gauze pad until leakage has stopped.

IV. Complications
A. Hypotension. Hypotension is caused by removing too much fluid or removing fluid too rapidly. To minimize this possibility, take only the amount needed for studies or what is needed to improve ventilation. *Always* remove fluid slowly.

B. Infection. The risk of peritonitis is minimized by using strict sterile technique.

C. Perforation of the intestine. To help prevent perforation, use the shortest needle possible and take careful note of landmarks (see **III.B,** p 157). If perforation occurs, broad-spectrum antibiotics may be indicated with close observation for signs of infection.

D. Perforation of the bladder. Perforation of the bladder is normally self-limited and requires no specific treatment.

E. Persistent fluid leak. The "Z-track" technique, as described above in **III.E,** usually prevents the problem of persistent leakage of fluid. Persistent fluid leaks may have to be bagged to quantify the volume of drainage.

FIGURE 25-1. Recommended sites for abdominal paracentesis.

26 Pericardiocentesis

I. Indications

A. To remove air from the pericardial sac in infants with pneumopericardium and associated cardiac tamponade.

B. To obtain pericardial fluid for diagnostic studies in infants with pericardial effusion.

C. To remove pericardial fluid for the treatment of pericardial effusion with associated cardiac tamponade.

II. Materials required.
Povidone-iodine solution, sterile gloves and gown, 22- or 24-gauge 1-inch catheter-over-needle assembly, sterile drapes, 10-mL syringe, connecting tube, and underwater seal for use if the catheter is to be left indwelling.

III. Procedure

A. Prepare the area (xiphoid and precordium) with antiseptic solution. Put on sterile gloves and gown.

B. Drape the area, leaving the xiphoid and a 2-cm circular area around it exposed.

C. Prepare the needle by attaching the syringe to it. If you want to leave an indwelling catheter, a 3-way stopcock and tubing should be attached to the needle in addition to the syringe.

D. Identify the area where the needle is to be inserted. The area most commonly used is approximately 0.5 cm to the left of and just below the infant's xiphoid (Fig 26–1).

E. Insert the needle at about a 30-degree angle, aiming toward the midclavicular line on the left (Fig 26–1).

F. Apply constant suction on the syringe while advancing the needle.

FIGURE 26–1. Recommended sites for pericardiocentesis.

G. Once air or fluid is obtained (depending on which is to be evacuated), remove the needle from the catheter. Withdraw the necessary amount of air or fluid, ie, enough to relieve symptoms or obtain sufficient fluid for laboratory studies.

H. If an indwelling catheter is to be left in place, secure it with tape and attach the tubing to continuous suction.

I. Obtain a chest x-ray film to confirm the position of the catheter and the effectiveness of drainage.

IV. Complications

A. **Puncturing the heart.** Avoid this complication by advancing the needle only far enough to obtain fluid or air. Another technique to avoid puncturing the heart is to attach the ECG anterior chest lead to the needle with an alligator clip. If changes are seen on the ECG (eg, ectopic beats, changes in the ST segment, or increase in the QRS voltage), the needle has contacted the myocardium and should be withdrawn. Avoid leaving a metal needle indwelling for continuous drainage.

B. **Pneumothorax or hemothorax.** This can occur if landmarks are not used and "blind" punctures are done. If this complication has occurred, a chest tube on the affected side is usually needed.

C. **Infection.** Strict sterile technique must be followed to avoid infection.

27 Venous Access

PERCUTANEOUS VENOUS CATHETERIZATION

I. **Indications**
   A. To administer intravenous medications and fluids.
   B. To give intravenous fluids when patient is NPO.
   C. to administer parenteral nutrition.

II. **Materials required.** Arm board, adhesive tape, tourniquet, alcohol swabs, normal saline for flush ($\frac{1}{2}$ normal saline preferred if concerned about hypernatremia), povidone-iodine ointment, needle (23- or 25-gauge scalp vein needle or 22- to 24-gauge catheter-over-needle [Angiocath]).

III. **Procedure**
   A. **Scalp vein needle**
      1. **Select the vein to use.** The following can be used in the neonate (Fig 27–1). It is useful to select the "Y" region of the vein, where 2 veins join together. The needle can be inserted in the crotch of the veins.
         a. **Scalp.** Supratrochlear, superficial temporal, or posterior auricular vein.
         b. **Back of hand.** Dorsal arch vein.
         c. **Forearm.** Median antebrachial or accessory cephalic vein.
         d. **Foot.** Dorsal arch vein.
         e. **Antecubital fossa.** Basilic or cubital vein.
         f. **Ankle.** Greater saphenous vein.
      2. **Shave the area if a scalp vein is to be used.**
      3. **Restrain the extremity** on an armboard or have an assistant help hold the extremity or the head.
      4. **Apply a tourniquet** proximal to the puncture site. If a scalp vein is to be used, a rubber band can be placed around the head, just above the eyebrows.
      5. **Clean the area with alcohol swabs.**
      6. **Fill the tubing with flush.** Detach the syringe from the needle.
      7. **Grasp the plastic wings** and, using your free index finger, **pull the skin taut** to help stabilize the vein.
      8. **Insert the needle** through the skin and advance approximately 0.5 cm prior to entry of the side of the vessel. Alternatively, the vessel can be entered directly after puncture of the skin, but this often results in the vessel being punctured "through and through" (Fig 27–2).
      9. **Advance the needle** until blood appears in the tubing.
      10. **Gently inject some of the flush** to assure patency and proper positioning of the needle.
      11. **Connect the intravenous tubing and fluid** and **tape the needle in position.**
   B. **Catheter-over-needle assembly (Angiocath)**
      1. **Steps 1-5 above, as for scalp vein needle.**
      2. **Fill the needle and hub with flush** via syringe; then remove the syringe.
      3. **Pull the skin taut** to stabilize the vein.

FIGURE 27-1. Sites for venous access frequently used in the neonate.

4. **Puncture the skin;** then enter the side of the vein in a separate motion. Alternately, the skin and the vein can be entered in one motion.
5. **Carefully advance the needle** until blood appears in the hub.
6. **Withdraw the needle** while advancing the catheter.
7. **Remove the tourniquet** and gently inject some normal saline into the catheter to verify patency and position.
8. **Connect the intravenous tubing and fluid** and **tape securely in place.**

IV. **Complications**
   A. **Infection.** The risk of infection can be minimized by using sterile technique, including antiseptic prep.
   B. **Phlebitis.** The risk of phlebitis is increased the longer a catheter is left in place.
   C. **Vasospasm.** Vasospasm rarely occurs when veins are accessed and usually resolves spontaneously.

FIGURE 27-2. Two techniques for for entering the vein for intravenous access. **A:** Direct puncture. **B:** Side entry.

D. Hematoma. Hematoma at the site can often be managed effectively by gentle manual pressure.

E. Embolus (air or clot). *Never* allow the end of the catheter to be open to the air, and make sure that the intravenous line is flushed free of air bubbles before it is connected.

F. Infiltration of subcutaneous tissue. Intravenous solution may leak out into the subcutaneous tissue as a result of improper catheter place-ment or damage to the vessel. To help prevent this, confirm placement of the catheter with the flush solution before the catheter is connected to the intravenous solution. Infiltration often means that the catheter needs to be removed.

VENIPUNCTURE (PHLEBOTOMY)

I. Indications
  A. To obtain a blood sample for analysis or culture.
  B. To give medications.

II. Materials required. A 23- or 25-gauge scalp vein needle, alcohol and povidone-iodine swabs, specimen containers (eg, red-topped tube), tourniquet or rubber band (for scalp), 4 x 4 sterile gauze pads, syringe.

III. Procedure
  A. Have an assistant restrain the infant.
  B. Decide which vein to use (see Fig 27-1 to help with vein selection).
  C. If an assistant is not available, **restrain the specific area selected** for venipuncture. For example, tape the extremity on an armboard.
  D. "Tourniquet" the extremity to occlude the vein. Use either a rubber band (for the head), a tourniquet, or an assistant's hand to encircle the area proximal to the vein.
  E. Prepare the site with antiseptic solution.
  F. With the bevel up, puncture the skin, and then **direct the needle into the vein at a 45-degree angle.**
  G. Once blood enters the tubing, **attach the syringe** and **collect the blood slowly** (or administer the medication).
  H. Remove the tourniquet.
  I. Remove the needle and **apply gentle pressure** on the area until hemo-stasis has occurred. If blood has been collected, distribute it to the appropriate containers to send to the laboratory.

IV. Complications

A. **Infection** is a rare complication that can be minimized by using sterile technique.

B. **Venous thrombosis** is often unavoidable, especially when multiple punctures are performed on the same vein.

C. **Hematoma or hemorrhage** is avoided by applying pressure to the site long enough after the needle is removed to assure hemostasis.

UMBILICAL VEIN CATHETERIZATION

I. **Indications**

A. Central venous pressure monitoring.

B. Immediate access for intravenous fluids, emergency medications.

C. Exchange transfusion, partial exchange transfusion.

II. **Materials required.** Same as for umbilical artery catheterization (see p 134), except that a 5F catheter should be used for infants weighing less than 2 kg and an 8F catheter for infants over 2 kg.

III. **Procedure**

A. **Place the infant supine** with a diaper wrapped around both legs to help stabilize the infant.

B. **Prep the area** around the umbilicus with povidone-iodine solution. Put gown and gloves on.

C. **Prepare the tray** as you would for the umbilical artery catheterization procedure (see p 134).

D. **Put sterile drapes on,** leaving the umbilical area exposed.

E. **Tie a piece of umbilical tape** around the base of the umbilicus.

F. **Cut the excess umbilical cord** with a scalpel or scissor, leaving a stump of about 0.5–1.0 cm. Identify the umbilical vein. The umbilical vein is thin-walled, larger than the 2 arteries, and is close to the periphery of the stump (Fig 16–3B).

G. **Grasp the end of the umbilicus with the curved hemostat** to hold it upright and steady (Fig 27–3A).

H. **Open and dilate the umbilical vein with the forceps.**

I. Once the vein is sufficiently dilated, **insert the catheter** (Fig 27–3B).

J. **To determine the specific length of catheter needed,** see Appendix K. Another method is to measure the length from the xiphoid to the umbili-

FIGURE 27-3. Umbilical vein catheterization. **A:** The umbilical stump is held upright before the catheter is inserted. **B:** The catheter is passed into the umbilical vein.

cus and add 0.5–1.0 cm. This number is how far the venous line should be inserted.

K. **Connect the catheter to the fluid and tubing.** Place a piece of silk tape on the catheter, and secure it to the base of the umbilicus with silk sutures (see Fig 16–4).

L. **Obtain an x-ray film** to confirm the position (see Fig 9–6). The correct position for a central venous pressure line is with the catheter tip 0.5–1.0 cm above the diaphragm.

M. **Never advance a catheter once it is secured in place.**

N. **Occasionally, a catheter will enter the portal vein.** (Fig 27–4.) You should suspect that you have entered the portal vein if you meet resistance and cannot advance the catheter the desired distance or if you detect a "bobbing" motion of the catheter. To correct this, you can do several things.

1. Try injecting flush as you advance the catheter. Sometimes this makes it easier to pass the catheter through the ductus venosus.

2. Pass another catheter (smaller size, usually 3.5F) through the same opening. Sometimes this allows one catheter to go through the ductus venosus while the other enters the portal system. The one in the portal system can then be removed.

IV. Complications

A. **Infection.** Use strict sterile technique, and never advance a catheter that has already been positioned.

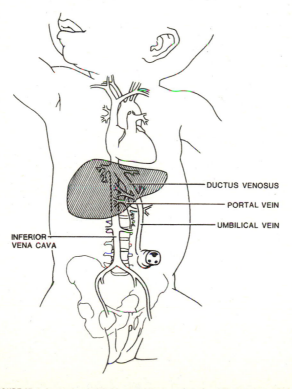

DUCTUS VENOSUS

PORTAL VEIN

UMBILICAL VEIN

INFERIOR VENA CAVA

FIGURE 27–4. Anatomic relationships used in placement of umbilical venous catheter.

B. **Thrombolic or embolic phenomenon.** Never allow air to enter the end of the catheter. A nonfunctioning catheter should be removed. Never try to flush clots from the end of the catheter.
C. **Hepatic necrosis.** Do not allow a catheter to remain in the portal system. In case of emergency placement, the catheter should be advanced only 3 cm (just until blood returns) to avoid hepatic infusion.
D. **Cardiac arrhythmias.** Arrhythmias are usually caused by a catheter that is inserted too far and is irritating the heart.
E. **Portal hypertension.** Portal hypertension is caused by a catheter that is positioned in the portal system.
F. **Necrotizing enterocolitis.** NEC is thought to be a complication of umbilical vein catheters, especially if left in place over 24 hours.

INTRAOSSEOUS INFUSION

I. **Indications.** Immediate vascular access (for administration of fluids and medications) in management of emergencies when other methods of vascular access have been attempted and have failed. (*Note:* This procedure is well described for use in term infants and older children but has not been well studied in premature infants.)
II. **Materials required.** Povidine-iodine solution, 4 x 4 sterile gauze pads, syringe, sterile towels, gloves, 18-gauge disposable iliac bone marrow aspiration needle or 18- to 20-gauge short spinal needle.
III. **Procedure.** The **proximal tibia** is the preferred site.
   A. **Restrain the lower leg.**
   B. **Place a small sandbag or intravenous bag behind the knee** for support.
   C. **Select the area** in the midline on the flat surface of the anterior tibia, 1–3 cm below the tibial tuberosity.
   D. **Clean the area** with betadine. Sterile drapes can be placed around the area that is going to be used.
   E. **Insert the needle** at an angle of 60–90 degrees away from the growth plate.
   F. **Advance the needle** until a lack of resistance is felt, at which point entry into the marrow space should have occurred. (*Note:* At this point, aspiration of bone marrow for laboratory studies can be done, if needed. Bone marrow aspirates can be sent for blood chemistry values, carbon dioxide level, pH, hemoglobin level, culture and sensitivity, and blood typing and cross-matching.)
   G. **Secure the needle to the skin** with tape to prevent it from dislodging.
   H. **Attach the needle to intravenous fluids.** Hypertonic and alkaline solutions should be diluted 1:2 with normal saline.
   I. **Withdraw the needle** and **apply pressure over the puncture site.**
   J. To avoid the risk of infectious complications, this method of vascular access should optimally be used for less than 2 hours.
IV. **Complications**
   A. Fluid infiltration of subcutaneous tissue (most common).
   B. Subperiosteal infiltration of fluid.
   C. Localized cellulitis.
   D. Formation of subcutaneous abscesses.
   E. Clotting of bone marrow, resulting in loss of vascular access.
   F. Osteomyelitis (rare).

This section outlines common problems encountered in the neonatal intensive care unit (NICU) or newborn nursery. Guidelines for rapid diagnosis and treatment are given. Clinical situations and institutional guidelines may vary extensively, and recommendations for treatment should be modified based on these factors. If a treatment approach is designated "controversial," it signifies that the approach has been useful at some institutions but may not have been confirmed in randomized trials.

28 Arrhythmia

I. **Problem.** An infant has an abnormal tracing on the heart rate monitor.
II. **Immediate questions**
   A. **What is the heart rate?** Heart rate in newborns vary from 70 to 190 beats/min (bpm). It is normally 120–140 bpm but may decrease to 70–90 bpm during sleep and increase to 170–190 bpm with increased activity such as crying. See Table 28–1 for normal heart rate values.
   B. **Is the abnormality continuous or transient?** Transient episodes of sinus bradycardia, tachycardia, or arrhythmias (usually lasting less than 15 seconds) are benign and do not require further workup. Episodes lasting longer than 15 seconds usually require full electrocardiographic assessment.
   C. **Is the infant symptomatic?** A symptomatic infant may need immediate treatment. Signs and symptoms of some pathologic arrhythmias include tachypnea, poor skin perfusion, hepatomegaly, and rales on pulmonary examination. All of these signs and symptoms may signify congestive heart failure, which may accompany arrhythmias.
III. **Differential diagnosis**
   A. **Heart rate abnormalities**
      1. **Tachycardia.** Tachycardia is a heart rate greater than 2 standard deviations above the mean for age (Table 28–1).
         a. **Benign causes**
            (1) Postdelivery.
            (2) Heat or cold stress.
            (3) Painful stimuli.
            (4) Medications (eg, atropine, theophylline (aminophylline), epinephrine, intravenous glucagon, pancuronium bromide [Pavulon], tolazoline, and isoproterenol) can cause tachycardia.
         b. **Pathologic causes**
            (1) **More common:** fever, shock, hypoxia, anemia, sepsis, patent ductus arteriosus, congestive heart failure.
            (2) **Less common:** hyperthyroidism, metabolic disorders, cardiac arrhythmias, hyperammonemia.

TABLE 28-1. MINIMUM AND MAXIMUM HEART RATES IN NORMAL NEWBORNS

Age	Minimum	Mean	Maximum	SD[a]
0–24 hours	85	119	145	16.1
1–7 days	100	133	175	22.3
8–30 days	115	163	190	19.9

[a] Standard deviation.
Reproduced, with permission, from Hastreiter AR, Abella JB: The electrocardiogram in the newborn period. I. The normal infant. *J Pediatr* 1971;**78**:146.

2. **Bradycardia.** Bradycardia is a heart rate greater than 2 standard deviations below the mean for age (Table 28-1).
   a. **Benign causes**
      (1) Defecation.
      (2) Vomiting.
      (3) Micturition.
      (4) Gavage feedings.
      (5) Suctioning.
      (6) Medications: propranolol, digitalis, atropine, and infusion of calcium.
   b. **Pathologic causes**
      (1) **More common:** hypoxia, apnea, convulsions, airway obstruction, air leak (eg, pneumothorax), congestive heart failure, intracranial bleeding, severe acidosis, severe hypothermia.
      (2) **Less common:** hyperkalemia, cardiac arrhythmias, pulmonary hemorrhage, diaphragmatic hernia, hypothyroidism, hydrocephalus.
B. **Arrhythmias**
   1. **Benign** arrhythmias include any transient episode (less than 15 seconds) of sinus bradycardia and tachycardia and any of the benign causes of sinus tachycardia and bradycardia noted above in **A.1, 2.** Sinus arrhythmia, which is a phasic variation in the heart rate often associated with respiration, is also benign.
   2. **Pathologic**
      a. Supraventricular tachycardia.
      b. Atrial flutter.
      c. Atrial fibrillation.
      d. Wolff-Parkinson-White syndrome (short PR interval and delta wave, slow upstroke of the QRS complex).
      e. Ectopic beats.
      f. Ventricular tachycardia.
      g. Atrioventricular block.
   3. **Secondary to extracardiac disease**
      a. Sepsis (usually tachycardia).
      b. Diseases of the central nervous system (usually bradycardia).
      c. Hypoglycemia.
      d. Drug toxicity
         (1) Digoxin. The effect of this drug is potentiated by hypokalemia, alkalosis, hypercalcemia, and hypomagnesemia.
         (2) Quinidine.
         (3) Theophylline.
      e. Adrenal insufficiency.
      f. Electrolyte (potassium, sodium, magnesium, calcium) abnormalities.
      g. Metabolic acidosis or alkalosis.
IV. **Data base**
   A. **Physical examination.** Perform a complete physical examination.

Check for signs of congestive heart failure (tachypnea, rales on pulmonary examination, enlarged liver, and cardiomegaly). Vomiting and lethargy may be seen in patients with digoxin toxicity. Hypokalemia can cause ileus.

B. **Laboratory studies**
   1. **Electrolyte, calcium, and magnesium levels.**
   2. **Blood gas levels** may reveal acidosis or hypoxia.
   3. **Drug levels** to evaluate for toxicity:
      a. **Digoxin.** Normal serum levels are 0.5–2.0 ng/mL, (sometimes up to 4 ng/mL). Elevated levels of digoxin alone are not diagnostic of toxicity; clinical and ECG findings consistent with toxicity are also needed.
      b. **Quinidine.** Normal serum levels are 3–7 mg/mL. Toxicity is associated with levels greater than 7 mg/mL.
      c. **Theophylline.** Normal levels are 4–12 μg/mL. Toxicity is associated with levels greater than 15–20 μg/mL.

C. **Radiologic and other studies**
   1. **Electrocardiography.** Full electrocardiographic evaluation should be performed in all infants who have an abnormal ECG tracing that lasts longer than 15 seconds or is not related to a benign condition.
      a. **Supraventricular tachycardia**
         (1) Ventricular rate of 180–300/min.
         (2) No change in heart rate with activity or crying.
         (3) Abnormal P wave or PR interval.
         (4) Fixed RR interval.
      b. **Atrial flutter**
         (1) Atrial rate is 220–400/min.
         (2) Sawtooth configuration seen best in leads V1,2,3.
         (3) QRS complex is usually normal.
      c. **Atrial fibrillation**
         (1) Irregular atrial waves that vary in size and shape from beat to beat.
         (2) Atrial rate is 350–600/min.
         (3) QRS complex is normal, but ventricular response is irregular.
      d. **Wolff-Parkinson-White syndrome**
         (1) Short PR interval.
         (2) Widened QRS complex.
         (3) Presence of delta wave.
      e. **Ventricular tachycardia**
         (1) Ventricular premature beats at a rate of 120–200/min.
         (2) Widened QRS complex.
      f. **Ectopic beats**
         (1) Abnormal P wave.
         (2) Widened QRS complex.
      g. **Atrioventricular block**
         (1) **First-degree block**
            (a) Prolonged PR interval (normal 0.08–0.12).
            (b) Normal sinus rhythm.
            (c) Normal QRS complex.
         (2) **Second-degree block**
            (a) **Mobitz type 1**
               (i) Prolonged PR interval with a dropped ventricular beat.
               (ii) Normal QRS complex.
            (b) **Mobitz type II.** Constant PR interval with dropped ventricular beats.
         (3) **Third-degree block**
            (a) Regular atrial beat.
            (b) Slower ventricular rate.

          (c) Independent atrial and ventricular beat.
    h. Hyperkalemia
        (1) Tall, tented T waves.
        (2) Widened QRS complex.
        (3) Flat and wide P wave.
        (4) Ventricular fibrillation and late asystole.
    i. Hypokalemia
        (1) Prolonged QT and PR interval.
        (2) Depressed ST segment.
        (3) Flat T wave.
    j. Hypocalcemia. Prolonged QT interval.
    k. Hypercalcemia. Shortened QT interval.
    l. Hypomagnesemia. Same as hyperkalemia.
    m. Hyponatremia
        (1) Short QT interval.
        (2) Increased duration of QRS complex.
    n. Hypernatremia
        (1) Prolonged QT interval.
        (2) Decreased duration of QRS complex.
    o. Metabolic acidosis
        (1) Prolonged PR and QRS interval.
        (2) Increased amplitude of P wave.
        (3) Tall, peaked T waves.
    p. Metabolic alkalosis. Inverted T wave.
    q. Digoxin
        (1) Therapeutic levels: prolonged PR interval, short QT interval.
        (2) Toxic levels: most common are sinoatrial (SA) block, second-degree atrioventricular (AV) block, multiple ectopic beats; also, atrioventricular block, bradycardia.
    r. Quinidine
        (1) Therapeutic levels: prolonged PR and QT intervals, decreased amplitude of P wave, widened QRS complex.
        (2) Toxic levels: prolonged PR interval, prolonged QRS complex; AV block, multifocal ventricular premature beats.
    s. Theophylline
        (1) Therapeutic levels: no effect.
        (2) Toxic levels: tachycardia, conduction abnormality.
  2. Chest x-ray studies should be obtained in all infants with suspected heart failure or air leak.
V. Plan
  A. General management. First decide if the arrhythmia is benign or pathologic. If it is pathologic, full electrocardiographic evaluation must be performed. Any acid-base disorder, hypoxia, or electrolyte abnormality needs to be corrected.
  B. Specific management
    1. Heart rate abnormalities
      a. Tachycardia
        (1) Benign. No treatment is necessary, as the tachycardia is usually secondary to a self-limited event.
        (2) Medications. With certain medications, such as theophylline, you can order a serum drug level to determine if it is in the toxic range. If it is, lowering the dosage may restore normal rhythm. Otherwise, a decision needs to be made to accept the tachycardia if the medication is needed or to discontinue the drug.
        (3) Pathologic conditions. The underlying disease needs to be treated.
      b. Bradycardia

      (1) Benign. No treatment is usually necessary.

      (2) Drug-related. Check serum drug level if possible; then consider lowering the dosage or discontinuing the drug unless it is necessary.

      (3) Pathologic

         (a) Treat the underlying disease.

         (b) In severe hypotension or cardiac arrest, check the airway and initiate breathing and cardiac compressions.

         (c) Administer atropine, epinephrine, or isoproterenol to restore normal rhythm (see Chap 75 for dosages and other pharmacologic information).

2. Arrhythmias. (See Chap 75 for dosages of drugs mentioned below and for other pharmacologic information; see p 172, **VI,** for technique of cardioversion.)

   a. Benign. Only observation is indicated (no other treatment).

   b. Pathologic. Treat any underlying acid-base disorders, hypoxia, or electrolyte abnormalities.

      (1) Supraventricular tachycardia

         (a) If the infant's condition is critical, electrical cardioversion is indicated, with digoxin started for maintenance therapy.

         (b) If the infant's condition is not critical, vagal stimulation (ice cold washcloth applied to the infant's face for a few seconds) can be tried. If this is ineffective, digoxin should be started. Other drugs that may be used instead of digoxin are propranolol and quinidine.

      (2) Atrial flutter

         (a) If the infant's condition is critical (severe CHF or unstable hemodynamic state), perform electrical cardioversion, with digoxin started for maintenance therapy.

         (b) If the infant is stable, start digoxin, which slows the ventricular rate. A combination of digoxin and quinidine may be used instead of digoxin alone.

      (3) Recurrent atrial flutter: Management is the same as that for atrial flutter.

      (4) Atrial fibrillation. Management is the same as that for atrial flutter.

      (5) Wolff-Parkinson-White syndrome. Treat any symptomatic arrhythmias that may occur. (High incidence of supraventricular tachycardia.)

      (6) Ventricular tachycardia. Perform electrical cardioversion (except in digitalis toxicity), with lidocaine started for maintenance therapy. Although lidocaine is the drug of choice, other drugs that may be used are procainamide, phenytoin, or bretylium.

3. Ectopic beats

   a. Asymptomatic. No treatment is necessary.

   b. Symptomatic. Underlying heart disease with ectopic beats that are compromising cardiac output: suppress with phenytoin, propranolol, or quinidine.

4. Atrioventricular block

   a. First degree. No specific treatment is usually necessary.

   b. Second degree. Treat underlying cause.

   c. Third degree (complete). Treat initially with transvenous pacemaker. Implantation of a permanent pacemaker will subsequently be necessary.

5. Arrhythmias secondary to extracardiac cause

   a. Pathologic conditions. Treat underlying disease.

   b. Digoxin toxicity. Check PR interval before each dose, obtain stat

serum digoxin level, and hold dose. Consider digoxin immune fab (ovine) (Digibind) (see pp 463–464).
   c. Quinidine toxicity. Discontinue medication.
   d. Theophylline toxicity. Reduce dosage or discontinue medication.
   6. Electrolyte abnormalities
      a. Check serum electrolyte levels with repeat determinations.
      b. Treat electrolyte abnormalities accordingly (see Chap 7).
VI. Technique of cardioversion. Place the paddles at the base (left lower chest in fifth intercostal space in the anterior axillary line) and apex of the heart (right of midline below clavicle). Remember to place a saline-soaked gauze pad beneath each paddle to ensure good electrical conduction. The dose is 1–4 joules/kg, which should be increased 50–100% each time an electrical charge is delivered. When cardioversion is used for infants with ventricular fibrillation, the synch switch should be off.

29 Apnea and Bradycardia ("A's and B's")

I. **Problem.** An infant has just had an apneic episode with bradycardia. Apnea is the absence of breathing for 20 seconds with or without a decrease in heart rate.

II. **Immediate questions**

   A. **What is the gestational age of the infant?** Apnea and bradycardia are common in premature infants. In term infants, they are uncommon and are usually associated with a serious disorder. Apnea in a term infant is almost never physiologic; it usually requires a full workup to determine the cause.

   B. **Was oxygen supplementation needed to return the heart rate to normal?** An infant requiring oxygen by bag-and-mask ventilation needs immediate evaluation and treatment. An infant who has had one episode of apnea and bradycardia not requiring oxygen supplementation may not need a full evaluation unless the infant is term.

   C. **If the patient is already receiving medication (eg, theophylline) for apnea and bradycardia, is the dosage adequate?** Determining the serum drug level is helpful.

   D. **Did the episode occur during or after feeding?** Insertion of a nasogastric tube may cause a vagal reflex, resulting in apnea and bradycardia. Gastroesophageal reflux may cause apnea and bradycardia during or shortly after feeding.

   E. **How old is the infant?** Apnea and bradycardia in the first 24 hours is usually pathologic, whereas if the infant is more than 3 days old, apnea of prematurity is high on the list of differential diagnoses.

III. **Differential diagnosis.** Causes of apnea and bradycardia can be classified according to diseases and disorders of various organ systems, gestational age, or neonatal age.

   A. **Diseases and disorders of various organ systems**
   1. **Head and central nervous system**
      a. Perinatal asphyxia.
      b. Intraventricular or subarachnoid hemorrhage.
      c. Meningitis.
      d. Hydrocephalus with increased intracranial pressure.
      e. Cerebral infarct with seizures.
      f. Seizures.
   2. **Respiratory system**
      a. Hypoxia.
      b. Airway obstruction.
      c. Lung disease.
      d. Inadequate ventilation or performing extubation too early.
   3. **Cardiovascular system**
      a. Congestive heart failure.
      b. Patent ductus arteriosus.
   4. **Gastrointestinal tract**
      a. Necrotizing enterocolitis (NEC).
      b. Gastroesophageal reflux.

      c. Feeding intolerance.
  5. Hematologic system
      a. Anemia. There is no specific hematocrit at which apnea and brady-cardia will occur. They have been seen in infants with anemia of prematurity. These infants have significant relief after transfusion.
      b. Polycythemia. This disorder is more common in term infants.
  6. Other diseases and disorders
      a. Temperature instability. Apnea and bradycardia may occur in patients with temperature instability, especially hyperthermia but also hypothermia. Note the incubator temperature. An infant may have a normal body temperature but have a rise in incubator temperature (meaning that the infant is hypothermic) or require a lower incubator temperature (meaning that the infant is hyperthermic).
      b. Infection (sepsis).
      c. Electrolyte imbalance. Hypoglycemia, hyponatremia, hypermagnesemia, hyperkalemia, and hypocalcemia can cause apnea and bradycardia.
      d. Vagal reflex. This may occur secondary to nasogastric tube insertion.
      e. Drugs. High levels of phenobarbital or other sedatives such as diazepam and chloral hydrate may cause apnea and bradycardia.
B. Gestational age. See Table 29–1.
C. Neonatal age
  1. Full-term infants. In full-term infants of any neonatal age, apnea and bradycardia are usually never due to physiologic causes. The disease or disorder causing apnea and bradycardia must be identified.
  2. Preterm infants. Causes of apnea and bradycardia in preterm infants at 1–2 days of life are shown in Table 29–1. In preterm infants at 3–5 days of life or more, the most likely cause is **apnea of prematurity.** Infants with this disorder usually weigh less than 1800 g and have no other identifiable cause of apnea and bradycardia.
IV. Data base. Determine whether there has been any prenatal risk of sepsis. The cord pH should be obtained to rule out birth asphyxia. A history of feeding intolerance will increase the suspicion of necrotizing enterocolitis.
A. Physical examination. Perform a complete physical examination, paying careful attention to the following signs.
  1. Head. Look for signs of increased intracranial pressure.
  2. Heart. Listen for a murmur or gallop.
  3. Lungs. Check for adequate movement of the chest if mechanical ventilation is being used.
  4. Abdomen. Check for abdominal distention, one of the earliest signs of NEC. Other signs of NEC are decreased bowel sounds and visible bowel loops.

TABLE 29–1. CAUSES OF APNEA AND BRADYCARDIA ACCORDING TO GESTATIONAL AGE

Full-Term Infant	Premature Infant
Infection (sepsis or meningitis)	Apnea of prematurity (usually at 3–5 days of life)
Hypoglycemia	Necrotizing enterocolitis
Polycythemia	Sepsis
Seizures	Patent ductus arteriosus
Cerebral infarction	Hypoxia
Cerebral hemorrhage	Hypoglycemia
	Intraventricular hemorrhage
	Electrolyte abnormalities

5. **Skin.** An infant with polycythemia has a ruddy appearance. Pallor is associated with anemia.

B. **Laboratory studies**
1. **Complete blood count and differential.** Findings may suggest infection or possible anemia or polycythemia.
2. **Serum electrolyte, calcium, and glucose levels** help rule out metabolic abnormality.
3. **Serum phenobarbital and/or theophylline levels** are obtained if indicated.
4. **Arterial blood gas levels** should be obtained to rule out hypoxia, acidosis, or hypocarbia.

C. **Radiologic and other studies**
1. **Chest x-ray study.** A chest x-ray study should be performed immediately if there is any suspicion of heart or lung disease.
2. **Electrocardiography.** If cardiac disease is suspected, electrocardiography should be performed.
3. **Abdominal x-ray study.** An abdominal x-ray study should be performed immediately if indicated. It may detect signs of NEC (see **A.4,** p 174).
4. **Ultrasonography of the head** is performed to rule out intraventricular hemorrhage or hydrocephalus.
5. **CT scanning of the head** will detect cerebral infarction and subarachnoid hemorrhage if present.
6. **Barium swallow** is performed to rule out gastroesophageal reflux only in cases of apnea and bradycardia associated with feeding.
7. **Lumbar puncture.** Lumbar puncture and CSF examination should be performed if meningitis is suspected or if increased intracranial pressure from hydrocephalus is causing apnea and bradycardia.
8. **Esophageal-pH probe testing (acid reflux test of Tuttle and Grossman)** is useful in determining whether gastroesophageal reflux is present. A small-caliber tube (to which a pH electrode is attached) is passed into the distal esophagus. Continuous monitoring can be carried out over 4–24 hours. If the pH is acidic, gastroesophageal reflux is occurring.
9. **Electroencephalography.** Because apnea and bradycardia may be a manifestation of seizure activity, an electroencephalogram (EEG) is obtained in any infant who may be having seizures.
10. **Pneumography, thermistor pneumography, and polysomnography.** See p 407, **E.2,** for a detailed discussion of these procedures.

V. **Plan**
A. **Determine the cause of apnea and bradycardia** and treat if possible.
B. **Apnea of prematurity**
1. **General measures**
a. Provide tactile stimulation.
b. Place the infant on a water bed or an oscillating bed if it is the practice of your institution. Randomized controlled studies have shown this measure not to be effective, but it is still used in some institutions.
2. **Specific treatment**
a. **Theophylline or caffeine** is used initially. Caffeine seems to have fewer side effects than theophylline, but the choice of drug depends on institutional preference and availability. Therapy can usually be discontinued by 37 weeks' postconceptional age. (See Chap 75 for dosages, side effects, and other pharmacologic information.)
b. If the above drug trial fails, use **continuous positive airway pressure (CPAP)** via nasal prongs at a rate of 2–4 cm of water and continue administration of the drug.

    c. If apnea persists, begin **doxapram.** Doxapram has had limited clinical use but appears to be efficacious. One concern regarding doxapram is that it contains benzyl alcohol as a preservative. (See Chap 75 for drug dosage, side effects, and other pharmacologic information.)

    d. Mechanical ventilation should be used if apnea and bradycardia cannot be controlled by drug therapy and/or nasal CPAP. Low pressures are used at the rate necessary to prevent apnea. (See p 46, **E.4.**)

  3. Long-term monitoring of respiratory function. See p 408, **C.**

C. Anemia. Most institutions do not treat anemia if the infant is asymptomatic and is feeding and growing and the reticulocyte count indicates that red cells are being made (> 5–6%). If the hematocrit is low ("low" is usually < 28%) and if the infant is symptomatic and not feeding well and the reticulocyte count is not appropriate for the low hematocrit (ie, reticulocyte is < 2–3%), transfusion is indicated *(controversial).*

D. Gastroesophageal reflux. Keep the infant in the prone position as much as possible; use small-volume thickened feedings. Reglan may also be tried (see Chap 75 for dosage and other pharmacologic information).

30 Bloody Stool

I. **Problem.** A newborn infant has passed a bloody stool.

II. **Immediate questions**

A. **Is it grossly bloody?** *This finding is usually an ominous sign; an exception is swallowed maternal blood, which is a benign condition.* A grossly bloody stool usually occurs in infants with a lesion in the ileum or colon or with massive upper gastrointestinal tract bleeding. Necrotizing enterocolitis is the most common cause of bloody stool in premature infants and should be strongly suspected in the differential diagnosis.

B. **Is the stool otherwise normal in color but with streaks of blood?** This description is more characteristic of a lesion in the anal canal, such as anal fissure.

C. **Is the stool positive only for occult blood?** Occult blood often signifies that the blood is from the upper gastrointestinal tract (proximal to the ligament of Treitz). Nasogastric trauma and swallowed maternal blood are common causes.

D. **Was the infant given vitamin K at birth?** Hemorrhagic disease of the newborn may present with bloody stools, as may any coagulopathy.

III. **Differential diagnosis**

A. **Occult blood only, no visible blood**
1. Swallowing of maternal blood during delivery or during breast-feeding may be the cause.
2. Nasogastric tube trauma.
3. Necrotizing enterocolitis.
4. Formula intolerance (cow's milk protein allergy).
5. Gastritis or ulcer.
6. Unknown etiology.

B. **Streaks of visible blood in the stool**
1. Anal fissure.
2. Rectal trauma. This is often secondary to temperature probes.

C. **Grossly bloody stool**
1. Necrotizing enterocolitis.
2. Disseminated intravascular coagulation. There may be bleeding from other sites.
3. Hemorrhagic disease of the newborn. This entity may also present with bleeding from other sites.
4. Other surgical diseases such as malrotation with midgut volvulus, intestinal duplications, and intussusception (rare in the neonatal period).
5. Intestinal infections such as *Shigella, Salmonella, Campylobacter, Yersinia,* and enteropathogenic strains of *E coli.*

IV. **Clinical findings.** The age of the infant is important. If the infant is less than 7 days old, swallowing of maternal blood is a possible cause; in older infants, it is an unlikely cause.

A. **Physical examination**
1. **Examination of peripheral perfusion.** Evaluate the infant's peripheral perfusion. An infant with necrotizing enterocolitis can be poorly perfused and may appear to be in early or impending shock.
2. **Abdominal examination.** Check for bowel sounds and tenderness.

If the abdomen is soft and nontender and there is no erythema, a pathologic process is probably not occurring. If the abdomen is distended, rigid, or tender, a pathologic process is likely to be present. Abdominal distention is the most common sign of necrotizing enterocolitis. If there are red streaks and erythema on the abdominal wall, suspect necrotizing enterocolitis with peritonitis.

3. **Anal examination.** If the infant's condition is stable, perform a visual examination of the anus to check for anal fissure or tear.

B. Laboratory studies

1. **Apt test.** If swallowed maternal blood is suspected, perform the Apt test, which differentiates maternal from fetal blood. The test is performed as follows: Mix equal parts of the bloody material with water and centrifuge it. Add 1 part 0.25–molar sodium hydroxide to 5 parts of the pink supernatant. If the fluid remains pink, the blood is fetal in origin because hemoglobin F stays pink. Hemoglobin A from maternal blood is hydrolyzed and changes color from pink to yellow brown.

2. **Stool culture.** Obtain a stool culture. Certain pathogens cause bloody stools, but they are rare in the neonatal nursery.

3. **Coagulation studies.** Coagulation studies should be performed to rule out disseminated intravascular coagulation or a bleeding disorder. The usual studies are partial thromboplastin time (PTT), prothrombin time (PT), fibrinogen level, and platelet count. Thrombocytopenia can also be seen with cow's milk protein allergy.

4. **If necrotizing enterocolitis is suspected, the following studies should be performed.**
   a. **Complete blood count with differential.** This test is done to establish an inflammatory response and to check for thrombocytopenia and anemia.
   b. **Serum potassium levels.** Hyperkalemia due to hemolysis may occur.
   c. **Blood gas levels.** Blood gases should be measured to rule out metabolic acidosis, which is often associated with sepsis or necrotizing enterocolitis.

C. Radiologic and other studies. A **plain x-ray film of the abdomen** is useful if necrotizing enterocolitis or a surgical abdomen is suspected. Look for an abnormal gas pattern, thickened bowel wall, or pneumatosis intestinalis. Pneumatosis can appear as a "soap bubble" area. If a suspicious area appears on the abdominal x-ray film in the right upper quadrant, it is usually never stool. A left lateral decubitus view of the abdomen may show free air if perforation has occurred. Surgical conditions usually show signs of intestinal obstruction.

V. Plan

A. Swallowed maternal blood. Only observation is necessary.

B. Anal fissure and rectal trauma. Observation is indicated. Petroleum jelly applied to the anus may promote healing.

C. Necrotizing enterocolitis. (See Chap 66.)

D. Nasogastric trauma. In most cases of bloody stool involving nasogastric tubes, trauma is mild and requires only observation. If the tube is too large, replacing it with a smaller one may resolve the problem. If there has been significant bleeding, gastric lavages are helpful; it is *controversial* whether tepid water or normal saline is best. Then, if possible, removal of the nasogastric tube is recommended.

E. Formula intolerance. This diagnosis is difficult to document, so it is usually made if the patient has remission of symptoms when the formula is eliminated.

F. Gastritis or ulcers. Treatment usually consists of ranitidine or cimetidine (see Chap 75 for dosages and other pharmacologic information).

Use of antacids is *controversial,* as some clinicians feel concretions may occur.

G. **Unknown etiology.** If no cause is found, the infant is usually closely followed, and in the majority of the cases, the bleeding will subside.

H. **Intestinal infections.** Antibiotic treatment and isolation are standard treatment. (See Chap 76 and Appendix H.)

I. **Hemorrhagic disease of the newborn.** Intravenous vitamin K is usually adequate therapy (see Chap 75).

J. **Surgical conditions.** Malrotation with midgut volvulus, intussusception, or intestinal duplications require immediate surgical evaluation.

31 Abnormal Blood Gas

I. **Problem.** An abnormal blood gas value is reported by the laboratory for a neonate on a ventilator.

II. **Immediate questions**

A. **What component of the blood gas is abnormal?** Accepted normal values for an arterial blood gas sample are pH between 7.35 and 7.45, $Paco_2$ between 35 and 45 (slightly higher values may be accepted if the blood pH remains normal), and Pao_2 between 55 and 65 on room air.

B. **Is this blood gas value very different from the patient's previous blood gas determination?** This is a key question. If the patient has had metabolic acidosis on the last 5 blood gas measurements and now has metabolic alkalosis, it might be best to repeat the blood gas measurements before initiating treatment. Do not treat the infant on the basis of one abnormal gas value, especially if the infant's clinical status has not changed.

C. **How was the sample collected?** Blood gas measurements can be reported on arterial, venous, or capillary blood samples. Arterial blood samples are the best indicator of pH, $Paco_2$, and Pao_2. Venous blood samples will give a lower pH value and a higher Pco_2 than arterial samples. Capillary samples will give a fair assessment of the infant's pH, Pco_2, and Pao_2. Capillary samples will give a fair assessment of the infant's pH, Pco_2. Capillary samples give a lower pH value (but not as low as the venous pH) and a slightly higher Pco_2 than arterial samples. An accurate capillary blood gas measurement cannot be obtained on an infant who is hypotensive or in shock.

D. **Is the infant on ventilatory support?** Management of abnormal blood gas levels is approached differently in an intubated infant than in a patient breathing room air.

III. **Differential diagnosis**

A. **Metabolic acidosis.** This is defined as a pH value ≤ 7.35 with a normal carbon dioxide value and a base deficit > 5.

1. **Common causes**
   a. Sepsis.
   b. Necrotizing enterocolitis.
   c. Hypothermia or cold stress.
   d. Intraventricular hemorrhage.
   e. Patent ductus arteriosus.
   f. Shock.
   g. Factitious acidosis (too much heparin in the syringe).
   h. Drugs (eg, acetazolamide [Diamox]).

2. **Less common causes**
   a. **Renal tubular acidosis.** This involves a defect in the reabsorption of bicarbonate or secretion of hydrogen ion and can present in 3 forms: proximal, distal, or mixed.
   b. **Inborn errors of metabolism.** See Table 61–4, p 319, to see which diseases present with metabolic acidosis.
   c. Maternal use of salicylates and maternal acidosis.
   d. Renal failure.
   e. Congenital lactic acidosis.

B. **Metabolic alkalosis.** This is defined as a pH value ≥ 7.45 with a base excess of > 5.
   1. **Common causes**
      a. Excess alkali administration (eg, sodium bicarbonate).
      b. Potassium depletion.
      c. Prolonged nasogastric suction.
      d. Diuretics (such as in patients with bronchopulmonary dysplasia [BPD]).
   2. **Less common causes**
      a. Bartter's syndrome.
      b. Primary hyperaldosteronism.
C. **Low CO_2, high O_2**
   1. Overventilation.
   2. Air bubble in the syringe.
D. **High CO_2, normal or high O_2**
   1. Obstructed endotracheal tube (eg, mucous plug).
   2. Endotracheal tube down the right main stem bronchus or at the carina.
   3. Pneumothorax.
   4. Patent ductus arteriosus. Clinical signs and symptoms include metabolic acidosis, congestive heart failure, bounding pulses, active precordium, deteriorating blood gases with an increase in the ventilator settings, and a large heart with increased pulmonary vascularity on chest x-ray film.
   5. Ventilator malfunction.
E. **High CO_2, low O_2**
   1. Pneumothorax.
   2. Improper endotracheal tube position. An endotracheal tube positioned in the oropharynx will cause this type of blood gas result.
   3. Increasing respiratory failure.
   4. Patent ductus arteriosus (PDA).
   5. Insufficient respiratory support.
   6. Atelectasis.
F. **Normal CO_2, low O_2**
   1. Agitation.
   2. Pneumothorax.
   3. Improper endotracheal tube position.
   4. Atelectasis.
   5. Pulmonary hypertension.
   6. Pulmonary edema.
IV. **Data base**
   A. **Physical examination.** Evaluate for signs of sepsis (eg, hypotension, poor perfusion). Check for equal breath sounds; asymmetric breath sounds suggest pneumothorax. Listen for breath sounds over the chest vs the epigastric region, which may help determine if the endotracheal tube is malpositioned. Listen to the heart for any murmur and palpate for cardiac displacement.
   B. **Laboratory studies**
      1. **Repeat blood gas measurement.** Especially if the result is unexpected or if a major clinical decision is to be made on the basis of venous or capillary blood gas values, an arterial blood sample should be obtained and sent to the laboratory for blood gas values.
      2. **Complete blood count and differential** are helpful if sepsis is being considered.
      3. **Serum potassium level.** Severe metabolic alkalosis can cause hypokalemia.
   C. **Radiologic and other studies**

1. **Transillumination of the chest** should be done if pneumothorax is suspected (see p 230, **IV.C.1**, for details on this procedure).
2. **Chest x-ray study.** A chest x-ray study should be performed if an abnormal blood gas value is reported by the laboratory, unless there is an obvious cause. An anteroposterior x-ray view should be obtained to check endotracheal tube placement, to rule out air leak (eg, pneumothorax), to check heart size and pulmonary vascularity (increased or decreased), and to determine if the infant is being hypoventilated or hyperventilated.
3. **Abdominal x-ray study.** An abdominal x-ray study should be done if necrotizing enterocolitis is suspected in a patient with severe metabolic acidosis.
4. **Ultrasonography of the head** will diagnose intraventricular hemorrhage if present.
5. **Echocardiography.** Patent ductus arteriosus or other cardiac abnormality may be detected with echocardiography.

V. **Plan**
   A. **Overall plan.** Verify the blood gas result, find the cause of the problem, and provide appropriate treatment for the specific cause. The first step is to examine the infant. If the infant's clinical status has not changed, repeat blood gas measurements to verify the report. If the clinical status has changed, the abnormal report is probably correct; repeat blood gas measurements can be obtained, but further evaluation of the infant should begin.
   B. **Specific management**
      1. **Metabolic acidosis**
         a. **General measures.** Most institutions treat acidosis with an alkali infusion if the base excess is greater than -5 to -10 or if the pH is equal to or less than 7.25–7.30. The alkali can be given as 1 dose over 20 to 30 minutes or it can be given as an 8- to 12-hour correction. If the acidosis is mild, usually only 1 dose is given and repeat blood gas measurements are obtained. If the acidosis is severe, a dose is given and correction is started at the same time. One of 3 medications is used.
            (1) **Sodium bicarbonate** can be used if the infant's serum sodium and P_{CO_2} are not high. If given as a one-time dose, it should be 1–2 meq/kg diluted 1:1 with sterile water. It should be given over 20–10 minutes unless the infant is unstable, in which case an intravenous push dose can be given at a rate of 1 mL/min. To calculate how much to give as an 8- to 12-hour correction:

            Bicarbonate dose (meq) = Base deficit $\times$ Body weight (kg) $\times$ 0.3

            is the total dose required to correct the base deficit. It should be added to the intravenous fluids, and the correction should be given over 8–12 hours.
            (2) **Tromethamine (THAM)** can be used in infants who have metabolic acidosis but have a high serum sodium and P_{CO_2}. *It should be used only in infants who have a good urine output.* (See Chap 75 for dosage and other pharmacologic information.)
            (3) **Polycitrate (Polycitra).** This alkali is especially useful in patients receiving acetazolamide (Diamox). It consists of 1 meq sodium, 1 meq potassium, and 2 meq citrate. Each meq of citrate equals 1 meq bicarbonate. The dose is 2–3 meq/kg/d polycitrate in 3–4 divided doses. Adjust the dosage to maintain a normal pH.

b. **The underlying cause should be treated** as outlined below.
   (1) **Sepsis.** Initiate a septic workup and consider broad-spectrum antibiotics. (See Chap 76 for specific antibiotic agents, dosages, and other pharmacologic information.)
   (2) **Necrotizing enterocolitis.** (See Chap 66.)
   (3) **Hypothermia or cold stress.** Gradual rewarming should be done at 0.5–1.0 °C per hour (see p 32).
   (4) **Intraventricular hemorrhage.** Weekly ultrasonographic examinations of the head and daily head circumferences are indicated. If hydrocephalus occurs, neurosurgic consultation should be obtained to detect possible shunting.
   (5) **Patent ductus arteriosus.** The patient who has clinically symptomatic PDA should be treated. Treatment includes furosemide, decreasing fluid intake, and a course of indomethacin. (See Chap 75 for drug dosages and other pharmacologic information.)
   (6) **Renal tubular acidosis.** Treatment consists of sodium bicarbonate therapy [see p 182, **a.(1)**].
   (7) **Inborn errors of metabolism.** (See Chap 61.)
   (8) **Maternal use of salicylates.** Acidosis usually resolves, without treatment.
   (9) **Renal failure.** (See p 424.)
   (10) **Congenital lactic acidosis.** Correction of the metabolic acidosis (see p 182, **1.a**) and megavitamin therapy are indicated.
2. **Metabolic alkalosis.** The treatment of metabolic alkalosis depends on the cause.
   a. **Excess alkali.** Adjust or discontinue the dose of THAM, sodium bicarbonate, or polycitrate.
   b. **Hypokalemia.** If the serum potassium level is low, metabolic alkalosis can occur because potassium is exchanged for hydrogen. The infant's potassium level should be corrected (see Chap 42).
   c. **Prolonged nasogastric suction** is treated with intravenous fluid replacement, usually with $\frac{1}{2}$ normal saline containing 20 meq potassium chloride, replaced milliliter for milliliter each shift.
   d. **Diuretics.** Mild alkalosis is sometimes seen; no specific treatment is usually necessary.
   e. **Bartter's syndrome** is treated with potassium replacement and adequate nutrition.
   f. **Primary hyperaldosteronism** is treated with dexamethasone. (See Chap 75 for dosage and other pharmacologic information.)
3. **Other causes of abnormal blood gases**
   a. **Pneumothorax.** (see p 230.)
   b. **Mucous plug.** If an infant has decreased breath sounds on both sides of the chest and has retractions, a plugged endotracheal tube is probably responsible. The infant can be suctioned and, if clinically stable, repeat blood gas measurements are obtained. If the infant is in extreme distress, the tube should be replaced.
   c. **Overventilation.** If the blood gas levels reveal overventilation, the ventilation parameters need to be adjusted. If the oxygen level is high, the following parameters can be decreased: oxygen, positive end-expiratory pressure (PEEP), peak inspiratory pressure (PIP), or inspiratory time (IT). If the patient's carbon dioxide level is low, the following parameters can be decreased: rate, positive inspiratory pressure (PIP), or expiratory time (ET). Deciding which parameter to wean depends on the patient's lung disease and the disease course. Ventilator changes are discussed on p 45, **F.**
   d. **Agitation.** An agitated infant may have a drop in oxygenation and may need to be sedated or have ventilator settings changed. One

may have to sit by the bedside and try different rates to see if he or she fights less. If sedation is chosen, phenobarbital, diazepam, chloral hydrate, meperidine, or morphine may be used. (See Chap 75 for dosages and other pharmacologic information.) Use the agent with which your institution has experience. **Remember, agitation can be a sign of hypoxia, so a blood gas level should be obtained prior to ordering sedation.** If there is documented hypoxia, attempts to increase oxygenation should be used.

e. **Problem with endotracheal tube placement.** An infant who has a tube down his right main-stem bronchus will have breath sounds on the right only. An infant with a tube that has dislodged or become plugged will have decreased or no breath sounds on chest auscultation. The patient needs to be reintubated.

f. **Ventilator malfunction.** Respiratory Therapy should be notified to check the ventilator and replace it if necessary.

g. **Increasing respiratory failure.** Ventilator settings need to be adjusted.

h. **Insufficient respiratory support.** If the infant's chest is not moving, the PIP is not high enough, and adjustment of the ventilator setting is needed.

i. **Atelectasis.** Treatment consists of percussion and postural drainage and possibly increased PIP or PEEP.

j. **Pulmonary edema.** Diuretics (eg, furosemide) (See Chap 75) and mechanical ventilation are indicated.

k. **Pulmonary hypertension.** (See p 284.)

32 Cyanosis

I. **Problem.** During a physical examination, an infant appears blue.
II. **Immediate questions**
   A. **Does the infant have respiratory distress?** If the infant has increased respiratory effort with increased rate, retractions, and nasal flaring, respiratory disease should be high on the list of differential diagnoses. Cyanotic heart disease usually presents without respiratory symptoms but can have effortless tachypnea. Blood disorders usually present without respiratory or cardiac symptoms.
   B. **Does the infant have a murmur?** A murmur usually implies heart disease. Transposition of the great arteries can present without a murmur.
   C. **Is the cyanosis continuous, intermittent, sudden in onset, or occurring only with feeding?** Intermittent cyanosis is more common with neurologic disorders, as these infants may have apneic spells alternating with periods of normal breathing. Continuous cyanosis is usually associated with intrinsic lung disease or heart disease. Cyanosis with feeding may occur with esophageal atresia and severe esophageal reflux. Sudden onset of cyanosis may occur with an air leak, such as pneumothorax. Cyanosis that disappears with crying may signify choanal atresia.
   D. **Is there differential cyanosis?** If there is cyanosis of the upper or lower part of the body only, it usually signifies serious heart disease. The more common pattern is cyanosis restricted to the lower half of the body, which is seen in patients with patent ductus arteriosus. Cyanosis restricted to the upper half of the body is seen occasionally in patients with pulmonary hypertension, patent ductus arteriosus, coarctation of the aorta and D-transposition of the great arteries.
   E. **What is the prenatal and delivery history?** An infant of a diabetic mother has increased risk for hypoglycemia, polycythemia, respiratory distress syndrome (RDS), and heart disease. Infection, such as that which can occur with premature rupture of the membranes, may cause shock and hypotension with resultant cyanosis. Amniotic fluid abnormalities, such as oligohydramnios (associated with hypoplastic lungs) or polyhydramnios (associated with esophageal atresia), may suggest a cause for the cyanosis. Cesarean section is associated with increased respiratory distress.
III. **Differential diagnosis.** The causes of cyanosis can be classified as respiratory, cardiac, central nervous system, or other disorders.
   A. **Respiratory diseases**
      1. **Lung diseases**
         a. Hyaline membrane disease.
         b. Transient tachypnea of the newborn.
         c. Pneumonia.
         d. Meconium aspiration.
      2. **Air leak syndrome.**
      3. **Congenital defects** (eg, diaphragmatic hernia and hypoplastic lungs).
   B. **Cardiac diseases**
      1. **All cyanotic heart diseases,** including transposition of the great arteries, total anomalous pulmonary venous return, Ebstein's anomaly,

tricuspid atresia, pulmonary atresia, pulmonary stenosis, tetralogy of Fallot, patent ductus arteriosus, and ventricular septal defect.
2. **Persistent pulmonary hypertension.**
C. **Central nervous system (CNS) diseases.** Intracranial hemorrhage or malformation, meningitis, and primary seizure disorder can all cause cyanosis.
D. **Other disorders**
1. **Methemoglobinemia.** May be familial.
2. **Polycythemia.**
3. **Hypothermia, hypoglycemia, sepsis, pseudocyanosis caused by fluorescent lighting.**
4. **Respiratory depression secondary to maternal medications (eg, magnesium sulfate and narcotics).**
5. **Shock.**
6. **Choanal atresia.** Nasal passage obstruction caused most commonly by a bony abnormality.

IV. **Data base.** Obtain a prenatal and delivery history (see p 185, **II.E**).
A. **Physical examination**
1. **Assess the infant for central vs peripheral cyanosis.** In central cyanosis, the lips and tongue will appear blue. In peripheral cyanosis, the oral mucous membranes will be pink. Check the nasal passage for choanal atresia.
2. **Assess the heart.** Check for any murmurs. Assess heart rate and blood pressure.
3. **Assess the lungs.** Is there retraction, flaring of nose, grunting?
4. **Assess the abdomen** for an enlarged liver. The liver can be enlarged in congestive heart failure and hyperexpansion of the lungs. Absence of bowel sounds may suggest a diaphragmatic hernia.
5. **Check the pulses.** In coarctation of the aorta, the femoral pulses will be decreased. In patent ductus arteriosus, the pulses will be bounding.
6. **Consider neurologic problems.** Check for apnea and periodic breathing, which may be associated with immaturity of the nervous system. Observe the infant for seizures, which can cause cyanosis if the infant is not breathing during seizures.
B. **Laboratory studies**
1. **Arterial blood gas measurements on room air.** If the patient is not hypoxic, it suggests methemoglobinemia, polycythemia, or CNS disease. If the patient is hypoxic, perform the 100% hyperoxic test, described below.
2. **Hyperoxic test.** Measure arterial oxygen on room air. Then place the infant on 100% oxygen for 10–20 minutes. With cyanotic heart disease the PaO_2 will not change, whereas in lung disease the arterial oxygen saturation should improve.
3. **Complete blood count and differential** may reveal an infection process. A central hematocrit of more than 65% confirms polycythemia.
4. **Serum glucose level** will detect hypoglycemia.
5. **Methemoglobin level.** A drop of blood exposed to air has a chocolate hue. To confirm the diagnosis, a spectrophotometric procedure should be done.
C. **Radiologic and other studies**
1. **Transillumination of the chest** (see p 230, **IV.C.1**) should be done on an emergent basis if pneumothorax is suspected.
2. **Chest x-ray** may be normal, suggesting CNS disease or another cause for the cyanosis (see **III.D,** above). It can verify lung disease, air leak, or diaphragmatic hernia. It can help diagnose heart disease by evaluating the heart size and pulmonary vascularity. The heart

size may be normal or enlarged in hypoglycemia, polycythemia, shock, and sepsis.

3. **Electrocardiography** should be done to help determine the cause of the cyanosis. The ECG is usually normal in patients with methemoglobinemia or hypoglycemia; it is normal but may show right ventricular hypertrophy in patients with polycythemia, pulmonary hypertension, or primary lung disease. It is very helpful in identifying patients with tricuspid atresia; it will show left axis deviation and left ventricular hypertrophy.

4. **Echocardiography** should be performed if cardiac disease is suspected or if the diagnosis is unclear.

V. Plan

A. **General management.** Act quickly and accomplish many of the diagnostic tasks at once.

1. **Perform a quick physical examination.** Transilluminate the chest (see p 230, **IV.C.1**), and if a tension pneumothorax is present, rapid needle decompression may be needed (see p 231, **V.A**).

2. **Order stat laboratory tests (eg, blood gas levels, complete blood count, and chest x-ray film).**

3. **Perform the hyperoxic test.** (See **IV.B.2**, p 186.)

B. **Specific management**

1. **Lung disease.** (See Chap 69.) Respiratory depression caused by narcotics is treated with naloxone (Narcan) (see Chap 75 for dosage and other pharmacologic information).

2. **Air leak (pneumothorax).** (See Chap 48.)

3. **Congenital defects.** Surgery is indicated for diaphragmatic hernia.

4. **Cardiac disease.** The use of prostaglandin E_1 (PGE_1) is indicated for right heart outflow obstruction (tricuspid atresia, pulmonic stenosis, and pulmonary atresia), left heart outflow obstruction (hypoplastic left heart syndrome, critical aortic valve stenosis, preductal coarctation of the aorta, and interrupted aortic arch), and transposition of the great arteries. PGE_1 is contraindicated for hyaline membrane disease, persistent pulmonary hypertension, and dominant left-to-right shunt (patent ductus arteriosus, truncus arteriosus, or ventricular septal defect). **If the diagnosis is uncertain,** a trial of PGE_1 can be given over 30 minutes in an effort to improve blood gas values.

5. **CNS disorders.** Treat the underlying disease (see Chap 67).

6. **Methemoglobinemia.** Treat the infant with methylene blue only if the methemoglobin level is severely increased and the infant is in cardiopulmonary distress (tachypnea and tachycardia). Administer intravenously 1–2 mg/kg of a 1% solution of methylene blue in normal saline. The cyanosis should clear within 1–2 hours.

7. **Shock.** (See Chap 44.)

8. **Polycythemia.** (See Chap 49.)

9. **Choanal atresia.** The infant usually requires surgery.

10. **Hypothermia.** Rewarming is necessary (see p 34).

11. **Hypoglycemia.** (See Chap 41.)

33 Eye Discharge (Conjunctivitis)

I. **Problem.** Eye discharge is noted.
II. **Immediate questions**
   A. **How old is the infant?** Age is an important factor in determining the cause of eye discharge. Within the first 24–48 hours of life, the most likely cause is conjunctivitis secondary to use of ocular silver nitrate drops immediately after birth to prevent gonococcal ophthalmia. At 2–5 days, a bacterial infection is most likely. The organisms that most commonly cause conjunctivitis in the neonatal period are *Neisseria gonorrhoeae* and *Staphylococcus aureus*. *Chlamydia trachomatis* conjunctivitis is usually seen after the first week of life; it often presents as late as the third week. *Pseudomonas aeruginosa* infections are typically seen between the 5th and 18th days of life.
   B. **Is the discharge unilateral or bilateral?** Bilateral conjunctivitis is seen with infection due to *C trachomatis* or *N gonorrhoeae* or use of silver nitrate. Unilateral conjunctivitis is seen with *S aureus* and *P aeruginosa.*
   C. **What are the characteristics of the discharge?** It is important to distinguish between purulent and watery discharge. Purulent discharge is more common with bacterial infection. Infection due to *Chlamydia* may be watery early in the course and purulent later on. A greenish discharge is more characteristic of *P aeruginosa.*
III. **Differential diagnosis**
   A. **Chemical conjunctivitis** is usually secondary to the use of silver nitrate ocular drops. Currently, it is not seen much, because many nurseries are using erythromycin ophthalmic ointment, which causes less ocular irritation and protects against chlamydial and gonococcal infections.
   B. **Gonococcal conjunctivitis** is most commonly transmitted from the mother. The incidence is low because of prophylactic treatment immediately after birth.
   C. **Staphylococcal conjunctivitis** is usually a nosocomial infection.
   D. **Chlamydial conjunctivitis** is transmitted from the mother.
   E. **Pseudomonal conjunctivitis** is usually a nosocomial infection and is becoming more common in neonatal nurseries. The organism thrives in moisture-filled environments such as respiratory equipment.
   F. **Lacrimal duct obstruction (dacryostenosis).** In this disorder, the nasolacrimal duct may fail to canalize completely at birth. The obstruction is usually at the nasal end of the duct. The symptoms are persistent tearing and a mucoid discharge in the inner corner of the eye. The disorder is usually unilateral.
   G. **Other bacterial infections** include infections due to *Haemophilus* species, streptococci, and pneumococci.
IV. **Data base**
   A. **Physical examination**
      1. Examine both eyes for swelling and edema of the eyelids and check the conjunctiva for injection (congestion of blood vessels). A purulent discharge, edema, and erythema of the lids as well as injection of the conjunctiva are suggestive of bacterial conjunctivitis.
      2. Perform a complete physical examination to rule out signs of systemic infection.
   B. **Laboratory studies**

1. ***Always* obtain a gram-stained smear of the discharge** to check for white blood cells (a sign of infection) and bacteria to identify the specific organism.
   a. *N gonorrhoeae* conjunctivitis: Gram-negative intracellular diplococci and white blood cells are seen.
   b. *S aureus* conjuctivitis: Gram-positive cocci in clusters and white blood cells are seen.
   c. *P aeruginosa* conjunctivitis: Gram-negative bacilli and white blood cells are found.
   d. Chemical conjunctivitis, lacrimal duct obstruction, and *C trachomatis* conjunctivitis: The gram-stained smear will be negative.
   e. Conjunctivitis caused by *Haemophilus* species: Gram-negative coccoid rods are seen.
   f. Streptococcal or pneumococcal conjunctivitis: Streptococci are gram-positive spherical cocci and pneumococci are gram-positive lancet-shaped encapsulated diplococci.
2. **If a chlamydial infection is suspected, material is gathered for Giemsa staining by scraping (*not swabbing*) the lower conjunctiva** with a wire loop or blunt spatula to obtain epithelial cells. If chlamydial infection is present, **inclusion bodies** will be seen within the epithelial cells.
3. **A sample of the discharge should be submitted for culture and sensitivity testing.** It will verify the specific organism seen on gram-stained smear and will indicate antibiotic sensitivities.

C. **Radiologic and other studies.** None are usually needed.

V. **Plan.** Based on the results of Gram's stain and Giemsa's stain, empiric treatment should be started after a specimen of the discharge is sent to the laboratory for culture rather than waiting for the results.

A. **Chemical conjunctivitis.** Observation only is needed. This disorder usually resolves within 48–72 hours.

B. **Gonococcal conjunctivitis**
   1. Isolate the infant during the first 24 hours of parenteral antibiotic therapy.
   2. New data suggests Ceftriaxone sodium 50 mg/kg/d IV or IM given once a day is recommended as initial therapy depending on culture if organism is penicillin sensitive. Or give penicillin G, 50,000 units/kg/d in 2 divided doses for 7–10 days.
   3. Irrigate the eyes with sterile isotonic saline solution every 1–2 hours until clear.
   4. Because gonococcal opthalmia can lead to blindness, an ophthalmologic consultation is usually requested.

C. **Staphylococcal conjunctivitis**
   1. Isolate the infant to prevent spread of infection.
   2. Treat the infant with either topical 10% sodium sulfacetamide or erythromycin ointment, 2–4 times per day for 7–10 days.

D. **Chlamydial conjunctivitis**
   1. Treat the infant with either 10% sulfonamide ophthalmic suspension or erythromycin ophthalmic ointment 4 times per day for 2 weeks.
   2. Erythromycin suspension, 40 mg/kg/d orally for 2 weeks, is often recommended because of the high recurrence rate of this infection.

E. **Pseudomonal conjunctivitis**
   1. Isolate the patient.
   2. Treat the conjunctivitis with gentamicin ophthalmic ointment 4 times per day for 2 weeks.
   3. Gentamicin (see Chap 76) should also be given intravenously because sepsis may follow pseudomonal conjunctivitis.
   4. Because this infection may be devastating, an ophthalmologist should be consulted.

be treated effectively with ocular sodium sulfacetamide drops for 7–10 days.

G. Lacrimal duct obstruction
   1. Most obstructions clear spontaneously without treatment.
   2. Massaging the inside corner of the eye over the lacrimal sac, with expression toward the nose, may help to establish patency.
   3. If the problem does not resolve in the first few months of life, the infant should be evaluated by an ophthalmologist.

34 Gastric Aspirate (Residuals)

I. **Problem.** The nurse alerts you that a gastric aspirate has been obtained in an infant. Gastric aspiration is a procedure by which the stomach is aspirated with an oral or nasogastric tube. The procedure is usually performed before each feeding to determine whether the feedings are being tolerated and digested.

II. **Immediate questions**

A. **What is the volume of the aspirate?** A volume of more than 30% of the total formula given at the last feeding may be abnormal and requires more extensive evaluation.

B. **What is the character of the aspirate (ie, bilious, bloody, undigested, digested)?** This is important in the differential diagnosis (see **III.A**).

C. **Are the vital signs normal?** Abnormal vital signs may indicate a pathologic process, possibly an intra-abdominal process.

D. **Is the abdomen soft, with good bowel sounds, or distended, with visible bowel loops?** Absence of bowel sounds, distention, tenderness, and erythema are signs of peritonitis. Absence of bowel sounds may also indicate ileus.

E. **When was the last stool passed?** Constipation resulting in abdominal distention may cause feeding intolerance and increased gastric aspirates.

III. **Differential diagnosis.** The characteristics of the aspirate can provide important clinical clues to the cause of the problem and are outlined below, followed by a differential listing of causes of increased gastric aspirates.

A. **Based on nature of aspirate**

1. **Bilious in color.** This type of aspirate is usually a serious problem, especially if it occurs in the first 72 hours of life. This type of aspirate may be secondary to bowel obstruction, ileus, or, less commonly, to misplacement of the nasogastric tube (too distally in the duodenum). It can also be idiopathic. One study found that 31% of infants with bilious vomiting in the first 72 hours of life had obstruction, of which 20% required surgery. The most common surgical lesion was malrotation of the intestine.

2. **Bloody in color.** This type of aspirate may be caused by trauma from nasogastric intubation, a bleeding disorder (vitamin K deficiency, disseminated intravascular coagulation), stress ulcer, or necrotizing enterocolitis.

3. **Reflux containing undigested formula** may be seen if the interval between feedings is too short.

4. **Aspirate containing digested formula** may be a sign of delayed gastric emptying or overfeeding. Also, if the osmolarity of the formula is increased by the addition of vitamins, retained digested formula may be seen.

B. **Causes of gastric aspirate**

1. **Gastrointestinal obstruction** (eg, pyloric stenosis, malrotation) may cause gastric aspirate.

2. **Sepsis** may produce ileus, which may be responsible for a gastric aspirate.

3. **Formula intolerance** is an uncommon cause of aspirate but should nonetheless be considered. Some infants do not tolerate the carbo-

hydrate source in some formulas. If the infant is receiving a lactose-containing formula (eg, Enfamil, Similac), a stool pH should be performed to rule out lactose intolerance. If the stool pH is acidic (< 5.0), lactose intolerance may be present. In these cases, there is usually a strong family history of milk intolerance.

4. **Problems with feeding regimen.** Undigested or digested formula may be seen in the aspirate if the feeding regimen is too aggressive. This problem is especially likely in small premature infants who are given a small amount of formula initially and then are given larger volumes too rapidly. **Reflux containing undigested formula** can be seen if the feeding interval is too short. **Reflux containing digested formula** suggests overfeeding or a problem with the use of a hyperosmolar formula, which is most often caused by the addition of vitamins to the formula.

5. **Constipation.** If the abdomen is full but soft and the infant has not passed a stool in 48–72 hours, constipation may be the problem. The aspirate is usually not bloody or bilious.

6. **Factitious.** Passage of a feeding tube into the duodenum instead of the stomach may cause a bilious aspirate.

7. **Hemorrhage.** Hemorrhage due to either traumatic tube insertion or another cause listed in **III.A.2, p 191,** may be responsible for a bloody aspirate.

IV. **Data base**

A. **Physical examination.** Perform a complete physical examination, paying particular attention to the abdomen. Check for bowel sounds (absent bowel sounds may indicate ileus or peritonitis), abdominal distention, tenderness to palpation and erythema of the abdomen (this may signify peritonitis), or visible bowel loops. Check for hernias, as they may cause obstruction.

B. **Laboratory studies**

1. **A complete blood count with differential** is performed to evaluate for sepsis if suspected. The hematocrit and platelet count may be checked if bleeding has occurred.

2. **Blood culture** is performed if sepsis is suspected and before antibiotics are started.

3. **Serum potassium level.** If ileus is present, a serum potassium level should be obtained to rule out hypokalemia.

4. **Stool pH.** If there is a family history of milk intolerance, a stool pH should be obtained to rule out lactose intolerance (stool pH will usually be < 5.0). It is more common to see diarrhea than gastric aspirates with lactose intolerance.

5. **Coagulation profile (prothrombin time [PT], partial thromboplastin time [PTT], fibrinogen and platelets).** A bloody aspirate may signify the presence of a coagulopathy, and in this case, coagulation studies should be obtained.

C. **Radiologic and other studies**

1. **Plain x-ray film (flatplate) of the abdomen.** A plain x-ray film of the abdomen should be obtained if the aspirate is bilious, if there is any abnormality on physical examination, or if aspirates continue. The x-ray film will show whether the nasogastric tube is in the correct position and will define the bowel gas pattern. Look for an unusual gas pattern, pneumatosis intestinalis, ileus, or evidence of bowel obstruction.

2. **Upright x-ray film of the abdomen.** If bowel obstruction is suspected on the film, obtain an upright x-ray film of the abdomen and look for air-fluid levels.

V. **Plan.** The approach to management of the neonate with increased gastric aspirates is most often initially based on the nature of the aspirate.

A. Bilious aspirate
   1. Bowel obstruction. A nasogastric tube should be placed for decompression of the stomach. Consultation with a pediatric surgeon should be obtained immediately.
   2. Ileus. If ileus is diagnosed, the patient is fed nothing orally and a nasogastric tube is placed for decompression of the stomach. Ileus in the neonate may be secondary to the following underlying causes, which should be treated if possible.
   a. Sepsis.
   b. Necrotizing enterocolitis.
   c. Prematurity.
   d. Hypokalemia.
   e. Effects of maternal drugs (especially magnesium sulfate).
   f. Pneumonia.
   g. Hypothyroidism.
B. Bloody aspirate
   1. Nasogastric trauma. (See p 196.)
   2. Gastrointestinal hemorrhage
   a. Stress ulcer
      (1) Stress ulcer is treated with **gastric lavages of tepid water, ½ normal saline, or normal saline**—5 mL/kg given by nasogastric tube until the bleeding has subsided. (**Note:** There is controversy about which fluid to use. Some clinicians feel that if water is used, hyponatremia may occur, and if normal saline is used, hypernatremia may occur. Follow your institution's guidelines. Never use cold water lavages, because they lower the infant's core temperature too rapidly.)
      (2) If the above lavages do not stop the bleeding, a **lavage of 0.1 mL of 1:10,000 epinephrine solution in 10 mL of sterile water** can be used. This recommendation is also controversial.
      (3) The infant is usually started on **ranitidine or cimetidine.** (See Chap 75 for dosages and other pharmacologic information.) Ranitidine is usually preferred because it has fewer side effects.
      (4) Antacids may be used (eg, Maalox 2–5 mL, depending on the size of the infant, placed in the nasogastric tube every 4 hours until bleeding has subsided), but this recommendation is also controversial; some clinicians feel that it may cause concretions in the gastrointestinal tract.
   b. Disseminated intravascular coagulation (DIC). If clotting studies are abnormal and if gastrointestinal hemorrhage and hemorrhage at other sites are occurring, the cause of the coagulopathy must be identified and treated. Immediate transfusion of blood or fresh-frozen plasma, or both, may be needed, depending on the amount of blood loss and blood pressure levels. Platelets may have to be given, depending on the platelet count.
   c. Vitamin K deficiency. Hemorrhage may occur if vitamin K injection was not given at birth. Vitamin K_1 (1 mg intramuscularly or intravenously) needs to be given.
   d. Necrotizing enterocolitis. See Chap 66.
C. Aspirate containing undigested formula. If the volume of undigested formula in the aspirate does not exceed 30% of the previous feeding and the physical examination and vital signs are normal, the volume can be replaced. The time interval between feedings may not be long enough for digestion to take place. If the infant is being fed every 2 hours and aspirates continue, the feeding interval may be increased to 3 hours. If aspirates still continue, the patient must be reevaluated. An

abdominal x-ray film should be obtained. The patient may have to be fed intravenously to allow the gut to rest.

D. Aspirate containing digested formula. This aspirate is usually discarded, especially if it contains a large amount of mucus. If the physical examination and vital signs are normal, continue feedings and aspiration of stomach contents. If reflux continues, the patient must be reassessed. An abdominal film must be taken, and oral feedings should be discontinued for a time to let the gut rest. The number of calories given should be calculated to make certain that overfeeding (usually > 130 kcal/kg/d) is not occurring.

E. Sepsis. If sepsis is likely, broad-spectrum antibiotics are started after a laboratory workup is performed. A penicillin (usually ampicillin) and an aminoglycoside (usually gentamicin) are given initially, until culture results are obtained (see Chap 75 for drug dosages and other pharmacologic information). The patient is usually not fed orally if this diagnosis is entertained; an infant with sepsis usually does not tolerate oral feedings.

F. Formula intolerance. A trial of lactose-free formula (eg, ProSobee, Isomil) can be instituted if lactose intolerance is verified.

G. Constipation. Anal stimulation can be attempted. If this fails, a glycerin suppository can be given. (See also Chap 45.)

35 Gastrointestinal Bleeding from the Upper Tract

I. **Problem**. Vomiting of bright red blood or active bleeding from the nasogastric tube is seen.

II. **Immediate questions**

A. **What are the vital signs?** If the blood pressure is dropping and there is active bleeding from the nasogastric tube, urgent colloid replacement is necessary.

B. **What is the hematocrit?** A spun hematocrit should be done as soon as possible. The result is used as a baseline value and to determine if blood replacement should be done immediately. Remember, with an acute episode of bleeding, the hematocrit may not reflect the blood loss for several hours.

C. **Is blood available in the blood bank should transfusion be necessary?** Verify that the infant has been typed and cross-matched so that blood will be quickly available if necessary.

D. **Is there bleeding from other sites?** Bleeding from other sites suggests disseminated intravascular coagulation or another coagulopathy. If bleeding is coming only from the nasogastric tube, disorders such as stress ulcer, nasogastric trauma, and swallowing of maternal blood are likely causes to consider in the differential diagnosis.

E. **How old is the infant?** During the first day of life, vomiting of bright red blood or the presence of bright red blood in the nasogastric tube is frequently secondary to swallowing of maternal blood during delivery. Infants with this problem are clinically stable, with normal vital signs.

F. **What medications are being given?** Certain medications are associated with an increased incidence of gastrointestinal bleeding. The most common of these medications are indomethacin (Indocin), tolazoline (Priscoline), and corticosteroids.

G. **Was vitamin K given at birth?** Failure to give vitamin K at birth may result in a bleeding disorder, usually at 3–4 days of life.

III. **Differential diagnosis**

A. **Idiopathic etiology.** More than 50% of cases have no clear diagnosis.

B. **Coagulopathy.** Hemorrhagic disease of the newborn and disseminated intravascular coagulation account for approximately 20% of cases.

C. **Swallowing of maternal blood.** This accounts for about 10% of cases. Typically, in these cases blood is swallowed during cesarean section delivery.

D. **Stress ulcer.**

E. **Nasogastric trauma.**

F. **Necrotizing enterocolitis.** This is a rare cause of upper GI tract bleeding.

G. **Drug-induced bleeding.** Indomethacin, corticosteroids, tolazoline, and other drugs may cause upper GI tract bleeding.

IV. **Data base**

A. **Physical examination.** A complete physical examination should be performed, paying particular attention to observation of other possible bleeding sites.

B. Laboratory studies

1. **Apt test.** The Apt test should be performed if swallowing of maternal blood is a possible cause (see p 178, **B.1**).
2. **Hematocrit** should be checked as a baseline and serially to gauge the extent of blood loss.
3. **Coagulation studies (prothrombin time [PT], partial thromboplastin time [PTT], fibrinogen, and platelets).** These studies should be done to rule out disseminated intravascular coagulation and other coagulopathies.

C. Radiologic and other studies. An **abdominal x-ray film** should be obtained to assess the bowel gas pattern and to rule out necrotizing enterocolitis. The x-ray film will also show the position of the nasogastric tube.

V. Plan

A. General measures. The most important goal is to stop the bleeding. This measure should be taken in every case except in infants who have swallowed maternal blood. (Infants with this problem are usually only a few hours old, are not sick, and have a positive Apt test result. Once stomach aspiration is performed, no more blood is obtained.) To help stop an acute episode of gastrointestinal bleeding, the following measures can be used.

1. **Gastric lavage.** The technique for gastric lavage is explained on p 193, **B.2.a(1)**.
2. **Epinephrine lavage** (1:10,000 solution), 0.1 mL diluted in 10 mL of sterile water, can be used if tepid water lavages do not stop the bleeding (*controversial*).
3. **Colloid replacement.** If the blood pressure is low or dropping, colloid (usually Plasmanate or albumin) can be given immediately.
4. **Blood replacement** may be indicated, depending on the result of hematocrit values obtained from the laboratory.

B. Specific measures

1. **Idiopathic.** In cases in which no cause is determined, the bleeding usually subsides and no other treatment is necessary.
2. **Swallowing of maternal blood.** Perform the Apt test to confirm maternal hemoglobin (see p 178, **B.1**). No treatment is necessary.
3. **Stress ulcer.** Stress ulcer is commonly diagnosed following an episode of gastrointestinal bleeding. This disorder is difficult to confirm by radiologic studies, and they are not often obtained. Remission usually occurs; recurrence is rare. Antacids (eg, Maalox) may be given, but it is considered a *controversial* treatment because of the possibility of concretion formation. If used, the dosage for Maalox is 2–5 mL given by nasogastric tube every 4 hours. Ranitidine (now preferred because of less central nervous system, hepatic, and platelet side effects) or cimetidine is often used during the period of bleeding (see Chap 75 for dosages and other pharmacologic information).
4. **Nasogastric trauma.** This may occur if the nasogastric tube is too large or insertion is traumatic. Use the smallest nasogastric tube possible. Observation is indicated.
5. **Necrotizing enterocolitis.** Severe cases of necrotizing enterocolitis will cause upper gastrointestinal bleeding. Treatment is discussed in Chapter 66.
6. **Coagulopathy**
   a. **Hemorrhagic disease of the newborn.** This is more common in infants who have not received vitamin K at birth. If the history of vitamin K administration is unknown, give 1 mg vitamin K_1 intramuscularly. Administer it intravenously if active bleeding is occurring.

   b. **Disseminated intravascular coagulation (DIC).** If DIC is present, bleeding from other sites is usually seen. Coagulation studies will be abnormal (increased PT and PTT and decreased fibrinogen levels). Treat the underlying condition and support blood pressure with multiple transfusions of colloid, as needed. Platelets may need to be given. The cause of DIC (eg, hypoxia, acidosis, bacterial or viral disease, toxoplasmosis, necrotizing enterocolitis, shock, erythroblastosis fetalis) must be investigated. Several obstetric disorders, including abruptio placentae, chorioangioma, eclampsia, and fetal death associated with twin gestation, may give rise to DIC.

7. **Drug-induced bleeding.** The drug responsible for the bleeding should be stopped if possible.

36 Conjugated (Direct) Hyperbilirubinemia

I. Problem. An infant's direct (conjugated) serum bilirubin level is 3 mg/dL. (A value greater than 1.5 or 2.0 mg/dL [or a fraction greater than 10% of the total serum bilirubin] is considered abnormal at any age.)

II. Immediate questions

A. Is the infant receiving total parenteral nutrition (TPN)? TPN may cause direct hyperbilirubinemia by an unknown mechanism. It usually does not occur until the infant has been on TPN for 3 to 4 weeks.

B. Is a bacterial or viral infection present? Infection may cause hepatocellular damage, leading to increased direct bilirubin levels.

C. Did direct hyperbilirubinemia occur only after feedings had been established? If this is the case, a metabolic disorder such as galactosemia may be present.

III. Differential diagnosis. This problem usually indicates a serious derangement in hepatic function; therefore it is necessary to pursue a workup for a persistent or increasing high direct bilirubin. (See also Chap 60.)

A. More common causes of direct hyperbilirubinemia. The most common causes are **biliary atresia** and **idiopathic neonatal hepatitis**. Other common causes are:

1. Hyperalimentation.
2. Infection (sepsis or urinary tract infection).
3. Intrauterine infection (TORCH).
4. Acute hemolytic disease.
5. Alpha$_1$-antitrypsin deficiency.
6. Choledochal cyst.
7. Galactosemia.

B. Less common causes of direct hyperbilirubinemia

1. Inspissated bile syndrome.
2. Dubin-Johnson syndrome.
3. Cystic fibrosis.
4. Hypothyroidism.
5. Rotor's syndrome.
6. Storage disease (Niemann–Pick disease, Gaucher's disease).

IV. Data base. A detailed history, including prenatal (to evaluate for intrauterine infection or hemolytic disease) and postnatal (feeding history as well as the presence of any acholic stools) should be obtained.

A. Physical examination. Particular attention should be given to examination of the abdomen. Palpate for an enlarged liver or spleen. Splenomegaly is more common in neonatal hepatitis but can be a late sign in biliary atresia. Check carefully for signs of sepsis.

B. Laboratory studies

1. **For the common causes,** the workup should be as follows:

   a. **Complete blood count and differential** may help to determine if infection is present.

   b. **Coombs' test** may indicate the possibility of hemolytic disease.

   c. **Reticulocyte count** may be elevated (ie, > 4–5%) if bleeding has occurred.

   d. **Liver function tests** should include AST (SGOT), ALT (SGPT), and alkaline phosphatase. Elevated levels of AST and ALT signify hepatocellular damage. Elevated alkaline phosphatase levels may signify biliary obstruction.

  e. **Blood and urine culture.** If sepsis is considered, blood and urine samples must be obtained for culture.

  f. **Testing for viral disease.** Test the serum IgM level. If high, test for TORCH infections (see p 339). Urine is tested for cytomegalovirus and a serum hepatitis profile is obtained (hepatitis surface antigen and IgM hepatitis A antibody).

  g. **Serum alpha$_1$-antitrypsin levels.** These levels are obtained to rule out alpha$_1$-antitrypsin deficiency.

  h. **Clinitest** may be positive in galactosemia.

2. **For the less common causes,** perform the following additional studies.

  a. **Serum thyroxine (T$_4$)** and **thyroid-stimulating hormone (TSH) levels** should be obtained if hypothyroidism is suspected.

  b. **Sweat chloride test.** A quantitative sweat chloride test should be done to rule out cystic fibrosis.

C. **Radiologic and other studies**

1. **Ultrasonography.** Ultrasound examination of the liver and biliary tract will rule out choledochal cyst and will also provide information on the gallbladder.

2. **^{131}I-labeled rose bengal excretion test** will differentiate biliary atresia and idiopathic neonatal hepatitis.

3. **Liver biopsy** is usually performed after all other tests have been done and a definitive diagnosis is still needed.

V. **Plan.** The cause of direct hyperbilirubinemia is determined. If the infant is receiving TPN, it should be stopped. If there are signs of sepsis, appropriate cultures should be sent and empiric antibiotic therapy should be initiated. Supportive measures are indicated for the treatment of idiopathic neonatal hepatitis. The treatment of biliary atresia includes exploratory laparatomy and corrective surgery. For a more detailed description of treatment, see Chapter 60.

37 Unconjugated (Indirect) Hyperbilirubinemia

I. **Problem.** An infant's indirect (unconjugated) serum bilirubin level is 10 mg/dL.

II. **Immediate questions**

A. **How old is the infant?** High indirect serum bilirubin levels during the first 24 hours of life are *never* physiologic. Hemolytic disease (Rh isoimmunization or ABO incompatibility) or infection is a likely cause. The age of the infant helps to determine the bilirubin level at which phototherapy should be initiated.

B. **Is the infant dehydrated?** If the infant is dehydrated, fluid administration may lower the serum bilirubin level. Fluids can be given orally if tolerated; otherwise, intravenous fluids should be given. An example is an infant who is being totally breast-fed, and at 3 days of age the mother's milk has not come in, so the infant becomes dehydrated.

C. **Is the infant being breast-fed?** Breast milk jaundice may be present; the cause is unknown.

III. **Differential diagnosis.** (See also Chap 60.)

A. **More common causes of indirect hyperbilirubinemia**
   1. Physiologic hyperbilirubinemia.
   2. ABO incompatibility.
   3. Breast milk jaundice.
   4. Rh isoimmunization.
   5. Infection.
   6. Subdural hematoma or cephalohematoma.
   7. Excessive bruising.
   8. Infant of diabetic mother.

B. **Less common causes of indirect hyperbilirubinemia**
   1. Glucose-6-phosphate dehydrogenase (G6PD) deficiency.
   2. Pyruvate kinase deficiency.
   3. Hereditary spherocytosis.
   4. Lucey-Driscoll syndrome (familial neonatal jaundice).
   5. Crigler-Najjar disease.
   6. Hypothryoidism.

IV. **Data base.** (See also Chap 60.)

A. **Physical examination.** Particular attention should be paid to signs of bruising, cephalohematoma, or intracranial bleeding.

B. **Laboratory studies**
   1. Total and direct serum bilirubin levels.
   2. Complete blood count and differential.
   3. Mother's blood type with Rh determination.
   4. Infants's blood type with Rh determination.
   5. Direct and indirect Coombs' tests.
   6. Reticulocyte count.
   7. Red blood cell smear. Fragmented red blood cells should be present in hemolysis.

C. **Radiologic and other studies.** None are usually necessary.

V. **Treatment.** (See also Chap 60.)

A. **Phototherapy.** Phototherapy should be initiated according to the guidelines in Appendix I. If phototherapy is used, perform the following additional procedures.

1. **Increase the maintenance infusion of intravenous fluids** by 0.5 mL/kg/h if the infant weighs less than 1500 g and by 1 mL/kg/h if the infant weighs more than 1500 g.
2. **Perform total bilirubin testing** every 6–8 hours.
3. **Attempt regular feedings,** if possible. Feeding increases bilirubin excretion by stooling and increasing the enterohepatic cycle.
4. **Phototherapy can be safely discontinued** once serum bilirubin levels have fallen 2 mg/dL or more below the level at which phototherapy was initiated. Once phototherapy is stopped, a rebound increase in the serum bilirubin level of approximately 2 mg/dL will occur.

B. **Drug therapy.** Phenobarbital has been shown to be effective in reducing the serum bilirubin level by increasing hepatic glucuronyl transferase activity and conjugation of bilirubin. It is usually used in severe cases of prolonged hyperbilirubinemia only. (See Chap 75 for dosage and other pharmacologic information.)

C. **Exchange transfusion** is performed based on the guidelines Appendix F. The procedure for exchange transfusion is outlined in Chapter 21.

38 Hyperglycemia

I. **Problem.** The glucose value is greater than 125 mg/dL on Dextrostix testing or greater than 120 mg/dL on Chemstrip-bG testing. (Hyperglycemia in infants is defined as serum blood glucose levels > 125–150 mg/dL.)

II. **Immediate questions**

A. **What is the serum glucose value on laboratory testing?** Dextrostix values are often inaccurate because the procedure is performed incorrectly or the Dextrostix strips are old and no longer reliable. Chemstrip-bG values are thought to be more reliable by some, but it is best to obtain a serum glucose level from the laboratory before initiating treatment.

B. **Is glucose being spilled in the urine?** A trace amount of glucose in the urine is accepted as normal. If the urinary glucose level is +1, +2, or greater, the renal threshold has been reached and there is an increased chance of osmotic diuresis. Some institutions accept a urinary glucose level of +1 without treating the patient (*controversial*).

C. **How much glucose is the patient receiving?** Normal maintenance glucose therapy in infants not being fed orally is 6 mg/kg/min. To calculate this, see p 59, II.

D. **Are there signs of sepsis?** Sepsis may cause hyperglycemia by inducing a stress response.

III. **Differential diagnosis**

A. **Excess glucose administration.** Incorrect calculation of glucose levels or errors in formulation of intravenous fluids may cause hyperglycemia.

B. **Inability to metabolize glucose** may occur with prematurity or secondary to sepsis or stress.

C. **Transient neonatal diabetes mellitus** is a rare disorder. Most patients with the disorder are term infants with evidence of intrauterine malnutrition. The disorder may present at any time from 2 days up to 6 weeks of age. The most common findings are hyperglycemia, dehydration, glycosuria, and acidosis.

D. **Medications** such as maternal use of diazoxide and theophylline use in the infant may cause hyperglycemia.

IV. **Data base**

A. **Physical examination.** Perform a complete physical examination. Look for subtle signs of sepsis (eg, temperature instability, changes in peripheral perfusion, or any changes in gastric aspirates if the infant is feeding).

B. **Laboratory studies**

1. **Serum glucose level.** Confirm the rapid paper-strip test result with a serum glucose level.

2. **Urine dipstick testing for glucose level.**

3. **Complete blood count and differential** are performed as screening tests for sepsis.

4. **Blood and urine cultures** are indicated if sepsis is suspected and if antibiotics are to be started.

5. **Serum electrolytes.** Hyperglycemia may cause osmotic diuresis, which may lead to electrolyte losses and dehydration. Therefore it is important to follow serum electrolyte levels in hyperglycemic patients.

C. **Radiologic and other studies.** None are usually required; however, a chest x-ray study may be useful in the evaluation of sepsis.

V. **Plan**

A. **Excess glucose administration**

1. **Positive urinary glucose level.** Decrease the amount of glucose being given by decreasing the concentration of dextrose in intravenous fluids or by decreasing the infusion rate. Most infants who are not feeding require approximately 6 mg/kg/min of glucose to maintain normal glucose levels. Use Dextrostix or Chemstrip-bG testing every 4–6 hours and check for glucose in the urine with each voiding.

2. **Negative urinary glucose level.** If glucose is being given to increase the caloric intake, it is acceptable to have a higher serum glucose level as long as glucose is not being spilled in the urine. Perform Dextrostix and urinary glucose testing every 4–6 hours.

B. **Inability to metabolize glucose.** Sepsis should always be considered in an infant with hyperglycemia. If the blood count looks suspicious or if there are clinical signs of sepsis, it is acceptable to treat the infant for 3 days with antibiotics and then stop if cultures are negative. Ampicillin and an aminoglycoside are usually given initially (see Chap 76 for dosages and other pharmacologic information). Treatment of infants unable to metabolize glucose for any reason is described below.

1. **Decrease the concentration of glucose or the rate of infusion until a normal serum glucose level is present.** Do not use a solution that has a dextrose concentration of less than 4.7%. Such a solution is hyposomolar and could cause hemolysis, with resulting hyperkalemia. If a glucose concentration of less than 4.7% is used, electrolytes should be added.

2. **Insulin.** Insulin administration is usually not recommended in neonates because of their erratic response. If insulin is used, it can be given in one of 2 ways.

a. An insulin **infusion** may be given at a rate of 0.1/units/kg/h. Albumin, which used to be added to the bag to prevent adherence of the insulin to the plastic tubing, is now considered unnecessary. It is currently thought that by simply flushing the solution with an adequate amount of the insulin-containing solution, all binding sites and the tubing will be saturated satisfactorily prior to the beginning the insulin infusion. Dexstrostix testing must be performed every 30 minutes until the level of glucose is stable.

b. Insulin may be given **subcutaneously,** 0.1 unit/kg. Chemstrip-bG testing (or Dextrostix testing) must be performed every 30 minutes until the glucose level is stable.

C. **Transient neonatal diabetes mellitus**

1. **Give intravenous (or oral) fluids** and follow the urine output, blood pH, and serum electrolyte levels.

2. **Give insulin,** either by constant infusion or subcutaneously, 1–2 units/kg/d. Follow glucose levels with Chemstrip-bG testing (or Dextrostix testing) every 4–6 hours. This disease usually resolves in a period of days to weeks.

D. **Medications**

1. If the infant is receiving **theophylline,** the serum theophylline level should be checked to detect possible toxicity, with resulting hyperglycemia. Other signs of theophylline toxicity include tachycardia, jitteriness, feeding intolerance, and seizures. If the level is high, the dosage must be altered or the drug discontinued.

2. With maternal use of **diazoxide,** the infant may have tachycardia and hypotension as well as hyperglycemia. Toxicity in the infant is usually self-limited, and only observation is usually necessary.

39 Hyperkalemia

I. **Problem.** The serum potassium level is greater than 5.5 meq/dL. (Normal potassium levels are 3.5–5.5 meq/dL.)
II. **Immediate questions**
   A. **How was the specimen collected and what is the central serum potassium level?** Blood obtained by heelstick may yield falsely elevated potassium levels secondary to hemolysis. Blood drawn through a tiny needle may cause hemolysis and falsely elevated potassium levels.
   B. **How much potassium is the infant receiving?** Normal amounts of potassium given for maintenance are 1–3 meq/kg/d.
   C. **Does ECG show cardiac changes characteristic of hyperkalemia?** Early cardiac changes include tall, "tented" T waves. Late signs include a wide QRS complex; wide, flat P waves; ventricular fibrillation; and cardiac arrest.
   D. **What are the blood urea nitrogen and creatinine levels? What is the urine output and weight?** Elevated blood urea nitrogen and creatinine measurements indicate renal insufficiency. Another indication of renal failure is decreasing or inadequate urine output with weight gain.
III. **Differential diagnosis**
   A. **Falsely elevated potassium level.** This is usually caused by hemolysis during phlebotomy or heelstick or by drawing of blood proximal to an intravenous site.
   B. **Excess potassium administration.**
   C. **Pathologic hemolysis of red blood cells.** This may be secondary to intraventricular hemorrhage, use of a hypotonic glucose solution (< 4.7% dextrose), or Rh incompatibility.
   D. **Renal failure.**
   E. **Metabolic acidosis.** Systemic acidosis causes potassium to move out of cells, resulting in hyperkalemia. For every 0.1 unit decrease in pH, the serum potassium will increase approximately 0.3–1.3 meq/L.
   F. **Tissue necrosis.** In certain disease states, such as necrotizing enterocolitis (NEC), tissue necrosis can occur and hyperkalemia may result.
IV. **Data base**
   A. **Physical examination.** Perform a complete physical examination, paying special attention to the abdomen for signs of NEC (abdominal distention, decreased bowel sounds, visible bowel loops).
   B. **Laboratory studies**
      1. **Serum potassium level.**
      2. **Serum ionized and total calcium levels.** Because hypocalcemia may potentiate the effects of hyperkalemia, maintain normal serum calcium concentrations.
      3. **Serum pH.** The serum pH is obtained to rule out acidosis, which may potentiate hyperkalemia.
      4. **Blood urea nitrogen and serum creatinine levels** may reveal renal insufficiency.
      5. **Urine specific gravity** is obtained to assess renal status.
   C. **Radiologic studies**
      1. **Abdominal x-ray study.** If necrotizing enterocolitis is suspected, an abdominal x-ray film should be obtained.
      2. **Electrocardiography.** ECG may reveal the cardiac changes charac-

teristic of hyperkalemia and will provide a baseline study (see **II.C**, p 204).

V. Plan

A. Hyperkalemia without ECG changes

1. Stop administration of potassium in intravenous fluids; also consider stopping any potassium-containing medications.
2. Check the serum potassium level frequently (every 4–6 hours).
3. Furosemide (Lasix) can be given if renal function is adequate; the usual dose is 1 mg/kg given intravenously (*controversial*). (See Chap 75.)
4. Sodium polystyrene sulfonate (Kayexalate), a potassium-exchange resin, can be given. The usual dose is 1 g/kg/dose orally every 6 hours or rectally every 2–6 hours. (See Chap 75.)
5. Insulin and glucose can be used (see **B.4**, below).

B. Hyperkalemia with ECG changes (See p 204, **II.C**.)

1. Stop administration of potassium in intravenous fluids.
2. Give sodium bicarbonate; the usual dose is 1 meq/kg intravenously. Inducing alkalosis will drive potassium ions into the cells.
3. Give calcium gluconate; the usual dose is 50 mg/kg/dose intravenously. Calcium provides some protection for the heart from the effects of hyperkalemia.
4. Glucose and insulin may be given to drive potassium into the cells. The usual dose is 250–500 mg/kg/dose of dextrose intravenously, followed by regular insulin, 0.2 unit/kg/dose intravenously over 1 hour. Monitor the infant for hypoglycemia.
5. Start administration of sodium polystyrene sulfonate (see **A.4**, above). It will lower the potassium level slowly and is therefore of limited value acutely.

C. Refractory hyperkalemia. If all of the above measures fail to lower the potassium level, other measures, such as exchange transfusion with freshly washed red blood cells, hemofiltration, and renal dialysis, must be considered.

40 Hypertension

I. **Problem.** An infant has a systolic blood pressure greater than 90 mm Hg. Hypertension is defined as a blood pressure greater than two standard deviations above normal values for age and weight. The values for normal blood pressure are given in Appendix C, Figure C–1.

II. **Immediate questions**

A. **How was the blood pressure taken?** Doppler flow ultrasonography is the most reliable noninvasive method of measurement. The size of the cuff is important. The cuff should encircle two-thirds of the length of the upper extremity. If the cuff is too narrow, the blood pressure will be falsely elevated. If measurements are taken by means of an umbilical artery catheter, be certain the catheter is free of bubbles or clots and the transducer is calibrated.

B. **Is an umbilical artery catheter in place, or has one been in place in the past?** Umbilical artery catheters are associated with an increased incidence of renovascular hypertension. There is no relation between the time the catheter is in and the development of hypertension. A catheter-related aortic thrombosis can also produce hypertension.

C. **Are symptoms of hypertension present?** Infants with hypertension may be asymptomatic or may have the following symptoms: tachypnea, cyanosis, seizures, lethargy, increased tone, apnea, abdominal distention, fever, and mottling. They may also present with congestive heart failure and respiratory distress.

D. **What is the blood pressure in the extremities?** The blood pressure in a normal infant should be higher in the legs than in the arms. If the pressure is lower in the legs, coarctation of the aorta may be the cause of the hypertension.

E. **What is the birth weight and postnatal age of the infant?** The normal blood pressure values increase with increasing birth weight and age. Values rise approximately 1–2 mm Hg per day during the first week of life and then approximately 1–2 mm Hg per week over the next 6 weeks.

F. **Is the infant in pain or agitated?** Pain (such as that from a surgical procedure), crying, agitation, or suctioning can all cause a temporary rise in blood pressure.

III. **Differential diagnosis**

A. **More common causes**
1. Renal artery thrombosis.
2. Aortic thrombosis.
3. Obstructive uropathy.
4. Infantile polycystic kidneys.
5. Renal failure.
6. Medications such as theophylline and corticosteroids.
7. Fluid overload.
8. Pain, agitation.
9. Bronchopulmonary dysplasia (BPD). Approximately 40% of patients with BPD have hypertension. The etiology is probably multifactorial (increased renin activity and catecholamine secretion may be associated with chronic lung disease).
10. Coartation of the aorta.

B. **Less common causes**

   1. Renal artery stenosis. The infant will be hypertensive from birth.
   2. Renal vein thrombosis.
   3. Hypoplasia or dysplasia of the kidneys.
   4. Pyelonephritis.
   5. Medications such as ocular phenylephrine, pancuronium, dopa-
      mine, and epinephrine.
   6. Primary hyperaldosteronism.
   7. Neuroblastoma or pheochromocytoma.
   8. Hyperthyroidism.
   9. Increased intracranial pressure secondary to intracranial hemor-
      rhage, hydrocephalus, meningitis, or subdural hemorrhage.
   10. Closure of abdominal wall defects.
   11. Seizures.

IV. Data base
A. Physical examination
   1. **Check the femoral pulse,** which is absent or decreased in coarcta-
      tion of the aorta.
   2. **Examine the abdomen** carefully for masses and to determine the
      size of the kidneys. An enlarged kidney may indicate tumor, poly-
      cystic kidneys, obstruction, or renal vein thrombosis.
B. Laboratory studies. See Figure 40–1 for complete evaluation.
   1. **Assessment of renal function.** To assess renal function, perform the
      following tests.
      a. **Serum creatinine and blood urea nitrogen levels.** Elevated serum
         creatinine and blood urea nitrogen levels may indicate renal in-
         sufficiency, which may be associated with hypertension.
      b. **Urinalysis.** Red cells in the urine suggest obstruction, infection,
         or renal vein thrombosis.
      c. **Urine culture.**
      d. **Serum electrolytes and carbon dioxide.** A low serum potassium
         level and high carbon dioxide level will be seen in primary hyper-
         aldosteronism.
   2. **Plasma renin levels** may be elevated in patients with renovascular
      disease. Levels will be low in patients with primary hyperaldos-
      teronism.
C. Radiologic and other studies
   1. **Abdominal ultrasonography.** The preferred screening test in neo-
      nates to detect abdominal masses as well as kidney obstruction.
      Doppler flow ultrasonography can screen for arterial or venous prob-
      lems.
   2. **Cranial ultrasonography.** To rule out intraventricular hemorrhage.
   3. **Echocardiography.** If a disease such as coarctation is suspected.
   4. **Intravenous pyelography.** Usually of limited value in the newborn
      due to poor renal concentrating ability.
   5. **Further studies.** The following invasive procedures and laboratory
      studies are sometimes done to further evaluate the infant with hy-
      pertension.
      a. **Arteriography** to evaluate renovascular disease **or venacavagra-**
         phy to evaluate renal vein thrombosis.
      b. **Renal vein renin level** to further evaluate renovascular disease.
      c. **Renal biopsy** to rule out any underlying renal disease.
      d. **24-Hour urinary catecholamines** to evaluate for pheochromocy-
         toma.
      e. **Urinary 17-hydroxysteroid and 17-ketosteroid levels** to evaluate
         for Cushing's syndrome and congenital adrenal hyperplasia.
      f. **Lumbar puncture and cerebrospinal fluid examination** to rule out
         meningitis.

V. Plan

FIGURE 40-1. Evaluation of hypertension in the newborn. (Modified and reproduced, with permission, from Adelman RD: Hypertension in infants. *Pediatr Ann* [Sept] 1989; **18**:568.)

*Urinalysis, urine culture, blood urea nitrogen, creatinine, electrolytes, carbon dioxide, plasma renin activity

A. **General.** Treat any obvious underlying condition. Stop medications if they are causing hypertension. Correct fluid overload by decreasing fluids and administering diuretics.

B. **Drug therapy.** To guide drug therapy, decide if the hypertension is mild, moderate, or life-threatening. (Dosages and other pharmacologic information for the following drugs are given in Chapter 75.)

1. **Life-threatening hypertension** (blood pressure extremely high and symptoms present). Give nitroprusside (Nipride) or diazoxide (Hyperstat).

2. **Moderate hypertension**
   a. Give hydralazine alone.
   b. Give hydralazine in combination with a diurectic or a beta blocker (propranolol).
   c. Give captopril alone. This drug is contraindicated in infants with bilateral renovascular disease.
   d. Either furosemide or chlorothiazide can be used in combination with hydralazine and/or captopril. Propranolol and methyldopa are other drugs that can be used in combination with hydralazine and/or captopril.

3. **Mild hypertension**
   a. Only observation is required for asymptomatic patients.
   b. Diuretics are necessary if nonpharmacologic measures fail.
   c. Hydralazine, a vasodilator, may be used if the above measures fail.

41 Hypoglycemia

I. **Problem.** An infant has a low blood glucose level on Dextrostix or Chemstrip-bG testing. (Hypoglycemia is defined as a blood sugar less than 40 mg/dL in a term or premature infant.)

II. **Immediate questions**

A. **Has the value been repeated, and has a serum blood sugar been sent to the laboratory?** Dextrostix or Chemstrip-bG strips can sometimes give incorrect values if the test is not done properly or if the strips used are too old. Send a serum sample to the laboratory before starting treatment.

B. **Is the infant symptomatic?** Symptoms of hypoglycemia include apnea, hypotonia, inadequate sucking reflex, cyanosis, high-pitched cry, jitteriness, seizures, lethargy, and temperature instability.

C. **Is the mother a diabetic?** Infants of diabetic mothers have approximately a 40% chance of having hypoglycemia. Diabetic mothers have fluctuating hyperglycemia that causes fetal hyperglycemia. This fetal hyperglycemia causes pancreatic B cell hyperplasia, which in turn causes hyperinsulinism. After delivery, hyperinsulinism persists and hypoglycemia results.

D. **How much glucose is the infant receiving?** The normal glucose requirement is 6 mg/kg/min. If the glucose order was written arbitrarily and not calculated on the basis of the body weight, the infant may not be getting enough glucose. (See p 59, **II,** for glucose calculations.)

III. **Differential diagnosis**

A. **Decreased glycogen stores**
   1. Intrauterine growth retardation (IUGR) or small for gestational age (SGA).
   2. Premature infants.
   3. Postmature infants.

B. **Increased circulating insulin**
   1. Infant of diabetic mother (IODM).
   2. Beckwith-Wiedemann syndrome (visceromegaly, macroglossia, and hypoglycemia).
   3. Maternal drugs such as beta-sympathomimetic agents (eg, terbutaline, ritodrine) or chlorpropamide.
   4. Islet cell dysplasias.
   5. Insulin-producing tumors such as nesidioblastoma.

C. **Insufficient amount of glucose administered.** See **II.D,** above.

D. **Endocrine disorders**
   1. Panhypopituitarism.
   2. Growth hormone deficiency.
   3. Hypothyroidism.
   4. Cortisol deficiency.
   5. Defects in metabolism.
      a. Amino-acid metabolism (maple syrup urine disease, methylmalonic acidemia, hereditary tyrosinemia, and propionicacidemia).
      b. Carbohydrate metabolism (galactosemia, fructose intolerance, and type 1 glycogen storage disease).

D. **Other causes**
   1. Sepsis.

    2. Asphyxia.
    3. Hypothermia.
    4. Polycythemia.
    5. Shock.
    6. Maternal use of propranolol.

IV. Data base
  A. History and physical examination. Evaluate the infant for symptoms of hypoglycemia (see p 210, II.B). Are there signs of sepsis, shock, or Beckwith-Wiedemann syndrome?
  B. Laboratory studies
    1. A serum glucose level should be obtained to confirm paper strip determination.
    2. Complete blood count and differential should be obtained to evaluate for sepsis and to rule out polycythemia.
    3. Serum laboratory studies. The following studies should be done on any infant with persistent hypoglycemia not responding to the usual management.
      a. Insulin.
      b. Growth hormone.
      c. Cortisol.
      d. Free fatty acids.
      e. Thyroxine (T_4) and thyroid-stimulating hormone (TSH).
      f. Glucagon.
      g. Uric acid.
      h. Lactate.
      i. Alanine.
      j. Ketones.
  C. Radiologic and other studies. None are usually necessary.

V. Plan
  A. Overall plan. Attempt to maintain normoglycemia. Infants at risk for hypoglycemia and those with established hypoglycemia should have glucose screening every 1–2 hours until glucose levels are stable, then every 4 hours. Once the glucose level is stable, the next step is the find out why the patient is hypoglycemic. Sometimes the cause is obvious, as in the case of an infant of a diabetic mother or one with intrauterine growth retardation. If the cause is not obvious, further workup is necessary.
    1. Asymptomatic hypoglycemia
      a. Draw a blood sample and send it to the laboratory for a stat baseline serum glucose level.
      b. For infants with Dextrostix values of less than 25 mg/dL or Chemstrip-bG values of less than 20 mg/dL. (confirmed by stat central serum level), **insert an intravenous line and start a glucose infusion** of 6 mg/kg/min (see calculation on p 59), even if the infant is asymptomatic. Initially, glucose levels should be checked every 30 minutes until stable. The infusion should be increased until normoglycemia is achieved. A bolus of glucose in the asymptomatic infant is contraindicated, because it is thought to result in hyperglycemia with rebound hypoglycemia (*controversial*).
      c. For infants with Dextrostix values of 25–45 mg/dL or Chemstrip-bG values of 20–40 mg/dL, if there are no risk factors for hypoglycemia and the infant is clinically stable, an **early feeding of D5W** can be given. The glucose levels are followed every 30 minutes until stable, then every 4 hours. If the glucose remains low, an intravenous line will have to be started with a glucose infusion of 6 mg/kg/min.
    2. Symptomatic hypoglycemia (transient)
      a. Draw a sample for a baseline serum glucose level.

    b. Insert an intravenous line and start a glucose infusion. Infuse 2–4 mL/kg of a 10% glucose solution over 2–3 minutes. Then give a continuous infusion of glucose at a rate of 6–8 mg/kg/min and increase the rate as needed to maintain a normal blood glucose (at least 40 mg/dL). The level should be followed every 30 minutes until stable. Remember, the highest concentration of glucose that can be infused through a peripheral line is 12.5%. If a more concentrated solution is required, a central line will have to be placed. Higher concentrations are hypertonic and may damage the veins.

    c. If an intravenous line cannot be started, glucagon (p 468) **can be given to infants with adequate glycogen stores.** This measure may be effective in infants of diabetic mothers. It is not effective in infants who have growth retardation or are small for gestational age, because they have poor glycogen stores.

  3. Persistent hypoglycemia. Endocrinologic consultation should be obtained.

    a. Continue administration of intravenous glucose. Continue to increase the rate of intravenous glucose administration to 16–20 mg/kg/min. Rates higher than 20 mg/kg/min are not usually helpful. If it is evident at this point that the infant still has problems with hypoglycemia, further workup should be done (see **b,** below).

    b. Perform a definitive workup. The definitive workup of an infant with persistent hypoglycemia consists in obtaining a set of laboratory determinations prior to and 15 minutes after the parenteral administration of glucagon (0.3 mg/kg/dose). Laboratory studies include serum glucose, ketones, free fatty acids, lactate, alanine, uric acid, insulin, growth hormone, cortisol, glucagon, T_4, and TSH. The results are interpreted as shown in Table 41–1. The following methods of treatment can be tried while waiting for results of the glucagon test.

      (1) Consider a trial of corticosteroids. The recommended drug is either hydrocortisone sodium succinate (Solu-Cortef), 5 mg/kg/d given intravenously in 4 divided doses, or prednisone, 2 mg/kg/d orally.

      (2) If hypoglycemia persists, the following can be tried for 3 days each (it is not necessary to stop corticosteroids).

        (a) Diazoxide, 8–15 mg/kg/d orally in 3–4 divided doses.

TABLE 41–1. DIAGNOSIS OF PERSISTENT HYPOGLYCEMIA BEFORE AND AFTER PARENTERAL GLUCAGON ADMINISTRATION[a]

	Hyperinsulinism		Hypopituitarism		Metabolic Defect	
	Before	After	Before	After	Before	After
Glucose	↓	↑↑↑	↓	↑/N	↓	↓/N
Ketones	↓	↓	N/↓	N	↑	↑
Free fatty acids	↓	↑	N/↓	N	↑	↑
Lactate	N	N	N	N	↑	↑↑
Alanine	N	?	N	N	↑	↑↑
Uric acid	N	N	N	N	↑	↑↑
Insulin	↑↑	↑↑↑	N/↑	↑	N	↑
Growth hormone	↑	↓	↓	↓	↑	↑
Cortisol	↑	↓	↓[b]	↓[b]	↑	↑
TSH and T_4	N	N	↓[b]	↓[b]	N	N

[a] N, normal or no change; ↑, elevated; ↓, lowered; ?, unknown.
[b] Response may vary, depending on the degree of hypopituitarism.
Courtesy of Marvin Cornblath, MD, Baltimore, Maryland.

      (b) Human growth hormone (Somatrem, Protropin) 0.1 unit/d intramuscularly.

      (c) Surgery to remove most of the pancreas is the treatment of choice in patients with B-cell hyperplasia or nesidioblastosis.

B. Specific treatment plans

  1. Neonatal hyperinsulinism. Pancreatectomy, removing at least 95% of the organ, is usually necessary.

  2. Congenital hypopituitarism usually responds to administration of cortisone and intravenous glucose. Administration of human growth hormone may be necessary. (See Chap 75 for dosages and other pharmacologic information.)

  3. Metabolic defects

    a. Type I glycogen storage disease. Frequent small feedings with fructose or galactose may be beneficial.

    b. Hereditary fructose intolerance. The infant should be put on a fructose-free diet.

    c. Galactosemia. The infant should be put on a galactose-free diet.

42 Hypokalemia

I. **Problem.** A serum potassium value is less than 3.5 meq/L. (Normal potassium is 3.5–5.5 meq/L.)

II. **Immediate questions**
   A. **What is the central serum potassium?** If a low value is obtained by heelstick, central values should be obtained because they may actually be lower than values obtained by heelstick.
   B. **Are potassium-wasting medications or digitalis being given?** Diuretics may cause hypokalemia. Hypokalemia may cause arrhythmias if digitalis is being given.
   C. **How much potassium is the infant receiving?** Normal maintenance dosages are 1–2 meq/kg/d.
   D. **Is diarrhea occurring or is a nasogastric tube in place?** Loss of large amounts of gastrointestinal fluids can cause hypokalemia.

III. **Differential diagnosis**
   A. **Inadequate maintenance infusion of potassium.**
   B. **Abnormal potassium losses**
      1. **Medications.** Amphotericin B can cause direct renal tubular damage with resulting hypokalemia. Any thiazide diuretic may cause hypokalemia. High and continuous doses of spironolactone with hydrochlorothiazide (Aldactazide) have also resulted in hypokalemia.
      2. **GI tract losses.** Diarrhea and loss of fluid via nasogastric tube may cause hypokalemia.
      3. **Bartter's syndrome,** a rare form of potassium wasting, is characterized by hypokalemia, normal blood pressure, and increased levels of aldosterone and renin.
   C. **Alkalosis (metabolic or respiratory).** An increase in pH by 0.1 unit causes a decrease in the potassium level by 0.3–1.3 meq/L. The decrease is less in respiratory than in metabolic alkalosis.

IV. **Data base**
   A. **Physical examination.** Hypokalemia may cause ileus. Symptoms of hypokalemia include muscle weakness and decreased tendon reflexes, but these are difficult to evaluate in an infant.
   B. **Laboratory studies**
      1. **Repeat measurement of serum potassium level.**
      2. **Spot checks of urinary electrolytes.** Perform periodic spot checks of urinary potassium levels to determine if urinary losses are high.
      3. **Blood gas levels.** Metabolic alkalosis may cause or aggravate hypokalemia (ie, as hydrogen ions leave the cells, potassium ions enter the cells, causing decreased serum potassium levels).
   C. **Radiologic and other studies**
      1. **Abdominal x-ray study.** If ileus is suspected, an abdominal x-ray film should be obtained.
      2. **Electrocardiography.** If hypokalemia is present and the infant is unstable, an ECG may show a prolonged QT interval, flat T wave, and depressed ST segment.

V. **Plan**
   A. **General measures.** Hypokalemia is increasingly becoming a problem in NICUs because of the widespread use of diuretics. The goal of treatment is to increase the potassium intake so that normal blood levels

are achieved and maintained. Short-term potassium administration may cause damage to the veins and, sometimes, hyperkalemia because the potassium does not rapidly equilibrate. Therefore, corrections are given slowly, often over 24 hours. If too large a bolus is given, cardiac arrest may result. Serum potassium levels should be followed every 4–6 hours until correction is achieved. Once levels reach high normal, decrease the amount of potassium given.

B. Specific measures

1. **Inadequate maintenance infusion of potassium.** Calculate the normal maintenance infusion of potassium that should be given and increase the amount accordingly (normal maintenance infusion is 1–2 meq/kg/d).

2. **Abnormal potassium losses**

    a. **Medications.** If the infant is receiving potassium-wasting medications, increase the maintenance dose of potassium. Abnormal potassium loss often occurs in patients with bronchopulmonary dysplasia who are receiving long-term furosemide therapy. Oral supplementation in the form of potassium chloride may be given, 1–2 meq/kg/d in 3–4 divided doses (with feedings). This amount may be increased or decreased, depending on serum potassium levels. Often, a potassium-sparing diuretic (eg, spironolactone) may decrease the amount of potassium supplementation needed.

    b. **Gastrointestinal losses.** Severe diarrhea leading to potassium losses in the stool can be corrected by treating the cause of the diarrhea, withholding oral feedings to allow the gut to rest, and giving intravenous fluids. Potassium supplementation may be given intravenously. The initial intravenous dosage of potassium chloride is 1–2 meq/kg/d. Serum potassium levels are followed, and the intravenous dosage is increased accordingly.

3. **Bartter's syndrome.** Potassium supplementation is given orally, usually at a starting dosage of 2–3 meq/kg/d, which is increased as necessary to maintain a normal serum potassium level.

C. Alkalosis. Determine the cause of metabolic or respiratory alkalosis and treat the underlying disorder.

43 Hyponatremia

I. **Problem.** The serum sodium level is 127 meq/L, below the normal accepted value of 135 meq/L.

II. **Immediate questions**

A. **Are seizures occurring?** Seizure activity is often seen in patients with extremely low serum sodium levels (usually < 120 meq/L). *This event is a medical emergency, and urgent sodium correction is needed.*

B. **How much sodium and free water is the patient receiving? Is weight gain or loss occurring?** Be certain that an adequate amount of sodium is being given and that free water intake is not excessive. The normal amount of sodium intake is 2–3 meq/kg/d. Weight gain with low serum sodium levels is most likely due to volume overload, especially in the first day or two of life, when weight loss is expected.

C. **What is the urine output?** With syndrome of inappropriate secretion of antidiuretic hormone (SIADH), urine output is decreased. If the urine output is increased (> 4 mL/kg/h), perform a spot check of urine sodium to determine if sodium losses are high.

D. **Are renal salt-wasting medications being given?** Diuretics such as furosemide may cause hyponatremia.

III. **Differential diagnosis**

A. **Volume overload (dilutional hyponatremia).**

B. **Inadequate sodium intake.**

C. **Increased sodium loss.** In very low birth weight infants, renal tubular sodium losses are high and an increased amount of sodium is needed (see Chap 7).

D. **Drug-induced hyponatremia** such as with diuretics.

E. **Syndrome of inappropriate secretion of antidiuretic hormone (SIADH).** SIADH is more commonly seen with central nervous system disorders such as intraventricular hemorrhage, hydrocephalus, and birth asphyxia but may also be seen with lung disease. SIADH is often considered in the differential diagnosis of ill patients, but it is not frequently encountered in neonatal nurseries.

IV. **Data base**

A. **Evaluation of bedside chart.** Evaluate the pertinent information on the bedside chart. First, check for **weight loss or gain.** Weight gain is more likely to be associated with dilutional hyponatremia. Next, assess the **urine output and specific gravity.** A low urine output with a high specific gravity is more commonly seen with SIADH. Check the **fluid intake and output** over a 24-hour period. Normally, infants retain two-thirds of the fluid administered, and the rest is lost in the urine or by insensible water loss. If the input is much greater than the output, the patient may be retaining fluid, and dilutional hyponatremia should be considered.

B. **Physical examination.** Perform a complete physical examination. Note signs of seizure activity (abnormal eye movements, jerking of the extremities, tongue thrusting) or volume overload.

C. **Laboratory studies**

1. Serum sodium and osmolality.

2. Urine spot sodium, osmolality, and specific gravity.

The **diagnosis of SIADH** is made by documenting the following on simultaneous laboratory studies: low urine output, urine osmolality greater than serum osmolality, low serum sodium level and low serum osmolality, high urinary sodium level and high specific gravity.

D. **Radiologic and other studies.** Usually, none are needed.

V. Plan

A. **Emergency measures.** If the infant is having **seizures due to hyponatremia** (usually sodium < 120 meq/dL), hypertonic saline solution (3% sodium chloride) should be given. The total body deficit of sodium (see **C.3,** below) is calculated, and half of that is given over 12–24 hours. Rapid corrections may result in brain damage.

B. **Volume overload (dilutional hyponatremia)** is treated with fluid restriction. The total maintenance fluids can be decreased by 20 mL/kg/d, and serum sodium levels should be followed every 6–8 hours.

C. **Inadequate sodium intake**

1. The maintenance sodium requirement for term infants is 2–4 meq/kg/d; it is higher in premature infants (see p 57, **B.2**). Calculate the amount of sodium the patient is receiving, using the equations on page 59, **III.** Readjust the intravenous sodium intake if it is the cause of hyponatremia.

2. If the infant is receiving oral formula only, check the formula being used. Low-sodium formulas include SMA 20 and PM 60/40. Use of supplemental sodium chloride or a formula with a higher sodium content may be necessary.

3. To calculate total sodium deficit the following equation can be used:

Sodium value desired (130–135) −

Infant's sodium value × Weight (kg) × 0.6

The result will be the amount of sodium needed to correct the hyponatremia. Usually only half of this amount is given over 12 to 24 hours.

D. **Increased sodium losses.** Increase sodium administered.

E. **Drug-induced hyponatremia.** If a renal salt-wasting medication such as furosemide (Lasix) is being given, serum sodium levels will be low even though an adequate amount of sodium is being given in the diet. An increase in sodium intake may be required, often the case in infants with bronchopulmonary dysplasia who are receiving furosemide. Most are also receiving oral feedings, so an oral sodium chloride supplement can be used. Start with 1 meq 3 times per day with feedings and adjust as needed. Some infants may require as much as 12–15 meq/d.

F. **Syndrome of inappropriate secretion of antidiuretic hormone (SIADH).** Restrict fluids, usually to 40–60 mL/kg/d. (This regimen does not allow for fluid loss that accompanies the use of a radiant warmer or phototherapy.) Follow the serum sodium level and osmolality and the urine output to determine if the patient is responding. The cause of SIADH is usually obvious, but if it is not, further investigation is needed—for example, ultrasonography of the head to diagnose or rule out intraventricular hemorrhage or hydrocephalus; chest x-ray studies to diagnose or rule out lung pathology.

44 Hypotension and Shock

I. **Problem.** The blood pressure is more than 2 standard deviations below normal for age. (For normal blood pressure values, see Appendix C.)

II. **Immediate questions**

   A. **What method of measurement was used?** If a cuff was used, be certain that it was the correct width (ie, covering two-thirds of the upper arm). A cuff that is too large will give falsely low readings. If measurements were obtained from an indwelling arterial line, a "dampened" waveform suggests there is air in the transducer or tubing or a clot in the system, and the readings may be inaccurate.

   B. **Are symptoms of shock present?** Symptoms of shock include tachycardia, poor perfusion, cold extremities with a normal core temperature, narrow pulse pressure, apnea, tachypnea, metabolic acidosis, and weak pulse.

   C. **Is the urine output acceptable?** Normal urine output is approximately 2 mL/kg/d. Urine output is decreased in shock because of decreased renal perfusion. If the blood pressure is low but the urine output is adequate, aggressive treatment may *not* be necessary, because the renal perfusion is adequate. (*Note:* An exception to this would be an infant with septic shock and hyperglycemia who has osmotic diuresis.)

   D. **Is there a history of birth asphyxia?** Birth asphyxia may be associated with hypotension.

   E. **At the time of delivery, was there maternal bleeding (eg, abruptio placentae or placenta previa) or was clamping of the cord delayed?** These factors may be associated with loss of blood volume in the infant.

III. **Differential diagnosis.** Hypotension, (diminished blood pressure) is distinct from shock, which is a clinical syndrome of inadequate tissue perfusion.

   A. **Hypovolemic shock** may be secondary to antepartum or postpartum blood loss.

      1. **Antepartum blood loss**
         a. Abruptio placentae.
         b. Placenta previa.
         c. Twin-twin transfusion.
      2. **Postpartum blood loss**
         a. Coagulation disorders.
         b. Vitamin K deficiency.
         c. Iatrogenic causes (eg, loss of arterial line).
         d. Birth trauma (eg, liver injury, adrenal hemorrhage).

   B. **Septic shock.** Endotoxemia occurs, with release of vasodilator substances and resulting hypotension. It usually involves gram-negative organisms such as *E. coli* and *Klebsiella* but can also occur with gram-positive organisms such as in group B streptococcal and staphylococcal infections.

   C. **Cardiogenic shock**
      1. **Birth asphyxia.**
      2. **Metabolic problems** (eg, hypoglycemia, hypocalcemia) can cause decreased cardiac output with a decrease in blood pressure.
      3. **Congenital heart disease** (eg, hypoplastic left heart, aortic stenosis).
      4. **Arrhythmias.**

5. **Any obstruction of venous return** (eg, tension pneumothorax).
D. **Neurogenic shock.** Birth asphyxia and intracranial hemorrhage can both cause hypotension.
E. **Drug-induced hypotension.** Certain drugs (eg, tolazoline, tubocurarine, magnesium sulfate, digitalis, barbiturates) will cause vasodilation and a drop in blood pressure.
F. **Endocrine disorders.** Complete 21-hydroxylase deficiency and adrenal hemorrhage are the most notable endocrine disorders that can cause hypotension and shock.

IV. **Data base**
A. **Physical examination.** Particular attention is given to signs of blood loss (eg, intracranial or intra-abdominal bleeding) or sepsis.
B. **Laboratory studies**
1. **Complete blood count with differential.** Decreased hematocrit will identify blood loss; however, the hematocrit can be normal in patients with acute blood loss. Elevated white blood count and differential may help identify sepsis as the cause.
2. **Coagulation studies (prothrombin time [PT] and partial thromboplastin time [PTT]) and platelet count** if disseminated intravascular coagulation is suspected.
3. **Serum glucose and calcium levels** may reveal a metabolic disorder.
4. **Cultures.** Obtain blood and urine for culture and antibiotic sensitivity testing.
5. **Kleihauer-Betke test** should be performed if fetomaternal transfusion is suspected. The test detects the presence of fetal erythrocytes in the mother's blood by a slide elution technique. A smear of maternal blood is fixed and incubated in an acidic buffer. It causes adult hemoglobin to be eluted from erythrocytes; fetal hemoglobin resists elution. After the slide is stained, fetal hemoglobin cells, if present, appear dark, whereas maternal erythrocytes appear clear.
6. **Arterial blood gases** to assess for hypoxia and/or acidosis.
C. **Radiologic and other studies**
1. **Chest x-ray study.** An anteroposterior chest x-ray study should be done to assess the heart and lungs and rule out any mechanical cause of shock (eg, pneumothorax).
2. **Ultrasonography of the head** is done in infants in whom intracranial hemorrhage is suspected.
3. **Electrocardiography** should be performed if an arrhythmia is suspected.
4. **Echocardiography** is performed in birth-asphyxiated infants to assess myocardial function. If there is myocardial failure, drug therapy is needed to improve cardiac output. Echocardiography is also useful to rule out a congenital heart lesion.
5. **Central venous pressure measurement.** A venous umbilical catheter can be placed above the diaphragm to obtain central venous pressure readings. Normal values are 4–6 mm Hg. If these readings are low, hypovolemia is present and transfusion is necessary.

V. **Plan**
A. **General measures**
1. **Rapidly assess the infant and determine what is causing the hypotension** in order to direct treatment accordingly. The basic decision is whether the infant needs volume replacement or administration of inotropic agents. The decision is not difficult in the majority of patients. Four parameters are useful in making this decision.
a. **History.** A history should be obtained to rule out birth asphyxia, blood loss (antepartum or postpartum), drug infusion, and birth trauma (adrenal hemorrhage or liver injury).

     b. Physical examination. A careful physical examination will often reveal which organ systems are involved.

     c. Chest x-ray. A small heart is seen in volume depletion; a large heart is seen in cardiac disease.

     d. Central venous pressure. If it is low (< 4 mm Hg), the infant is volume depleted. If it is high (eg > 6 mm Hg), the infant probably has cardiogenic shock.

  2. If you are still unsure of the cause, start empirical volume expansion with either intravenous colloid or crystalloid (10 mL/kg intravenously over 5–10 min).

     a. If there is a response, continue volume expansion.

     b. If there is no response, an inotropic agent (eg, dopamine) should be started (see p 221, **B.3**).

  3. Provide respiratory support as needed. Blood gas determinations and clinical examinations will dictate whether supplemental oxygen will suffice or whether intubation and mechanical ventilation are necessary.

B. Specific measures

  1. Hypovolemic shock

     a. Volume expansion using either intravenous crystalloid or colloid should be given (see **2,** above for dosage). Colloids such as albumin or plasma protein fraction (Plasmanate) are preferred, but agents such as normal saline or Ringer's lactate may be used in an emergency. The goal is to give a volume expander until adequate tissue perfusion is attained, as evidenced by good urine output and central nervous function. If blood loss has occurred and the patient is severely hypovolemic, immediate volume expansion with colloid or crystalloid is essential. Meanwhile a blood sample should be sent to the laboratory for a hematocrit value, which is used to determine the specific blood products that should be used in blood replacement therapy.

     b. Blood replacement therapy

       (1) Hematocrit less than 40%. Packed red blood cells should be given, 5–10 mL/kg over 30–40 minutes. The following formula may also be used to calculate the volume of packed red blood cells needed. This formula assumes that the total blood volume is 80 mL/kg and the hematocrit (Hct) of the packed red blood cells is 70%.

$$\text{Volume required} = \frac{(\text{Weight [kg]} \times \text{Total blood volume}) \times (\text{Desired Hct} - \text{Patient's Hct})}{\text{Hct of transfusion product}}$$

       (2) Hematocrit over 50%. Plasmanate, albumin, or fresh-frozen plasma (FFP) should be used. FFP is used only if clotting studies are also abnormal.

       (3) Hematocrit of 40–50%. Alternating transfusions of packed red blood cells and Plasmanate or albumin should be given.

  2. Septic shock

     a. Obtain cultures (blood and urine [unless in the first 24 hours of life, obtain only blood]); lumbar puncture for CSF culture and other culture studies as clinically indicated).

     b. Initiate empiric antibiotic therapy after culture specimens have been obtained. **Intravenous ampicillin and gentamicin** are recommended. **Vancomycin** may be substituted for ampicillin if staphylococcal infection is suspected (usually seen in infants more than 3 days old who have invasive monitoring lines or chest tubes in place). Some institutions are advocating the use of **cefotaxime**

with vancomycin instead of gentamicin to avoid the nephrotoxicity. (See Chap 76 for dosages.)

   c. **Use volume expansion and inotropic agents as needed** to maintain adequate tissue and renal perfusion (see p 220, **B.1.a**, and **3**, below).

   d. **Use of corticosteroids.** Intravenous corticosteroid therapy for sepsis is *controversial.* Agents such as dexamethasone have been used, however (see p 462).

   e. **Use of naloxone.** Naloxone has been used in patients with septic shock and persistent hypotension, but its use is *controversial* (see p 474 for dosage).

3. **Cardiogenic shock.** In cardiogenic shock, the goal is to improve cardiac output. Inotropic agents should be used intravenously (see Chap 75 for dosages and other pharmacologic information).

   a. **Dopamine.** Dopamine is the drug of first choice. Previous studies have suggested that higher than traditionally used dosages may be used without causing alpha-adrenergic side effects such as decreased renal perfusion and decreased urine output.

   b. **Dobutamine.** If dopamine fails to improve blood pressure, dobutamine is recommended as a second-line drug. In neonates, it is usually given together with dopamine infusion.

   c. **Other agents.** Epinephrine and isoproterenol are sometimes used.

4. **Neurogenic shock.** Neurogenic shock is treated with volume expansion (see p 220, **B.1.a**) and inotropic agents (see **3**, above).

5. **Drug-induced hypotension.** Volume expansion (see p 220, **B.1.a**) will usually maintain the blood pressure in cases of drug-induced vasodilatation. If the blood pressure cannot be maintained, the drug causing hypotension may need to be discontinued.

6. **Endocrine disorders.**

   a. **Adrenal hemorrhage** is treated with volume expansion and blood replacement (see p 220, **B.1.a,b**) and corticosteroids (see Chap 75).

   b. **Congenital adrenal hyperplasia** is treated with corticosteroids (see Chap 75).

45 No Stool in 48 Hours

I. **Problem.** No stool has been passed in 48 hours.
II. **Immediate questions**
   A. **Has a stool been passed since birth?** If a stool has been passed since birth but not in the last 48 hours, constipation may be the cause. If a stool has never been passed, imperforate anus or some degree of intestinal obstruction may be present. Table 45–1 shows the time after birth at which the first stool is passed. In the first 48 hours of life, 94% of infants will pass a stool.
   B. **What is the gestational age?** Prematurity may be associated with delayed passage of stool because of immaturity of the colon.
   C. **Were maternal drugs used that could cause a paralytic ileus with delayed passage of stool?** Magnesium sulfate, which is used to slow the premature onset of labor, may cause paralytic ileus. Use of heroin by the mother may also cause delayed passage of stool in the infant.
III. **Differential diagnosis**
   A. **Constipation.**
   B. **Anorectal abnormalities such as imperforate anus.**
   C. **Bowel obstruction**
      1. **Meconium plug.** A meconium plug is an obstruction in the lower colon and rectum caused by meconium. It is more common in infants of diabetic mothers (as seen in neonatal small left colon syndrome where the plug extends to the splenic flexure) and in premature infants. (*Note:* A rectal biopsy should be done in all these patients, as they have an increased incidence of Hirshsprung's disease [10–15%].)
      2. **Meconium ileus** occurs when meconium becomes obstructed in the terminal ileum. It is the most common presentation of cystic fibrosis in the neonatal period.
      3. **Hirschsprung's disease** accounts for approximately 15% of infants who have delayed passage of stool. A functional obstruction is caused by aganglionosis of cells in Meissner's and Auerbach's plexus of the colon. The affected segment of colon is aperistaltic.
      4. **Ileal atresia** can occur secondary to meconium ileus, Hirshsprung's

TABLE 45-1. PASSAGE OF FIRST STOOL

	Premature Infant		Term Infant	
	Percentage	Cumulative Percentage	Percentage	Cumulative Percentage
Delivery room	13	13	27.2	27.2
0–24 hours	31.5	44.5	41.8	69
12–24 hours	35.5	80	25	94
24–48 hours	14	94	5.8	99.8
Over 48 hours	6	100	1	100

Based on data from Sherry SN, Kramer I: *J Pediatr* 1955;**46**:158; and Kramer I, Sherry SN: *J Pediatr* 1957;**51**:373.

disease, incarcerated hernia, or intussception. Signs include abdominal distention, bilious vomiting, and failure to pass meconium.

5. **Inspissated milk syndrome.** In this syndrome, milk curds form and obstruct the gut. The infant initially has a normal stooling pattern and is being fed and then has abdominal distention, vomiting, and no stooling.

6. **Adhesions.** Postoperatively, such as after surgery for necrotizing enterocolitis, there is a 30% chance of having adhesions.

7. **Incarcerated hernia.** A hernia is obstructed when its contents cannot be reduced and the bowel is obstructed. Signs include irritability, cramps, bilious vomiting, and abdominal distention. Neonates have a 15–20% risk of incarcerated hernia.

8. **Malrotation.** Malrotation is the failure of the GI tract to properly rotate and adhere. Volvulus is a specific malrotation of the gut and is a **surgical emergency** because it can cause ischemia of the gut, with resulting shock and possibly death. Malrotation without volvulus formation may present with intermittent episodes of vomiting and abdominal distention. The stooling pattern can be normal.

D. **Other causes**
   1. **Ileus** can be secondary to:
      a. Sepsis.
      b. Necrotizing enterocolitis.
      c. Hypokalemia.
      d. Pneumonia.
      e. Maternal use of magnesium sulfate or narcotics.
      f. Hypothyroidism.
   2. **Prematurity** (see II.B, p 222).

IV. **Data base**
   A. **Physical examination.** First, document the patency of the anus. Check for abdominal distention or rigidity, bowel sounds, and evidence of a mass. A rectal examination will determine whether muscle tone is adequate, and it may reveal hardened stool in the colon.
   B. **Laboratory findings**
      1. **A complete blood count and differential and blood culture** should be done to rule out sepsis. A sterile urine culture should also be done.
      2. **Urinary drug screening** should be performed for mother and infant to detect maternal use of narcotics.
      3. **The serum magnesium level** should be determined to detect hypermagnesemia.
      4. **The serum thyroxine (T_4) level and thyroid-stimulating hormone (TSH) level** should be determined to detect hypothyroidism.
      5. **Serum electrolytes** should be measured, especially to rule out hypokalemia.
   C. **Radiologic and other studies**
      1. **Plain-film abdominal x-rays.** A flat plate and upright film of the abdomen should be obtained to look for ileus or bowel obstruction in any infant who has not passed stool within 48 hours of birth. With Hirschsprung's disease or meconium plug, distention of the colon with multiple air-fluid levels is seen.
      2. **Abdominal x-rays with barium enema** should be obtained in all cases of delayed passage of stool if the patient is symptomatic. It will help to define the disease process and may be therapeutic. Specific findings for each disease are described below under **V.**

V. **Plan**
   A. **Constipation**
      1. Digital rectal stimulation can be tried first.

    2. Glycerin suppositories can be used if digital rectal stimulation is unsuccessful.

B. Anorectal abnormality: imperforate anus
1. Obtain pediatric surgical consultation immediately.
2. Insert a nasogastric tube for decompression.
3. Look for other congenital anomalies. Genitourinary tract abnormalities are frequently seen with imperforate anus.

C. Bowel obstruction
1. **Meconium plug**
   a. Barium enema is performed to verify meconium plug. In infants with this problem, the study usually reveals a normal-sized colon with filling defects.
   b. If meconium plug is verified by barium enema, repeated water-soluble enemas are usually given every 4–6 hours.
   c. If water-soluble enemas are ineffective, a dilute 4% solution of acetylcysteine (Mucomyst) and water can be used as an enema to break down the meconium so that it can be passed.
   d. If normal stooling occurs, no further workup is needed. However, some clinicians recommend rectal biopsy in these infants because up to 15% have Hirschsprung's disease.
   e. If an abnormal pattern of stooling occurs, further workup (eg, rectal biopsy) is necessary to rule out Hirschsprung's disease.
2. **Meconium ileus**
   a. Barium enema may reveal microcolon. Evidence of perforation, volvulus, or atresia may also be seen.
   b. Mild obstruction can be treated with Mucomyst enemas (see **1.c,** above).
   c. Complete obstruction may be relieved by Gastrograffin enema. Adequate fluid and electrolyte replacement must be given.
   d. Operative management may be necessary in cases not relieved by enemas.
3. **Hirschsprung's disease**
   a. Barium enema examination usually shows a narrowed, aganglionic segment leading to a dilated proximal segment.
   b. Rectal biopsy is performed to confirm aganglionosis.
   c. Once the diagnosis is confirmed, a colostomy is usually indicated.
4. **Inspissated milk syndrome**
   a. Barium enema reveals a narrow colon with filling defects.
   b. Gastrograffin enema often relieves the obstruction.
   c. Surgery may be necessary in rare cases.
5. **Adhesions.** Surgery is necessary to lyse the adhesions.
6. **Incarcerated hernia** is a surgical emergency.
7. **Malrotation**
   a. Barium enema reveals an abnormally placed cecum.
   b. Surgical correction is necessary.
8. **Volvulus**
   a. Barium enema reveals obstruction at the midtransverse colon.
   b. Surgery should be an immediate intervention.

D. Ileus
1. **Ileus caused by sepsis**
   a. Broad-spectrum antibiotics are started after a septic workup (see p 223, **B.1**) is performed. Intravenous ampicillin and gentamicin are recommended. Vancomycin may be substituted for ampicillin if staphylococcal infection is suspected (see Chap 75 for dosages).
   b. A nasogastric tube should be placed to decompress the bowel. The infant should not be fed orally.

    2. Ileus caused by necrotizing enterocolitis (see Chap 66).

    3. Ileus caused by hypokalemia

        a. Treat underlying metabolic abnormalities.

        b. Place a nasogastric tube to rest the bowel.

E. Prematurity. Conservative treatment is usually recommended in infants who are not vomiting but have progressive abdominal distention, even if microcolon is seen. Treatment consists of a hyperosmolar contrast enema for passage of the stool. (**Note:** Some institutions are advocating the use of low-osmolality contrast enemas because of fewer side effects. Low-osmolality contrast media include metrizamide, iohexol, iopamidol, and ioxaglate.)

F. Hypothyroidism. If the serum T_4 and TSH levels confirm the presence of hypothyroidism, thyroid replacement therapy is indicated. However, consultation with an endocrinologist should be obtained before starting this therapy.

46 No Urine Output in 48 Hours

I. **Problem.** Urine output has been scant or absent for 48 hours.

II. **Immediate question**

A. **Is the bladder distended?** If distention is present, there is urine in the bladder. The Credé maneuver (manual compression of the bladder) may initiate voiding, especially in infants receiving medications causing muscle paralysis.

B. **Has bladder catheterization been performed?** It will determine whether urine is present in the bladder.

C. **What is the blood pressure?** Hypotension can cause decreased renal perfusion and urine output.

D. **Has the infant ever voided?** If the infant has never voided, consider bilateral renal agenesis, renovascular accident, or obstruction. Table 46–1 shows the time after birth at which the first voiding occurs.

III. **Differential diagnosis.** See Chapter 70 for a complete discussion of acute renal failure. *Oliguria* is defined as urine output of less than 20 mL/kg in a 24-hour period.

A. **Prerenal causes (inadequate blood supply to the kidneys)**
1. Sepsis.
2. Hemorrhage.
3. Hypotension.
4. Asphyxia.
5. Hypokalemia.
6. Heart failure.

B. **Intrinsic renal failure (kidney failure because of intrinsic renal disease)**
1. Renal agenesis.
2. Hypoplastic or dysplastic kidneys.
3. Pyelonephritis.
4. Vascular accident.
5. Nephritis.

C. **Postrenal causes** (urine is formed but not voided)
1. Neurogenic bladder.
2. Urethral stricture.
3. Posterior urethral valves (males only).

IV. **Data base**

TABLE 46–1. TIME TO FIRST VOIDING

	Premature Infant		Term Infant	
	Percentage	Cumulative Percentage	Percentage	Cumulative Percentage
Delivery room	21.5	21.5	17	17
0–12 hours	43	64.5	50.6	67.6
12–24 hours	26	90.5	24.8	92.4
24–48 hours	9.5	100	7	99.4
Over 48 hours			0.6	100

Based on data from Sherry SN, Kramer I: *J Pediatr* 1955;**46**:189; and Kramer I, Sherry SN: *J Pediatr* 1957;**51**:374.

A. **Physical examination.** Physical examination may reveal bladder distention, abdominal masses, or ascites. Signs of renal disorders (eg, Potter's facies) should be noted. Urinary ascites may be seen with posterior urethral valves.

B. **Laboratory studies.** The following laboratory tests should be obtained to help establish the diagnosis. Interpret the results as outlined in Table 70–1, page 425.

   1. **Urine osmolality.**
   2. **Urine sodium (meq/L).**
   3. **Urine/plasma creatinine ratio.**
   4. **Fractional excretion of sodium** (see p 425, **B.2**).
   5. **Renal failure index** (see p 425, **B.2**).
   6. **Serum creatinine.**

C. **Radiologic and other studies**

   1. **Ultrasonography of the abdomen and kidneys** will rule out urinary tract obstruction.
   2. **Abdominal x-ray studies** may reveal spina bifida or absent sacrum, suggesting neurogenic bladder.

V. **Plan.** See Chapter 70 for management of renal failure.

47 Pneumoperitoneum

I. **Problem.** A pneumoperitoneum (abnormal collection of air in the peritoneal cavity) is seen on an abdominal x-ray film.

II. **Immediate questions**

A. **Is mechanical ventilation being given?** High peak inspiratory pressures (PIP) (mean of 34 cm water) are more likely to be associated with pneumoperitoneum.

B. **Are signs or symptoms of pneumoperitoneum present?** These findings can include abdominal distention, respiratory distress, deteriorating blood gas levels, and a decrease in blood pressure.

C. **Are signs or symptoms of necrotizing enterocolitis present?** If so, the pneumoperitoneum is likely to be associated with gastrointestinal tract perforation.

D. **Is a pneumomediastinum present?** If a pneumomediastinum is present, the peritoneal air collection is more likely to be of respiratory tract origin.

E. **Did the infant recently undergo abdominal surgery?** Intra-abdominal air is normal in the immediate postoperative period. It usually resolves without treatment.

III. **Differential diagnosis.** Pneumoperitoneum develops secondary to air leak from the chest or from a perforated viscus.

A. **Pneumoperitoneum associated with respiratory disorder (eg, pneumomediastinum, pneumothorax)**

B. **Pneumoperitoneum associated with gastrointestinal perforation**

1. **Spontaneous perforation** occurs most commonly in the stomach. It may be due to a misplaced nasogastric tube. Perforation of the appendix and Meckel's diverticulum have also been reported.

2. **Necrotizing enterocolitis** may also be associated with perforation.

C. **Iatrogenic pneumoperitoneum** may be caused by improperly performed suprapubic bladder aspiration, paracentesis, or postexploratory laparotomy.

IV. **Data base**

A. **Physical examination.** Perform a complete physical examination. Clinical evaluation will not help in differentiating whether the pneumoperitoneum is of respiratory or gastrointestinal tract origin.

B. **Laboratory studies**

1. **Preoperative laboratory testing** should be performed, including **serum electrolyte levels** and a **complete blood count.** Elevation of the white blood cell count or a left shift may signify a gastrointestinal tract perforation.

2. **Arterial blood gas levels** should be obtained. They may reveal hypoxemia and increasing Pco_2 levels.

C. **Radiologic and other studies**

1. **Anteroposterior x-ray study of the abdomen** may show signs of necrotizing enterocolitis or ileus. Air-fluid levels in the peritoneal cavity usually indicate bowel perforation.

2. **Lateral decubitus x-ray study of the abdomen** with the right side up is the best examination for free abdominal air. Air rises anteriorly, so that a lucency will be seen over the liver if a perforation has occurred.

3. **Paracentesis.** Air obtained by paracentesis (see Chap 25) may be tested for its oxygen level. If the oxygen level is high, the air is probably from a respiratory tract leak. Fluid may be obtained by paracentesis if the diagnosis is still undetermined. If more than 0.5 mL of green or brown fluid is obtained, the air is probably of gastrointestinal tract origin.

V. Plan

A. **General measures.** A nasogastric tube should be placed.
B. **Specific measures**
   1. **Pneumoperitoneum of respiratory tract origin**
      a. **For asymptomatic patients,** observation is the treatment of choice, with follow-up x-ray studies usually performed every 8–12 hours but more frequently if the patient's clinical course changes.
      b. **For symptomatic patients,** paracentesis can be performed (see Chap 25).
   2. **Pneumoperitoneum of gastrointestinal tract origin.** Unless the pneumoperitoneum is iatrogenic in origin, **immediate surgical evaluation is necessary. Exploratory laparotomy** is usually the treatment of choice.
      a. **Preoperative laboratory values** should be available.
      b. **The infant should be stabilized** as much as possible before taken to the operating room.
      c. **The surgical team may request a study with a water-soluble contrast medium given through the nasogastric tube** to try to localize the perforation (see below).
   3. **Iatrogenic pneumoperitoneum**
      a. **Pneumoperitoneum caused by suprapubic bladder aspiration or** paracentesis may require surgical exploration.
      b. **Pneumoperitoneum associated with uncomplicated postexploratory laparotomy** usually resolves spontaneously.
   4. **If the cause of the pneumoperitoneum is in doubt, a low-osmolality water-soluble contrast medium (such as metrizamide) can be given through a nasogastric tube.** If there is a pneumoperitoneum due to bowel perforation, contrast material will pass into the peritoneal cavity.

48 Pneumothorax

I. **Problem.** An infant may have a pneumothorax (an accumulation of air in the pleural space).
II. **Immediate questions**
   A. **Are symptoms of tension pneumothorax present?** Tension pneumothorax presents as a **medical emergency,** and the patient's status will deteriorate acutely. The following signs and symptoms may be seen with tension pneumothorax: cyanosis, hypoxia, tachypnea, sudden decrease in heart rate with bradycardia, sudden increase in systolic blood pressure followed by narrowing pulse pressure and hypotension, asymmetric chest (bulging on the affected side), distention of the abdomen (secondary to downward displacement of the diaphragm), decreased breath sounds on the affected side, and shift of the cardiac apical impulse away from the affected side.
   B. **Is the patient asymptomatic?** Asymptomatic pneumothorax is present in 1–2% of neonates. Most of these cases are discovered on chest x-ray at admission. Up to 15% of these infants were meconium-stained at birth.
   C. **Is mechanical ventilation being used?** The incidence of pneumothorax in patients receiving positive-pressure ventilation is 15%–20%.
III. **Differential diagnosis.** A pneumothorax may be spontaneous or it may develop secondary to mechanical ventilation causing barotrauma.
   A. **Pneumothorax**
      1. **Symptomatic** pneumothorax (includes tension pneumothorax).
      2. **Asymptomatic** pneumothorax.
   B. **Pneumomediastinum**
   C. **Congenital lobar emphysema.** Overdistention of one lobe secondary to air trapping occurs most commonly in the left upper lobe (47%). Other lobe involvement is 20% right upper lobe, 28% right middle lobe, and rare in the lower lobes. The causes of congenital lobar emphysema are probably multifactorial.
   D. **Atelectasis with compensatory hyperinflation.** Compensatory hyperinflation may appear as a pneumothorax on a chest x-ray film.
   E. **Pneumopericardium.** In neonates, pneumopericardium and tension pneumothorax can both present as sudden and rapid clinical deterioration. In pneumopericardium, the blood pressure drops and heart sounds are distant or absent. In tension pneumothorax, the blood pressure may initially increase. The chest x-ray film easily differentiates between the two. A pneumopericardium has a halo of air around the heart.
IV. **Clinical findings**
   A. **Physical examination.** Perform a thorough examination of the chest. Specific findings are discussed in **II.A,** above.
   B. **Laboratory studies.** Blood gas levels may show decreased Pao_2 and increased Pco_2, with resultant respiratory acidosis.
   C. **Radiologic and other studies**
      1. **Transillumination.** Transillumination of the chest will define the pneumothorax. The room lights are lowered, and a fiberoptic transilluminator is placed along the posterior axillary line on the side on which pneumothorax is suspected. If pneumothorax is present, the

chest will "light up" on that side. The transilluminator may be moved up and down along the posterior axillary line and may also be placed above the nipple. Transilluminate both sides of the chest and then compare the results. If severe edema is present, transillumination may be falsely positive. Therefore, always verify the diagnosis of pneumothorax by chest x-ray studies.

2. **Chest x-ray studies** are the best method of defining pneumothorax. The following films will help in making the diagnosis.

   a. **Anteroposterior view** of the chest will show the following:
      (1) A shift of the mediastinum away from the side of pneumothorax (with tension pneumothorax).
      (2) Depression of the diaphragm on the side of the pneumothorax (with tension pneumothorax).
      (3) The lung on the affected side will be displaced away from the chest wall by a radiolucent band of air.

   b. **Cross-table lateral view** will show a rim of air around the lung ("pancaking"). It will *not* help to identify the affected side. This film must be considered together with the anteroposterior view to identify the involved side.

   c. **Lateral decubitus view.** The infant should be positioned so that the side of the suspected pneumothorax is up (eg, if pneumothorax is suspected on the left side, the film is taken with the left side up). This view will detect even a small pneumothorax not seen on a routine chest x-ray film.

V. Plan

A. **Symptomatic (tension) pneumothorax is an emergency! A 1- to 2-minute delay could be fatal. If a tension pneumothorax is suspected, act immediately and take the "heat" if it turns out there is no pneumothorax.** If the patient's status is deteriorating rapidly, a needle or Angiocath can be placed for aspiration, followed by chest tube placement.

   1. The site of puncture should be at the second or third intercostal space along the midclavicular line. Cleanse this area with antibacterial solution (Betadine).

   2. Connect a 21- or 23-gauge scalp vein needle or a 22- or 24-gauge Angiocath to a 20-mL syringe with a stopcock attached. Have an assistant hold the syringe and withdraw the air.

   3. Palpate the third rib at the midclavicular line. Insert the needle above the rib and advance it until air is withdrawn from the syringe. The needle may be removed before the chest tube is placed if the infant is relatively stable, or it may be left in place for continuous aspiration while the chest tube is being placed. If an Angiocath is used, the needle may be removed and the catheter left in place.

B. **Asymptomatic pneumothorax**

   1. **If positive-pressure mechanical ventilation is the cause of asymptomatic pneumothorax,** a chest tube *must* be inserted because the pressure being given by the ventilator will prevent resolution of the pneumothorax, and tension pneumothorax may develop. If a pneumothorax develops in a patient who is ready to be extubated, clinical judgment must be used in deciding whether a chest tube should be placed.

   2. **If positive-pressure mechanical ventilation is *not* being given,** one of 2 treatments may be used:

      a. Close observation with follow-up chest x-ray studies every 8–12 hours, or sooner if the infant becomes symptomatic. The pneumothorax will probably resolve within 48 hours.

      b. For more rapid resolution of the pneumothorax, give the infant 100% oxygen for 8–12 hours, a procedure known as **nitrogen washout therapy.** Less nitrogen is able to enter the lungs, and, at the same time, absorption of nitrogen from the extrapleural space is increased and then exhaled. The total gas tension is decreased, which also facilitates absorption of nitrogen by the blood. *It should be used only in full-term infants in whom retinopathy of prematurity will not be a problem.*

C. **Pneumomediastinum** may progress to a pneumothorax or pneumopericardium. Close observation is required.

D. **Congenital lobar emphysema**
   1. **Asymptomatic.** Conservation management with observation is advocated.
   2. **Symptomatic.** If respiratory failure is occurring, the treatment is usually surgical excision of the affected lobe.

E. **Atelectasis with compensatory hyperinflation**
   1. Chest physiotherapy and postural drainage should be initiated.
   2. Treatment with bronchodilators is indicated (see p 47, **H.2**).
   3. Positioning the infant with the affected side (hyperinflated side) down may speed resolution.

F. **Pneumopericardium** should be treated emergently by pericardiocentesis (see Chap 26).

49 Polycythemia

I. **Problem.** The hematocrit is 68% in a newborn. (The upper limit of normal is 65%.)
II. **Immediate questions**
   A. **What is the central hematocrit?** In blood obtained by heelstick, the hematocrit may be falsely elevated by 5–15%. Therefore, treatment should not be initiated based on heelstick hematocrit values alone; a central hematocrit is needed.
   B. **Is the infant dehydrated?** Dehydration may cause hemoconcentration, resulting in a high hematocrit. It usually occurs in infants more than 48 hours old.
   C. **Does the infant have symptoms of polycythemia?** Symptoms and signs of polycythemia include respiratory distress, tachypnea, hypoglycemia, lethargy, irritability, apnea, seizures, jitteriness, weak sucking reflex, poor feeding, and cyanosis.
   D. **Is the mother diabetic?** Poor control of diabetes during pregnancy leads to chronic fetal hypoxia, which results in increased neonatal erythropoiesis.
   E. **What is the infant's age?** The hematocrit reaches a peak at 2–4 hours of age. After 48 hours of age, hemoconcentration due to dehydration may be present.
III. **Differential diagnosis.** (See also Chap 56.)
   A. **Falsely elevated hematocrit.** This finding occurs most often when blood is obtained by heelstick.
   B. **Dehydration.** Weight loss and decreased urine output are sensitive indicators of dehydration.
   C. **True polycythemia**
      1. **Placental transfusion** occurs with delayed cord clamping, twin-twin transfusion, or fetomaternal transfusion.
      2. **Intrauterine hypoxia** may be caused by placental insufficiency. It may be seen in postmature or small-for-gestational-age (SGA) infants, preeclampsia-eclampsia, and with maternal use of the drug propranolol. Maternal smoking and severe maternal heart disease may also cause intrauterine hypoxia.
      3. **Other causes**
         a. Maternal diabetes.
         b. Chromosomal abnormalities such as Down's syndrome and trisomies 13 and 18.
         c. Beckwith-Wiedemann syndrome.
         d. Neonatal thyrotoxicosis.
         e. Congenital adrenal hyperplasia.
IV. **Data base**
   A. **Physical examination**
      1. **Hemoconcentration secondary to dehydration.** If more than 8–10% of the birth weight has been lost, dehydration is likely to be present. It usually occurs in the second or third day of life. The mucous membranes will be dry. Increased skin turgor is usually *not* seen.
      2. **True polycythemia.** True polycythemia is often, but not always, associated with visible skin changes. Ruddiness, plethora, or "pink on blue" or "blue on pink" coloration may be present. In males, priap-

ism may be seen secondary to sludging of red blood cells. Clinical signs are listed on page 233, **II.C.**

B. Laboratory studies

1. A **central hematocrit value** must be obtained.
2. **The serum glucose level** should be checked because hypoglycemia is commonly seen with polycythemia.
3. **Serum bilirubin level.** Infants with polycythemia have problems with hyperbilirubinemia because of the increased turnover of red blood cells.
4. **Serum sodium and blood urea nitrogen levels.** These levels should be obtained if dehydration is being considered. They are usually high, or higher than baseline values, if dehydration is present.
5. **Urine specific gravity.** A high specific gravity (> 1.015) is usually seen with dehydration.
6. **Blood gas levels.** Blood gas levels should be obtained to rule out inadequate oxygenation.

C. Radiologic and other studies. Other studies are usually not indicated.

V. Plan

A. Falsely elevated hematocrit (> 65%). If the central hematocrit is normal, no further evaluation is needed. If the central hematocrit is high, either dehydration of true polycythemia is present (see **B** and **C** below for treatment).

B. Hemoconcentration secondary to dehydration. If the infant is dehydrated and does not have symptoms or signs of polycythemia, a trial of rehydration over 6–8 hours can be attempted. The type of fluid used depends on the infant's age and serum electrolyte status (see Chap 7). Usually 130–150 mL/kg/d is given. The hematocrit is checked every 6 hours. It usually decreases with adequate rehydration.

C. True polycythemia

1. **Central hematocrit of 65–70% in asymptomatic infant.** If the central hematocrit is 65–70% and the infant is asymptomatic, only observation may be needed. Many of these patients respond to increased fluid therapy; increases of 20–40 mL/kg/d can be tried. The central hematocrit must be checked every 6 hours. The hematocrit normally reaches a peak at 2–4 hours of age. If the hematocrit is 70% at birth, it may be 5–10% higher at 2–4 hours of age.
2. **Central hematocrit greater than 65% in symptomatic infant.** Partial exchange transfusion should be given. To calculate the volume of Plasmanate that must be exchanged, use the following formula (blood volume = 80 mL/kg).

$$\text{Volume exchanged} = \frac{(\text{Weight [kg]} \times \text{Blood volume}) \times (\text{Hct of patient} - \text{Desired Hct})}{\text{Hct of patient}}$$

Partial exchange transfusion may be administered via a low or high umbilical venous catheter *(care must be taken not to place it in the liver).* A low umbilical artery catheter may also be used. The fluid that can be used for a partial exchange transfusion is Plasmanate, 5% albumin, normal saline, or fresh-frozen plasma (usually not recommended because of the risk of HIV transmission). The decision about which fluid to use depends on a particular institution's preference. The exchange procedure is discussed in detail in Chapter 21. Serial hematocrits should be obtained following transfusion.
3. **Central hematocrit greater than 70% in asymptomatic infant.** Most neonatologists agree that partial exchange transfusion should be given, although some controversy still exists. Institutional guidelines should be followed.

D. **Infants who have a central hematocrit between 60-65% but symptoms of polycythemia.** If all other disease entities are ruled out, these infants may indeed be polycythemic and hyperviscous. In these cases, management is *controversial.* Use clinical judgment and institutional guidelines to decide whether or not this infant should have a partial exchange transfusion.

50 Poor Perfusion

I. **Problem.** The infant "doesn't look good," looks "mottled" or "washed out," "perfusion is poor."

II. **Immediate questions**

A. **What is the age of the infant?** Hypoplastic left heart syndrome may cause poor perfusion and a mottled appearance. It may be seen at days 1–21 of life (more commonly, day 2 or 3). In an infant less than 3 days old, sepsis may be a cause. Associated risk factors are premature rupture of the membranes or maternal infection and fever.

B. **Are congenital anomalies present?** Persistent cutis marmorata may be seen in de Lange syndrome and trisomies 18 and 21.

C. **What are the vital signs?** If the temperature is lower than normal, cold stress or hypothermia associated with sepsis may be present. Hypotension may cause poor perfusion (see normal blood pressure values in Appendix C). Decreased urine output (< 2 mL/kg/h) may indicate depleted intravascular volume or shock.

D. **Is the liver enlarged and are metabolic acidosis, a poor peripheral pulse rate, and gallop present?** These problems are signs of failure of the left side of the heart (**such as hypoplastic left heart syndrome**). Poor perfusion occurs because of reduced blood flow to the skin.

E. **If mechanical ventilation is being used, are chest movements adequate and are blood gas levels improving?** Inadequate ventilation can result in poor perfusion. Pneumothorax may also be a cause.

III. **Differential diagnosis**

A. **Sepsis.**

B. **Cold stress** (in general, a skin temperature < 36.5 °C).

C. **Hypotension, usually with shock.**

D. **Hypoventilation.**

E. **Pneumothorax.**

F. **Necrotizing enterocolitis.**

G. **Left-sided heart lesions** such as hypoplastic left heart syndrome, coarctation of the aorta, and aortic stenosis.

H. **Cutis marmorata,** a marbling pattern of the skin (infant appears poorly perfused), may occur in a normal infant, especially when it is exposed to cold stress. Persistent cutis marmorata may be seen in de Lange syndrome and trisomies 18 (Edwards' syndrome) and 21 (Down's syndrome).

IV. **Data base**

A. **Physical examination.** Note temperature and vital signs. Look for signs of sepsis. The cardiovascular and pulmonary examinations are important. Signs of trisomy 18 include micrognathia and overlapping digits; signs of trisomy 21 include single palmar transverse crease and epicanthal folds.

B. **Laboratory studies**

1. **CBC and differential.** These studies suggest the presence of sepsis or decreased hematocrit.

2. **Blood gas levels.** These studies reveal inadequate ventilation or the presence of acidosis, which may be seen in sepsis or necrotizing enterocolitis.

3. **Cultures.** If sepsis is suspected, a complete workup should be con-

sidered, especially if antibiotics are to be started. This workup includes cultures of blood, urine, and spinal fluid (if indicated).

C. **Radiologic and other studies**

   1. **Transillumination of the chest.** This study can be performed quickly to help determine whether or not pneumothorax is present (see p 230, **IV.C.1**).

   2. **Chest x-ray study.** A chest x-ray study should be obtained if pneumonia, pneumothorax, congenital heart lesion, or hypoventilation is suspected. In left-sided heart lesions, the x-ray film shows cardiomegaly with pulmonary venous congestion (except in hypoplastic left heart syndrome, when the size of the heart may be normal). If a view taken during lung expansion shows that the lungs are down only to the sixth rib or less, hypoventilation should be considered. With hyperventilation, lung expansion will be down to the ninth or tenth rib.

   3. **Abdominal x-ray study.** A flat-plate x-ray film of the abdomen should be obtained if necrotizing enterocolitis is suspected.

   4. **Echocardiography** should be performed if a congenital heart lesion is suspected. In hypoplastic left heart syndrome, a large right ventricle and a small left ventricle is seen on the echocardiogram, and there is failure to visualize the mitral or aortic valve. In aortic stenosis, the echocardiogram reveals a deformed aortic valve. In coarctation of the aorta, it reveals decreased aortic diameter.

   5. **Karyotyping** is performed if trisomy 18 or 21 is suspected.

V. **Plan**

A. **General plan.** A quick workup should initially be done. While checking vital signs and quickly examining the patient, order stat blood gas levels and a chest x-ray study. Initiate oxygen supplementation.

B. **Specific plans**

   1. **Sepsis.** If sepsis is suspected, a septic workup is indicated. Empiric antibiotic therapy may be started at the discretion of the physician.

   2. **Cold stress.** Gradual rewarming is necessary, usually at a rate of no more than 1 °C per hour. It can be accomplished by means of a radiant warmer or incubator, heat shield, heating pad, or plastic wrap draped over the infant. (See also Chap 5.)

   3. **Hypotension/shock.** If the blood pressure is low because of depleted intravascular volume, give colloid, 10 mL/kg IV 5–10 min.

   4. **Hypoventilation.** If hypoventilation is suspected, it may be necessary to increase the pressure being given by the ventilator. The amount of pressure must be decided on an individual basis. One method is to increase the pressure by 2–4 cm water and then obtain blood gas levels in 20 minutes. Another method is to use bag-and-mask ventilation, observing the manometer to determine the amount of pressure needed to move the chest.

   5. **Pneumothorax.** (See Chap 48.)

   6. **Necrotizing enterocolitis.** (See Chap 66.)

   7. **Left-sided heart lesions.** Treat with oxygen, possibly diuretics and digoxin if congestive heart failure is present, and infusion of prostaglandin E_1. Surgery is usually indicated in all these patients except those with hypoplastic left heart syndrome, for whom it is *controversial.*

   8. **Cutis marmorata.** If this condition has occurred secondary to cold stress, treat the patient as described in **2,** above. If the condition persists, chromosomes may need to be obtained to rule out trisomies 18 and 21.

51 Premature Rupture of the Membranes

I. **Problem.** A newborn whose mother had premature rupture of the membranes is admitted to the nursery. Should a sepsis workup be done and should antibiotics be started?

II. **Immediate questions**

A. **How long before delivery did the membranes rupture?** Rupture of the membranes occurring 24–48 hours before delivery is associated with an increased incidence of neonatal sepsis. If the rupture occurs 24 hours or less before delivery, there is no increased risk.

B. **Did the mother show signs of infection?** Fever, urinary tract infection, amnionitis, pneumonia, or sepsis in the mother increase the risk of sepsis in the infant.

C. **Are signs of sepsis present in the infant?** Signs of sepsis include apnea and bradycardia, temperature instability (hypothermia or hyperthermia), feeding intolerance, tachypnea, jaundice, cyanosis, poor peripheral perfusion, hypoglycemia, lethargy, poor sucking reflex, and irritability.

D. **Was the infant monitored during labor?** Fetal tachycardia and decelerations (usually late) can be associated with neonatal infection. A biophysical profile score of less than 6 (see Table 1–1) can be associated with an increased incidence of infection.

III. **Differential diagnosis**

A. **Sepsis.**

B. **Infant at increased risk for sepsis.**

C. **Infant at low risk for sepsis.**

IV. **Data base**

A. **Physical examination.** Perform a complete physical examination, looking for signs of sepsis (see **II.C,** above).

B. **Laboratory studies**

1. **Complete blood count and platelet count.** *An abnormally low or high white blood cell count is worrisome. Values less than 6000 μL or greater than 30,000 μL in the first 24 hours of life are abnormal.* A band neutrophil count greater than 20% is abnormal. A normal white blood cell count does not rule out sepsis. The total neutrophil count can be calculated and plotted on the White Cell Count Graph in Appendix M.

2. **Peripheral blood cultures.** Resin bottles should be used for antibiotic removal if the mother has been receiving antibiotics.

3. **Suprapubic aspiration of urine for urinalysis and culture** (*controversial*). Many institutions do not insist on this procedure in newborn infants with possible sepsis on day 1 of life, because newborns rarely present with urinary tract infection in the first day.

4. **Maternal endocervical culture.** Requested from obstetric service.

5. **Arterial blood gas levels.**

6. **Baseline bilirubin and serum glucose levels.**

C. **Radiologic and other studies**

1. **Chest x-ray study.** If there are signs of respiratory infection, obtain a chest x-ray film to rule out pneumonia.

2. **Lumbar puncture** for cerebrospinal fluid examination is indicated if a decision is made to give antibiotics. This measure is *controver-*

sial—some institutions perform a lumbar puncture only if the infant has signs of CNS infection.

V. Plan

A. **General measures.** For the majority of cases, a decision about whether an infant requires a septic workup and antibiotics is usually straight-forward. These infants are either clinically sick or have such a positive history of an increased risk for sepsis and some clinical signs of sepsis that the decision is easily made. However, if an infant does not have a clear-cut history and clinical presentation, the decision is difficult. Once the decision is made to treat the infant, treatment usually involves 3 days of antibiotics after obtaining cultures. The following guidelines can be used to help make the decision to treat.

1. **Use of scoring systems.** Some institutions have devised their own septic scoring systems to help decide which infants should be treated. Listed below are 2 scoring systems.

   a. Five tests whose results are available in less than 1 hour are used. If 2 or more of these 5 tests are positive, the score is positive and the infant should receive a septic workup and antibiotics.
      (1) Total white blood count less than 5000/mm^3.
      (2) Immature neutrophils (bands) divided by total neutrophils $\geq$ 0.2.
      (3) Latex C-reactive protein positive.
      (4) Latex haptoglobin positive.
      (5) Mini-erythroctye sedimentation rate > 15 mm/h.

   b. The second scoring system includes 7 findings with a score of 1 for each; a total score of greater than or equal to 3 identifies a high-risk infant. In such cases, a workup should be done and antibiotics started.
      (1) Abnormal white blood count (< 5000 mm^3 or > 25,000 mm^3 at birth, > 30,000 mm^3 at 12–24 hours of age, > 21,000 mm^3 at 2 days of age or more).
      (2) Abnormal total neutrophil count (see Appendix M).
      (3) Elevated immature PMN (band) count (see Appendix M).
      (4) Elevated immature to total PMN ratio (see Appendix M).
      (5) Immature to mature PMN ratio > 0.3.
      (6) Platelet count < 150,000 mm^3.
      (7) Degenerative changes in PMNs ($\geq$ +3 for vacuolization, toxic granulation, or Döhle's bodies when quantified on 0 to 4+ scale).

2. **If no septic scoring system is used,** a few guidelines should be followed when deciding whether or not to treat the infant.

   a. **Send culture specimens to the laboratory and initiate empiric antibiotic therapy:**
      (1) If symptoms of infection are present, regardless of the history or laboratory value results.
      (2) If the white blood count is obtained and shows neutropenia.
      (3) If there is documented sepsis in the mother and she is receiving antibiotics.
      (4) If the membranes ruptured more than 48 hours before delivery and there is evidence of infection in the mother.
      (5) If the membranes ruptured 24–48 hours before delivery and the mother is asymptomatic, obtain a white blood count on the infant. If the count is abnormal, if the infant is symptomatic, or if there are perinatal risk factors for infection, obtain cultures and begin antibiotics.

   b. **Observe the infant:**
      (1) If the white blood cell count is elevated and the infant has no clinical signs of sepsis. However, a repeat white blood count

        must be obtained in 4–6 hours. The infant must be *closely* observed for any changes in clinical status.

    (2) If the membranes ruptured less than 24 hours before delivery and the mother is afebrile or is not receiving antibiotics and is doing well.

    (3) If the membranes ruptured more than 24 hours before delivery and the mother is asymptomatic, obtain a white blood count on the infant. If the count is normal, observe the infant.

B. Specific therapy

  1. If the decision is to treat

    a. Obtain cultures of the blood, urine, and spinal fluid (cultures of urine and spinal fluid are *controversial*).

    b. Ampicillin and gentamicin are the antibiotics most commonly used for initial therapy. (See Chap 76 for dosages and other pharmacologic information.)

  2. Discontinuing antibiotics is another *controversial* topic. The following guidelines may be used.

    a. If the cultures are negative and the patient is doing well, antibiotics are usually stopped after 3 days.

    b. If the cultures are negative but the infant had signs of sepsis, some clinicians treat the infant for 5–10 days.

    c. If the cultures are positive, treat accordingly (see Chap 76 for antibiotic agents, dosages, and other pharmacologic information).

52 Pulmonary Hemorrhage

I. **Problem.** Gross bleeding is seen in the endotracheal tube.
II. **Immediate questions**
   A. **Are any other signs or symptoms abnormal?** Typically, an infant with pulmonary hemorrhage is a low birth weight infant, 2–4 days old, who suddenly develops pallor, shock, apnea, bradycardia, and cyanosis.
   B. **Is the infant hypoxic? Has a blood transfusion recently been given?** Hypoxia or hypervolemia (usually caused by overtransfusion) may cause an acute rise in the pulmonary capillary pressure and lead to pulmonary hemorrhage.
   C. **Is bleeding occurring from other sites?** If there is bleeding from multiple sites, coagulopathy may be present, and coagulation studies should be obtained. Volume replacement with colloid or blood may be needed.
III. **Differential diagnosis**
   A. **Direct trauma to the airway** is usually due to nasogastric or endotracheal intubation.
   B. **Aspiration of gastric or maternal blood** is usually seen following cesarean section. The majority of blood is usually obtained from the nasogastric tube, but blood may be seen in the endotracheal tube.
   C. **Coagulopathy.**
   D. **Other disorders associated with pulmonary hemorrhage**
      1. **Hypoxia.**
      2. **Hypervolemia** (usually caused by overtransfusion).
      3. **Congestive heart failure** (especially in pulmonary edema caused by patent ductus arteriosus).
      4. **Respiratory distress syndrome.**
      5. **Severe Rh incompatibility.**
      6. **Pneumonia.**
      7. **Hemorrhagic disease of the newborn** (failure to administer vitamin K).
IV. **Data base**
   A. **Physical examination.** Note the presence of other bleeding sites, signs of pneumonia or other infection, or congestive heart failure.
   B. **Laboratory studies**
      1. **Complete blood count with differential and platelet count.** With pneumonia or other infection, results of these studies may be abnormal. Thrombocytopenia may be seen. The hematocrit should be checked to determine whether excessive blood loss has occurred.
      2. **Coagulation profile (prothrombin time [PT], partial thromboplastin time [PTT], thrombin time [TT], and fibrinogen level)** will reveal coagulation disorders.
      3. **Arterial blood gas levels** will detect hypoxia.
      4. **Apt test** if aspiration of maternal blood is suspected (see p 178).
   C. **Radiologic and other studies.** A chest x-ray study will rule out pneumonia, respiratory distress syndrome, and congestive heart failure. With massive pulmonary hemorrhage, the chest x-ray film shows a complete white-out.
V. **Plan**
   A. **General measures**

1. Support blood pressure with volume expansion and colloids (see p 220, **B.1.a**).
2. Treat the underlying cause. The following measures may help to stop the bleeding.
   a. If mechanical ventilation is being used when the bleeding begins:
      (1) Increase the positive end-expiratory pressure (PEEP) to 4–8 cm water; it may cause tamponade of the capillaries.
      (2) Consider giving epinephrine through an endotracheal tube (*controversial*). This may cause constriction of the pulmonary capillaries.
   b. If mechanical ventilation is not being used, consider initiating its use in providing the treatments outlined in **a,** above.
B. **Specific therapy**
   1. **Direct nasogastric or endotracheal trauma.** If there is significant bleeding immediately after an endotracheal or nasogastric intubation, trauma is the most likely cause; surgical consultation is indicated.
   2. **Aspiration of maternal blood.** If the infant is stable, no treatment is needed, since the condition is self-limited.
   3. **Coagulopathy**
      a. **Hemorrhagic disease of the newborn.** Vitamin K_1, 1 mg intravenously, should be given.
      b. **Other coagulopathies.** Fresh frozen plasma, 10 mL/kg every 12–24 hours, should be given. If the platelet count is low, give 1 unit/5 kg. Monitor the thrombin time (TT), partial thromboplastin time (PTT), platelet count, and fibrinogen level.

53 Seizure Activity

I. **Problem.** The nurse reports that an infant is having abnormal movements of the extremities consistent with seizure activity.

II. **Immediate questions**

A. **Is the infant really seizing?** This question is very important and is often initially difficult to answer. **Jitteriness** is sometimes confused with seizures. In a jittery infant, eye movements are normal. The hands will stop moving if they are grasped, and movements are of a fine nature. In an infant who is seizing, eye movements can be abnormal (staring, blinking, nystagmoid jerks, or tonic horizontal eye deviation). The hands continue to move if grasped, and movements are of a coarser nature.

B. **Is there a history of birth asphyxia or risk factors for sepsis?** Asphyxia and sepsis with meningitis may cause neonatal seizures.

C. **What is the blood glucose level?** Hypoglycemia is an easily treatable cause of seizures in the neonatal period.

D. **How old is the infant?** The age of the infant is often the best clue to the cause of the seizures. Common causes for specific ages are given below.

At birth. Maternal anesthetic agents.

Day 1. Metabolic abnormalities such as hypoglycemia, hypocalcemia, hypoxic-ischemic encephalopathy (presenting at 6–18 hours after birth and getting more severe in the next 24–48 hours).

Days 2–3. Drug withdrawal, meningitis.

Day 5 or greater. Hypocalcemia, TORCH infections, developmental defects.

More than 1–2 weeks. Methadone withdrawal.

III. **Differential diagnosis.** (See also Chap 67.)

A. **Seizure activity** may be secondary to the following conditions.

1. **Hypoxic-ischemic injury.**

2. **Intracranial hemorrhage (subarachnoid, intraventricular, subdural).**

3. **Metabolic abnormality**

   a. Hypoglycemia.

   b. Hypocalcemia or hypercalcemia.

   c. Hypomagnesemia.

   d. Hyponatremia or hypernatremia.

   e. Pyridoxine dependence.

4. **Infection**

   a. Meningitis.

   b. Sepsis.

   c. TORCH infections.

5. **Neonatal drug withdrawal** (see Chap 59).

6. **Inborn errors of metabolism** (see Chap 61).

   a. Maple syrup urine disease.

   b. Methylmalonic acidemia.

   c. Nonketotic hyperglycinemia.

7. **Maternal anesthetic agents.** If mepivacaine is accidentally injected into the infant, seizures can occur at birth.

8. **Drug toxicity.** Theophylline overdose causes seizures.

9. **Developmental abnormalities.** Cerebral malformations can cause

seizures. Often, the infant will have obvious anomalies of the face or head if developmental abnormalities are present.

B. Jitteriness. This benign condition is differentiated from seizures as described in **II.A,** p 243.

C. Benign myoclonic activity. These isolated jerky, nonrepetitive movements of an extremity or other part of the body occur mainly during sleep and are benign.

IV. Data base

A. History. A detailed history will help in diagnosing seizure activity. The nurse or physician observing the activity should record a complete description of the event on the chart.

B. Physical examination. Perform a complete physical examination, with close attention to the neurologic status.

C. Laboratory studies

  1. Metabolic workup

   a. Serum glucose level. If the glucose level on paper-strip testing is less than 25 mg/dL, obtain a serum glucose value from the laboratory.

   b. Serum sodium level.

   c. Serum ionized and total calcium levels. Only an ionized calcium level is usually necessary, but if that test cannot be done, a total calcium study should be ordered. Ionized calcium is the most accurate measurement of calcium.

   d. Serum magnesium level.

  2. Infection workup

   a. Complete blood count and differential.

   b. Blood, urine, and CSF cultures.

   c. Serum IgM- and Igm-specific TORCH titers. The serum IgM titer may be elevated in TORCH infections.

  3. Urine drug screening if drug withdrawal is suspected.

  4. Theophylline level if the infant is on this medication and toxicity is suspected.

  5. Blood gas levels to rule out hypoxia or acidosis.

D. Radiologic and other studies

  1. Ultrasound examination of the head will confirm intraventricular hemorrhage (IVH). (*Note:* The coexistence of IVH and seizures does not necessarily mean they are related.)

  2. CT scan of the head. A CT scan can be done to diagnose subarachnoid or subdural hemorrhage. It may also reveal a congenital malformation.

  3. Lumbar puncture. The presence of blood in the cerebrospinal fluid suggests intraventricular hemorrhage. Cultures of the fluid should be done to diagnose infection. (See Chap 24.)

  4. Electroencephalography. It is usually not possible to perform electroencephalography during the episode of seizure activity. This study should be done at some time after seizure activity has been documented. It may confirm seizure activity and may also be used as a baseline study.

V. Plan

A. General measures. Once it is determined that the infant is having seizures, because the other two diagnoses (jitteriness and benign myoclonic activity) are benign conditions, the following measures should be taken.

  1. Rule out hypoxia. Send blood sample to the laboratory for measurement of blood gases and start oxygen therapy. Assess the infant's airway and breathing.

  2. Check glucose level. A Dextrostrix or Chemstrip-bG paper-strip test should be done to rule out hypoglycemia. Also, send a blood sample to the laboratory for a **stat serum glucose level** for confirmation of the paper-strip test result. If the paper-strip test shows low blood glucose, it is acceptable to give 10% glucose, 2–4 mL/kg intravenous push before obtaining results from the laboratory.

3. **Send a blood sample to the laboratory for stat serum calcium and sodium levels.** If these levels were low on earlier values and a metabolic disorder is strongly suspected to be the cause of the seizures, it is acceptable to go ahead and treat the infant before new laboratory values are available.

4. **Anticonvulsant therapy.** If hypoxia and all metabolic abnormalities have been treated or if blood gas and metabolic workup values are normal, start anticonvulsant therapy. See p 386, **VI.C,D,** and Chapter 75 for detailed pharmacologic information.

   a. Give **phenobarbital** as the first-line drug.

   b. If seizures persist and the phenobarbital level is satisfactory, (> 40 μg/mL), give **phenytoin** (Dilantin).

   c. If seizures still persist, the following drugs may be used: paraldehyde, lorazapam, or diazepam, depending on institutional preference.

B. **Specific measures**

1. **Hypoxic ischemic injury.** Seizures secondary to birth asphyxia usually present anywhere from 6 to 18 hours of age.

   a. Careful observation by the physician and nursing staff are required to detect seizure activity.

   b. Some institutions give prophylactic phenobarbital (*controversial*).

   c. Restrict fluids to approximately 60 mL/kg/d.

   d. If seizures begin, follow guidelines given in **A.4,** above.

2. **Hypoglycemia.** Treat and determine the cause, as outlined in Chapter 41.

3. **Hypocalcemia.** Slowly give 100–200 mg/kg calcium gluconate intravenously. Make certain the infant is receiving maintenance calcium therapy (usually 50 mg/kg every 6 hours). Monitor the heart rate continuously and make certain that the intravenous line is correctly positioned.

4. **Hypomagnesemia.** Give 0.2 meq/kg magnesium sulfate intravenously every 6 hours until magnesium levels are normal or symptoms resolve.

5. **Hyponatremia.** See Chapter 43.

6. **Hypernatremia.** Treat the seizure activity as described in **A.4,** above. If hypernatremia is secondary to decreased fluid intake, increase the rate of free water. The amount of sodium needs to be decreased; it should be reduced over 48 hours to decrease the possibility of cerebral edema.

7. **Hypercalcemia.** Usual treatment plans include:

   a. Increase intravenous fluids by 20 mL/kg/d.

   b. Administer a diuretic, eg, furosemide (Lasix), 1–2 mg/kg/dose every 12 hours.

   c. Administer phosphate, 30–40 mg/kg/d orally or intravenously.

8. **Pyridoxine dependence.** Pyridoxine, 100 mg, is given intravenously. If the seizures stop immediately, it is diagnostic.

9. **Infection.** If sepsis is suspected, a complete workup should be performed and empiric broad-spectrum antibiotic therapy started. A complete septic workup includes white blood count and differential, blood culture, urine and serum Wellcogen, lumbar puncture (if indicated), and urinalysis and urine culture (if indicated).

10. **Drug withdrawal syndrome.** Supportive therapy and anticonvulsants are used. See Chapter 59.

11. **Subarachnoid hemorrhage.** Only supportive therapy is necessary.
12. **Subdural hemorrhage.** Only supportive therapy is necessary unless the infant has lacerations of the falx and tentorium or hemorrhage over cerebral convexities. Rapid surgical correction is necessary for lacerations of the falx and tentorium. Hemorrhage over cerebral convexities is treated by repeated subdural taps.

54 Vasospasm of Leg

I. **Problem.** An infant with an indwelling umbilical artery catheter develops vasospasm in one leg.

II. **Immediate questions**

   A. **Can the umbilical artery catheter be removed?** Evaluate the need for the catheter. If the catheter can be removed, this is the treatment of choice. **Vasospasm is most commonly related to the use of umbilical artery catheters.**

   B. **Was a medication given recently through the catheter?** The majority of medications, if given too rapidly, can cause vasospasm.

III. **Differential diagnosis**

   A. **Vasospasm.** Vasospasm is a muscular contraction of a vessel, manifested by acute color change (white or blue) in the lower extremity, sometimes only on the toes, sometimes over the entire extremity. Occasionally the color change extends to the buttocks and abdomen. The change in color may be transient or persistent. It may be caused by prior injection of medication or a thromboembolic phenomenon.

   B. **Thromboembolic phenomenon.** A **thrombus** is a clot formation at a specific site in a vessel. It can cause complete obstruction, resulting in loss of pulses and an extremity that is white. An **embolus** is a clot that lodges in a blood vessel and may cause obstruction or vasospasm.

IV. **Data base**

   A. **Physical examination.** The severity of the vasospasm must be assessed, as it dictates treatment. The areas on involvement, appearance of the skin over the involved areas, and pulses of the affected extremity are measures of severity.

   1. **Severe vasospasm** involves a large area of one or both legs, the abdomen, or the buttocks. The skin may be completely white. Pulses of the affected extremity are present.

   2. **Less severe vasospasm** involves a small area of one of both legs (usually some of the toes and part of the foot). The skin has a mottled appearance. Pulses of the affected extremity are present.

   3. **Thrombosis.** If pulses are absent, thrombosis (a **medical emergency**) is likely.

   B. **Laboratory studies.** Laboratory tests are not usually needed. However, the following laboratory tests should be obtained if thrombosis is suspected and streptokinase is to be used.

   1. **Thrombin time (TT).**
   2. **Activated partial thromboplastin time (PTT).**
   3. **Prothrombin time (PT).**
   4. **Hematocrit.**
   5. **Platelet count.**

   C. **Radiologic and other studies**

   1. **Real-time ultrasonography** can be used to diagnose thrombosis.
   2. **Angiography** performed through the umbilical artery catheter can be used to diagnose aorto-iliac thrombosis. (In one study, this procedure was found to be the most effective diagnostic technique.)
   3. **An x-ray study of the abdomen** should be done to determine catheter placement.

V. **Plan**

A. **Vasospasm.** *(Note:* Treatment is highly controversial and guidelines vary extensively. Check with your institutions's guidelines prior to initiating treatment.)
   1. **Severe vasospasm**
      a. **If possible, remove the catheter.** The vasospasm should then resolve spontaneously.
      b. **Tolazoline** (Priscoline), 0.1 mg/mL by continuous infusion at a rate of 0.25 mg/kg/h, until the catheter is removed. This dosage was used in one series of 3 cases with success.
      c. **Tolazoline,** 0.1 mg/h through the catheter as a continuous infusion for 3–4 hours. If the vasospasm resolves, the infusion may be stopped. If the vasospasm does not resolve, remove the catheter. *This treatment is highly controversial!*
   2. **Less severe vasospasm**
      a. **Conservative.** Wrap the entire *unaffected* leg in a warm—not hot—washcloth. This measure will cause reflex vasodilation of the vessels in the affected leg, and the vasospasm may resolve. Alternatively, immerse the affected leg in a sterilized container filled with warm water *(controversial).* A possible side effect of this method is increased oxygen consumption in the extremity. With either method, treatment should continue for 15–30 minutes before a beneficial effect will be seen.
      b. **Papaverine.** If the above treatment does not work, give papaverine hydrochloride, 1 mg intramuscularly, in the unaffected leg *(controversial).* Papaverine is a mild vasodilator; if it is going to work, the effect is usually apparent within 30 minutes.
      c. **Tolazoline.** If both of the above treatments fail, tolazoline may be given as described above in **1.b,c** for severe vasospasm.
      d. **Catheter removal.** If all of the above treatments fail, it is best to remove the catheter.
B. **Thromboembolic phenomenon.** If thrombosis is suspected and there is loss of pulses in the affected extremity, it is a **medical emergency.** *Management is highly controversial.*
   1. **Don't remove the catheter.** Leave the catheter in place to facilitate arteriography and streptokinase infusion, if needed.
   2. **Emergency consultation** with a vascular surgeon is recommended.
   3. **Infusion of intra-arterial streptokinase** has been successful in some infants. See p 481 for dosage and other pharmacologic information.
   4. **Immediate surgery** may be indicated.

55 Ambiguous Genitalia

I. **Definition.** Ambiguous genitalia are present (1) when the sex of an infant is not readily apparent after examination of the external genitalia or (2) when a gender role cannot be assigned on the basis of the appearance of the external genitalia alone (eg, microphallus in an apparent male, labial gonads in an apparent female, or bifid penis and scrotum as part of exstrophy of the bladder).

II. **Embryology.** Sexual differentiation of the external genitalia begins at 6–8 weeks' gestation and is virtually complete by 16 weeks. Differentiation of the external genitalia depends solely on the presence or absence of **androgen.** Adequate androgen will cause the external genitalia to differentiate along male lines. Absence of androgen causes a division of the urogenital sinus into the urethra and vagina with no further differentiation.

A. In the normal male, androgen production is determined by differentiation of the gonad as testes or ovary. Gonadal differentiation is determined by the **Y chromosome** and is either closely linked to or directly caused by the presence of the HY antigen, an HLA cell surface antigen expressed on all male cells. If the gonad differentiates as testis, chorionic gonadotropins drive it to produce and release **testosterone.** Testosterone is taken into the target-organ cells and converted there to **dihydrotestosterone,** the most potent of the androgens involved with sexual differentiation. At each step of this process, developmental or metabolic disorders may cause inadequate androgen production and incomplete male differentiation or pseudohermaphroditism.

B. In the female fetus, excessive androgen production mimics the effects of testosterone and dihydrotestosterone in the male, but the effect is usually partial, leading to phallic (clitoral) enlargement, incomplete fusion of the labioscrotal folds, and incomplete separation of the urethra and vagina.

III. **Pathophysiology**

A. **Virilization of female infants**

1. The **most common cause** of excess fetal androgen is an **enzymatic deficiency in the cortisol pathway** leading to excessive ACTH stimulation, adrenal hyperplasia, and excessive production of adrenal androgens (dihydroepiandrosterone and androstenedione) and testosterone. Virilization is most commonly caused by **absence of the 21-hydroxylase enzyme.** Relative or absolute **aldosterone deficiency** is usually present, producing salt loss and subsequent shock. **11-Hydroxylase enzyme deficiency** is less common and is not associated with salt loss.

2. **Other less common causes** are virilizing maternal or fetal tumors or inadvertent maternal androgen ingestion.

B. **Inadequate virilization of male infants.** This problem can be caused by inadequate androgen production or incomplete end-organ response to androgen. All of these abnormalities are uncommon, and most require extensive laboratory investigation before a final diagnosis can be confirmed.

1. **Decreased androgen production** can be caused by one of 5 rare enzyme defects. Three of these defects also cause cortisol deficiency and **nonvirilizing adrenal hyperplasia,** and 2 are specific to the testosterone pathway. The association of **micropenis** and **hypoglycemia** suggests **pituitary deficiency** with absence of gonadotropins, adrenocorticotropic hormone (ACTH), and/or growth hormone.

2. **Decreased end-organ response to androgen** is often called **testicular feminization** and can be caused by a defect in the androgen receptor or an unknown defect with normal receptors. It can be total (labial testes with otherwise normal-appearing female genitalia) or partial (incomplete virilization of a male).

C. **True hermaphroditism.** The presence of both testis and ovary (or ovotestes) in the same individual is a rare cause of ambiguous genitalia. Most individuals with true hermaphroditism have a 46,XX karyotype, but mosaics of 46,XX, 45,X, 46,XY, and multiple X/multiple Y have all been reported. Sixty percent of true hermaphrodites are unambiguously male at birth, but the remainder can have varying degrees of genital ambiguity or nearly normal female genitalia.

D. **Chromosome abnormalities** do not usually lead to ambiguous genitalia.

1. **Turner syndrome** (45,X chromosomes) and its variants do not cause an increase in androgen production, so differentiation of the genitalia is unambiguously female.

2. **Klinefelter syndrome** (47,XXY) and its variants cause differentiation of the gonad as a testes followed by male differentiation of the external genitalia.

3. **Mixed gonadal dysgenesis,** the presence of a normal or partially differentiated testis and an undifferentiated or streak gonad, is usually associated with 45,X/46,XY mosaicism and ambiguity of the external genitalia. Mixed gonadal dysgenesis is associated with a high incidence of gonadal malignancy in mid to late childhood, and it should be recognized and treated (with removal of the dysfunctional gonads) as early as possible to reduce the risk of future malignancy.

IV. **Risk factors.** Ingestion of some oral contraceptives during pregnancy is associated with ambiguous genitalia. Most other causes are chromosomal defects, either sporadic or familial.

V. **Clinical presentation.** Ambiguous genitalia usually are noted immediately at birth, when the first person to see the infant cannot readily assign a sex to the child. Occasionally the abnormality of genital development is noted later when a careful examination discloses the presence of labial gonads (suggesting testes and testicular feminization) or a micropenis (usually defined as less than 2.0 cm in length, pubis to tip) or perineoscrotal hypospadius.

VI. **Diagnosis**

A. **Laboratory studies**

1. **Chromosome analysis.** Most laboratories can now determine sex chromosome status from a blood sample in 24–48 hours, and it is the most appropriate test to use. Buccal smears provide a fast answer but are notoriously unreliable and are not frequently used today. The remainder of the diagnostic evaluation depends on the sex chromosome status; accuracy is paramount.

a. **Normal 46,XX karyotype.** This finding implies virilization of a genetic female and is caused by excessive maternal or fetal androgen. If the mother is not virilized, the infant almost always has **virilizing adrenal hyperplasia.** To confirm the diagnosis, measure:

(1) **17-hydroxyprogesterone (17-OHP).** This is the immediate precursor to the enzyme defect in 21-hydroxylase enzyme deficiency and two steps prior to that in 11-hydroxylase enzyme deficiency. In infants with either defect, the serum or plasma level of 17-OHP will be 100 to 1000 times the normal infant level.

(2) **Daily serum measurements of sodium and potassium.** Infants with 21-hydroxylase enzyme deficiency will usually have relative or absolute aldosterone deficiency and will begin to demonstrate hyperkalemia at days 3–5 and hyponatremia a day or two later. If hyperkalemia becomes clinically significant before the 17-OHP result is available, begin treatment empirically with intravenous saline, cortisol, and Florinef, since the diagnosis is virtually certain (see p 252, **C.1.b**).

(3) **Serum testosterone.** About 3% of infants with ambiguous genitalia will be true hermaphrodites and most will have 46,XX chromosomes. If the 17-OHP is not elevated and there is no maternal virilization, elevated testosterone suggests hermaphroditism or fetal testosterone-producing tumor.

b. **Normal 46,XY karyotype.** The differential diagnosis of an **incompletely virilized genetic male** is extremely complex and includes in utero testicular damage, defects of testosterone synthesis, end-organ resistance, or an enzymatic defect in conversion of testosterone to dihydrotestosterone. The laboratory evaluation is correspondingly complex and usually proceeds through a number of steps before the results of the preceding step become available.

(1) **Testosterone (T) and dihydrotestosterone (DHT).** These hormone levels should be measurable and higher in newborns than later in childhood. The T:DHT ratio should be between 5:1 and 20:1 when expressed in similar units. High T:DHT ratio suggests 5_α-reductase deficiency.

(2) **Luteinizing hormone (LH) and follicle-stimulating hormone (FSH).** These hormones are also higher in infancy than they are in childhood. A diagnosis of gonadotropin deficiency is suspected if these values are low in a reliable assay but can be confirmed in infancy only if there are other pituitary hormone deficits. Remember, growth hormone and ACTH deficiency are manifested in the newborn period as hypoglycemia.

(3) **Human chorionic gonadotropin.** Human chorionic gonadotropin should be administered. Recommendations vary, but a dose of 500–1000 units every day or every other day for 3 doses is most common. Then measure T and DHT again to demonstrate adequate gonadal response.

(4) **Testosterone.** Depo-Testosterone should be administered. The usual dose is 25 mg intramuscularly at 3–4 week intervals for 3 doses. This regimen is followed to demonstrate adequate growth of the phallus and is essential before a final decision is made to raise an ambiguous child as a male.

c. **Abnormal karyotype.** Mixed gonadal dysgenesis with a dysplastic gonad is the great risk for infants with abnormal karyotype and ambiguous genitalia. Hormone studies are likely to be unrevealing in this circumstance. Sex of rearing should be determined by the appearance of the external genitalia after consultation with a pediatric or urologic surgeon and detailed discussion with the family. Surgical exploration should be done

before age 2 to look for dysplastic gonads and remove gonadal tissue incompatible with the sex of rearing.
  B. **Radiographic studies.** Ultrasonography of the pelvis sometimes demonstrates the presence of a uterus. Contrast studies to outline the internal anatomy (sinography, urethrography, intravenous urography) should be done prior to any reconstructive surgery.
VII. **Management**
  A. **General considerations.** The most important aspect of the treatment of ambiguous genitalia in an infant is to protect the privacy of the parents and child while diagnostic studies are in progress. Once a diagnosis has been established, gender identity can be unambiguously assigned and steroid replacement, gonadal removal, and reconstructive surgery can be started to make the appearance and function of the child fit the gender assignment.
  B. **Initial measures**
    1. **Early instructions for the parents.** As soon as the abnormality is noted, a physician responsible for the infant should be identified and the parents should be informed. The family should be told their infant is generally healthy (if it is true) but that the genitalia are "incompletely developed" and that it is not possible, at present, to identify the sex of their child. It is best to use gender-nonspecific nouns such as baby, infant, or child rather than gender-specific pronouns such as he or she, him or her at this point to avoid showing your biases to the parents. All attempts to identify the sex of the child on the basis of appearance should be resisted, although there is likely to be great pressure to do so from parents, relatives, and professional personnel. It is important not to complete the birth certificate or make any reference to gender in any of the permanent medical records of mother or child.
    2. **Isolation of the infant.** The next objective should be to isolate the child from the inquiries of the community. *Tell the parents not to send out birth announcements and not to tell anyone outside the immediate family that the baby has been born until a gender assignment has been made.* Whatever the final gender assignment of the child, he or she will probably live the majority of its life in the community of birth, and confusion about gender assignment because of premature release of information will never be completely forgotten.
    3. **Early referral.** It is advisable to seek consultation from a specialist in the evaluation of children with ambiguous genitalia (usually an endocrinologist or geneticist) as soon as feasible. It is never acceptable to discharge a child from the nursery prior to detailed evaluation of the causes of ambiguous genitalia. In most cases, complete diagnosis, assignment of sex of rearing, and some surgical reconstruction should be initiated before discharge to home.
  C. **Medical management.** Most causes of ambiguous genitalia are not acute medical or surgical emergencies, and therapy is variable.
    1. **Congenital adrenal hyperplasia.** All forms of adrenal hyperplasia have absolute or relative cortisol deficiency and require early diagnosis and replacement therapy to prevent vascular collapse.
      a. **Glucocorticoid therapy.** Standard replacement therapy is **cortisone acetate,** 10–25 mg intramuscularly daily for 2–3 days followed by 37.5 mg/M^2 intramuscularly every 3 days. Oral hydrocortisone is erratically absorbed in infants but is the common agent for children after 6 months of age.
      b. **Mineralocorticoid therapy.** Deoxycorticosterone actetate (DOCA) is no longer being manufactured. **9$_\alpha$-Fluorocortisol (Florinef)** is the drug of choice. The usual dose is 0.05–0.1 mg orally daily.

Most endocrinologists also give 15–20 meq oral sodium daily as 25% sodium chloride or 1 g table salt (about $\frac{1}{4}$ tsp) added to the formula.

2. **Incompletely virilized genetic male.** See p 251, **b.(3),(4).**

D. **Gender assignment.** Gender assignment is beyond the scope of this brief discussion, but in general, the sex of rearing should be determined only when the final diagnosis is secure. The decision is generally made primarily on the basis of external anatomy. If the phallic length is less than 2.0 cm, it is best to raise the child as a female, whatever the chromosomal and gonadal sex. In the very rare circumstances of 5_α-reductase deficiency, or pituitary deficiency with concomitant growth hormone deficiency, the child may be raised as a male even with a very small phallus in infancy. In androgen resistance syndromes, the phallus may not enlarge with the increasing androgen levels of adolescence, and a final decision on the sex of rearing may have to await the results of a 2–3 month trial of testosterone therapy (see p 251, **b(4)**). In any case, the decision must be made in conjunction with surgical colleagues and with the goal of appropriate sexual function, if not fertility, as an adult. The parents must have a complete understanding of the options, and achieving this understanding can be a very time-consuming process.

VIII. **Prognosis.** Morbidity and mortality are largely dependent on associated anomalies. Although most children with ambiguous genitalia are fertile as adults, in some cases the gonads are dysplastic or must be removed to prevent malignant degeneration or to allow normal functional development compatible with assigned sex of rearing. Despite gonadal dysfunction or absence, anyone with a normal uterus is now a candidate for pregnancy using the steadily advancing techniques of in vitro fertilization.

REFERENCES

Donahoe PK: The diagnosis and treatment of infants with intersex abnormalities. *Pediatr Clin North Am* 1987;**34:**1333.

Griffen JE, Wilson JD: The syndromes of androgen resistance. *N Engl J Med* 1980;**302:**198.

Grumbach MM, Conte FA: Disorders of sexual differentiation. Pages 312–401 in: *Williams Textbook of Endocrinology,* 7th ed. Wilson JD, Foster DW (editors). Saunders, 1985.

Pagon RA: Diagnostic approach to the newborn with ambiguous genitalia. *Pediatr Clin North Am* 1987;**34:**1019.

White PC, New MI, DuPont B: Congenital adrenal hyperplasia. *N Engl J Med* 1987;**316:**1519, 1580.

56 Blood Abnormalities

ABO INCOMPATIBILITY

I. **Definition.** Isoimmune hemolytic anemia may result when ABO incompatibility occurs between the mother and the newborn infant. This disorder is most common with blood type A or B infants born to type O mothers. The hemolytic process begins in utero and is the result of active placental transport of maternal isoantibody. In type O mothers, isoantibody is predominantly 7S-IgG and is capable of crossing the placental membranes. Because of its larger size, the 19S-IgM isoantibody found in type A or type B mothers cannot cross. Symptomatic clinical disease, which usually does not present until after birth, is a compensated mild hemolytic anemia with reticulocytosis, microspherocytosis, and early-onset unconjugated hyperbilirubinemia.

II. **Incidence.** Risk factors for ABO incompatibility are present in 12–15% of pregnancies, but evidence of fetal sensitization (positive direct Coombs' test) occurs in only 3–4%. Symptomatic ABO hemolytic disease occurs in less than 1% of all newborn infants but accounts for approximately two-thirds of observed cases of hemolytic disease in the newborn.

III. **Pathophysiology.** Transplacental transport of maternal isoantibody results in an immune reaction with the A or B antigen on fetal erythrocytes, which produces characteristic **microspherocytes.** This process eventually results in complete extravascular hemolysis of the end-stage spherocyte. The ongoing hemolysis is balanced by compensatory reticulocytosis and shortening of the cell-cycle time, so that there is overall maintenance of the erythrocyte indices within physiologic limits. A paucity of A or B antigenic sites on the fetal (in contrast to the adult) erythrocytes and competitive binding of isoantibody by soft tissues may explain the often mild hemolytic process that occurs and the usual absence of progressive disease with subsequent pregnancies.

IV. **Risk factors**
   A. **A_1 antigen in infant.** Of the major blood group antigens, the A_1 antigen has the greatest antigenicity and is associated with a greater risk of symptomatic disease.
   B. **Elevated isohemagglutinins.** Antepartum intestinal parasitism or third-trimester immunization with tetanus toxoid or pneumococcal vaccine may stimulate isoantibody titer to A or B antigens.
   C. **Birth order.** Birth order is not considered a risk factor. Maternal isoantibody exists naturally and is independent of prior exposure to incompatible fetal blood group antigens. First-born infants have a 40–50% risk for symptomatic disease. Progressive severity of the hemolytic process in succeeding pregnancies is a rare phenomenon.

V. **Clinical presentation**
   A. **Symptoms and signs**
      1. **Jaundice.** Icterus is often the sole physical manifestation of ABO incompatibility with a clinically significant level of hemolysis. The onset is usually within the first 24 hours of life. The jaundice

evolves at a faster rate over the early neonatal period than nonhe-molytic physiologic pattern jaundice.

2. **Anemia.** Because of the effectiveness of compensation by reticulo-cytosis in response to the ongoing mild hemolytic process, erythro-cyte indices are maintained within a physiologic range that is nor-mal for asymptomatic infants of the same gestational age. Additional signs of clinical disease (hepatosplenomegaly, hydrops fetalis) are extremely unusual but may be seen with a more progres-sive hemolytic process (see Rh Incompatibility, p 266).

Exaggerated physiologic anemia may occur at 8–12 weeks of age, particularly when treatment during the neonatal period re-quired phototherapy or exchange transfusion.

VI. **Diagnosis.** Obligatory screening for infants with unconjugated hyperbili-rubinemia include the following studies.

A. **Blood type and Rh factor in mother and infant.** These studies estab-lish risk factors for ABO incompatibility.

B. **Reticulocyte count.** Elevated values following adjustment for gesta-tional age and degree of anemia, if any, will support the diagnosis of hemolytic anemia. For term infants, normal values are 4–5%; for pre-term infants of 30–36 weeks' gestational age, 6–10%. In ABO hemo-lytic disease of the newborn, values range from 10% to 30%.

C. **Direct Coombs' test.** The direct Coombs test (see definition under Rh incompatibility, p 267, **VI.C**) is usually weakly positive. If negative, it may raise doubt about ABO incompatibility as the cause of clinical disease or may indicate a lack of analytic sensitivity of the test. A strongly positive test is distinctly unusual and would direct attention to other isoimmune or autoimmune hemolytic processes.

D. **Blood smear.** The blood smear typically demonstrates **microsphero-cytes, polychromasia** proportionate to the reticulocyte response, and **normoblastosis** above the normal values for gestational age.

E. **Bilirubin levels** (fractionated or total and direct). Indirect hyperbili-rubinemia is mainly present and provides an index of the severity of disease. The rate at which unconjugated bilirubin levels are increas-ing suggests the required frequency of testing, usually every 4–8 hours until values plateau.

F. **Additional laboratory studies.** Supportive diagnostic studies may be indicated on an individual basis if the nature of the hemolytic process remains unclear.

1. **Antibody identification (indirect Coombs' test).** The indirect Coombs test is more sensitive than the direct Coombs test in de-tecting the presence of maternal isoantibody and will identify anti-body specificity. The test is performed on an eluate of neonatal erythrocytes, which is then tested against a panel of type-specific adult cells.

2. **Maternal IgG titer.** The absence in the mother of elevated IgG titers against the infant's blood group will tend to exclude a diagnosis of ABO incompatibility.

VII. **Management**

A. **Antepartum treatment.** Because of the low incidence of moderate to severe ABO hemolytic disease, invasive maneuvers before term is reached (eg, amniocentesis, early delivery) are usually not indicated.

B. **Postpartum treatment**

1. **General measures.** The maintenance of adequate hydration (see Chap 7) and evaluation for potentially aggravating factors (eg, sep-sis, drug exposure, or metabolic disturbance) should be consid-ered.

2. **Phototherapy.** Once a diagnosis of ABO incompatibility is estab-lished, phototherapy may be initiated before exchange transfusion

is given. Because of the usual mild to moderate hemolysis, photo-therapy may entirely obviate the need for exchange transfusion or may reduce the number of transfusions required. See Appendix I for guidelines on phototherapy.

3. **Exchange transfusion.** See Chapter 21 and Appendix F.

VIII. **Prognosis.** For infants with ABO incompatibility, the overall prognosis is excellent. Timely recognition and appropriate management of the rare infant with aggressive ABO hemolytic disease may avoid any potential morbidity or severe hemolytic anemia and secondary hyperbilirubinemia and the inherent risks associated with exchange transfusion and with the use of blood products.

ANEMIA

I. **Definition.** Anemia developing during the neonatal period (0–28 days of life) in infants older than 34 weeks' gestational age is indicated by a central venous hemoglobin less than 13 g/dL or a capillary venous hemoglobin less than 14.5 g/dL.

II. **Normal physiology.** At birth, normal values for the central venous hemoglobin in infants older than 34 weeks' gestational age are 14–20 g/dL, with an average value of 17 g/dL. In term infants, these values remain unchanged until 3 weeks of age, when hemoglobin begins to decline. In preterm infants of 30–36 weeks' gestational age, a similar process begins slightly earlier, at the end of the second week. Fetal **stress erythropoiesis** present at birth is reflected by reticulocytosis and macrocytic red cell indices. In anemia of prematurity, there is a similar physiologic adaptation in hemoglobin, but the lowest levels (7–9 g/dL) are reached earlier in the postnatal period (4–8 weeks). In the absence of clinical complications associated with prematurity, infants will remain asymptomatic during this process.

III. **Pathophysiology.** Anemia in the newborn infant results from one of 3 processes: (1) loss of red blood cells, or hemorrhagic anemia, the most common cause; (2) increased destruction of red blood cells, or hemolytic anemia; or (3) underproduction of red blood cells, or hypoplastic anemia.

A. **Hemorrhagic anemia**

1. **Antepartum period** (1:1000 live births).

a. **Loss of placental integrity.** Abruptio placentae, placenta previa, or traumatic amniocentesis (acute or chronic) may result in loss of placental integrity.

b. **Anomalies of umbilical cord or placental vessels.** Velamentous insertion of the umbilical cord occurs in 10% of twin gestations and almost all gestations with 3 or more fetuses. Communicating vessels (vasa previa), umbilical cord hematoma (1:5500 deliveries), or entanglement of the cord by the fetus may also cause hemorrhagic anemia.

c. **Twin-twin transfusion.**

2. **Intrapartum period**

a. **Fetomaternal hemorrhage.** Fetomaternal hemorrhage occurs in 30–50% of pregnancies. The risk is increased with preeclampsia-eclampsia, with the need for instrumentation, and with cesarean section. In approximately 8% of pregnancies, the volume of the hemorrhage is more than 10 mL.

b. **Cesarean section.** In elective cesarean deliveries, there is a 3% incidence of anemia. The incidence is increased in emergency cesarean deliveries. Delay in cord clamping beyond 30 seconds is associated with an increased risk of fetomaternal hemorrhage.

c. **Traumatic rupture of the umbilical cord.** Rupture may occur if delivery is uncontrolled or unattended.

d. **Failure of placental transfusion.** Failure is usually caused by umbilical cord occlusion (nuchal cord, entangled or prolapsed cord) during vaginal delivery. Blood loss may be 25–30 mL in the newborn.

e. **Obstetric trauma.** During a difficult vaginal delivery, occult visceral or intracranial hemorrhage may occur. It may not be apparent at birth. Difficult deliveries are more common with large-for-gestational-age (LGA) infants, breech presentation, or difficult extraction.

3. **Neonatal period**
   a. **Enclosed hemorrhage.** Hemorrhage severe enough to cause neonatal anemia suggests obstetric trauma, perinatal distress, or a defect in hemostasis.
      (1) **Caput succedaneum** is relatively common and may result in benign hemorrhage.
      (2) **Cephalohematoma** is found in up to 2.5% of births. It is associated with vacuum extraction and primiparity (5% risk of associated linear nondepressed skull fracture).
      (3) **Intracranial hemorrhage** may occur in the subdural, subarachnoid, or subependymal space.
      (4) **Visceral parenchymal hemorrhage** is uncommon. It is usually the result of obstetric trauma to an internal organ, most commonly the liver but also the spleen, kidneys, or adrenal glands.
   b. **Defects in hemostasis.** Defects in hemostasis may be congenital, but more commonly hemorrhage occurs secondary to consumption coagulopathy, which may be caused by:
      (1) Congenital coagulation factor deficiency.
      (2) Consumption coagulopathy
         (a) Disseminated congenital or viral infection.
         (b) Bacterial sepsis or hypotension.
         (c) Intravascular embolism of thromboplastin (due to dead twin, maternal toxemia, necrotizing enterocolitis (NEC), others).
      (3) **Deficiency of vitamin K–dependent coagulation factors** (factors II, VII, IX, and X).
         (a) Failure to administer vitamin K at birth usually results in a bleeding diathesis at 3–4 days of age.
         (b) Use of antibiotics may interfere with the production of vitamin K by normal gastrointestinal flora.
      (4) **Thrombocytopenia**
         (a) Immune thrombocytopenia may be isoimmune or autoimmune.
         (b) **Congenital thrombocytopenia with absent radii** is a syndrome frequently associated with hemorrhagic anemia in the newborn.
   c. **Iatrogenic blood loss.** Anemia may occur if blood loss due to repeated venipuncture is not replaced routinely. Symptoms may develop if a loss of 20% or more occurs within a 48-hour period.

B. **Hemolytic anemia**
   1. **Immune hemolysis**
      a. **Isoimmune hemolytic anemia** is due to ABO, Rh, or minor blood group incompatibility.
      b. **Autoimmune hemolytic anemia.**
   2. **Nonimmune hemolysis**
      a. Bacterial sepsis may cause primary microangiopathic hemolysis.
      b. Congenital TORCH infections (see p 339).
   3. **Congenital erythrocyte defect**
      a. Metabolic enzyme deficiency.

      (1) Glucose-6-phosphate dehydrogenase (G6PD) deficiency.
      (2) Pyruvate kinase deficiency.
   b. Thalassemia.
   c. Hemoglobinopathy may be characterized as unstable hemoglobins or congenital Heinz-body anemias.
   d. Membrane defects are usually autosomal dominant.
      (1) Hereditary spherocytosis (1:5000 neonates) commonly presents with jaundice and less often with anemia.
      (2) Hereditary elliptocytosis (1:2500 neonates) rarely presents in the newborn infant.
  4. Systemic diseases
   a. Galactosemia.
   b. Osteopetrosis.
  5. Nutritional deficiency. Vitamin E deficiency occurs in association with prematurity or chronic malabsorption but usually does not present until after the neonatal period.
 C. Hypoplastic anemia
  1. Congenital disease
   a. Diamond-Blackfan syndrome (congenital hypoplastic anemia).
   b. Atransferrinemia.
   c. Congenital leukemia.
   d. Sideroblastic anemia.
  2. Acquired disease
   a. Infection. Rubella and syphilis are the most common causes.
   b. Aplastic crisis.
   c. Aplastic anemia.
IV. Clinical presentation
 A. Symptoms and signs. The 3 major forms of neonatal anemia may be demonstrated by determination of the following factors: (1) age at presentation of anemia, (2) associated clinical features at presentation, (3) hemodynamic status of infant, and (4) presence or absence of compensatory reticulocytosis.
  1. Hemorrhagic anemia. Hemorrhagic anemia is often dramatic in clinical presentation when acute but may be more subtle when chronic. Both forms have significant rates of perinatal morbidity and mortality if they remain unrecognized. Neither form has significant elevation of bilirubin levels or hepatosplenomegaly.
   a. Acute hemorrhagic anemia presents at birth or with internal hemorrhage after 24 hours. There is pallor unassociated with jaundice and often without cyanosis (< 5 g deoxyhemoglobin) and unrelieved by supplemental oxygen. Tachypnea or gasping respirations are present. Vascular instability ranges from decreased peripheral perfusion (≤ 10% loss of blood volume) to hypovolemic shock (20–25% loss of blood volume). There is also decreased central venous pressure and poor capillary refill. Normocytic or normochromic red blood cell indices are present, with reticulocytosis developing within 2–3 days of the hemorrhagic event.
   b. Chronic hemorrhagic anemia presents at birth with unexplained pallor, often without cyanosis (< 5 g deoxyhemoglobin) and unrelieved by supplemental oxygen. Minimal signs of respiratory distress are present. The central venous pressure is normal or increased. Microcytic or hypochromic red blood cell indices are present, with compensatory reticulocytosis. Hydrops fetalis or stillbirth may occur with failure of compensatory reticulocytosis or intravascular volume maintenance.
   c. Asphyxia pallida (severe neonatal asphyxia) is not associated with hemorrhagic anemia at presentation. This disorder must be

distinguished clinically from acute hemorrhage because specific immediate therapy is needed for each disorder. Asphyxia pallida presents at birth with pallor and cyanosis that improves with supplemental oxygen delivery, respiratory failure, bradycardia, and normal central venous pressure.

2. **Hemolytic anemia.** Jaundice is often seen before diagnostic levels of hemoglobin are obtained, in part because of the compensatory reticulocytosis that is invariably present. The infant usually presents with pallor after 48 hours of age. However, severe Rh isoimmune disease or homozygous alpha thalassemia will present at birth with severe anemia and, in many cases, hydrops fetalis. Unconjugated hyperbilirubinemia exceeding 10–12 mg/dL, tachypnea, and hepatosplenomegaly may be seen with hemolytic anemia.

3. **Hypoplastic anemia.** Hypoplastic anemia is uncommon. It is characterized by presentation after 48 hours of age, absence of jaundice, and reticulocytopenia.

4. **Other forms of anemia**
   a. **Anemia associated with twin-twin transfusion.** If chronic hemorrhage is occurring, there is often more than a 20% difference in the birth weights of the 2 infants, with the donor being the smaller twin.
   b. **Occult (internal) hemorrhage**
      (1) **Intracranial hemorrhage.** Signs include a bulging anterior fontanelle and neurologic signs (eg, change in consciousness, apnea, or seizures).
      (2) **Visceral hemorrhage.** Most commonly, the liver has been injured. An abdominal mass or distention is seen.
      (3) **Pulmonary hemorrhage.** Partial or total radiographic opacification of a hemithorax and bloody tracheal secretions are seen.

B. **History**
   1. **Anemia at birth**
      a. **Hemorrhagic anemia.** There may be a history of third-trimester vaginal bleeding or amniocentesis. Hemorrhagic anemia may be associated with multiple gestation, maternal chills or fever postpartum, and nonelective cesarean section.
      b. **Hemolytic anemia** may be associated with intrauterine growth retardation (IUGR) and Rh-negative mothers.
   2. **Anemia presenting after 24 hours of age** is often associated with obstetric trauma, unattended delivery, precipitous delivery, perinatal fetal distress, or a low Apgar score.
   3. **Anemia presenting with jaundice** suggests hemolytic anemia. There may be evidence of drug ingestion late in the third trimester; IUGR; a family member with splenectomy, anemia, jaundice, or cholelithiasis; maternal autoimmune disease; or Mediterranean or Oriental ethnic background.

V. **Diagnosis**
   A. **Obligatory initial studies**
      1. **Hemoglobin**
      2. **Red blood cell indices**
         a. **Microcytic or hypochromic red blood cell** indices suggest fetomaternal or twin-twin hemorrhage or alpha thalessemia (MCV < 90 fl).
         b. **Normocytic or normochromic red blood cell indices** are suggestive of acute hemorrhage, systemic disease, intrinsic red cell defect, or hypoplastic anemia.
      3. **Reticulocyte count** (corrected). The following formula is used.

Corrected reticulocyte count =

$$\frac{\text{Observed reticulocyte count} \times \text{Observed hematocrit}}{\text{Normal hematocrit for age}}$$

An elevated reticulocyte count is associated with antecedent hemorrhage or hemolytic anemia. A low count is seen with hypoplastic anemia.

4. **Blood smear**
   a. Spherocytes are associated with ABO isoimmune hemolysis or hereditary spherocytosis.
   b. Elliptocytes are seen in hereditary elliptocytosis.
   c. Pyknocytes may be seen in G6PD deficiency.
   d. Schistocytes or helmet cells are most often seen with consumption coagulopathy.
5. **Direct antiglobin test (direct Coombs' test).** This test is positive in isoimmune or autoimmune hemolysis.
B. **Other selected laboratory studies**
   1. **Isoimmune hemolysis.** The blood type and Rh type should be determined, and an eluate of neonatal cells should be prepared
   2. **Fetomaternal hemorrhage.** The **Kleihauer-Betke test** should be performed. Using an acid elution technique, a maternal blood smear is stained with eosin. Fetal red blood cells stain darkly. Adult red blood cells do not stain and appear as "ghost cells." ABO incompatibility between mother and infant will result in increased clearance rate of fetal cells from the maternal circulation, giving a falsely low result.

   $$2400 \times \text{Ratio of fetal to maternal cells} =$$
   mL of fetal blood lost into maternal circulation

   3. **Pulmonary hemorrhage.** Perform the Apt test (see p 178, **B.1**).
   4. **Congenital hypoplastic or aplastic anemia.** Bone marrow aspiration is usually indicated.
   5. **TORCH infection**
      a. Skull and long bone films.
      b. IgM levels.
      c. Acute or convalescent serologic.
      d. Urine culture for cytomegalovirus.
   6. **Consumption coagulopathy**
      a. Prothrombin time (PT) and partial thromboplastin time (PTT).
      b. Platelet count.
      c. Thrombin time (TT) or fibrinogen assay.
      d. Factor V and factor VIII levels.
      e. Fibrin split products.
   7. **Occult hemorrhage**
      a. Pathologic examination of placenta.
      b. Cranial or abdominal ultrasonography will help identify the site of bleeding.
   8. **Intrinsic red blood cell defect**
      a. Red blood cell enzyme studies.
      b. Analysis of globin chain ratio.
      c. Studies of red blood cell membrane.
VI. **Management.** Treatment of neonatal anemia may involve, individually or in combination, simple replacement transfusion, exchange transfusion, nutritional supplementation, or treatment of the underlying primary disorder.
A. **Simple replacement transfusion**
   1. **Indications**
      a. Acute hemorrhagic anemia.
      b. Ongoing deficit replacement.
      c. Maintenance of effective oxygen-carrying capacity (hemoglobin,

15 g/dL) in high-risk infants with apnea, or compromised tissue oxygenation (eg, NEC, cardiopulmonary instability).

2. Emergency transfusion at birth only
  a. Use type O, Rh-negative packed red blood cells.
  (1) Adjust the hematocrit to 50%.
  (2) *If a medical emergency exists, blood that has not been cross-matched may be given.*
  (3) Blood drawn from the placental vein and heparinized (1 unit/mL) can be utilized if given through a blood filter. If time permits, blood may be cross-matched to the mother's blood.
  b. Alternative replacement fluids include fresh-frozen plasma, 5% albumin in saline, and dextran. Timely infusion of packed red blood cells or partial exchange transfusion should follow.
  c. Perform umbilical vein catheterization to a depth of 2–3 cm or until free blood flow is established (see p 164).
  d. Measure the central venous pressure, if time and technical capabilities allow, after advancing the catheter to the level of T6–T9.
  e. Draw initial blood samples for diagnostic studies. Obtain a hemogram and differential, blood type and Rh type, direct Coombs' test, and, if indicated, total bilirubin levels. In a medical emergency, transfusion may be started before the results of laboratory testing are known.
  f. Infuse 10–15 mL/kg of replacement fluid over 10–15 minutes if emergency measures are needed. Once the infant's status has stabilized, reassess the diagnostic studies, physical examination, and obstetric history.
  g. Calculate the red blood cell volume. Under controlled circumstances or if simple transfusion is indicated, calculate the volume of packed red blood cells needed to achieve the desired increase in red blood cell mass (see p 220).
  h. The volume of a single transfusion should not exceed 10 mL/kg unless the central venous pressure is monitored.

B. Exchange transfusion
  1. Indications
    a. Chronic hemolytic anemia or hemorrhagic anemia with increased central venous pressure.
    b. Severe isoimmune hemolytic anemia with circulating sensitized red blood cells and isoantibody.
    c. Consumption coagulopathy.
  2. Technique. See Chapter 21.

C. Nutritional replacement
  1. Iron. Iron replacement is useful in the following situations.
    a. Fetomaternal hemorrhage of significant volume.
    b. Chronic twin-twin transfusion (in the donor twin).
    c. Incremental external blood loss (if unreplaced).
    d. Preterm infant (< 36 weeks gestational age).
  2. Folate (especially with serum levels < 0.5 ng/mL).
    a. Premature infants weighing less than 1500 g or younger than 34 weeks' gestational age.
    b. Chronic hemolytic anemias or conditions involving "stress erythropoiesis."
    c. Infants receiving phenytoin (Dilantin).
  3. Vitamin E. Preterm infants younger than 34 weeks' gestational age, unless they are being breast-fed.

D. Prophylactic nutritional supplementation
  1. Elemental iron, 1–2 mg/kg/d, beginning at 2 months of age and continuing through 1 year of age.
  2. Folic acid, 1–2 mg/wk for preterm infants; 50 μg/d for term infants.

3. **Vitamin E,** 25 IU/d, until a corrected age of 4 months is reached.
E. **Treatment of selected disorders**
   1. **Consumption coagulopathy**
      a. Treat the underlying cause, eg, sepsis.
      b. Give blood replacement therapy. Perform exchange transfusion or give fresh-frozen plasma, 10 mL/kg every 12–14 hours. Platelet concentrate, 1 unit, may be used as a substitute for plasma transfusion.
      c. Perform coagulation studies. Monitor the PTT, TT, and fibrinogen levels and the platelet count.
   2. **Immune thrombocytopenia**
      a. **Isoimmune thrombocytopenia**
         (1) Consider performing cesarean section if the diagnosis has been confirmed and there is an older sibling with immune thrombocytopenia (75% risk of recurrence).
         (2) Give maternal washed platelets when indicated for bleeding diathesis in an infant with a platelet count less than 20,000–30,000/μL. Exchange transfusion may be used as an alternative.
         (3) Corticosteroid therapy is *controversial*.
      b. **Autoimmune thrombocytopenia**
         (1) Consider performing cesarean section if the maternal platelet count is less than 100,000/μL or the fetal platelet count is less than 50,000/μL.
         (2) Use of corticosteroids is *controversial*. Under the above conditions, consider giving corticosteroids to the mother several weeks before delivery.
         (3) Transfusion of random donor platelets may be given when indicated.

POLYCYTHEMIA AND HYPERVISCOSITY

I. **Definitions.** Polycythemia is increased total red blood cell mass. Polycythemic hyperviscosity is increased viscosity of the blood resulting from increased numbers of red blood cells.
   A. **Polycythemia.** Polycythemia of the newborn is defined as a central venous hematocrit of 65% or more. The clinical significance of this value results from the curvilinear relationship between the circulating red cell volume (hematocrit) and whole blood viscosity. Above a hematocrit of 65%, blood viscosity rises exponentially.
   B. **Hyperviscosity.** Hyperviscosity is a more direct cause of clinical symptoms in most polycythemic infants. Factors other than hematocrit may sometimes exacerbate or occur independently of increased red cell volume, causing hyperviscosity. The terms *polycythemia* and *hyperviscosity* are thus not interchangeable. Although most polycythemic infants are also hyperviscous, it is not invariably the case.
II. **Incidence**
   A. **Polycythemia.** Polycythemia occurs in 2–4% of the general newborn population; half of these patients are symptomatic. Determining the hematocrit only in symptomatic newborn infants tends to underestimate the incidence of polycythemia.
   B. **Hyperviscosity.** Hyperviscosity without polycythemia occurs in an additional 1% of normal newborns. In infants with a hematocrit of 60–64%, one-fourth have hyperviscosity.
III. **Pathophysiology.** Symptomatic clinical disease in a polycythemic infant results from the regional effects of hyperviscosity, including tissue hypoxia, acidosis, and hypoglycemia, and from the formation of microthrombi within the microcirculation. More commonly involved structures

include the central nervous system, the kidneys and adrenal glands, the cardiopulmonary system, and the gastrointestinal tract. The degree to which clinical disease is expressed depends on the interaction of frictional forces in the whole blood. These forces are defined as **shear stress** and **shear rate,** a measure of blood flow velocity. The frictional forces identified within whole blood and their relative contributions to hyperviscosity in the newborn include the following.

A. **Hematocrit.** Increase in the hematocrit is the most important single factor contributing to hyperviscosity in the neonate. An increased hematocrit results from either an absolute increase in circulating red blood cell volume or a decrease in plasma volume.

B. **Plasma viscosity.** A direct linear relationship exists between plasma viscosity and the concentration of plasma proteins, particularly those of high molecular weight, such as fibrinogen. Term infants and, to a greater degree, preterm infants have low plasma fibrinogen levels compared to those of adults. Consequently, except for the rare case of primary hyperfibrinogenemia, plasma viscosity does not contribute to increased whole blood viscosity in the neonate. Under normal conditions, low plasma fibrinogen levels and correspondingly low plasma viscosity actually may protect the microcirculation of the neonate by facilitating perfusion and contributing to low whole-blood viscosity.

C. **Red blood cell aggregation.** Aggregation of erythrocytes occurs only in areas of low blood flow and is usually limited to the venous microcirculation. Because fibrinogen levels are typically low in term and preterm infants, red cell aggregation does not contribute significantly to whole blood viscosity in newborn infants. There is some recent concern that the use of adult fresh-frozen plasma for partial exchange transfusion in neonates might critically alter the concentration of fibrinogen and limit the expected fall of whole blood viscosity within the microcirculation.

D. **Deformability of red blood cell membrane.** There are apparently no differences between term infants, preterm infants, and adults in terms of the membrane deformability of erythrocytes.

IV. **Risk factors**

A. **Conditions that alter incidence**

1. **Altitude.** There is an absolute increase in red blood cell mass as part of physiologic adaptation to high altitude.

2. **Neonatal age.** The normal pattern of fluid shifts during the first 6 hours of life is away from the intravascular compartment. The period of maximum physiologic increase in the hematocrit occurs at 2–4 hours of age.

3. **Obstetric factors.** A delay in cord clamping beyond 30 seconds or stripping of the umbilical cord, if that is the prevailing practice, will result in a higher incidence of polycythemia.

4. **High-risk delivery.** High-risk delivery is associated with an increased incidence of polycythemia, particularly if precipitous or uncontrolled.

B. **Perinatal processes**

1. **Enhanced fetal erythropoiesis.** Elevated erythropoietin levels result from a direct stimulus, usually related to fetal hypoxia, or from altered regulation of erythropoietin production.

a. **Placental insufficiency**

(1) Maternal hypertensive disease (preeclampsia-eclampsia) or primary renovascular disease.

(2) Abruptio placentae (chronic recurrent).

(3) Postmaturity.

(4) Cyanotic congenital heart disease.

(5) Intrauterine growth retardation.

(6) Maternal cigarette smoking.
  b. **Endocrine disorders.** Increased oxygen consumption is the suggested mechanism by which hyperinsulinism or hyperthyroxinemia creates fetal hypoxemia and stimulates erythropoietin production.
    (1) Infant of a diabetic mother (> 40% incidence of polycythemia).
    (2) Infant of a mother with gestational diabetes (> 30% incidence of polycythemia).
    (3) Congenital thyrotoxicosis.
    (4) Congenital adrenal hyperplasia.
    (5) Beckwith-Wiedemann syndrome (secondary hyperinsulinism).
  c. **Genetic trisomies** (trisomies 13,18, and 21).
2. **Hypertransfusion.** Conditions that enhance placental transfusion at birth may create hypervolemic normocythemia, which evolves into hypervolemic polycythemia as the normal pattern of fluid shift occurs. A larger transfusion may create hypervolemic polycythemia at birth, with acute symptoms present in the infant. Conditions associated with hypertransfusion include the following.
  a. **Delay in cord clamping.** Placental vessels contain up to one-third of the fetal blood volume, half of which will be returned to the infant within 1 minute after birth. Representative blood volumes for term infants with a variable delay in cord clamping are:
    (1) 15-second delay, 75–78 mL/kg.
    (2) 60-second delay, 80–87 mL/kg.
    (3) 120-second delay, 83–93 mL/kg.
  b. **Gravity.** Positioning the infant below the placental bed (> 10 cm below the placenta) enhances placental transfusion via the umbilical vein. Elevation of the infant more than 50 cm above the placenta will prevent placental transfusion.
  c. **Maternal use of medications.** Drugs that enhance uterine contractility—specifically oxytocin—do not significantly alter the gravitational effects on placental transfusion during the first 15 seconds after birth. With further delay in clamping of the cord, however, blood flow toward the infant will accelerate to a maximum at 1 minute of age.
  d. **Cesarean section.** In cesarean delivery, there is usually a lower risk of placental transfusion if the cord is clamped early because of the absence of active uterine contractions in most cases and because of gravitational effects.
  e. **Twin-twin transfusion.** Interfetal transfusion (**parabiosis syndrome**) is observed in monochorionic twin pregnancy with an incidence of 15%. The recipient twin, on the venous side of the anastomosis, becomes polycythemic and the donor, on the arterial side, becomes anemic. Simultaneous venous hematocrits obtained following delivery differ by more than 12–15%, and both twins will have a high risk of intrauterine or neonatal death.
  f. **Maternal-fetal transfusion.** Approximately 10–80% of normal newborn infants receive a small volume of maternal blood at the time of delivery. The "reverse" Kleihauer-Betke acid elution technique (see p 260) will document maternal red blood cell "ghosts" on a neonatal blood smear. With large transfusions, the test will be positive for several days.
  g. **Intrapartum asphyxia.** Prolonged fetal distress enhances the net umbilical blood flow toward the infant until cord clamping occurs.

V. Clinical presentation. *Clinical signs observed in polycythemia are non-specific and reflect the regional effects of hyperviscosity within a given microcirculation. The conditions listed below may occur independently of polycythemia or hyperviscosity and must be considered in the differential diagnosis.*

  A. **Central nervous system.** There is an altered state of consciousness, including lethargy and decreased activity or hyperirritability. Proximal muscle hypotonia, vasomotor instability, vomiting, seizures, thrombosis, and cerebral infarction may also be seen.

  B. **Cardiopulmonary system.** Respiratory distress syndrome may be present. Tachycardia and low-output congestive heart failure with cardiomegaly may be seen. There may be primary pulmonary hypertension.

  C. **Gastrointestinal tract.** Feeding intolerance, abdominal distention, or necrotizing enterocolitis may be present.

  D. **Genitourinary tract.** Oliguria, acute renal failure, renal vein thrombosis, or priapism may occur.

  E. **Metabolic disorders.** Hypoglycemia, hypocalcemia, or hypomagnesemia may be seen.

  F. **Hematologic disorders.** There may be hyperbilirubinemia, thrombocytopenia, or reticulocytosis (with enchanced erythropoiesis only).

VI. Diagnosis

  A. **Venous (not capillary) hematocrit.** Polycythemia is present when the central venous hematocrit is 65% or more.

  B. **The following screening studies may be used.**
  1. A cord blood hematocrit greater than 56% indicates polycythemia.
  2. A warmed capillary hematocrit greater than 65% indicates polycythemia.

VII. Management. Clinical management of the polycythemic infant is based on the presence of symptoms, the age of the infant, central venous hematocrit, and associated conditions.

  A. **Asymptomatic infants.** Only expectant observation is required for most asymptomatic infants. The exceptions are infants with a central venous hematocrit over 70%, in which case partial exchange transfusion is recommended. Meticulous clinical examination is necessary to detect subtle clinical signs of polycythemia or hyperviscosity. The absence of even subtle signs does not preclude some risk of neurologic sequelae, however.

  B. **Symptomatic infants.** When the central venous hematocrit is 65% or more, partial exchange transfusion is indicated at any age. When the central venous hematocrit is 60–64% and the infant is less than 2 hours of age, monitor the hematocrit closely and consider partial exchange transfusion in anticipation of physiologic fluid shifts and further decrease in plasma volume. See p 150, **V.C,** for the procedure for partial exchange transfusion. The efficacy of partial exchange transfusion in polycythemic infants remains controversial.

VIII. Prognosis. The long-term outcome of infants with polycythemia or hyperviscosity and response to partial exchange transfusion is as follows.

  A. A causal relationship exists between partial exchange transfusion and an increase in gastrointestinal tract disorders and necrotizing enterocolitis.

  B. Randomized controlled prospective studies of polycythemic and hyperviscous infants indicate that partial exchange transfusion may reduce but not eliminate the risk of neurologic sequelae.

  C. Infants with "asymptomatic" polycythemia have an increased risk for neurologic sequelae.

  D. The natural spectrum of neurologic sequelae observed in polycythemic infants not undergoing partial exchange transfusion includes abnormalities in speech, delay in acquiring both fine and gross motor control, and general neurologic deficits.

Rh INCOMPATIBILITY

I. **Definition.** Isoimmune hemolytic anemia of variable severity may result when Rh incompatibility develops between an Rh-negative mother previously sensitized to the Rh antigen and her Rh-positive fetus. The onset of clinical disease begins in utero as the result of active placental transfer of maternal IgG-Rh antibody. It is manifested as a partially compensated, moderate to severe hemolytic anemia at birth, with unconjugated hyperbilirubinemia developing in the early neonatal period.

II. **Incidence.** Historically, Rh hemolytic disease of the newborn accounted for up to one-third of symptomatic cases seen and was associated with detectable antibody in approximately 15% of Rh-incompatible mothers. The use of Rh immunoglobulin (RhoGAM) prophylaxis has reduced the incidence of Rh sensitization to less than 1% of Rh-incompatible pregnancies. Isoimmunization may still occur when incompatibility for Rh antigens other than the D antigen exists, notably C and E, which occur in low frequency in the population and cannot be prevented by the use of D-antigen-specific Rh immunoglobulin.

III. **Pathophysiology.** Initial exposure of the mother to the Rh antigen occurs most often during parturition, miscarriage, or abortion or following traumatic amniocentesis. If recognition of the antigen by the immune system ensues following initial exposure, reexposure to the Rh antigen will induce a maternal anamnestic response and elevation of specific IgG-Rh antibody. Active placental transport of this antibody and immune attachment to the Rh antigenic sites on the fetal erythrocyte are followed by extravascular hemolysis of erythrocytes within the fetal liver and spleen. The rate of the hemolytic process is proportionate to the levels of the maternal antibody titer but is more accurately reflected in the antepartum period by elevation of the amniotic fluid bilirubin concentration, and in the postpartum period by the rate of rise of unconjugated bilirubin. In contrast to ABO incompatibility, the greater antigenicity and density of the Rh antigen loci on the fetal erythrocyte will facilitate progressive, rapid clearance of fetal erythrocytes from the circulation. A demonstrable phase of spherocytosis will be absent. Compensatory reticulocytosis and shortening of the erythrocyte generation time, if unable to match the often high rate of hemolysis in utero, will result in anemia in the newborn infant and a risk of multiple systemic complications.

IV. **Risk factors**

A. **Birth order.** The first-born infant is at minimum risk (< 1%) unless sensitization has occurred previously. Once sensitization has occurred, subsequent pregnancies are at a progressive risk for fetal disease.

B. **Fetomaternal hemorrhage.** The volume of fetal erythrocytes entering the maternal circulation correlates directly with the risk of sensitization. The risk is approximately 8% with each pregnancy but ranges from 3% to 65%, depending on the volume of fetal blood (0.1 mL to > 5 mL) that passes into the maternal circulation.

C. **ABO incompatibility.** Coexistent incompatibility for either the A or B blood group antigen will reduce the risk of maternal Rh sensitization to 1.5–3.0%. Rapid immune clearance of these fetal erythrocytes following their entry into the maternal circulation exerts a protective effect that decreases with increasing parity.

D. **Obstetric factors.** Cesarean section or trauma to the placental bed during the third stage of labor increases the risk of significant fetomaternal transfusion and subsequent maternal sensitization.

E. **Gender.** Male infants are reported to have an increased risk of more severe disease than females, although the basis for this observation is unclear.

F. **Ethnicity.** Approximately 15% of Caucasians are Rh-negative compared to 5.5% of blacks. The risk to the fetus varies accordingly. Rh-negativity is not seen in Orientals.

G. **Maternal immune response.** A significant proportion of Rh-negative mothers (10–50%) fails to develop specific IgG-Rh negative antibody despite repeated exposure to Rh antigen.

V. **Clinical presentation**
   A. **Symptoms and signs**
      1. **Jaundice.** Unconjugated hyperbilirubinemia is the most common presenting neonatal sign of Rh disease, usually appearing within the first 24 hours of life.
      2. **Anemia.** A low cord blood hemoglobin at birth reflects the relative severity of the hemolytic process in utero and is present in approximately 50% of cases.
      3. **Hepatosplenomegaly.** Enlargement of the liver and spleen are seen in severe hemolysis, sometimes occurring in association with ascites, with an increased risk for splenic rupture.
      4. **Hydrops fetalis.** Severe Rh disease has an historical association with hydrops fetalis and at one time was its most common cause. Clinical features in the fetus include progressive hypoproteinemia with ascites or pleural effusion, or both; severe chronic anemia with secondary hypoxemia; and cardiac failure. There is an increased risk of late fetal death, stillbirth, and intolerance of active labor. The neonate frequently has generalized edema, notably of the scalp, which can be detected by antepartum ultrasound; cardiopulmonary distress often involving pulmonary edema; congestive heart failure; hypotension and peripheral perfusion defects; cardiac rhythm disturbances; and severe anemia with secondary hypoxemia and metabolic acidosis. Currently, nonimmune conditions are more commonly associated with hydrops fetalis. Severe anemia per se is not the controlling factor in the clinical development of fetal hydrops. It may be that several systemic disturbances must be present in combination to produce the clinical expression of disease. Secondary involvement of other organ systems may result in hypoglycemia or thrombocytopenic purpura.

VI. **Diagnosis.** Obligatory screening in an infant with unconjugated hyperbilirubinemia includes the following studies.
   A. **Blood type and Rh type (mother and infant).** These studies establish the likelihood of Rh incompatibility and will exclude the diagnosis if the infant is Rh-negative, with one exception (see direct Coombs' test, below).
   B. **Reticulocyte count.** Elevated reticulocyte levels, adjusted for the degree of anemia and gestational age in preterm infants, reflect the degree of compensation and support a diagnosis of an ongoing hemolytic process. Normal values are 4–5% for term infants, and 6–10% for preterm infants (30–36 weeks' gestational age). In symptomatic Rh disease, expected values are 10–40%.
   C. **Direct Coombs' test.** A strongly positive direct Coombs test on fetal red blood cells, indicative of an active immune reaction occurring against fetal erythrocytes, is diagnostic of Rh incompatibility in the presence of the appropriate setup and an elevated reticulocyte count. If Rh immunoglobulin was given at 28 weeks' gestation, subsequent passive transfer of antibody will result in a false-positive direct Coombs test, without associated reticulocytosis. Rarely, a falsely Rh-negative infant will present with a strongly positive direct Coombs

test, resulting from blockage of the Rh antigenic sites by high-titer maternal antibody.

D. Blood smear. Polychromasia and normoblastosis proportionate to the reticulocyte count are typically present. Hypochromia in proportion to the severity of the hemolytic process and anemia are seen. Spherocytes are not usually present.

E. Bilirubin levels. Progressive elevation of unconjugated bilirubin on serial testing provides an index of the severity of the hemolytic process. In severe disease, an elevated direct fraction may be secondary to a laboratory artifact or coexisting hepatobiliary damage.

F. Bilirubin-binding capacity is currently investigational.

G. Glucose and blood gas levels should be followed closely.

H. Supplementary laboratory studies. Supportive diagnostic studies may be required when the basis of the hemolytic process remains unclear.

    1. Direct Coombs' test in mother. This study will be negative in Rh disease but often is positive if maternal autoimmune hemolytic disease is present, particularly collagen vascular disease.

    2. Antibody identification (indirect Coombs' test in infant). An eluate of antibody attached to neonatal erythrocytes is tested against a type-specific panel of adult erythrocytes to determine the antibody specificity.

VII. Management

A. Antepartum treatment. Verification of the Rh-negative status at the first prenatal visit may be obtained by the following measures.

    1. Maternal antibody titer (indirect Coombs' test). Detection of specific IgG-Rh antibody will document prior sensitization. Serial antibody titer determinations are required every 1–4 weeks (depending on gestational age) during pregnancy. A negative indirect Coombs test signifies absence of sensitization. This test should be repeated at 28–34 weeks' gestation.

    2. Rh immunoglobulin (RhoGAM). Current obstetric guidelines suggest giving immunoprophylaxis at 28 weeks' gestation in the absence of sensitization.

    3. Amniocentesis. If maternal antibody titers indicate a risk of fetal death (usual range, 1:16–1:32), amniocentesis should be performed. To reasonably predict the risk of moderate to severe fetal disease, serial determinations of amniotic fluid bilirubin levels present photometrically at 450 nm are plotted on standard graphs according to gestational age.

    4. Ultrasonography. As a screening study in pregnancies at risk, serial fetal ultrasound examinations allow detection of scalp edema, ascites, or other signs of developing hydrops fetalis.

    5. Intrauterine transfusion. Based on the above studies, intrauterine transfusion may be indicated because of possible fetal demise or the presence of fetal hydrops. This procedure must be performed by an experienced team. The goal is maintenance of effective erythrocyte mass within the fetal circulation and maintenance of the pregnancy until there is a reasonable chance for successful extrauterine survival of the infant.

B. Postpartum treatment

    1. Resuscitation. Moderately to severely anemic infants with or without hydropic features are at risk for high-output cardiac failure, hypoxemia secondary to decreased oxygen-carrying capacity, and hypoglycemia. These infants may require immediate single-volume exchange blood transfusion at delivery to improve oxygen-carrying capacity, mechanical support of ventilation, and an extended period of monitoring for hypoglycemia.

    2. Cord blood studies. A cord blood bilirubin level greater than 4 mg/

dL or a cord hemoglobin less than 12 g/dL, or both, usually suggests moderate to severe disease. The cord blood is used for these and initial screening studies, including blood typing, Rh typing, and Coombs' test.

3. **Serial unconjugated bilirubin studies.** Determination of the rate of increase in unconjugated bilirubin levels will provide an index of the severity of the hemolytic process and the need for exchange transfusion. Commonly used guidelines include a rise of more than 0.5 mg/dL/h or more than 5 mg/dL over 24 hours within the first 2 days of life, or projection of a serum level that will exceed a predetermined "exchange level" for a given infant (usually 20 mg/dL in term infants).

4. **Phototherapy.** In Rh hemolytic disease, because of its frequently severe course, phototherapy is used only as an adjunct to exchange transfusion and should not be instituted until a decision has been made regarding exchange transfusion. Phototherapy may reduce the number of total exchange transfusions required.

5. **Exchange transfusion.** (See Chap 21 for procedure.) Exchange transfusion is indicated if the unconjugated bilirubin level is likely to reach a predetermined "exchange level" for that patient (see Appendix F). Optimally, exchange transfusion is done well before this "exchange level" is reached, to minimize the entry of unconjugated bilirubin into soft tissues. Consideration should be given to irradiation of blood before the transfusion is given, particularly in preterm infants or infants expected to require multiple transfusions, to reduce the risk of graft vs host disease.

C. **Rh immunoglobin (RhoGAM) prophylaxis.** Most cases of incompatibility involve the D antigen. RhoGAM given at 28 weeks' gestation or within 72 hours of suspected Rh antigen exposure, or both, will reduce the risk of sensitization to less than 1%; the recommended dosage should be well in excess of the amount of Rh antigen transfused. In massive fetomaternal hemorrhage, however, conventional doses may be insufficient. The amount of fetal blood entering the maternal circulation may be estimated using the Kleihauer-Betke acid elution technique (p 260) during the immediate postpartum period.

No treatment equivalent to RhoGAM is available for maternal Rh sensitization to non-D antigens, notably C and E antigens. These antigens, however, are significantly less antigenic than the D antigen, and clinical manifestations of incompatibility are frequently milder and the risk of severe disease considerably less.

D. **Hydrops fetalis.** Skilled resuscitation and anticipation of selective systemic complications may prevent early neonatal death.

1. **Isovolumetric partial exchange transfusion** with type O Rh-negative packed erythrocytes will raise the hematocrit and improve the oxygen-carrying capacity (see p 150, **D**).

2. **Central arterial and venous catheterization** may be performed to provide the following measures.
   a. Isovolumetric exchange transfusion.
   b. Monitoring of arterial blood gas levels and central venous and systemic blood pressures.
   c. Monitoring of fluid and electrolyte balance, particularly renal and hepatic function, the calcium:phosphorus ratio, and serum albumin levels as well as appropriate hematologic studies and serum bilirubin levels.

3. **Positive-pressure mechanical ventilation.** This measure may include increased levels of positive-end expiratory pressure, if pulmonary edema is present, as a means of stabilizing alveolar ventilation.

4. **Therapeutic paracentesis or thoracentesis** may be performed to remove fluid that may further compromise respiratory effort. Attention to the volume removed and progressive systemic hypotension is important.

5. **Volume expanders** may be necessary in addition to erythrocytes to improve peripheral perfusion defects. Only **fresh-frozen plasma containing high-molecular-weight proteins** should be used. *Albumin is contraindicated* and may aggravate existing ascites or pleural effusion. Transfused volumes should be small to avoid further cardiac embarrassment.

6. **Drug treatment** may include diuretics such as furosemide for pulmonary edema and pressor agents including dopamine, which may also benefit renal perfusion (for dosages, see Chap 75). In the case of cardiac rhythm disturbances, appropriate drugs may be used if indicated.

7. **Electrocardiography or echocardiography** may be needed to determine whether cardiac abnormalities are present.

VIII. **Prognosis.** Prenatal mortality for infants at risk of anti-DRH isoimmunization is currently approximately 1.5% and has decreased significantly over the past 2 decades. Antenatal immune prophylaxis and improved management techniques including amniotic fluid spectrophotometry, intrauterine transfusion, and advances in neonatal intensive care have been largely responsible for this reduction. Isolated cases of severe isoimmunization still occur due to isoimmunization by other than anti-D antibody or failure to receive immune prophylaxis and may exhibit the full spectrum of disease, including an increased risk of stillbirths and early neonatal morbidity and mortality.

THROMBOCYTOPENIA AND PLATELET DYSFUNCTION

I. **Definition.** Thrombocytopenia is defined as a platelet count less than $150,000/\mu L$, although a few normal neonates may have counts as low as $100,000/\mu L$ in the absence of clinical disease. The best measure of platelet function is the standardized (Ivy) bleeding time. Normal values for the Ivy bleeding time are the same as for older children (1.5–5.5 minutes).

II. **Normal platelet physiology.** The rate of platelet production and turnover in neonates is similar to that of older children and adults. The platelet life span is approximately 8 days, and the mean platelet count is greater than $200,000/\mu L$. Platelet counts are slightly lower in low birth weight infants, in whom platelet counts less than $100,000/\mu L$ have occasionally been observed in the absence of a clinical disorder. Low platelet counts should nonetheless be investigated in low birth weight infants. Platelet counts vary according to the method of determination. Phase microscopy determinations are generally $25,000–50,000/\mu L$ lower than those obtained by direct microscopy.

III. **Etiology**

A. **Thrombocytopenia**

1. **Maternal disorders causing thrombocytopenia in infant**

a. Drug use (eg, quinine, quinidine, digoxin, chlorothiazide, sulfonamide derivatives).

b. Infections (eg, TORCH infections, bacterial or viral infections).

c. Disseminated intravascular coagulation (DIC).

d. Severe hypertension.

e. Antiplatelet antibodies.

(1) Antibodies against maternal platelets (autoimmune thrombocytopenia).

(a) Idiopathic thrombocytopenic purpura (ITP).

(b) Drug-induced thrombocytopenia.

        (c) Systemic lupus erythematosus.
     (2) Antibodies against fetal platelets (isoimmune thrombocytopenia).
        (a) Isolated isoimmune thrombocytopenia.
        (b) Isoimmune thrombocytopenia associated with erythroblastosis fetalis.

2. **Placental disorders causing thrombocytopenia in infant (rare)**
   a. Chorioangioma.
   b. Vascular thrombi.
   c. Placental abruption.
3. **Neonatal disorders causing thrombocytopenia**
   a. Decreased platelet production or congenital absence of megakaryocytes.
      (1) Isolated.
      (2) Thrombocytopenia–absent radius syndrome.
      (3) Fanconi's anemia.
      (4) Rubella syndrome.
      (5) Congenital leukemia.
      (6) Trisomies 13, 18, or 21.
   b. **Increased platelet destruction**
      (1) Bacterial sepsis.
      (2) TORCH infections.
      (3) DIC.
      (4) Necrotizing enterocolitis.
      (5) Platelet destruction associated with giant hemangiomas (**Kasabach-Merritt syndrome**).

B. **Platelet dysfunction**
   1. Drug-induced platelet dysfunction.
      a. Maternal use of aspirin.
      b. Indomethacin.
      c. Perhaps penicillins, furosemide, theophylline.
   2. Metabolic disorders.
      a. Hyperbilirubinemia.
      b. Phototherapy-induced metabolic abnormalities.
      c. Acidosis.
      d. Fatty acid deficiency.
      e. Maternal diabetes.
   3. Inherited thrombasthenia (Glanzmann's disease).
IV. **Clinical presentation**
   A. **Symptoms and signs**
      1. Generalized superficial petechiae are often present, particularly in response to minor trauma or pressure or increased venous pressure.
      2. Platelet counts are usually less than 60,000/μL.
      3. Mucosal bleeding and spontaneous hemorrhage may be occurring from other sites with platelet counts less than 20,000/μL.
      4. Intracranial hemorrhage may occur with severe thrombocytopenia.
      5. Large ecchymoses and muscle hemorrhages are more likely to be due to coagulation disturbances than to platelet disturbances.
      6. Petechiae in normal infants tend to be clustered on the head and upper chest, do not recur, and are associated with normal platelet counts. They are a result of a transient increase in venous pressure during birth.
   B. **History**
      1. There may be a family history of thrombocytopenia.
      2. Maternal drug ingestion may be a factor.
      3. A history of infection should be noted.
      4. Previous episodes of bleeding may have occurred.

   C. The placenta should be carefully examined for evidence of choriangioma, thrombi, or abruptio placentae.

   D. Physical examination
     1. Petechiae and bleeding should be noted.
     2. Physical malformations may be present in thrombocytopenia—absent radius syndrome, rubella syndrome, giant hemangioma, or trisomy syndromes.
     3. Hepatosplenomegaly may be caused by viral or bacterial infection or congenital leukemia.

V. Diagnosis
   A. Laboratory studies
     1. Test for maternal thrombocytopenia. A low maternal count suggests autoimmune thrombocytopenia or inherited thrombocytopenia (X-linked recessive thrombocytopenia or autosomal dominant thrombocytopenia).
     2. Neonatal platelet count.
     3. Complete blood count.
     4. Blood typing.
     5. Coombs' test.
     6. Coagulation studies.
     7. Other studies (if indicated).
       a. TORCH titers.
       b. Bacterial cultures.
       c. Bone marrow studies if decreased platelet production is present.

   B. Decreased platelet production vs increased platelet destruction
     1. Decreased platelet production
       a. Platelet size is normal.
       b. Platelet survival time is normal.
       c. Megakaryocytes are decreased in a bone marrow sample.
       d. A sustained increase in the platelet count over a period of 4–7 days is seen following platelet transfusion.
     2. Increased platelet destruction
       a. Platelet size is increased.
       b. Platelet survival time is decreased.
       c. Megakaryocytes in the bone marrow are normal or increased.
       d. There is little or no sustained increase in platelet count following platelet transfusion.

   C. Evaluation of platelet function as indicated by prolonged Ivy bleeding time caused by:
     1. Platelet dysfunction.
     2. Thrombocytopenia with platelet counts less than 80,000/μL.

VI. Management
   A. Obstetric management of maternal autoimmune thrombocytopenia
     1. Treatment is aimed at prevention of intracranial hemorrhage during vaginal delivery.
     2. There is an increased risk of severe neonatal thrombocytopenia and intracranial hemorrhage if antibody is present in the maternal plasma or if fetal scalp platelet counts are less than 75,000–100,000/μL.
     3. Cesarean delivery may be indicated.
     4. Administering corticosteroids to the mother have been beneficial in preliminary studies.

   B. Management of isoimmune thrombocytopenia
     1. Transfuse platelets lacking the incompatible antigen. Although these platelets are usually obtained from the mother, transfusion of unmatched platelets from a random donor may be helpful if matched platelets cannot be obtained.

2. Intravenous gamma globulin is useful (see Chap 75 for dosage and other pharmacologic information).
3. The risk of recurrence in siblings is greater than 75%. In subsequent pregnancies, the administration of intravenous gamma globulin weekly during the third trimester may be effective (see Chap 75 for dosage and other pharmacologic information). These infants are usually delivered by cesarean section.

C. **Treatment of infants with thrombocytopenia**
   1. Treat the underlying cause (eg, sepsis). If drugs are the cause, stop administration.
   2. **Platelet transfusions** are indicated (1) if active bleeding is occurring with any degree of thrombocytopenia or (2) if there is no active bleeding but platelet counts are less than $20,000/\mu L$. Random donor platelets are given in a dosage of 1 unit/5 kg. The platelet count should increase to over $50,000/\mu L$. Failure to achieve or sustain such a rise suggests a destructive process.
   3. **Exchange transfusion** is given for immune thrombocytopenia. The platelet count may rise only transiently. There is considerable risk involved.
   4. Prednisone, 2 mg/kg/d, may also be beneficial in immune thrombocytopenia.

REFERENCES

Black VD, Lubchenco LO: Neonatal polycythemia and hyperviscosity. *Pediatr Clin North Am* 1982;**29**:1137.
Black VD, Lubchenco LO et al: Neonatal hyperviscosity: Randomized study of effect of partial plasma exchange transfusion on long-term outcome. *Pediatrics* 1985;**75**:1048.
Bowman, JM: Rh erythroblastosis fetalis 1975. *Semin Hematol* 1975;**12**:189.
Bussel JB et al: Antenatal treatment of neonatal alloimmune thrombocytopenia *N Engl J Med* 1988;**319**:1374.
Castle V et al: Frequency and mechanism of neonatal thrombocytopenia. *J Pediatr* 1986;**108**:749.
Dickerman JF: Anemia in the newborn infant. *Pediatr Rev* 1984;**6**:131.
Glader BE: Erythrocyte disorders in infancy. In: *Schaffer's Diseases of the Newborn*, 5th ed. Avery ME, Taeusch HW (editors). Saunders, 1984.
Gross S, Shurin SB, Gordon EM: The blood and hematopoietic system. Pages 708–752 in: *Behrman's Neonatal Perinatal Medicine*, 3rd ed. Fanaroff AA, Martin RJ (editors). Mosby, 1983.
Klemperer MR: Hemolytic anemias: Immune defects. In *Blood Diseases of Infancy and Childhood*, 5th ed. Miller DR, Baehner RL, McMillan CW (editors). Mosby, 1984.
Linderkamp O: Placental transfusion: Determinants and effects. *Clin Perinatol* 1982;**9**:559.
Linderkamp O et al: Contributions of red cells and plasma to blood viscosity in preterm and full-term infants and adults. *Pediatrics* 1984;**74**:45.
Martin JN, Morrison JC, Files FC: Autoimmune thrombocytopenic purpura: Current concepts and recommended practices. *Am J Obstet Gynecol* 1984;**150**:86.
Mentzer WC: Polycythemia and hyperviscosity syndrome in newborn infants. *Clin Haematol* 1978;**7**:63.
Miller DR (editor): Normal values and examination of the blood: Perinatal period, infancy, childhood, and adolescence. Pages 22–47 in: *Blood Diseases of Infancy and Childhood*, 5th ed. Miller DR, Baehner RL, McMillan CW (editors). Mosby, 1984.
Naiman JL: Disorders of the platelets. In: *Hematologic Problems in the Newborn*, 3rd ed. Oski FA, Naiman JL (editors). Saunders, 1982.
Naiman JL: Erythroblastosis fetalis. In: *Hematologic Problems in the Newborn*, 3rd ed. Oski FA, Naiman JL (editors). Saunders, 1982.
Oh W: Neonatal polycythemia and hyperviscosity. *Pediatr Clin North Am* 1986;**33**:523.
Oski FA: Hematologic problems. In: *Neonatology Pathophysiology and Management of the Newborn*, 2nd ed. Avery GB (editor). Lippincott, 1981.
Oski FA: Hydrops fetalis. In: *Schaffer's Diseases of the Newborn*, 5th ed. Avery ME, Taeusch HW (editors). Saunders, 1984.
Oski FA, Naiman JL: Polycythemia and hyperviscosity in the neonatal period. In: *Hematologic Problems in the Newborn*, 3rd ed. Saunders, 1982.
Pearson HA: Posthemorrhagic anemia in the newborn. *Pediatr Rev* 1982;**4**:40.

Pearson HA, McIntosh S: Neonatal thrombocytopenia. *Clin Haematol* 1978;**7**:111.

Peddle LJ: The antenatal management of the Rh sensitized woman. *Clin Perinatol* 1984;**11**:251.

Polesky HF: Diagnosis, prevention and therapy in hemolytic diseases of the newborn. *Clin Lab Med* 1982;**2**:107.

Shohat M, Merlob P, Reisner S: Neonatal polycythemia: I. Early diagnosis and incidence related to time of sampling. *Pediatrics* 1984;**73**:7.

Stuart MJ: Platelet function in the neonate. *Am J Pediatr Hematol Oncol* 1979;**1**:227.

57 Cardiac Abnormalities

CONGENITAL HEART DISEASE

The diagnostic dilemma of the newborn with congenital heart disease must be resolved quickly since therapy may prove lifesaving for some of these infants. Congenital heart disease occurs in approximately 1% of live-born infants. Nearly half of all cases of congenital heart disease are diagnosed during the first week of life. The most frequently occurring anomalies seen during this first week are patent ductus arteriosus, D-transposition of the great arteries, hypoplastic left heart syndrome, tetralogy of Fallot, and pulmonary atresia.

- I. **Classification.** Symptoms and signs in newborns with heart disease permit grouping according to levels of arterial oxygen saturation. Further classification (based on other physical findings and laboratory tests) facilitates delineation of the exact cardiac lesion present.
  - A. **Cyanotic heart disease.** Infants with cyanotic heart disease are usually unable to achieve a PaO_2 above 100 mm Hg after breathing 100% inspired oxygen for 10–20 minutes.
  - B. **Acyanotic heart disease.** Infants with acyanotic heart disease will achieve PaO_2 levels of over 100 mm Hg under the same conditions as noted in **A**, above.
- II. **Cyanotic heart disease** (Table 57–1)
  - A. **100% oxygen test.** Because of intracardiac right-to-left shunting, the newborn with cyanotic congenital heart disease (in contrast to the infant with pulmonary disease) is unable to raise the arterial saturation, even in the presence of increased ambient oxygen.
    1. Determine PaO_2 while infant is on room air.
    2. Give 100% oxygen for 10–20 minutes by mask, hood, or endotracheal tube.
    3. Obtain an arterial blood gas level while the infant is breathing 100% oxygen.
  - B. **Cyanosis.** Care must be taken in evaluating cyanosis by skin color, since polycythemia, jaundice, racial pigmentation, or anemia may make clinical recognition of cyanosis difficult.
  - C. **Murmur.** The infant with cyanotic congenital heart disease often does not have a distinctive murmur. In fact, the most serious of these anomalies may not be associated with a murmur at all.
  - D. **Other studies.** Cyanotic infants may be further classified on the basis of pulmonary circulation on chest x-ray and electrocardiographic findings.
  - E. **Diagnosis and treatment.** Table 57–1 outlines the diagnosis and treatment of cyanotic heart disease.
  - F. **Specific cyanotic heart disease abnormalities**
    1. **D-Transposition of the great arteries** is the most common cardiac cause of cyanosis in the first year of life, with a male:female ratio of 2:1. The aorta comes from the right ventricle and the pulmonary artery from the left ventricle. With modern newborn care, 1-year survival approaches 80%.
       a. **Physical examination.** Typical presentation is a large, vigorous

TABLE 57-1. CYANOTIC CONGENITAL HEART DISEASE(PaO₂ < 100 mm Hg in 100% FiO₂)*

	Decreased blood flow with small heart (or normal heart)		Decreased pulmonary blood flow with large heart		Increased pulmonary blood flow with small heart	Increased pulmonary blood flow with large heart		Normal pulmonary blood flow, with normal-sized heart. No thymus
Chest x-ray								
ECG	RVH	LVH, LAD	LVH, normal axis	RBBB	RVH	RVH or normal	LVH or normal	Normal
Differential diagnosis	Pulmonary atresia with VSD, TOF	Tricuspid atresia	Pulmonary atresia with intact septum	Ebstein's anomaly	TAPVR	HLHS	TGA with VSD Truncus arteriosus	TGA
Physical examination	Short, soft ejection murmur may only be heard in back	Faint PDA murmur or systolic murmur of sm VSD	Systolic and diastolic murmurs at xiphoid TS/TI	Widely split S₂, scratchy diastolic murmur at xiphoid	No murmur. Quadruple rhythm often due to pulmonary ejection sound, split S₂, diastolic filling sound	Poor peripheral pulses	Systolic murmur	No murmur
Treatment	If PaO₂ low, start PGE₁ infusion. Then perform further cardiac evaluation. Operation may or may not be needed				Consider PGE₁ infusion. Then perform further cardiac evaluation. Operation may or may not be needed			Immediate balloon septostomy

* AS, aortic stenosis; EFE, endocardial fibroelastosis; HLHS, hypoplastic left heart syndrome; LAD, left axis deviation; LVH, left ventricular hypertrophy; PDA, patent ductus arteriosus; PS, pulmonary stenosis; RBBB, right bundle branch block; RVH, right ventricular hypertrophy; SEM, systolic ejection murmur; TAPVR, total anomalous pulmonary venous return; TGA, transposition of great arteries; TI, tricuspid incompetence; TOF, tetralogy of Fallot; TS, tricuspid stenosis; VSD, ventricular septal defect.

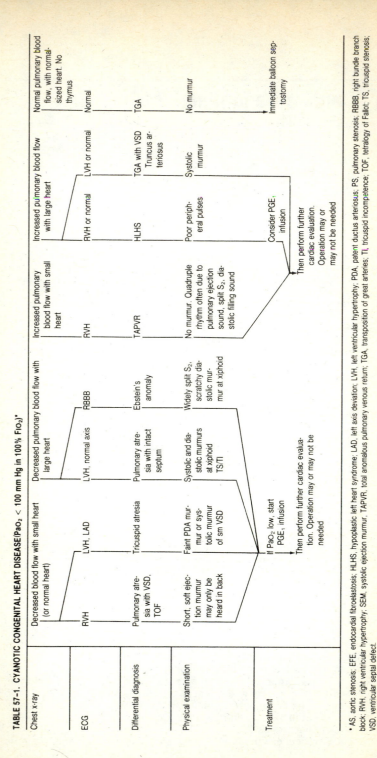

infant with cyanosis but little or no respiratory distress. There may be no murmur or a soft, systolic ejection murmur.

   b. Chest x-ray study. This study may be normal, but typically it reveals a very narrow upper mediastinal shadow ("egg on a stick" appearance).

   c. Electrocardiography. There are no characteristic ECG findings.

   d. Echocardiography is diagnostic. Typical findings are branching of the anterior great vessel into the inominate, subclavian, and carotid vessels and branching of the posterior great vessel into the right and left pulmonary arteries.

   e. Cardiac catherization. Like echocardiography, this study is diagnostic and often therapeutic as outlined in **f,** below.

   f. Treatment. Urgent cardiac catherization with balloon septostomy and later Mustard or Senning procedures (transposing venous return via an intra-arterial baffle) or early arterial switch operation are the methods of treatment.

2. Tetralogy of Fallot (TOF). TOF is characterized by 4 anomalies: pulmonary stenosis, ventricular septal defect, overriding aorta, and right ventricular hypertrophy (RVH). There is a slight male predominance. Cyanosis usually signifies complete or partial atresia of the right ventricular overflow tract or extremely severe pulmonary stenosis with hypoplastic pulmonary arteries. The degree of right ventricular outflow obstruction is inversely proportional to pulmonary blood flow and directly proportional to the degree of cyanosis. TOF with absent pulmonary valve may present later in infancy due to poor feeding (due to very large pulmonary arteries causing esophageal compression).

   a. Physical examination. The patient is cyanotic with a systolic ejection murmur along the left sternal border. Loud murmurs are associated with more flow across the right ventricular outflow tract, and softer murmurs, with less flow.

   b. Chest x-ray study. A small, often "boot-shaped" heart, with decreased pulmonary vascular markings. A right aortic arch is seen in about 20% of these infants.

   c. Echocardiography. The echocardiogram may be normal or demonstrate right ventricular hypertrophy (RVH). The only sign of RVH may be an upright T wave in V4R or V1 after 72 hours of age.

   d. Echocardiography is usually diagnostic, with the demonstration of an overriding aorta, ventricular septal defect (VSD), and small right ventricular outflow tract.

   e. Treatment. Pulmonary blood flow may be ductal-dependent with severe cyanosis and may respond to ductal dilation using prostaglandin E_1 (see Chap 75). This measure allows more flexibility for planning cardiac catherization and surgical correction. Surgery (shunting or total correction) may be palliative.

III. Acyanotic heart disease. (Table 57–2.)

   A. 100% oxygen test. (See **II.A,** above.)

   B. Murmur. The infant who is not cyanotic will present with either a heart murmur or symptoms of congestive heart failure.

   C. Diagnosis and treatment. (Table 57–2.)

   D. Specific acyanotic heart disease abnormalities

      1. Ventricular septal defect (VSD) is the most common congenital heart abnormality, with equal sex distribution. Murmurs are not heard at birth but typically appear between 3 days and 3 weeks of age. Congestive heart failure is unusual before 4 weeks of age but may develop earlier in premature infants. Symptoms and physical findings vary with the age of the patient and the size of the defect.

TABLE 57-2. ACYANOTIC CONGENITAL HEART DISEASE(PaO₂ > 100 mm Hg in 100% FiO₂)*

	Normal pulmonary blood flow with normal-sized heart		Normal pulmonary blood flow with large heart				Increased pulmonary blood flow with large heart
Chest x-ray							
ECG	RVH or normal	LVH or normal	Normal arrhythmia or complete heart block	LVH	RVH or LVH	RVH	LAD
Differential diagnosis	Valvar PS	Noncritical valvar AS, VSD, PDA	Intrauterine arrhythmia	AV malformation Common sites are head, liver, placenta; AS, critical	AV valve insufficiency Primary myocardial disease (including EFE)	HLHS, coarctation of aorta	AV canal
Physical examination	SEM	SEM-AS, VSD, no murmur, PDA, continuous murmur	May be hydropic or normal	AVM, usually continuous murmur over site Increased pulses; Critical AS, decreased pulses Not much murmur	Ti; MI Pansystolic murmur with rumble EFE, gallop	HLHS; poor pulses, perfusion, and color; gallop; Coarctation of aorta, decreased femoral pulses	SEM, diastolic rumble
Treatment	Observe	Observe	Treat arrhythmia with drugs or cardioversion May need furosemide; Congenital complete heart block may need pacemaker	AVM, ultrasound, CT scanning, angiography; AS: PGE, infusion Digoxin, furosemide	Digoxin, furosemide	Anticongestives if in heart failure; HLHS, consider PGE, infusion	Observe Anticongestives if in heart failure

Further cardiac evaluation

* Abbreviations are explained in Table 57–1 footnote.

Spontaneous closure occurs in half. Surgical correction is reserved for large, symptomatic VSD only.

2. **Atrial septal defect (ASD)** is not an important cause of morbidity or mortality in infancy. Occasionally, congestive heart failure can occur in infancy but not usually in the neonatal period.

3. **Endocardial cushion defects** include ostium primum–type ASD with or without cleft mitral valve and atrioventricular (AV) canal. These defects are commonly associated with multiple congenital anomalies, especially Down's syndrome. If marked AV-valve insufficiency is present, the patient may present with congestive heart failure at birth or in the neonatal period.

   a. **Physical examination.** A systolic murmur due to AV-valve insufficiency. Cyanosis may be present but is often not severe.

   b. **Chest x-ray study.** Variable findings may include a dilated pulmonary artery or a large heart due to atrial dilatation.

   c. **Electrocardiography.** Left axis deviation (left superior vector) is *always* found; the PR interval may be long or there may be a R-S-R' pattern in V4R and V1.

   d. **Echocardiography** is usually diagnostic; the echocardiogram usually demonstrates a common AV valve with inlet ventricular septal defect in the AV canals or a defect in the septum primum with an abnormal mitral valve.

   e. **Treatment.** Congestive heart failure is treated with diuretics and digoxin (see Chap 75); early cardiac catheterization with corrective surgery may be needed to prevent the development of pulmonary vascular obstructive disease.

IV. **Hypoplastic left heart syndrome (HLHS)** occurs in both cyanotic and acyanotic forms. In 15% of cases, the foramen ovale is intact and thus prevents mixing at the atrial level, causing cyanosis. The infants with free mixing at the atria are acyanotic. Hypoplastic left heart syndrome accounts for 25% of all cardiac deaths during the first week of life.

A. **Physical examination.** The baby is typically pale, tachypneic with poor perfusion, and poor to absent peripheral pulses. A loud single S2 is present, usually with a gallop and no murmur. There is hepatomegaly, and metabolic acidosis is usually present by 48 hours of age.

B. **Electrocardiography** demonstrates a small or absent left ventricular vector.

C. **Chest x-ray study.** Moderate cardiomegaly is present, often with large main pulmonary artery shadow.

D. **Echocardiography.** A diagnostic study demonstrates a small or slit-like left ventricle with a hypoplastic ascending aorta.

E. **Treatment.** Systemic blood flow is ductal dependent; therefore prostaglandin E_1 may be of value. Surgical correction is done in 2 stages. The first is palliation (Norwood procedure), redirecting the blood flow so that the right ventricle serves as the "systemic ventricle," and is high-risk intervention. The second stage (Fontan procedure) is directing systemic venous return directly to the pulmonary circulation and then closing the ASD. The second stage has variable results; survival is only fair after both procedures. Infant transplantation is available, with good results at some centers, but shortage of donors is a problem.

V. **Associated anomalies and syndromes** (Table 57–3). No discussion of heart disease in neonates would be complete without the inclusion of common multiple congenital anomaly (MCA) syndromes associated with heart defects. Many times, recognition of MCA syndrome will facilitate identification of the heart defect. Syndromes that tend to present after the newborn period have not been included.

VI. **Teratogens and heart disease.** Several teratogens associated with con-

TABLE 57-3. CONGENITAL ANOMALIES ASSOCIATED WITH HEART DEFECTS

Congenital Anomaly	Heart Defect
CHROMOSOMAL ANOMALY	
Trisomy 21 (Down's syndrome)	Atrioventricular canal, ventricular septal defect
Trisomy 13, 15, 18	Ventricular septal defect, patent ductus arteriosus
Syndrome associated with 4p—	Atrial septal defect, ventricular septal defect
Syndrome associated with 5p— (cri du chat syndrome)	Variable
XO (Turner's syndrome)	Coarctation of aorta, aortic stenosis
SYNDROMES WITH PREDOMINANTLY SKELETAL DEFECTS*	
Ellis-van Creveld syndrome	Atrial septal defect, single atrium
Laurence-Moon-Biedl syndrome	Tetralogy of Fallot, ventricular septal defect
Carpenter's syndrome	Patent ductus arteriosus, ventricular septal defect
Holt-Oram syndrome	Atrial septal defect, ventricular septal defect
Fanconi's syndrome	Patent ductus arteriosus, ventricular septal defect
Thrombocytopenia-absent radius syndrome	Atrial septal defect, tetralogy of Fallot
SYNDROMES WITH CHARACTERISTIC FACIES*	
Noonan's syndrome	Pulmonary stenosis
DiGeorge's syndrome	Tetralogy of Fallot, aortic arch anomalies
Smith-Lemli-Opitz syndrome	Ventricular septal defect, patent ductus arteriosus
de Lange's syndrome	Tetralogy of Fallot, ventricular septal defect
Goldenhar's syndrome	Tetralogy of Fallot, variable
William's syndrome	Supravalvular aortic stenosis, peripheral pulmonary artery stenosis
Asymmetric crying facies	Variable

*Not all infants with these syndromes have heart defects.

genital heart disease have been identified (Table 57–4), although there is not a 100% relationship between exposure and heart defects. A history of teratogen exposure may help in the diagnosis.

VII. **Abnormal situs syndromes.** Syndromes of abnormal situs relationships are associated with congenital heart disease. For example, an infant with situs inversus totalis and dextrocardia has the same incidence of congenital heart disease as the general population. If, however, there is disparity between thoracic and abdominal situs, the incidence of congenital heart disease is more than 90%. (Check the chest x-ray film to see if the cardiac apex and the stomach bubble are on the same side.) Some of these syndromes involve bilateral left-sidedness (2 bilobed lungs, multiple spleens) and complex cyanotic congenital heart disease, while others have bilateral right-sidedness (2 trilobed lungs, absent spleen) and complex cyanotic congenital heart disease.

VIII. **General principles of management**
    A. **Fetal echocardiography**

TABLE 57-4. TERATOGENS ASSOCIATED WITH HEART DEFECTS

Teratogen	Heart Defect
DRUGS	
Alcohol	Ventricular septal defect, tetralogy of Fallot, atrial septal defect
Phenytoin	Variable
Thalidomide	Tetralogy of Fallot, truncus arteriosus
Trimethadione	Ventricular septal defect, tetralogy of Fallot
OTHER TERATOGENS	
Maternal diabetes	Variable
Maternal systemic lupus erythematosus	Congenital heart block
Rubella syndrome	Patent ductus arteriosus, peripheral pulmonary stenosis

1. **General considerations.** Fetal echocardiography is now possible in many centers. The optimal gestational age to perform echocardiography is between 18 and 24 weeks, when structural abnormalities and arrhythmias can be detected. With early detection of cardiac abnormalities, arrangements can be made for delivery at a center with pediatric cardiac and surgical facilities. If the anomaly is not consistent with life, some families may elect termination of pregnancy.

2. **Indications**
   a. **Maternal factors.** Oligo- or polyhydramnios, diabetes, collagen vascular disease or teratogen exposure (Table 57–4).
   b. **Fetal factors.** Suspected cardiac abnormality on obstetric ultrasound examination, pleural fluid, pericardial fluid, heart rate abnormalities, intrauterine growth retardation, or other abnormality on obstetric ultrasound examination.
   c. **Genetic factors.** Familial history of chromosomal disorders or congenital heart disease.

B. **Emergency therapy.** Once the specific lesion has been identified as emergent, a decision about therapy must be made. If, for example, one is confronted with a very cyanotic infant with no murmur, a normal chest x-ray film, and a normal ECG and believes the diagnosis of D-transposition of the great arteries is likely, it is necessary to prepare the catheterization laboratory for a **balloon septostomy.**

C. **Prostaglandins.** As a general principle, if an infant is cyanotic and has decreased pulmonary blood flow, the Pao_2 will be improved by promoting flow through the ductus arteriosus via a drip of **prostaglandin E_1** (Alprostadil, Prostin VR Pediatric). Maintaining patency of the ductus will enable stabilization of the infant and allow cardiac catheterization and subsequent surgery to be planned on an urgent rather than emergent basis. Similarly, if poor peripheral pulses and acidosis from poor perfusion are present, infusion of prostaglandin, utilizing the same dose, will open the ductus arteriosus and allow right ventricular blood flow to augment the systemic circulation. This measure is beneficial in critical aortic stenosis, coarctation of the aorta, and hypoplastic left heart syndrome. (See Chap 75 for dosage and other pharmacologic information.)

D. **Antiarrhythmic drugs.** Arrhythmias may occur during intrauterine life or after delivery. They are a cause of fetal hydrops and intrauterine death; most often the rhythm disturbance is a rapid supraventricular tachycardia with a 1:1 ventricular response. Occasionally, atrial flutter with 2:1 block presents before or just after birth. **Digitalis** (see Chap 75) has been a successful antiarrhythmic agent in this situation, but electrical cardioversion is also sometimes necessary.

E. **Pacemaker.** In congenital complete heart block with imminent cardiovascular demise, **temporary transvenous ventricular pacing may be lifesaving.** It should be followed by urgent surgical placement of a permanent pacemaker.

PATENT DUCTUS ARTERIOSUS

I. **Definition.** Patent ductus arteriosus (PDA) results from failure of the ductus arteriosus to close or from its reopening after functional closure. The ductus arteriosus is an artery that normally closes functionally at birth. In the fetus, the majority of the blood supply bypasses the pulmonary circulation, going from the pulmonary artery to the aorta via the ductus. After birth, if the ductus remains patent, a left-to-right shunt develops, sometimes creating pulmonary overload and left ventricular failure.

II. **Incidence**

A. **Prematurity.** There is an increased incidence of PDA in premature infants weighing less than 1500 g, especially in those weighing less than 1000 g.

B. **Congenital rubella.** PDA is present in 60–70% of infants with congenital rubella syndrome.

C. **Other forms of congenital heart disease.** The overall incidence of congenital heart disease ranges from 0.3–0.6% of live births. The most common lesions are simple ventricular septal defect, PDA, coarctation of the aorta, pulmonic stenosis with intact septum, tetralogy of Fallot, aortic stenosis, and transposition of the great vessels. PDA is common in infants with these and other forms of congenital heart disease. PDA in the term infant is a distinct lesion with an incidence of about 0.05%.

III. Pathophysiology

A. **Increased oxygen concentration.** The most important factor stimulating functional closure of the ductus arteriosus at birth is the increased oxygen concentration, which has a direct action on smooth muscle in the wall of the ductus. This response increases with increasing gestational age.

B. **Other factors affecting closure of the ductus** are **levels of circulating prostaglandins** and the **available muscle mass.** The fetus has high levels of circulating prostaglandins (eg, PGE_2, PGI_2) as compared to the adult. These are products of arachidonic acid metabolism and have been shown to cause opening of an oxygen-constricted ductus arteriosus.

C. **Physiology of PDA.** At birth, there is a decrease in pulmonary vascular resistance and an increase in systemic resistance. If there is a PDA, the shunt thus becomes left-to-right. A small PDA may be of minimal significance, but a moderate size ductus may produce a significant shunt. The result is increased left ventricular end-diastolic volume and pressure, increased left atrial pressure and, eventually, if untreated, congestive heart failure.

IV. **Risk factors.** The major risk factor for PDA is prematurity. There is a slightly higher incidence in females and in infants born at higher altitudes. Congenital rubella and other forms of congenital heart disease are also risk factors (see **II**, above).

V. **Clinical presentation.** The initial presentation may be at birth or after the first few days of life, depending on the hemodynamics. In neonates, the cardiopulmonary signs and symptoms are as follows.

A. **Heart murmur.** The murmur is usually systolic and is heard best in the second or third intercostal space at the left sternal border. There may be a mid-diastolic flow rumble as well because of increased flow across the mitral valve in diastole. The presentation may vary with the degree of shunting, and in a collaborative PDA study, a murmur was found in only 20% of the cases.

B. **Hyperactive precordium.** The increased left ventricular stroke volume results in a hyperactive precordium.

C. **Bounding peripheral pulses.** A PDA results in a widened pulse pressure that produces bounding peripheral pulsations.

D. **Other signs.** The disease, if untreated, may progress to left ventricular failure with tachycardia, tachypnea, rales, and congestive hepatomegaly. Subsequent respiratory failure may require increasing ventilatory support.

VI. Diagnosis

A. **Laboratory studies.** In the presence of an increasing left-to-right shunt, **arterial blood gas determinations** will demonstrate progressive hypercarbia and metabolic acidosis.

B. **Radiologic studies.** The chest x-ray in an infant with a moderate to large shunt will often show cardiomegaly with prominence of the left ventricle and left atrium. Increased pulmonary vascular markings may be seen and may eventually lead to gross pulmonary edema.

C. **Echocardiography.** Two-dimensional and pulsed Doppler echocardiography are highly sensitive and specific in making the diagnosis of PDA. Hemodynamic significance may be estimated by documenting the left atrial and ventricular enlargement along with evidence of respiratory distress. However, the most sensitive method of detecting a shunt is with the use of real-time Doppler color flow mapping.

VII. Management

A. **Ventilatory support.** If the infant has deteriorating blood gases and is in respiratory distress, ventilatory support may be needed or increased if the infant has been on mechanical ventilation.

B. **Medical therapy.** Medical therapy may be tried initially.

1. **Fluid restriction and diuretics.** This measure attempts to minimize the effects of the cardiovascular volume overload by restricting fluid intake, sometimes in association with diuretics. Furosemide (Lasix) is often considered the drug of choice for short-term management (see Chap 75). If the infant is on mechanical ventilation, increasing the positive end-expiratory pressure may also help.

2. **Indomethacin (Indocin).** Indomethacin is a prostaglandin synthetase inhibitor that blocks the effect of arachidonic acid metabolites on the ductus. In multiple clinical trials, it has proved to be safe and effective. Closure rates as high as 79% have been reported. (See Chap 75 for full dosage information.) Indomethacin should be given if fluid management and ventilator changes fail to significantly lessen the degree of left-to-right ductal shunting. Some clinicians advocate prophylactic indomethacin therapy after initial echocardiographic demonstration of a PDA in the absence of an associated ductal-dependent cyanotic heart lesion.

   a. **Contraindications.** Contraindications to the use of indomethacin, as defined by a multicenter collaborative study, are as follows.
      (1) Blood urea nitrogen levels > 30 mg/dL.
      (2) Serum creatinine levels > 1.8 mg/dL.
      (3) Urine output of ≤ 0.6 mL/kg/h for the preceding 8 hours.
      (4) Platelet count < 60,000/μL.
      (5) Stool Hematest > 3+ (or "moderate to large").
      (6) Evidence of bleeding diathesis.
      (7) Necrotizing enterocolitis.

   b. **Complications.** There is some short-term toxicity associated with indomethacin treatment.
      (1) **Transient renal effects.** Increased BUN and creatinine concentrations and decreased urine output may occur.
      (2) **Gastrointestinal tract effects.** The few reports of gastrointestinal tract bleeding with indomethacin are not statistically significant. Bleeding has usually been transient, without an increased incidence of necrotizing enterocolitis.
      (3) **Intracranial hemorrhage.** Despite early reports to the contrary, there is no increased incidence of intracranial hemorrhage after indomethacin therapy.

C. **Surgical therapy.** Surgical ligation should be performed if medical treatment fails or if the ductus reopens to a significant degree. Depending on the condition of the patient, a second course of indomethacin may be considered prior to surgery. Ligation is done through a thoracotomy incision and requires a general anesthetic and placement of a chest tube. There is a higher incidence of pneumothorax and grades III and IV cicatricial retinopathy of prematurity in surgically treated infants.

VIII. **Prognosis.** The outcome is related to many factors, including the degree of prematurity, the underlying lung disease, the ease with which the ductus responds to medical therapy, and other events such as intraventricular hemorrhage. Because there often are associated problems, the mortality rate for the effects of PDA alone cannot be determined.

PERSISTENT PULMONARY HYPERTENSION (PERSISTENT FETAL CIRCULATION)

I. **Definition.** Persistent pulmonary hypertension (PPH) evolves when pulmonary vasoconstriction occurs, causing pulmonary hypertension. This, in turn, causes a right-to-left shunt through the ductus arteriosus and foramen ovale. This condition usually lasts 3–5 days. If the patient can be managed through this acute period, persistent fetal circulation will usually resolve spontaneously.

II. **Incidence.** Because of the many underlying causes of pulmonary artery hypertension and the clinical settings from which it may evolve, the incidence varies from center to center and is broad.

III. **Pathophysiology.** At birth, a sequence of events occurs, causing transition from fetal to adult circulation. Normally, there is expansion and oxygenation of the lungs, a decrease in pulmonary vascular resistance, and an increase in PaO_2, which constricts the ductus arteriosus. The systemic vascular resistance increases, and the foramen ovale closes functionally. However, if pulmonary hypertension occurs during this normal process, the foramen ovale and ductus arteriosus will remain open because the pulmonary vascular resistance remains higher than the systemic vascular resistance, allowing a right-to-left shunt to develop. Hypoxia and acidosis result, further constricting the pulmonary vessels and causing more pronounced pulmonary hypertension. The following factors are involved in the pathogenesis of pulmonary artery hypertension.

A. **Pulmonary vasoconstriction.** Pulmonary vasoconstriction may be caused by hypoxia, acidosis, or premature closure of the ductus arteriosus, which may be due to intrauterine exposure to prostaglandin synthetase inhibitors such as aspirin or indomethacin.

B. **Pathologic changes in the pulmonary arterial smooth muscle.** Abnormal muscularization and proliferation may occur secondary to abnormal development or intrauterine hypoxia or stress.

C. **Humoral agents.** Thromboxane A_2, a powerful pulmonary vasoconstrictor and a product of the lipoxygenase pathway of arachidonic acid metabolism, may play a role in the development of pulmonary artery hypertension.

IV. **Risk factors.** The following factors or conditions may be associated with an increased risk of persistent fetal circulation.

A. **Lung disease or meconium aspiration syndrome.** Hypoxia, hypercarbia, and acidosis may result from lung disease or from meconium aspiration.

B. **Decreased pulmonary vascular bed** may occur as primary congenital pulmonary hypoplasia as a result of chronic oligohydramnios (Potter syndrome), or it may be secondary to a diaphragmatic hernia, for example.

C. **Hyperviscosity (polycythemia)** may cause functional obstruction of the pulmonary vascular bed with resultant increased arterial pressures.

D. **Congenital heart disease.** Any cardiac disease that produces increased pulmonary blood flow (eg, D-transposition of the great arteries), pulmonary venous obstruction (eg, left ventricular failure), or even decreased pulmonary blood flow (eg, pulmonic stenosis) may be a cause.

E. Sepsis. Septic infants frequently develop severe metabolic acidosis with secondary pulmonary vasoconstriction.

F. Hypocalcemia or hypoglycemia. These metabolic abnormalities may cause decrease in cardiac output, leading to hypoxia and acidosis.

G. Perinatal factors

1. **Gestational age.** The muscular layers of the small pulmonary arterioles develop near term. This developmental change causes a decrease in the cross-sectional area of the pulmonary vascular bed and subsequent increase in resistance to blood flow to the lung.

2. **Fetal distress.** Intrauterine fetal distress, manifested by decelerations, may be a result of acute or chronic hypoxia.

3. **Repeat elective cesarean section.** Labor acts as a stimulus for reduction of pulmonary vascular resistance, resorption of lung fluid, lung maturation, and release of surfactant. If labor is bypassed by cesarean section, these mechanisms fail to occur, which may result in pulmonary hypertension.

V. Clinical presentation

A. Signs and symptoms. The following signs and symptoms are found in infants with pulmonary artery hypertension.

1. Increasing alveolar-arterial gradient (A-aDO_2). Normal values are < 20 mm Hg. Values in the range of 250–650 mm Hg may be seen, depending on the degree of the shunt. The A-aDO_2 is discussed on p 127, **8.a.**

2. Marked lability, ie, cyanosis. Readings on transcutaneous oxygen monitoring or the pulse oximeter fall during routine nursing care or drawing of blood or during periods of stress, loud noise, movement, or crying.

3. Progressive hypoxia leading to fixed hypoxemia with Pao_2 < 40 mm Hg.
   a. Intermittent cyanosis gives way to persistent cyanosis.
   b. Fixed acidemia (pH < 7.25) may develop.

4. Usually, difficulty in maintaining adequate intravascular volume. Central venous and systemic blood pressure are low even with continuous infusion of colloid. Urine output decreases.

VI. Diagnosis

A. Laboratory studies. The following tests should be closely monitored in a patient with persistent fetal circulation.

1. **Arterial blood gas levels.** Without adequate ventilation, blood gas levels will demonstrate fixed hypoxemia, progressive hypercarbia, and metabolic acidosis. Close monitoring of blood gas values is necessary to calculate the alveolar-arterial gradient and to define metabolic acidosis, carbon dioxide retention, and hypoxia.

2. **Total and ionized calcium levels.** Hypocalcemia, if present, may cause decreased cardiac output, hypoxia, and systemic hypotension.

3. **Serum glucose levels.** Hypoglycemia also potentiates hypoxia from decreased cardiac output.

B. Radiologic studies. A chest x-ray study will help detect lung disease. It is often said that oxygen requirements in persistent fetal circulation are out of proportion to the degree of disease seen on a chest x-ray film. Findings may include pneumonia, air leak syndrome (pneumothorax, pulmonary interstitial emphysema, pneumomediastinum, pneumopericardium), or wet lung. The lungs may also appear normal.

C. Echocardiography. Echocardiography is necessary to rule out congenital cyanotic heart disease. Once congenital heart disease has been excluded, the test is not diagnostic in persistent fetal circulation as the echocardiogram can be normal. Abnormalities may included right ventricular dilatation, hypertrophy, and poor contractility with bowing of the interventricular septum.

D. Differential oximeter readings. Oximetry helps to diagnose the presence of a right-to-left shunt, which is suggestive of persistent fetal circulation. Two transcutaneous oximeters are used, with one sensor placed on the right upper chest wall (preductal) and the other on the left lower abdomen (postductal). Alternately, a pulse oximeter can be used with one sensor on the right thumb (preductal) and a sensor on the left great toe (postductal). If there is a difference of 20 mm Hg in the two readings (correlated to simultaneous blood gases via the right radial and umbilical arteries), a right-to-left shunt should be expected.

E. Response to hyperventilation. The right-to-left shunt may be reversed by hyperventilation or infusion, or both, of alkali (bicarbonate) to increase the pH > 7.50. A significant increase in Pao_2 (generally to > 100 torr) with hyperventilation and alkalinization favors the diagnosis of pulmonary artery hypertension rather than cyanotic heart disease, in which the Pao_2 usually does not increase significantly.

VII. Management

A. Drug therapy. For dosages, see Chapter 75.

1. **Fluids and electrolytes.** Normal glucose and calcium levels are essential for maintaining cardiac output. Alkali is frequently needed to maintain a normal blood pH, since acidosis is a major cause of pulmonary vasoconstriction. The decision to use sodium bicarbonate or tromethamine (THAM) will depend on serum electrolyte levels, respiratory status, and urinary output. THAM is usually preferred if the serum sodium is high and the serum Pco_2 is high. To use THAM, the urine output must be satisfactory.

2. **Sedatives.** Sedation is often used in infants exhibiting marked lability and resistance to ventilation. Phenobarbital or lorazepam is useful in stabilizing the infant and reducing the incidence of air leak problems.

3. **Paralyzing agents.** The use of these agents is *controversial.* They may be tried in infants who have not responded to sedation and are still labile and resisting the ventilator. Pancuronium (Pavulon) has been used, since it does not have the hypotensive effects seen with curare. Some infants, however, will worsen with paralysis because of increased ventilation-perfusion mismatch.

4. **Volume expanders.** Blood pressure should be maintained by frequent colloid transfusions (5% albumin or whole blood, depending on the hematocrit). Use whole blood if the hematocrit is low. Maintenance of blood pressure increases the systemic vascular resistance, which helps to decrease the right-to-left shunt.

5. **Pressor agents.** Dopamine is used when the blood pressure is difficult to maintain and there is decreased renal perfusion. Dopamine in higher doses may increase the pulmonary vascular resistance (shown in animal studies), which will increase the right-to-left shunt.

6. **Pulmonary vasodilators.** Tolazoline (Priscoline) is an alpha-adrenergic blocking agent and should be used only when oxygenation is difficult to maintain. It is thought to cause dilation of the pulmonary vascular bed. A test dose is usually given, and if there is an increase in oxygenation (usually > 10–25, torr), a drip infusion is started. It is, however, a systemic vasodilator and may cause severe systemic hypotension. Colloid and pressor agents should be readily available if hypotension occurs.

B. Mechanical ventilation

1. **Ventilatory support** is instituted when the alveolar-arterial gradient

is high (usually > 250 mm Hg) and adequate ventilation can no longer be maintained. The goal is to provide ventilation using the **lowest mean airway pressure possible.** Ideally, blood gas levels should be maintained within the following ranges: pH, 7.40–7.50; $Paco_2$, 25–30 mm Hg; Pao_2, over 50 mm Hg. Initially, 100% inspired oxygen should be used, since most of these infants are term, and retinopathy of prematurity is not of major concern. With clinical improvement, the oxygen may then be slowly decreased to maintain acceptable Pao_2 with oxygen saturation > 90%.

2. **Rapid-rate ventilation** may be used in an attempt to hyperventilate the patient and achieve the critical $Paco_2$ (ie, pulmonary artery vasodilatation and a secondary rise in Pao_2). It must be remembered, however, that overventilation may reduce venous return and pulmonary blood flow. Pulmonary vasodilatation may be attained with ventilation in the normal range in conjunction with alkali infusions. Recent work has shown that high-frequency jet ventilation and high-frequency oscillatory ventilation may be used successfully if maximal conventional therapy fails. In approximately 30–40% of patients treated with high-frequency jet ventilation, the need for extracorporeal membrane oxygenation (ECMO) therapy can be averted. High-frequency ventilation should be attempted when conventional ventilation fails (ie, Pao_2 cannot be maintained at a level $\geq$ 50 mm Hg). (See Chap 14.)

3. **Air leaks** occur frequently when high mean airway pressures are used. Close monitoring for pneumothorax and other forms of barotrauma is essential.

4. **Bag-and-mask ventilation,** using different rates and pressures to determine which combination gives the best oxygenation, is often helpful.

C. **Extracorporeal membrane oxygenation (ECMO).** (See Chap 15.) ECMO has now been used in more than 1800 newborns at over 50 institutions. It is recommended for infants less than 7 days old, greater than 34 weeks' gestation, and greater than 2 kg in weight. It involves cannulation of the internal jugular vein and common carotid artery and placing the infant on cardiopulmonary bypass. There is currently an 86% rate of successful outcome. The decision to send an infant to an ECMO center depends on many factors; ECMO should be considered when:

1. The infant is unable to maintain adequate oxygenation (Pao_2 50 mm Hg).

2. The A-aDO_2 gradient is increasing.

3. Increasing support is required to maintain blood pressure.

4. The infant meets the ECMO criteria specified on page 127.

VIII. **Prognosis.** Prognosis depends on the underlying condition; for example, an infant with RDS usually does better than one with pulmonary hypoplasia. For all causes, survival is now in the range of 50–70%. Outcome also depends on other factors such as the presence of asphyxia, duration of hyperventilation, and central nervous system dysfunction. The condition of infants seen at follow-up can range from normal to severe neurodevelopmental delay.

REFERENCES

Barst RJ, Gersony WM: The pharmacological treatment of patent ductus arteriosus: A review of the evidence. *Drugs* 1989;**38**:249.

Beck R et al: Criteria for extracorporeal membrane oxygenation in a population of infants with persistent pulmonary hypertension of the newborn. *J Pediatr Surg* 1986;**21**:297.

Bender HW Jr et al: Repair of atrioventricular canal malformation in the first year of life. *J Thorac Cardiovasc Surg* 1982;**84**:515.

Bifano EM, Pfannenstiel A: Duration of hyperventilation and outcome in infants with persistent pulmonary hypertension. *Pediatrics* 1988;**81**:657.

Carlo WA et al: High frequency jet ventilation in neonatal pulmonary hypertension. *Am J Dis Child* 1989;**143**:233.

Clyman RI, Campbell D: Indomethacin therapy for patent ductus arteriosus: When is prophylaxis not prophylactic? *J Pediatr* 1987;**111**:718.

Copel JA, Pilu G, Kleinman CS: Congenital heart disease and extra-cardiac anomalies: Associations and indications for fetal echocardiography. *Am J Obstet Gynecol* 1986;**154**:1121.

Coster DD et al: Surgical closure of the patent ductus arteriosus in the neonatal intensive care unit. *Ann Thorac Surg* 1989;**48**:386.

Davis JM et al: Predicting survival in infants with persistent pulmonary hypertension of the newborn. *Pediatr Pulmonol* 1988;**5**:6.

Fyler DC et al: Reports of the New England Regional Infant Cardiac Program. *Pediatrics* 1980;**65**:377.

Garson A Jr et al: Surgical decision in tetralogy of Fallot: Weighing the risks and benefits with decision analysis. *Am J Cardiol* 1980;**45**:108.

Hammerman C et al: Prostaglandins and echocardiography in the assessment of patent ductus arteriosus. *Crit Care Med* 1986;**14**:462.

Hammerman C, Komar K, Abu-Khudair H: Hypoxic vs septic pulmonary hypertension. Selective role of thromboxane mediation. *Am J Dis Child* 1988;**142**:319.

Kohelet D et al: High frequency oscillation in the rescue of infants with persistent pulmonary hypertension. *Crit Care Med* 1988;**16**:510.

Kraus AN et al: Pulmonary function in preterm infants following treatment with intravenous indomethacin. *Am J Dis Child* 1989;**143**:78.

Mahoney LT et al: Atrial septal defects that present in infancy. *Am J Dis Child* 1986;**140**:1115.

Marx CR, Hougen TJ, Norwood WI: Transposition of the great arteries with intact ventricular septum. Results of Mustard and Senning operations in 123 consecutive patients. *J Am Col Cardiol* 1983;**1**:476.

Miller GA: Congenital heart disease in the first week of life. *Br Heart J* 1974;**36**:1160.

Moe DG, Guntheroth WG: Spontaneous closure of uncomplicated ventricular septal defect. *Am J Cardiol* 1987;**60**:674.

Perloff JK: *The Clinical Recognition of Congenital Heart Disease,* 3rd ed. Saunders, 1987.

Rabinovitch M: Structure and function of the pulmonary vascular bed: An update. *Cardiol Clin* 1989;**7**:227.

Reece EA et al: Persistent pulmonary hypertension: Assessment of perinatal risk factors. *Obstet Gynecol* 1987;**70**:696.

Rennie JM, Doyle J, Cooke RW: Early administration of indomethacin to preterm infants. *Arch Dis Child* 1986;**61**:233.

Rudolph A: Page 239 in: *Congenital Diseases of the Heart.* Year Book, 1974.

Siils JH, Cvetnic WG, Pietz J: Continuous negative pressure in the treatment of infants with pulmonary hypertension and respiratory failure. *J Perinatol* 1989;**9**:43.

Swensson RE et al: Real-time Doppler color flow mapping for detection of patent ductus arteriosus. *J Am Coll Cardiol* 1986;**8**:1105.

Tiefenbrunn LJ, Riemenschneider TA: Persistent pulmonary hypertension of the newborn. *Am Heart J* 1986;**111**:564.

58 Common Multiple Congenital Anomaly Syndromes

The intensive care newborn nursery is a busy place where quick decisions must often be made. For many disorders, treatment is the same regardless of the underlying problem. However, in the management of multiple congenital anomaly (MCA) syndromes, the neonatologist must deal with complex clinical issues calling for a wide range of diagnostic skills. Without a correct diagnosis of MCA syndrome, many available forms of therapy go underutilized and others may be tried when they will be relatively ineffective. Furthermore, unrealistic counseling may be given about prognosis and recurrence risk.

Only a few MCA syndromes are life-threatening in the neonatal period. It is important to note, however, that malformations are second only to prematurity as a cause of death at this critical point in the life span.

I. **Clinical presentation.** Table 58–1 lists symptoms and signs that should alert the clinician to the possibility of cryptogenic malformations or disorders. Obviously, if overt malformations are present, an MCA syndrome will be immediately recognized and diagnostic efforts will shortly follow. However, if external features of the disorder are subtle or nonspecific and the usual procedures associated with intensive newborn support have been started, findings may go unrecognized early. Each manifestation listed in Table 58–1 is more common in infants with MCA syndromes.

Tables 58–2 through 58–5 list the more common neonatal MCA syndromes, many of which share some of the features set forth in Table 58–1.

II. **General approach to diagnosis.** The diagnostic approach to malformations in neonates is no different from that in older children except that the effects of delivery and excess baby fat must be considered. Because so many of these children are intubated and have protective eye patches, the face may be obscured. Early and accurate documentation of physical char-

---

TABLE 58–1. SYMPTOMS AND SIGNS IN NEONATES THAT MIGHT INDICATE CRYPTIC MULTIPLE CONGENITAL ANOMALY SYNDROME

Prenatal
Oligohydramnios
Polyhydramnios
Decreased or unusual fetal activity
Abnormal fetal problem

Postnatal
Abnormalities of size: SGA or LGA, microcephaly or macrocephaly, large or irregular abdomen, small chest, limb-trunk disproportion, asymmetry
Abnormalities of tone: Hypotonia, hypertonia
Abnormalities of position: Joint contractures, fixation of joints in extension, hyperextension of joints
Midline aberrations: Hemangiomas, hair tufts, dimples or pits
Problems of secretion, excretion, or edema: No urination, no passage of meconium, chronic nasal or oral secretions, edema (nuchal, pedal, generalized, ascites)
Symptoms: Unexplained seizures, resistant or unexplained respiratory distress
Metabolic disorders: Resistant hypoglycemia, unexplained hypo- or hypercalcemia, polycythemia

acteristics, including photographs, is essential. If the infant is critically ill, confirmatory tests (chromosome studies, renal ultrasonography, echocardiography) become a priority equal in importance to ongoing therapy. **The basis of diagnosis of MCA syndromes in the neonate is knowing which disorders are most common plus documentation of the physical manifestations and appropriate exclusion tests such as chromosomal analysis.** This somewhat "overkill" approach is necessary because a significant percentage of infants with MCA syndromes die in the neonatal period, often before a diagnosis is made, and because the parents in such cases often refuse to permit autopsy. Diagnostic problems also occur because immediate efforts tend to emphasize therapy. Nevertheless, diagnosis will often facilitate or guide therapy in a more efficient manner. If clinical geneticists or dysmorphologists are locally available, they should be asked to examine the infant as soon after delivery as possible. If specialists in these fields are not available, a phone call to a university medical center asking for expert advice is often useful.

III. **Chromosomal syndromes** (Table 58–2). Chromosomal syndromes are by far the most common MCA syndromes diagnosed in the neonatal period.

A. **Trisomy 21 (Down's syndrome)**
1. **Incidence.** Trisomy 21 is by far the most common MCA syndrome, occurring in about 1:600 live births. Only about 80% of cases are diagnosed accurately in the newborn nursery, which means that there is a 20% rate of diagnostic error for this most common cause of MCA and mental retardation. The reason for missing the diagnosis is probably that most of the features of trisomy 21 may occur as isolated features in otherwise normal infants.
2. **Physical findings.** Findings include epicanthus, hypotelorism, a tendency to protrude the tongue, Brushfield's spots, single transverse palmar crease, and mongoloid slant of the palpebral fissures. Although each of these features may occur in normal individuals, it is the combination of features forming a recognizable pattern that usually permits early diagnosis.
3. **Associated anomalies** include congenital heart defects and increased frequency of duodenal atresia, esophageal atresia, and imperforate anus. Patients may have many immediate medical problems because of these anomalies.
4. **Hyptonia** may be associated with breathing difficulties, poor swallowing, and aspiration.

B. **Trisomy 18 (Edwards' syndrome)**
1. **Incidence.** About 1:5000 live births.
2. **Morbidity.** Highly lethal within the first 3 months of life.
3. **Physical findings.** Manifested by micrognathia, overlapping digits, rockerbottom feet, congenital heart disease (usually VSD or PDA), abnormal ears, short sternum, ptosis, and generalized hypertonicity.

C. **Trisomy 13 (Patau's syndrome)**
1. **Incidence.** About 1:7000 live births.
2. **Morbidity.** Highly lethal within the first 3 months of life.
3. **Physical findings.** Manifested by cleft lip and palate, polydactyly, microphthalmia, and congenital heart disease (usually VSD or PDA).

TABLE 58–2. MOST COMMON CHROMOSOME DISORDERS DIAGNOSED IN THE NEONATAL PERIOD

Trisomy 21 (Down's syndrome)
Trisomy 18
Trisomy 13
45,X (Turner's) syndrome

D. 45,X (Turner's) syndrome
1. **Incidence.** About 1:10,000 live-born females.
2. **Morbidity.** The 45,X syndrome is usually compatible with survival if the child reaches term.
3. **Physical findings.** Neck webbing, pedal and nuchal edema, and short stature are the hallmarks of this disorder.

IV. Nonchromosomal syndromes (Table 58–3)

A. Oligohydramnios sequence (Potter's oligohydramnios sequence)
1. **Incidence.** This syndrome is the second most common MCA (1:3000 live births). Most cases are nonsyndromic and have a 2–7% recurrence risk, depending on the specific urinary tract defect. Some may be associated with the prune belly syndrome (absent abdominal musculature, urinary tract abnormalities, cryptorchidism) if the kidneys were hydronephrotic early in gestation and later decompress, leaving a wrinkled abdomen and the effects of oligohydramnios (pulmonary hypoplasia and Potter' sequence). About 5% of cases are part of an MCA syndrome with primary defects outside the urinary system.
2. **Morbidity.** Almost all of these infants die.
3. **Pathophysiology.** Renal agenesis leads to decreased production of amniotic fluid (oligohydramnios). Deficient amniotic fluid is believed to be responsible for associated pulmonary hypoplasia.
4. **Clinical presentation**
   a. **History.** The history of oligohydramnios must be solicited from the obstetrician. Anuria is typically present in the newborn.
   b. **Placental examination.** The placenta must be examined for yellowish plaques ("**amnion nodosum**").
   c. **Physical findings.** Unexplained and highly refractory respiratory distress coupled with pneumothoraces, club feet, hyperextensible fingers, large cartilage-deficient ears, lower inner eye folds, and a beak nose are classic manifestations associated with prolonged and severe oligohydramnios.
5. **Diagnosis** is usually confirmed by renal ultrasonography and autopsy disclosure of the urinary tract abnormality. It is advisable to do chromosome studies on the propositus to exclude a chromosomal basis for the disorder. The recurrence risk depends on the specific syndrome diagnosis. In either case, future pregnancies should be monitored by ultrasonography unless the risk of recurrence is definitely ruled out.

B. Amniotic band syndrome
1. **Incidence.** About 1:4000 live births. Because in some newborns many body areas are involved and because the bands dissipate before delivery in 90% of cases, the diagnosis is often missed or a misdiagnosis is made.
2. **Pathophysiology.** This syndrome is poorly understood, but the effects of early amnion rupture with entanglement of body parts in bands or strands of amnion are well appreciated. The resulting biomechanical forces can cause deformities of the limbs, digits, and craniofacies. Viscera that are normally outside the fetus in early em-

TABLE 58–3. MOST COMMON NONCHROMOSOMAL DEFORMATION/DISRUPTION SEQUENCES DIAGNOSED IN THE NEONATAL PERIOD

Potter's oligohydramnios sequence
Amniotic band syndrome
Arthrogryposis
Pierre Robin sequence

bryologic development may be hindered in their return, giving rise to omphalocele and other anomalies.

3. **Physical findings**
   a. **Extremities.** Limb and digit amputations, constrictions, distal swellings.
   b. **Craniofacies.** Facial clefts, encephaloceles.
   c. **Viscera.** Omphalocele, gastroschisis, ectopia cordis.
4. **Placental examination.** It is always important to examine the placenta, but especially in these cases. The amnion is often small, absent, or rolled into strands. Not all amniotic bands cause intrauterine problems. Recent ultrasound studies of routine pregnancies have identified amniotic bands that were not attached to the fetus. Follow-up of these pregnancies has revealed normal newborns.
5. **Management.** Surgical removal of the constricting band and plastic surgical reconstruction should be done if possible.

C. **Arthrogryposis (multiple joint fixations)**
1. **Incidence.** About 1:3000 live births.
2. **Pathophysiology.** Ninety percent of children with arthrogryposis have a neurologic (brain, spinal cord) basis for the disorder. Many syndromes associated with fetal inactivity (akinesia) may be characterized by arthrogryposis also, because normal fetal joint development depends on adequate fetal movement.
3. **Clinical presentation.** The newborn infant is afflicted by a combination of joint contractures, joint extensions, and joint dislocations. Those with arthrogryposis of central nervous system origin are at increased risk for aspiration and inadequate respiratory movement.
4. **Management.** Early treatment and rehabilitation can result in remarkable improvement.

D. **Pierre Robin sequence**
1. **Incidence.** About 1:8000 live births.
2. **Pathophysiology.** The basis of this sequence is severe hypoplasia of the mandible, which does not support the tongue. The accompanying glossoptosis results in severe upper airway obstruction and early intrauterine cleft palate.
3. **Clinical presentation.** These infants present with a short jaw or receding chin associated with cleft palate. Respiratory distress due to upper airway obstruction may occur.
4. **Differential diagnosis.** Many syndromes (eg, **Stickler, Catel-Manzke**) have the craniofacial features of Pierre Robin sequence. If noncraniofacial primary defects (malformations) are present, an MCA syndrome other than Pierre Robin sequence is present. Some syndromes (eg, Stickler syndrome) may be manifested only by craniofacial features in infancy. Examinations for myopia and malar flattening should be done to support a diagnosis of Stickler syndrome rather than Pierre Robin sequence.
5. **Management.** Intubation, obturators, tracheostomy, and suturing of the tongue tip to the lower gingiva are effective temporary measures for glossoptosis. As the mandible grows out, the glossoptosis eventually will resolve. Oral feedings may result in choking or respiratory distress, and gavage feedings or gastrostomy tube feedings may be needed. Most cases of Pierre Robin sequence are nonsyndromic and have little or no recurrence risk.

V. **Miscellaneous syndromes** (Table 58–4)
A. **VATER association**
1. **Incidence.** About 1:5000 live births.
2. **Clinical presentation.** Major features include **V**ertebral anomalies, **A**nal atresia, **T**racheoesophageal fistula, **E**sophageal atresia, and

TABLE 58-4. OTHER MCA SYNDROMES OF SPECIAL INTEREST IN THE NEONATE

VATER association
CHARGE association
Lethal short-limb, short-rib dwarfism
DiGeorge association
Beckwith syndrome

Radial defects. The **V** in VATER can also represent vascular (cardiac) defects and the **R** renal defects, since these 2 areas are also commonly involved. The presence of additional features, except for atresia of the small intestine, rules out a diagnosis of VATER association. This nonrandom association is usually not of genetic origin and requires exclusion of other similar disorders, including chromosomal syndromes.

B. CHARGE association
  1. **Incidence.** While not as common as the VATER association, CHARGE often presents as a medical emergency because about half the patients have choanal atresia.
  2. **Clinical presentation**
     a. **CHARGE** stands for **C** coloboma, **H** heart disease, **A** choanal atresia, **R** retarded growth and development with or without CNS anomalies, **G** genital anomalies with or without hypogonadism, and **E** ear abnormalities and/or deafness.
     b. **Choanal atresia.** The infant may present with unexplained respiratory distress.
     c. **Associated anomalies.** Patients with CHARGE association also have heart defects, small ears, and retinal colobomas; males have micropenis. A smaller percentage have unilateral facial palsies and swallowing difficulties, the latter potentially as lethal as choanal atresia. Postnatal growth deficiency and psychomotor delay round out the major features of this nonrandom and nongenetic association.
  3. **Diagnosis.** Any newborn with unexplained breathing difficulties should have nasogastric tubes passed through its nasal passages, particularly if there are multiple congenital anomalies. Exclusion of other similar entities and chromosomal disorders is essential before the diagnosis of CHARGE association can be accepted.
C. Lethal short-limb, short-rib dwarfism
  1. **Incidence.** About 1:5000 live births.
  2. **Pathophysiology.** The 3 most common lethal dwarfing conditions are **achondrogenesis, thanatophoric dysplasia,** and **type II osteogenesis imperfecta.** However, at least 7 other disorders can be lethal in neonates. All of these disorders are of genetic origin.
  3. **Clinical presentation.** These conditions commonly present clinical and diagnostic difficulties in neonates. Recognition of disproportionate parameters in a newborn with respiratory distress should immediately suggest the possibility of a lethal dwarfing condition. Because many newborns have a lot of fat, chest size may be difficult to assess.
  4. **Diagnosis.** If the babygram (chest and abdominal x-ray film) shows a small chest and long bone metaphyseal or epiphyseal abnormalities, a potentially lethal dwarfing condition is present and accurate diagnosis is essential for prognosis estimation of recurrence risk. A full skeletal x-ray study is mandatory in all cases.
D. DiGeorge association
  1. **Clinical presentation**

    a. Physical findings include heart defects; small, abnormally shaped ears; and mild nonspecific facial dysmorphology.

    b. Laboratory findings usually consist of hypocalcemia secondary to absence or hypoplasia of the parathyroid glands. Hypocalcemia is often diagnosed before other features are recognized, and this finding should immediately stimulate a search for abnormalities of the heart and craniofacial area. A decreased lymphocyte count may also be seen.

  2. Associated anomalies. Total or partial **thymic absence** is a hidden feature of the DiGeorge association that should be investigated because it may be the most serious of all the abnormalities.

E. Beckwith's syndrome

  1. Clinical presentation

    a. Physical findings typically include macroglossia and omphalocele, but about 20% of patients have only one or neither of these 2 features. Unilateral limb hypertrophy may also be seen.

    b. Laboratory findings. Refractory hypoglycemia is frequently present regardless of the presence of external features and should immediately raise the possibility of Beckwith's syndrome.

  2. Management. Making the diagnosis early in the postnatal period and immediate institution of aggressive hypoglycemic therapy may prevent mental retardation.

VI. Teratogenic malformations (Table 58–5)

A. Fetal alcohol syndrome may be suspected on the basis of the phenotype alone or may present only as an SGA infant. It may also present with microcephaly, microphthalmia, and a flattened maxillary area. A thorough history of maternal drug intake is important to rule out a teratogenic cause of malformations.

B. Fetal hydantoin syndrome is characterized by a typical facies (broad, low nasal bridge, hypertelorism, epicanthal folds, ptosis, and prominent malformed ears), and these infants also have a high incidence of absence or hypoplasia of the fifth fingernail and toenail.

C. Fetal cocaine syndrome is characteristically seen in small-for-gestational-age (SGA) infants, who may show hyperirritability or withdrawal symptomatology. There is an increased incidence of genitourinary tract anomalies such as hydronephrosis, hypospadias, and prune belly sequence and central nervous system abnormalities such as microcephaly, porencephaly, and infarction. There have been reports of gastrointestinal and cardiac anomalies. No well-established facial phenotype is known at this time.

D. Infants of diabetic mothers

  1. Incidence. These infants are at 3 times the risk for malformations compared with the offspring of nondiabetic mothers. Infants of diabetic mothers present with anomalies in approximately 1:2000 consecutive deliveries.

  2. Clinical presentation. The well-known malformations are sacral agenesis, femoral hypoplasia, heart defects, and cleft palate. Others include preaxial radial defects, microtia, cleft lip, microphthalmia, holoprosencephaly, microcephaly, anencephaly, spina bifida, hemi-

---

TABLE 58–5. TERATOGENIC SYNDROMES COMMONLY SEEN IN NEONATES

Fetal alcohol syndrome
Fetal cocaine syndrome
Fetal hydantoin syndrome
Infant of diabetic mother

vertebra, urinary tract defects, and hallical polydactyly. Some infants of diabetic mothers have many anomalies, which may not be recognized as related to maternal diabetes.

REFERENCES

Hall BD: The twenty-five most common multiple congenital anomaly syndromes. Pages 141–150 in: *Genetic Issues in Pediatric, Obstetric, and Gynecologic Practice.* Kaback MM (editor). Year Book, 1981

Myrianthopoulos NC, Chung CS: Congenital malformations in singletons: Epidemiologic survey. *Birth Defects* 1974;**10**:1.

Smith DW: *Recognizable Patterns of Human Malformations*, 3rd ed. Saunders, 1982.

Van Regemorter N et al: Congenital malformations in 10,000 consecutive births in a university hospital: Need for genetic counseling and prenatal diagnosis. *J Pediatr* 1984;**104**:386.

59 Infant of Drug-Abusing Mother

I. **Definition.** The infant of a drug-abusing mother (IDAM) is one who may suffer withdrawal symptoms after birth due to the mother's use of a substance, or substances, during pregnancy.

II. **Incidence.** Maternal drug usage or addiction has increased dramatically over the past decade. As a result, the incidence of neonatal withdrawal syndrome has also increased rapidly.

III. **Pathophysiology.** Because of their low molecular weight, heroin, cocaine, and other substances of abuse cross the placenta and are distributed throughout fetal tissues. Potential benefits, such as diminished incidence of jaundice, have been described, and there is conflicting information regarding a decreased incidence of respiratory distress syndrome (RDS). The many adverse effects of drug usage during pregnancy outweigh the benefits, however. Overall complications include decreased birth weight and intrauterine growth retardation (IUGR). Sudden infant death syndrome (SIDS) is more than 5–15 times more prevalent in IDAM than in the general population. A decreased sensitivity to carbon dioxide in IDAM infants may contribute to this high incidence.

The prevalence of multiple drug abuse, such as a combination of smoking and alcohol consumption, complicates the attempt to study any single agent producing the withdrawal syndrome. Many drugs that are abused during pregnancy (eg, LSD, amphetamines) have not been associated with physical dependence and neonatal withdrawal syndrome.

Currently, cocaine use is a widespread problem. Use of **"crack" cocaine** has increased to epidemic proportions over recent years. Crack is derived from regular cocaine, but by a special process it is made more potent. A smaller quantity is required to get "high." As crack has become more popular, the adverse effect of its use in neonates has been better studied. Complications from maternal use of cocaine and other drugs during pregnancy, which were previously more controversial, have been documented (Table 59–1).

IV. **Risk factors**
   A. **Maternal drug use.** Drugs that have been reported to cause neonatal withdrawal are listed in Table 59–2.
   B. **Lower socioeconomic groups.**
   C. **Teenage or unwed mothers.**
   D. **Lack of education.**

V. **Clinical presentation.** Both mother and infant are at risk; the antenatal, intrapartum, and postnatal problems associated with maternal drug usage are summarized in Table 59–1. Table 59–3 summarizes most manifestations of neonatal withdrawal syndrome. Clinical presentation is usually within 24–48 hours after delivery, except for withdrawal 2 or more weeks later in the case of methadone, a liposoluble drug, and for withdrawal in the delivery room after the administration of naloxone (Narcan) to an infant of an opiate-abusing mother. Fever, tachypnea, high-pitched cry, tremors, increased muscle tone and Moro reflex, frequent yawning, nasal stuffiness, diarrhea (often watery), excoriation, or frantic sucking of the fists may be seen. Table 59–3 also gives an objective method of scoring the infant's daily withdrawal status for better dosage titration. Scoring is

TABLE 59–1. PERINATAL PROBLEMS ASSOCIATED WITH MATERNAL DRUG USAGE

Antenatal and Intrapartum Problems
Fetal asphyxia (meconium-stained amniotic fluid, low Apgar scores, cesarean section for fetal distress)
Anemia (mother and infant)
Premature rupture of the membranes
Infertility
Maternal infections
Prematurity
Low birth weight (SGA infant, IUGR)
Stillbirth
Cocaine- and "crack"-related problems
　　Lower gestational age at delivery
　　Increased preterm labor and delivery
　　Lower birth weight
　　Delivery of small for gestational age infants
　　Abruptio placentae
　　Microcephaly
　　Infections (especially sexually transmitted diseases)
　　Small intracranial bleeding episodes
　　Birth defects secondary to vasoconstriction, antenatal cerebral infarction (rare)

Postnatal Problems
Respiratory distress syndrome (conflicting information about whether increased or decreased aspiration pneumonia [meconium aspiration])
Thrombocytosis
Congenital malformations (perhaps drug related)
Neonatal withdrawal syndrome
Delayed motor development
Growth disturbances (poor weight gain)
Behavioral disturbances (hyperactivity/learning difficulties)
Sudden infant death syndrome (SIDS)
Cocaine-related problems
　　Withdrawal
　　SIDS (15% incidence)
　　Behavioral abnormalities
　　Neurobehavioral problems
　　Poor feeding
　　Myocardial infarction or ischemia (rare)

---

very important, since among different observers the degree of withdrawal will always differ. With this standardized method it is more difficult to over- or undertreat the symptoms of withdrawal syndrome.

VI. Diagnosis

　　A. Obtain maternal drug history. This history is frequently not honestly given by mothers.

　　B. Physical examination using modified Finnegan's Scoring System (Table 59–3).

TABLE 59–2. DRUGS CAUSING NEONATAL WITHDRAWAL SYNDROME

Opiates	**Miscellaneous**
Codeine	Alcohol
Heroin	Cocaine or "crack"
Meperidine	Chlordiazepoxide (Librium)
Methadone	Desmethylimipramine
Morphine	Diazepam (Valium)
Pentazocine	Diphenhydramine (Benadryl)
Pentazocine and Tripelennamine	Ethchlovynol (Placidyl)
Barbiturates	Glutethimide (Doriden)
Phenobarbital	Hydroxyzine (Atarax)
Secobarbital	Phencyclidine (PCP)
	Propoxyphene (Darvon)

TABLE 59–3. MODIFIED FINNEGAN'S SCORING SYSTEM FOR NEONATAL WITHDRAWAL[a,b]

Signs and symptoms are scored between feedings.

Cry:	High-pitch (2)													
	Continuous (3)													
Sleep hours after feed:	1 hour (3)													
	2 hours (2)													
	3 hours (1)													
Moro reflex:	Hyperactive (2)													
	Marked (3)													
Tremors when disturbed:	Mild (2)													
	Marked (3)													
Tremors when un-disturbed:	Mild (3)													
	Marked (4)													
Muscle tone increased:	Mild (3)													
	Marked (6)													
Convulsions:	(8)													
Feedings:														
Frantic sucking of fists	(1)													
Poor feeding ability	(1)													
Regurgitation	(1)													
Projectile vomiting	(1)													
Stools:	Loose (2)													
	Watery (3)													
Fever:	100–101 °F (2)													
	Over 101 °F (2)													
Respiratory rate:	> 60/minute (1)													
	Retractions (2)													
Excoriations:	Nose (1)													
	Knees (1)													
	Toes (1)													
Frequent yawning:	(1)													
Sneezing:	(1)													
Nasal stuffiness:	(1)													
Sweating:	(1)													
Total scores per day														

[a] Initiated by Loretta Finnegan, MD, and modified by J. Yoon, MD

[b] Once an objective score had been attained a dose for treatment can be decided upon. Table 59–4 indicates the dosage necessary for treatment of withdrawal.

Reproduced with permission.

C. Laboratory studies

1. **Urine drug screening (toxicology).** Opiate breakdown products as well as other drugs of abuse are excreted in the newborn's urine and may be detected by chromatography. Although the result of urine screening does not establish whether the infant should be treated, in many cases it serves as a helpful tool in assessing the mother's honesty regarding her use of drugs. Because it is used in the preparation of heroin, quinine may be found in the urine of heroin-addicted individuals.

2. **Blood gas levels.** Respiratory alkalosis has been seen in some newborns.

3. **Thyroid function tests.** Elevated levels of T_3 and T_4 have been seen in infants of mothers who use methadone.

4. **Platelet abnormality.** Thrombocytosis with increased platelet aggregation has been described in methadone-maintained mothers.

5. **Other laboratory tests.** The infant's sodium, calcium, magnesium, and glucose levels and the hematocrit are usually normal during withdrawal, but these studies should be obtained prior to starting any pharmacologic therapy to rule out imbalances as the cause of the infant's signs and symptoms.

VII. **Management**
   A. **Rule out other causes** of tremors, convulsions, hypernatremia, and diarrhea that may coexist, such as electrolyte imbalance, hypocalcemia, hypoglycemia, hypomagnesemia, hyperthyroidism, CNS hemorrhage, and infections, before starting pharmacologic therapy.
   B. **Examine the infant.** Use Table 59–3 as a guide. Ideally, the same person should serially examine the infant, determine the score for the infant, and treat when the total score is 6 or more.
   C. **Supportive care**
      1. Attempt to keep the infant quiet in a darkened and noise-controlled environment.
      2. Swaddle the infant loosely.
      3. To prevent excessive crying, use a pacifier if necessary.
      4. Attempt oral administration of fluids if possible.
      5. Monitor vital signs and platelet counts.
   D. **Drug treatment.** When supportive treatment alone is not sufficient and an infant has severe tachypnea, hypertension, or respiratory alkalosis, or fails to thrive because of increased oxygen consumption, pharmacologic therapy is required. All currently used pharmacologic agents have some disadvantages. Some of the drugs used and dosages are given in Table 59–4.
      1. **General principles of drug treatment**
         a. **Initiative therapy** when the withdrawal score (Table 59–3) is 6 or more and the clinical status is otherwise consistent with drug withdrawal syndrome.
         b. **Reevaluate symptoms** between feedings on every shift.
         c. **Taper dose gradually** if the scores are decreasing.
         d. **Increase the dose** if the scores remain the same or increase.
         e. **Observe for recurrence of symptoms** about 7 days after discontinuation of therapy.
      2. **Pharmacologic agents**
         a. **Phenobarbital (sedative).** Phenobarbital has been shown effective in controlling signs of withdrawal syndrome. However, recent studies have shown a greater number of seizures in infants on phenobarbital vs paregoric. Phenobarbital is an effective

TABLE 59–4. INITIAL DOSES OF MEDICATIONS USED IN DRUG TREATMENT OF NEONATES

Total Score (from Table 59–3)	Phenobarbital[a] (mg/kg/d)	Paregoric[b] (drops)	Diazepam[c] (mg/kg/dose)
6–9	6	1	0.1
10–13	8	2	0.2
14–18	11	3	0.4
19–22	15	4	0.6
23 or more	18–20	4	0.8

[a] Give dose IM or PO, divided q6–8h.
[b] Give dose PO q6h.
[c] Give dose IM or IV q6–8h as needed.

CNS depressant and impairs sucking and bonding. The dosage and serum level of phenobarbital necessary to control withdrawal vary; adequate serum concentrations to control withdrawal have not been determined.

b. Tincture of paregoric (narcotic). Tincture of paregoric contains 0.4 mg/mL morphine-equivalent paregoric. It has proved superior for the treatment of diarrhea and seizures. It rapidly normalizes sucking behavior, but it also has been associated with complications from its composition (CNS depression from alcohol; CNS stimulation from camphor; acidosis, CNS depression, respiratory distress, renal failure, and death from benzoic acid). Kandall and colleagues (1983) have found that phenobarbital is superior to paregoric in suppressing gross signs of drug abstinence. It is also important to exercise caution in the use of opiates in withdrawal from nonopiate drugs.

c. Tincture of opium (narcotic). Tincture of opium is **probably the best option** since it lacks the additive of paregoric. It should be diluted to the same dosage as paregoric. Tincture of opium has 10 mg/mL morphine equivalent, whereas paregoric has 0.4 mg/mL (no additives and less alcohol than paregoric).

d. Diazepam (Valium) (neuroleptic). Diazepam offers no advantage over the previously listed drugs. It decreases nutritive sucking behavior. With jaundice, parenteral diazepam is contraindicated owing to the preservative benzoate, which competes with bilirubin for albumin-binding sites and predisposes to kernicterus. It also contains propylene glycol and ethyl alcohol, which may give rise to cerebral and hepatic complications.

E. Duration of therapy. Because recurrence is common, infants should be observed for 5–7 days after discontinuation of any medication. The duration of therapy required is variable, depending on the degree of addiction as well as on the type of drug used. For example, the duration of therapy required for heroin withdrawal varies from 4 days to 6 weeks; with methadone therapy, it can be as long as 4 months.

F. Long-term management

1. Frequent follow-up visits and close involvement of social services are required.

2. Home monitoring is managed differently at each institution. Some favor home monitoring of apnea for every infant whose mother has a history of drug abuse. Others base the decision on the results of pneumography performed on infants who have had withdrawal syndromes. However, pneumograms have been shown to be predictive of future problems with apnea.

VIII. Prognosis. Generally, infants of drug-abusing mothers do well in the NICU during the neonatal period, but they usually have difficult home situations and, to aggravate matters, they usually are not easy to handle. The medical complications compounding these problems are as follows.

A. Acquired immune deficiency syndrome (AIDS). Intravenous drug users as well as methadone-maintained mothers have been reported to have an increased incidence of AIDS, which may be transmitted to the fetus during pregnancy.

B. Behavior and learning problems. An increased incidence of hyperactivity, learning, and behavioral disorders has been reported in children born to mothers who used methadone during pregnancy.

C. Child abuse. An increased incidence of child abuse is associated with parental drug abuse.

D. Seizures. If withdrawal symptoms in infants are improperly treated and, sometimes, even with adequate treatment, seizures may develop. The long-term prognosis for infants with seizures is unknown.

    E. Behavioral disturbances. Impaired growth and lower developmental scores have also been reported.

REFERENCES

Dixon SD, Bresnhan K, Zuckerman B: Cocaine babies: Meeting the challenge of management. *Contemp Pediatr* 1990;**7**:70.

Fricker HS, Segal S: Narcotic addiction, pregnancy, and the newborn. *Am J Dis Child* 1978;**132**:360.

Gawin FH, Ellinwood EH: Cocaine and other stimulants: Actions, abuse, and treatment. *N Engl J Med* 1988;**318(18)**:1173.

Glass L, Rajegowda BK, Evans HE: Absence of respiratory distress syndrome in premature infants of heroin-addicted mothers. *Lancet* 1971;**2**:685.

Hadeed AJ, Siegel SR: Maternal cocaine use during pregnancy: Effect on the newborn infant. *Pediatrics* 1989;**84(2)**:205.

Kahn EJ, Neuman LL, Polk GA: The course of the heroin withdrawal syndrome in newborn infants treated with phenobarbital or chlorpromazine. *J Pediatr* 1969;**75**:495.

Kandall SR et al: Opiate versus CNS depressant therapy in neonatal abstinence syndrome. *Am J Dis Child* 1983;**137**:378.

LeBlanc P et al: Effects of intrauterine exposure to alkaloidal cocaine ('crack'). *Am J Dis Child* 1987;**141**:937.

Olsen GD, Lees MH: Ventilatory response to carbon dioxide of infants following chronic prenatal methadone exposure. *J Pediatr* 1980;**96**:983.

Ostrea EM, Chavez CJ. Perinatal problems (excluding neonatal withdrawal) in maternal drug addiction: A study of 830 cases. *J Pediatr* 1979;**94**:292.

Shannon M et al: Cocaine exposure among children at a pediatric hospital. *Pediatrics* 1989;**83(3)**:337.

60 Hyperbilirubinemia

Hyperbilirubinemia is a common finding in the majority of newborn premature and full-term infants. An elevation of serum bilirubin concentration > 2 mg/dL is found in most newborns in the first several days of life.

Bilirubin is the end product of the catabolism of heme and is produced chiefly by the breakdown of red cell hemoglobin. Other sources of heme include myoglobin and certain liver enzymes. Bilirubin exists in several forms in the blood but is predominantly bound to serum albumin. In this form, unconjugated bilirubin cannot cross the blood-brain barrier. Free unconjugated bilirubin, and possible other forms, may enter the central nervous system and become toxic to cells. The precise mechanism is unknown.

Inside liver cells, unconjugated bilirubin is bound to ligandin, Z-protein, and other proteins; it is conjugated by uridine disphophate glucuronyl transferase. In the fetus, most unconjugated bilirubin crosses the placenta and is metabolized by the maternal liver. The capacity of the fetal liver to conjugate bilirubin is limited.

Conjugated bilirubin is water soluble and can be excreted in the urine, but most of it is rapidly excreted as bile into the intestine. In children and adults, conjugated bilirubin is further metabolized by bacteria in the intestine and excreted in the feces. Newborns have increased β-glucuronidase in the intestine and lack bacterial flora. β-glucuronidase hydrolyzes conjugated bilirubin to unconjugated bilirubin. Therefore, the newborn intestine contains excessive amounts of unconjugated bilirubin and, through enterohepatic uptake, contributes to the serum unconjugated bilirubin load.

Hyperbilirubinemia presents in one of 2 forms in the neonate: unconjugated hyperbilirubinemia or conjugated hyperbilirubinemia. The 2 forms have different causes and potential complications; their treatment will be discussed separately.

UNCONJUGATED (INDIRECT) HYPERBILIRUBINEMIA

I. **Definition.** Unconjugated hyperbilirubinemia is the most common form in the newborn. Elevations of indirect serum bilirubin are related to bilirubin load less bilirubin excretion and are therefore dependent on the gestational age and chronologic age of the infant.

II. **Classification and pathophysiology.** The causes of unconjugated hyperbilirubinemia are listed in Table 60-1.

   A. **Physiologic jaundice.** In almost every newborn infant, elevation of serum unconjugated bilirubin develops during the first week of life and resolves spontaneously. This form is referred to as physiologic jaundice.

   1. **Bilirubin levels**

      a. **In normal term infants,** levels of unconjugated bilirubin rise slowly and peak at 6–8 mg/dL by about the third to fourth day of life. In premature infants, liver function is less mature and jaundice is more frequent and more pronounced than in term infants. The bilirubin level may peak at 10–12 mg/dL, usually by the fifth day of life.

      b. **Physiologic jaundice** is defined as serum bilirubin not exceeding 12 mg/dL in full-term infants or 15 mg/dL in premature infants

TABLE 60-1. CAUSES OF UNCONJUGATED HYPERBILIRUBINEMIA

PHYSIOLOGIC JAUNDICE

HEMOLYTIC ANEMIA
Congenital: hereditary spherocytosis, infantile pyknocytosis, pyruvate kinase deficiency, G6PD deficiency, sickle cell disease (rarely seen in newborn period)
Acquired: ABO or Rh incompatibility, infection, drugs

POLYCYTHEMIA
Placental hypertransfusion: twin-twin transfusion, maternal-fetal transfusion, delayed cord clamping
Placental insufficiency: postmaturity, pregnancy-induced hypertension, SGA infant
Endocrine disorders: maternal diabetes, congenital adrenal hyperplasia, neonatal thyrotoxicosis
Other disorders: Down's syndrome, Beckwith-Wiedemann syndrome

BLOOD EXTRAVASATION

GLUCURONYL TRANSFERASE DEFECT
Congenital: Crigler-Najjar syndrome (type I deficiency), type II deficiency, Gilbert's syndrome
Acquired: Lucey-Driscoll syndrome

BREAST MILK AND BREAST-FEEDING JAUNDICE

METABOLIC DISORDERS: galactosemia, hypothyroidism, maternal diabetes

INCREASED ENTEROHEPATIC CIRCULATION: ileus, intestinal obstruction, swallowing of blood during delivery

DRUGS: Aspirin, sulfonamides, furosemide, and chloral hydrate

during the first week of life. Criteria that would rule out physiologic jaundice include clinical jaundice in the first 24 hours of life, conjugated bilirubin levels exceeding 2 mg/dL, total serum bilirubin concentrations increasing by more than 5 mg/dL/d, and clinical jaundice persisting for longer than 1 week in full-term or 2 weeks in preterm infants (Maisels, 1982).

2. **Mechanisms.** A number of mechanisms have been suggested.
    a. **An increased bilirubin load** owing to the larger red blood cell volume, the shorter life span of red blood cells, and increased enterohepatic circulation in newborn infants.
    b. **Defective uptake** of bilirubin by the liver.
    c. **Defective conjugation.**
    d. **Impaired excretion into bile.**
    e. **Overall impairment of liver function.**
B. **Hemolytic anemia**
    1. **Red blood cell defects.** Hemolytic anemia may result from a congenital red blood cell defect such as hereditary spherocytosis, infantile pyknocytosis, pyruvate kinase deficiency, glucose-6-phosphate dehydrogenase (G6PD) deficiency, thalassemia, or vitamin K-induced hemolysis.
    2. **Acquired hemolytic anemia** may be seen in ABO or Rh incompatibility (eg, erythroblastosis fetalis) between infant and mother. It may also be associated with the use of certain drugs (eg, oxytocin) or with infection.
C. **Polycythemia.** Polycythemia in the newborn infant may cause hyperbilirubinemia because the liver may not have the capacity to metabolize the increased bilirubin load (see p 262).
D. **Blood extravasation.** A large hematoma in the newborn period **may overload the bilirubin degradation pathway.** It may be seen with cephalohematoma, intraventricular and pulmonary hemorrhage, subcapsular hematoma of the liver, excessive ecchymoses or petechiae, or occult hemorrhaging.
E. **Defects of conjugation**
    1. **Congenital deficiency of glucuronyl transferase**
        a. **Type 1 deficiency (Crigler-Najjar syndrome)** is an autosomal recessive disorder with a poor prognosis.

     b. Type II glucuronyl transferase is an autosomal dominant benign deficiency.

     c. Gilbert's syndrome is autosomal dominant, benign, and relatively common.

  2. Glucuronyl transferase inhibition

     a. Drugs such as novobiocin.

     b. Lucey-Driscoll syndrome. In this syndrome, a maternal gestational hormone found in the infant's serum interferes with the conjugation of bilirubin. This problem appears to resolve spontaneously.

F. Breast milk jaundice (late onset) is characterized by a higher peak and slower decline in the serum bilirubin concentration and rarely appears before the end of the first week of life for term or preterm infants (Sirota, 1988). Factors associated with an abnormality of the milk itself include pregnanediol in the milk that inhibits glucuronyl transferase, increased concentration of fatty acids, and increased enteric absorption of unconjugated bilirubin. Levels of unconjugated bilirubin may be elevated for weeks to several months. Interruption of breast-feeding for 24–48 hours at unacceptable bilirubin levels results in a rapid decline in bilirubin levels. Resumption of breast-feeding increases bilirubin levels slightly but usually below previous levels. Breast milk jaundice may recur in 70% of future pregnancies (Schneider, 1986). There are no reported cases of kernicterus related to breast jaundice.

G. Metabolic disorders. Galactosemia, hypothyroidism, and maternal diabetes may be associated with unconjugated hyperbilirubinemia.

H. Increased enterohepatic circulation of unconjugated bilirubin may result in jaundice. It may be seen with **pyloric stenosis, duodenal atresia, annular pancreas, cystic fibrosis, and any form of gastrointestinal obstruction or ileus.** Blood swallowed during delivery and decreased caloric intake may also be contributing factors.

I. Substances and disorders affecting binding of bilirubin to albumin. Certain drugs occupy bilirubin-binding sites on albumin and increase the amount of free unconjugated bilirubin that can cross the blood-brain barrier. Drugs in which this effect may be significant include aspirin and sulfonamides. Fatty acids in nutritional products (eg, Intralipid) may also influence bilirubin-binding to albumin, as may asphyxia, acidosis, sepsis, hypothermia, hyperosmolality, and hypoglycemia. Chloral hydrate is shown to compete for hepatic glucuronidation with bilirubin and thus increase serum unconjugated bilirubin.

J. Kernicterus. Kernicterus, a postmortem diagnosis, is characterized by yellow pigmentation of the brain, which occasionally occurs when the amount of free unconjugated (indirect) bilirubin (from various causes) increases to the extent that it crosses the blood-brain barrier and is deposited in the central nervous system. The basal ganglion, hippocampus, and the cerebral and bulbar nuclei stain with the greatest intensity. The specific form of bilirubin that crosses the blood-brain barrier, the mechanisms of entry, and the causes of neuron damage are unclear. Bilirubin interferes with the function of many intracellular organelles (eg, mitochondria), but the specific metabolic and biochemical pathways interrupted by bilirubin are not completely known. Bilirubin toxicity is not confined to the central nervous system and can result in damage to other organ tissues, although encephalopathy is the most common symptom of toxicity.

    Controversy exists over what level of unconjugated bilirubin is associated with a significant risk of kernicterus. Most authors agree that clinical manifestations of kernicterus are unlikely to occur if the serum bilirubin level is kept lower than 20 mg/dL in full-term infants with hemolytic disease. The "magic number" in full-term infants without hemolysis or for preterm infants is less clear. Most clinicians try to keep serum bilirubin levels below 15 mg/dL in preterm infants (Maisels, 1982).

K. Prolonged indirect hyperbilirubinemia may be due to Crigler-Najjar syndrome, intestinal obstruction, ongoing hemolytic disease, breast milk jaundice, or hypothyroidism.

III. Clinical presentation

A. History

1. **Family history.** A family history of jaundice, anemia, splenectomy, or metabolic disorders is significant. A history of a previous sibling with jaundice may suggest blood group incompatibility, breast milk jaundice, or G6PD deficiency.

   A familial nature of neonatal hyperbilirubinemia is present regardless of breast-feeding and other risk factors, and the excess risk of neonatal hyperbilirubinemia in siblings is most notable for severe neonatal jaundice (Khoury, 1988).

2. **Maternal history.** Neonatal jaundice is increased with a history of maternal diabetes or infection. Use of oxytocin, sulfonamides, antimalarials, and nitrofurantoins by the mother may initiate hemolysis in G6PD deficient infants. Delivery trauma, asphyxia, delayed cord clamping, and prematurity are associated with an increased risk of hyperbilirubinemia in the infant.

3. **Infant's history.** Factors associated with the gastrointestinal tract may affect the bilirubin level. These factors include the history and frequency of breast-feeding. Poor breast-feeding may be associated with lethargy or abnormalities of the face and mouth, leading to a weak or absent suck. Poor caloric intake by the infant may increase the enterohepatic uptake of bilirubin. Vomiting may be an early presentation in sepsis, intestinal obstruction, or metabolic disorders, all of which may increase the risk of bilirubin load and toxicity. Delayed passage of meconium and infrequent stooling are seen with intestinal obstruction.

B. Symptoms and signs.
Clinical jaundice is visible when the serum bilirubin level approaches 5–7 mg/dL. Jaundice is often apparent first in the face, especially the nose, then descending to the torso and lower extremities as the degree of jaundice increases. Some infants appear "orange" in color because of the combination of "red" from a high neonatal hemoglobin concentration and "yellow" from the bilirubin. Jaundice can be demonstrated in some infants by pressing lightly on the skin with a finger. The yellow color is seen more easily in the "fingerprint" area than in the surrounding skin.

Besides confirming the presence of jaundice, physical examination may also be helpful in determining the cause of hyperbilirubinemia. Areas of bleeding such as cephalohematoma, petechiae, or ecchymoses indicate blood extravasation. Hepatosplenomegaly may signify hemolytic disease, liver disease, or infection. Physical signs of prematurity, intrauterine growth retardation (IUGR), and postmaturity may be helpful in elucidating a cause for hyperbilirubinemia. Plethora is seen with polycythemia, pallor with hemolytic disease, and large infants with maternal diabetes—all associated with hyperbilirubinemia. Omphalitis, chorioretinitis, microcephaly, and petechial and purpuric lesions all suggest infectious causes of increased serum bilirubin.

C. Kernicterus.
Three clinical phases occur in the neonate with kernicterus.

First phase: hypotonia, lethargy, poor feeding, vomiting, high-pitched cry, and seizures.

Second phase: spasticity, muscle rigidity, irritability, opisthotonus, hyperpyrexia, and irregular respirations.

Third phase: spasticity diminishes and those that survive have residual neurologic sequelae (particularly the athetoid form of cerebral palsy, high-frequency nerve deafness, mental retardation, and paralysis of upward gaze), and dental enamel dysplasia.

IV. Diagnosis

A. Laboratory studies.
Hyperbilirubinemia should be investigated whenever pathologic causes are suspected. The presence of a serum bilirubin level of 13 mg/dL or higher in any infant requires initial evaluation.

1. **Total and direct bilirubin**
   a. **Direct bilirubin** = conjugated.
   b. **Indirect bilirubin** = unconjugated.
   c. **Total minus direct** = indirect fraction.

2. **Hemoglobin or hematocrit.** Hemolytic anemia can be detected by a low hemoglobin or hematocrit associated with a high reticulocyte count and the presence of nucleated red blood cells. Polycythemia is defined as venous blood hematocrit greater than 65%. **Use of capillary blood samples may cause underestimation of venous bilirubin values when the latter exceeds 10 mg/dL.** This may be explained by the increased **light penetration and photoisomerization** of capillary unconjugated bilirubin and less penetration in the deeper venous vascular beds.

3. **Peripheral blood smear.** The peripheral blood smear aids in the diagnosis of hereditary spherocytosis and other red blood cell defects.

4. **Reticulocyte count.**

5. **Blood type and Rh status in mother and infant.** ABO and Rh incompatibility can be easily diagnosed by comparing infant and maternal blood types.

6. **Direct Coombs' test in the infant.** The direct Coombs test is usually positive in isoimmunization disorders.

7. **Measurement of serum albumin** may help to assess total bilirubin-binding sites available and whether there is a need for an albumin infusion.

8. **Other laboratory tests.** The white blood cell count or platelet count can be helpful in suggesting infection. The urine should be tested for reducing substances to rule out galactosemia if the infant is receiving a galactose-containing formula. If hemolysis is present in the absence of ABO or Rh incompatibility, hemoglobin electrophoresis, G6PD screening, or osmotic fragility testing may be required to diagnose red blood cell defects. Persistent jaundice (> 2 weeks of life) may call for further investigation into possible causes. Thyroid and liver function tests, blood and urine cultures, direct Coombs' test and a blood smear, and serum and urine amino acids and organic acid measurements may help in this search.

B. Radiologic studies.
Radiologic studies for suspected intestinal obstruction or blood extravasation into internal organs and ultrasonography of the head to document intraventricular or subdural hemorrhage may be indicated.

C. Transcutaneous bilirubinometry.
The transcutaneous bilirubinometer measures the degree of yellow color in the skin and subcutaneous tissues by selective wavelength reflection. Standardization has not been achieved, which makes correlation with serum bilirubin levels difficult to interpret.

V. Management.
Three methods of treatment are commonly used to decrease the level of unconjugated bilirubin: exchange transfusion, phototherapy, and phenobarbital therapy.

A. Phototherapy
1. **Indications.** Most infants with pathologic jaundice are treated initially with phototherapy. Phototherapy is usually started when it is

felt that bilirubin levels could enter the toxic range. The **exchange index** refers to the level of bilirubin at which exchange transfusion would be performed for a particular infant to decrease toxicity. **Phototherapy may be started when the bilirubin level is 5 mg/dL below the exchange index.** In very small premature infants or infants with hemolytic disease, phototherapy may be started earlier. The level of indirect bilirubin is used to determine if therapy is necessary. See Appendix I to determine when to begin phototherapy.

2. **Technique**
   a. **Light source and dosage.** The infant is exposed to light in the blue part of the spectrum (410–460 nm). The light causes a photochemical reaction in the skin **(photoisomerization)** that changes unconjugated bilirubin into photobilirubin, which is excreted by the liver into the bile. In addition, photooxidation produces bilirubin products that are excreted in the urine; however, this is not the mechanism by which phototherapy exerts its major effect. The effectiveness of phototherapy is related to the amount of **irradiation** to which the skin is exposed. Blue lamps are most efficient, but a combination of blue and cool white lamps is also effective; furthermore, this combination does not cause overheating and does not cause the infant to appear cyanotic. Bulbs must be changed regularly to ensure adequate irradiance. A radiometer may be used to measure the exact amount of irradiance delivered. The desired amount is 5–9 μW/cm^2/nm at 425–475 nm (Maisels, 1982). The infant's eyes are covered with opaque patches, because animal experiments have shown that retinal damage can occur from phototherapy. Phototherapy is usually given continuously, although irradiation for 15 minutes per hour may be just as effective. To maximize the surface area, exposed infants should be naked, except for eye patches.
   b. **Supportive management.** Small infants require use of a servocontrolled incubator to maintain body temperature. Fluid balance and temperature must be monitored closely. Tungsten bulbs have been shown to decrease insensible water loss. Phototherapy may be interrupted for feedings and parental visits. Once phototherapy is started, skin color cannot be used as a guide to the presence of hyperbilirubinemia. Since melanin and bilirubin both strongly absorb the blue end of the visible spectrum, increased pigmentation in the epidermis lowers the effectiveness of treatment. Moist skin is less translucent to light therapy and reduces its penetrance.

      Other simple measures to aid in elimination of bilirubin during phototherapy include maintenance of hydration status to ensure adequate urine output and encouragement of stooling to decrease enterohepatic uptake of bilirubin.

3. **Fluid management during phototherapy.** Use of phototherapy increases insensible water loss, and increased fluids must therefore be given to maintain fluid balance. For infants weighing less than 1500 g, increase fluid by 0.5 mL/kg/h; for those weighing more than 1500 g, increase by 1 mL/kg/h.

4. **Termination of phototherapy.** Phototherapy is stopped when the following criteria are met.
   a. The bilirubin level is low enough to eliminate the risk of kernicterus.
   b. The risk factors for the infant have resolved.
   c. The infant is old enough to handle the bilirubin load.

5. **Side effects.** No major toxicity has been associated with phototherapy thus far. Side effects include diarrhea, lactose intolerance,

hemolysis, skin burns, dehydration, skin rashes, and tanning. The eye shields may obstruct the airway and must be closely observed. If conjugated hyperbilirubinemia is present and phototherapy is used, a dark gray to brown discoloration may appear on the skin and in the serum and urine (**"bronze baby syndrome"**). The presence of cholestasis causes elevated copper and porphyrin serum concentrations. Copper porphyrins are sensitized by bilirubin and, under phototherapy, undergo photodestruction to degradation products, which are responsible for the brown discoloration of the skin.

B. Exchange transfusion. Exchange transfusion is used when the risk of kernicterus for a particular infant is significant. A double-volume exchange replaces 85% of the circulating red blood cells and decreases the bilirubin level to about half of the preexchange value. Besides removing bilirubin, an exchange transfusion can be used to correct anemia.

1. General guidelines. It appears that no specific level of bilirubin can be considered safe or dangerous for all infants, since variations in the permeability of the blood-brain barrier exist (Maisels, 1982). The current recommendation (from *Guidelines for Perinatal Care,* American Academy of Pediatrics and American College of Obstetrics and Gynecologists) is that both aggressive approaches (keeping bilirubin levels at 10 mg/dL with exchange transfusion) and conservative approaches (allowing bilirubin levels to approach 20 mg/dL before performing exchange transfusion) are acceptable for low birth weight infants. Furthermore, the guidelines state that in certain neonates, kernicterus is essentially not preventable. Bilirubin stains necrotic cells, and in the aftermath of hypoxic injury, cerebral staining cannot be attributed to the bilirubin toxicity alone (Rutledge, 1989).

2. Indications

a. Early exchange transfusions in term infants

(1) Cord bilirubin levels greater than 4.5 mg/dL and hemoglobin less than 11 g/dL.

(2) Bilirubin levels rising over 0.5 mg/dL/h.

(3) Bilirubin levels of 20 mg/dL or a likelihood that bilirubin levels will reach 20/mg/dL.

(4) Intrauterine exchange transfusions may reduce bilirubin levels in severe blood incompatibilities. Percutaneous umbilical blood sampling (PUBS) and amniotic fluid bilirubin levels are used to monitor fetal bilirubin levels. Umbilical vessel catheterization for intrauterine exchange transfusions is now routinely used at centers to reduce bilirubin levels in the fetus with severe blood incompatibility.

b. Indications for later exchange transfusion. If there is no hemolytic process or if hemolysis is mild, exchange transfusion is used to reduce toxicity from hyperbilirubinemia that is not being adequately controlled by phototherapy. In these cases, indications for exchange transfusion are:

(1) Unconjugated bilirubin levels approaching 20 mg/dL in a full-term infant with no evidence of acidosis or respiratory distress.

(2) Bilirubin levels of 10–15 mg/dL in a premature infant with hypoxia, acidosis, or respiratory distress.

(3) Clinical signs of kernicterus at any bilirubin level.

3. Factors that may affect the decision to perform exchange transfusion include the infant's maturity, birth weight, age, the rate of rise in bilirubin levels, and the presence of hypoxia, acidosis, sepsis, or hypoproteinemia.

4. Albumin infusions may be advocated if bilirubin levels are high, serum albumin levels are low, and blood for exchange transfusion is delayed. These infusions may prevent free bilirubin from crossing the blood-brain barrier by binding to the albumin.

5. **Technique.** See Chapter 21 and Appendix F.

C. **Phenobarbital therapy**

1. **Action.** Phenobarbital affects the metabolism of bilirubin by increasing the concentration of ligandin in liver cells, inducing production of glucuronyl transferase, and enhancing bilirubin excretion. Since it takes 3–7 days to become effective, phenobarbital is usually not helpful in treating unconjugated hyperbilirubinemia in the newborn infant.

2. **Indications**

   a. **Prenatal indications.** It may be useful to give phenobarbital 1–2 weeks before delivery to a mother whose fetus has **documented hemolytic disease** to aid in reducing bilirubin levels in the affected neonate.

   b. **Other indications.** Phenobarbital is also used to treat type II glucuronyl transferase deficiency and Gilbert's syndrome in the infant.

3. **Dosage.** See Chapter 75 for dosage and other pharmacologic information.

D. **Interruption of breast-feeding.** In full-term breast-fed infants with bilirubin levels approaching 20 mg/dL, interruption of breast-feeding for 25–48 hours may be helpful. If breast milk jaundice is the cause of hyperbilirubinemia, the bilirubin levels will fall with cessation of breast-feeding. When breast-feeding is restarted, the bilirubin levels will again rise but usually not as high as the previous levels. Kernicterus has not been reported in term infants with hyperbilirubinemia as a result of breast milk jaundice alone.

CONJUGATED (DIRECT) HYPERBILIRUBINEMIA

I. **Definition.** Conjugated hyperbilirubinemia is a sign of hepatobiliary dysfunction. It usually appears in the newborn infant during the first weeks of life, when the indirect hyperbilirubinemia of physiologic jaundice is receding. **When the direct bilirubin level exceeds 2.0 mg/dL and is greater than 10% of the total serum bilirubin, it is clinically significant.**

II. **Classification and pathophysiology.** Conjugated hyperbilirubinemia results from inability to remove bilirubin that has been conjugated from the body. This excretion process normally involves the liver, the biliary system, and the small intestine. **Cholestasis** refers to disorders of bile excretion that result in retention of conjugated bilirubin, bile acids, and other bile components. It is helpful diagnostically to separate extrahepatic biliary obstruction from intrahepatic biliary disease. Causes of conjugated hyperbilirubinemia are listed in Table 60–2.

A. **Intrahepatic biliary obstruction.** Most cases of conjugated hyperbilirubinemia in newborn infants are due to disorders involving the liver. These may be further divided into disorders of intrahepatic cholestasis with a paucity of bile ducts and disorders not associated with anatomic abnormalities.

1. **Intrahepatic cholestasis with paucity of bile ducts**

   a. Arteriohepatic dysplasia.

   b. Syndromatic paucity of interlobular bile ducts.

   c. Alagille's syndrome. Infants with this syndrome have cardiovascular anomalies, vertebral arch defects, and, in some cases, a characteristic facies. The disease is usually benign and is not associated with the development of cirrhosis.

2. **Intrahepatic cholestasis with normal bile ducts**

TABLE 60–2. CAUSES OF CONJUGATED HYPERBILIRUBINEMIA

EXTRAHEPATIC BILIARY OBSTRUCTION
Biliary atresia: polysplenia syndrome, trisomies 13 and 18
Choledochal cyst
Spontaneous rupture of bile duct
External compression of bile duct: enlarged lymph nodes, tumors, annular pancreas, hepatic cyst, pancreatic cyst
Others: hemangioendothelioma of pancreas or liver, inspissation of bile from cystic fibrosis, severe erythroblastosis fetalis

INTRAHEPATIC CHOLESTASIS WITH PAUCITY OF BILE DUCTS
Alagille's syndrome, nonsyndromatic form, biliary atresia

INTRAHEPATIC CHOLESTASIS WITH NORMAL BILE DUCTS
Infection
Viral: hepatitis B virus, non-A, non-B hepatitis virus, cytomegalovirus, herpes simplex virus, coxsackievirus, Epstein-Barr
    virus, adenovirus
Bacterial: *Treponema pallidum, Escherichia coli,* group B streptococcus, *Staphylococcus aureus, Listeria;* urinary tract infec-
    tion caused by *E coli* or *Proteus* sp, pneumococcus
Other: *Toxoplasma gondii*
Genetic disorders and inborn errors of metabolism: Dubin-Johnson syndrome, Rotor's syndrome, galactosemia, heredi-
    tary fructose intolerance, tyrosinemia, alpha₁-antitrypsin deficiency, Byler disease, recurrent cholestasis with lymph-
    edema, cerebrohepatorenal syndrome, congenital erythropoietic porphyria, Niemann–Pick disease, Menkes' kinky hair
    syndrome
Idiopathic neonatal hepatitis (giant cell hepatitis)

TPN-INDUCED CHOLESTASIS

a. **Total parenteral nutrition (TPN)** may cause cholestasis. The mean
   time from starting TPN to the onset of cholestasis is 42 days. The
   pathologic process is not clearly defined, although amino acids
   may directly influence bile flow. Although cirrhosis may occur,
   most abnormalities resolve once TPN is stopped.

b. **Idiopathic neonatal hepatitis (giant cell hepatitis)** may account
   for up to two-thirds of cases of cholestasis in newborn infants. It
   is a histologic diagnosis; there is no known explanation for the
   inflammatory process. If hepatitis is seen only on liver biopsy, the
   long-term prognosis is good. However, some infants may develop
   fulminant hepatic failure. Chronic liver disease develops in 20–
   40% of these infants (Gartner, 1983).

c. **Infection**

   (1) **Hepatitis.** Hepatitis B virus, rubella virus, non-A, non-B hepati-
       tis, cytomegalovirus, herpes simplex virus, coxsackievirus,
       Epstein-Barr virus, and adenovirus are all viruses that can
       cause hepatitis.

   (2) **Congenital syphilis or toxoplasmosis** may rarely present with
       cholestasis.

   (3) **Direct bacterial infection of the liver** may occur with over-
       whelming sepsis. Toxic cholestasis with no direct invasion of
       the liver by microorganisms may be seen with urinary tract
       infection.

d. **Genetic disorders and inborn errors of metabolism**

   (1) **Alpha₁-antitrypsin deficiency** is the most common genetic
       cause of cholestasis.

   (2) **Dubin-Johnson syndrome** is due to a genetic defect in the
       canalicular transport system. It is a relatively benign autoso-
       mal recessive disorder characterized by jaundice and dark
       gray pigmentation of the liver.

   (3) **Rotor's syndrome** is also inherited in an autosomal recessive
       manner but is believed to involve a defect in hepatic uptake
       and storage of organic anions, such as bilirubin. There is no
       abnormal pigmentation of the liver.

(4) **Inborn errors of metabolism** include galactosemia, hereditary fructose intolerance, and tyrosinemia.

(5) **Byler disease, or recurrent familial cholestasis,** is a progressive autosomal recessive disorder characterized by recurring episodes of cholestasis, each of which increases scarring of the liver and leads to cirrhosis and death. It has a high incidence in Amish populations.

(6) **Recurrent cholestasis with lymphedema** may be benign, or cirrhosis may develop.

(7) **Cerebrohepatorenal (Zellweger's) syndrome, Niemann–Pick disease, and Menkes' syndrome** may also be causes.

(8) **Congenital erythropoietic porphyria** presents with anemia and conjugated hyperbilirubinemia in the first month of life. Bullous skin lesions may form on areas exposed to light because of sensitization by accumulated porphyrins.

e. **Extracorporeal membrane oxygenation (ECMO).** Infants on ECMO support show an increase in prevalence and severity of cholestasis (Shneider, 1989).

B. Extrahepatic biliary obstruction

1. **Biliary atresia.** Biliary atresia accounts for 90% of cases of extrahepatic obstruction in neonates. The lumen of all or a portion of the bile duct system, including the gallbladder, is absent. The exact cause of this disease is unknown, but it does not appear to be an embryologic malformation. Recent evidence suggests a process of obliterative inflammation that begins in utero or after birth and then progresses.

2. **Choledochal cyst.** Choledochal cyst is dilatation of a portion of the extrahepatic biliary tree in association with complete or nearly complete segmental biliary obstruction.

3. **Spontaneous rupture of bile duct** may occur with ascites. The clinical presentation is identical to that of biliary atresia.

4. **External compression of the bile duct.** Enlarged lymph nodes, tumors, annular pancreas, or hepatic or pancreatic cysts can also cause extrahepatic biliary obstruction.

5. **Hemangioendothelioma** of the pancreas or liver may be a cause.

6. **Cystic fibrosis** may produce true inspissation of bile.

7. **Severe erythroblastosis fetalis** may present with elevated direct bilirubin levels at birth or later in the first week of life.

III. Clinical presentation

A. General findings

1. **Age.** Infants with conjugated hyperbilirubinemia tend to become jaundiced after 5–7 days of life. Alternatively, physiologic jaundice may not disappear as usual, and the infant may become increasingly icteric.

2. **Urine.** The urine is dark because of the presence of bilirubin.

3. **Stools** tend to be pale because bilirubin is not excreted into the small intestine. However, even in total extrahepatic obstruction, there may be some stool pigmentation. Persistence of acholic stools in an otherwise healthy infant is characteristic of biliary atresia or choledochal cyst.

4. **Liver and spleen.** The liver is usually enlarged. The spleen may also be enlarged, depending on the cause of cholestasis.

B. Specific findings in selected diseases

1. **Biliary atresia.** Hepatomegaly may be present but is not prominent. Splenomegaly is often absent. These infants are usually of normal birth weight, with good initial weight gain. Approximately 75% will

have acholic stools, which may not be seen until 1–2 weeks after the appearance of conjugated hyperbilirubinemia.

Biliary atresia may be isolated or may occur with a choledochal cyst. Ten percent of cases of biliary atresia are associated with malformations such as **polysplenia syndrome.** In these cases, the infants have multiple right-sided spleens, a midline liver, absent inferior vena cava, a preduodenal portal vein, and cardiac malformations. About half of infants with polysplenia have extrahepatic biliary atresia. Trisomies 13 and 18 are also associated with biliary atresia.

2. **Spontaneous rupture of the bile duct** may present with early ascites. There may be greenish-yellow discoloration of the scrotum, hernia sac, or umbilicus. Other causes of extrahepatic biliary obstruction have no specific clinical characteristics.

3. **Hepatitis.** Hepatomegaly may or may not be present, and acholic stools may be absent. There may be splenomegaly if a congenital infection such as cytomegalovirus is involved. Such infants may also have petechiae because of thrombocytopenia. Congenital infections may also cause microcephaly and chorioretinitis.

4. **Alagille's syndrome.** Facial features consisting of a prominent forehead, deep-set eyes, mild hypertelorism, a straight nose, and a small pointed chin may be seen. The face has a triangular shape. Butterfly vertebrae and cardiac anomalies such as peripheral pulmonic stenosis, pulmonary valve stenosis, and ventricular septal defect occur. An abnormality in the anterior chamber of the eye (posterior embryotoxon) may be seen.

5. **Metabolic disorders**
   a. **Galactosemia and hereditary fructose intolerance** are associated with failure to thrive, vomiting, diarrhea, hypoglycemia, hemolysis, hepatosplenomegaly, ascites, and bacterial sepsis. These disorders present only after sugar that cannot be metabolized is introduced into the diet.
   b. **Tyrosinemia** is characterized by failure to thrive, vomiting, diarrhea, hepatosplenomegaly, and rickets. The urine has an odor of decaying cabbage.
   c. **Alpha$_1$-antitrypsin deficiency.** The presentation is variable. There may be acholic stools and hepatomegaly, as in biliary atresia, or the symptoms may be very mild.

IV. **Diagnosis**
   A. **Laboratory studies**
      1. **Bilirubin levels (total and direct)** must be obtained.
      2. **Liver function tests.** SGOT (AST), SGPT (ALT), and alkaline phosphatase may be helpful in following the course of the disease.
      3. **Prothrombin time (PT) and partial thromboplastin time (PTT)** may be reliable indicators of liver function.
      4. **Gamma-glutamyl transpeptidase, 5'-nucleotidase, and serum bile acids** are also usually elevated in cholestasis. Once the diagnosis of cholestasis is made, measurement of these markers of cholestasis may not add any further information (Spivak, 1983).
      5. **A complete blood count and reticulocyte count** may be helpful if hepatitis is a possibility, since hemolysis may be found.
      6. **Serum cholesterol, triglycerides, and albumin levels.** Triglyceride and cholesterol levels may aid in nutritional management. Albumin is a long-term indicator of hepatic function.
      7. **Ammonia levels** should be checked if liver failure is suspected.
      8. **Serum glucose levels** should be checked if the infant appears ill.

9. **Urine testing for reducing substances** is a simple screening test that should always be performed to detect for metabolic disease.
10. **TORCH titers.** The use of TORCH titers (see p 339) should be guided by the clinical presentation, keeping in mind that cytomegalovirus infection may be asymptomatic and congenital syphilis is treatable.
11. **Other tests.** More specific tests are indicated in the investigation of the specific causes of conjugated hyperbilirubinemia.
    a. **Hepatitis.** The maternal HBsAg status should be known, and the infant should also be tested. Cytomegalovirus IgM and IgG, Venereal Disease Research Laboratory (VDRL), and IgM-specific titers for herpes simplex, rubella, and toxoplasmosis may be useful in some cases.
    b. **Sepsis.** If bacterial sepsis or urinary tract infection is suspected, appropriate cultures should be obtained.
    c. **Metabolic disorders**
        (1) **Galactosemia and hereditary fructose intolerance.** The urine should be tested for nonglucose-reducing substances. Enzymes involved in these disorders can also be assayed in the blood.
        (2) **Tyrosinemia.** High concentrations of tyrosine and methionine, and their metabolic derivatives, will be seen in the urine.
        (3) **Alpha$_1$-antitrypsin deficiency.** The serum alpha$_1$-antitrypsin level can be measured.
        (4) **Cystic fibrosis.** A sweat test may diagnose cystic fibrosis.
B. **Radiologic studies.** Diagnosis of biliary atresia and other forms of extrahepatic biliary obstruction by 8 weeks of age is required to prevent progression of the disease.
    1. **Ultrasonography** is the method of choice, especially because it is noninvasive and can be done at the bedside. It can be used to view the liver parenchyma and to diagnose dilatation of the biliary tree. In extrahepatic obstruction, half of the infants will have dilated proximal ducts within the liver. Choledochal cysts are seen. Inability to identify the gallbladder on ultrasonography may be due to obliteration of its lumen in biliary atresia. However, the presence of a gallbladder does not rule out biliary atresia.
    2. **Hepatobiliary imaging (scintigraphy).** Contrast agents are taken up by the liver and excreted into the bile. HIDA (hepatobiliary iminodiacetic acid), EHIDA (ethyl hepatobiliary iminodiacetic acid), and PIPIDA (*p*-isopropylacetanilido iminodiacetic acid) are technetium-labeled and provide a clear image of the biliary tree after intravenous injection. Neonatal hepatitis, hyperalimentation, and septo-optic dysplasia are reported causes of absent gastrointestinal contrast excretion and must be considered in the diagnosis or exclusion of biliary atresia. Administration of phenobarbital, 5 mg/kg/d for 5 days, in conjunction with hepatobiliary scanning, may be helpful in distinguishing infants who do not have biliary atresia, since excretion of the contrast medium may improve after this maneuver.
C. **Other studies**
    1. **Intubation of the duodenum** for collection of a 24-hour sample of fluid may be helpful. In this procedure an 8F radiopaque feeding tube is positioned between the second and third portions of the duodenum by fluoroscopy. Fluid is withdrawn from the tube every 2 hours and visually examined for the presence of bile pigment. If bile pigment is not observed in 24 hours, biliary atresia is a strong possibility. The presence of any amount of bile pigment rules out extrahepatic biliary atresia. This study may be repeated after a course of phenobarbital (Maisels, 1982).

2. **Percutaneous liver biopsy,** using a Menghini-type suction needle, is a safe procedure in experienced hands (Spivak, 1983). Biopsy findings must be correlated with clinical and laboratory date. Repeat biopsies are sometimes indicated.

3. **Exploratory laparotomy** is sometimes indicated to correct biliary atresia as soon as possible if the above tests are not diagnostic.

V. Management

A. Medical management

1. **General plan.** In cholestatic jaundice, promotion of bile flow and prevention of malnutrition, vitamin deficiencies, and bleeding are goals of treatment.

2. **Phenobarbital and cholestyramine** will promote bile flow and decrease serum bilirubin and bile salt levels. Cholestyramine is a non-absorbable anion exchange resin that irreversibly binds salts in the intestine. This leads to increased fecal excretion of bile salts and increased hepatic synthesis of bile salts from cholesterol, which may lower serum cholesterol levels. Therapy with phenobarbital and cholestyramine is helpful in Alagille's syndrome and the nonsyndromic form of paucity of the bile ducts. See Chapter 75 for dosages and other pharmacologic information.

B. Dietary management

1. **Medium-chain triglycerides.** Long-chain triglycerides are poorly absorbed in the absence of sufficient bile salts. Therefore, infants with cholestasis often require a diet that includes medium-chain triglycerides, which can be absorbed without the action of bile salts. Formulas containing medium-chain triglycerides include Portagen and Pregestimil.

2. **Vitamin supplementation.** Fat malabsorption will also interfere with maintenance of adequate levels of fat-soluble vitamins in these infants. Supplementation of vitamins A, D, E, and K is suggested. Extra vitamin K supplementation may be necessary if a bleeding tendency develops.

3. **Dietary restrictions.** Removal of galactose plus lactose and fructose plus sucrose may prevent the development of cirrhosis and other manifestations of galactosemia and hereditary fructose intolerance, respectively. Dietary restrictions may also be used to treat tyrosinemia but usually are less successful. Most other metabolic causes of cholestatic jaundice have no specific therapy.

C. Surgical management

1. **Laparotomy with biopsy.** If extrahepatic biliary obstruction is strongly suspected after completion of an appropriate evaluation, exploratory laparotomy should be performed with operative cholangiography and liver biopsy. Other causes of extrahepatic biliary obstruction that may be diagnosed and treated during exploratory laparotomy include choledochal cyst, spontaneous rupture of the bile duct, lymph node enlargement, tumors, annular pancreas, pancreatic and hepatic cysts, and hemangioendothelioma of the pancreas or liver. Inspissated bile syndrome caused by cystic fibrosis also requires surgical removal of tenacious bile from the bile ducts.

2. **Kasai procedure.** Attempts should be made to establish biliary drainage with the use of hepatic portoenterostomy (Kasai procedure). Optimal results are obtained before 8 weeks of age. Even if the Kasai procedure is successful, however, most infants will eventually progress to cirrhosis and death as a result of the ongoing intrahepatic inflammatory sclerosing process. The procedure is now used as a bridge to transplantation.

3. **Liver transplantation.** When end-stage liver disease is inevitable,

liver transplantation may be performed. Currently, 50–70% of infants with liver transplants are alive 1 year after operation (Gartner, 1983).

D. Other treatments
   1. Infectious diseases. Some of the infectious causes of hepatitis such as hepatitis B virus, herpes simplex virus, congenital syphilis, and bacterial infections have specific therapeutic regimens. Most other forms of infectious hepatitis resolve with no specific therapy.
   2. Total parenteral nutrition (TPN)–induced conjugated hyperbilirubinemia will usually resolve once TPN is stopped. Occasionally, infants will die of chronic liver disease while being maintained in TPN. The decision to continue TPN in an infant with cholestasis must be carefully considered.

REFERENCES

Auerbach KG, Gartner LM: Breastfeeding and Human milk: Their association with jaundice in the neonate. *Clin Perinatol* 1987;**14(1)**:89.

Broderson R: Bilirubin transport in the newborn infant reviewed with relation to kernicterus. *J Pediatr* 1980;**96**:349.

Ferry GD et al: Guide to early diagnosis of biliary obstruction in infancy: Review of 143 cases. *Clin Pediatr* 1985;**24**:305.

Gartner L: Cholestasis of the newborn. *Pediatr Rev* 1983;**5**:163.

Gollan JL, Knapp AB: Bilirubin metabolism and congenital jaundice. *Hosp Pract* 1985;**20**:83.

Khoury et al: Recurrence risk of neonatal hyperbilirubinemia in siblings. *Am J Dis Child* 1988;**142**:1065.

Lascari AD: "Early" breastfeeding jaundice: Clinical significance. *J Pediatr* 1986;**108(1)**:156.

Maisels MJ: Jaundice in the newborn. *Pediatr Rev* 1982;**3**:305.

Perlman M, Frank J: Bilirubin beyond the blood brain barrier. *Pediatrics* 1988;**81(2)**:304.

Reimche LD et al: Chloral hydrate sedation in neonates and infants: Clinical and pharmacologic considerations. *Dev Pharmacol Ther* 1981;**12**:57.

Rubaltelli FF et al: Bronze baby syndrome: New insights on bilirubin photosensitization of copper-porphyrins. Pages 265–275 in: *Neonatal Jaundice. New Trends in Phototherapy.* Rubaltelli FF, Jori G (editors). Plenum, 1983.

Salamy A, Eldredge L, Tooley WA: Neonatal status and hearing loss in high-risk infants. *J Pediatr* 1989;**114(5)**:847.

Schneider AP: Breast milk jaundice in the newborn. *JAMA* 1986;**255**:3270.

Schneider B et al: Cholestasis in infants supported with extracorporeal membrane oxygenation *J Pediatr* 1988;**115(3)**:462.

Sirota L et al: Breast milk jaundice in preterm infants. *Clin Pediatr* 1988;**27(4)**:195.

Spivak W, Grand RJ: General configuration of cholestasis in the newborn. *J Pediatr Gastroenterol Nutr* 1983;**2**:381.

Stevenson DK, Rodgers PA, Vreman HJ: Use of metalloporphyrins for the chemoprevention of neonatal jaundice. *Am J Dis Child* 1989;**143**:353.

Watchko JF, Oski FA: Bilirubin 20 mg/dL = vigintiphobia. *Pediatrics* 1983;**71**:660.

61 Inborn Errors of Metabolism With Acute Neonatal Onset

The concept of an inborn error of metabolism was first advanced by Garrod in 1908 to explain the clinical findings in alkaptonuria. That suggestion eventually evolved into the one gene–one enzyme hypothesis that united the fields of biochemistry and genetics. Since Garrod's time, a discrete error of metabolism has been identified as the underlying cause of a host of diseases that differ in severity, symptomatology, and time of onset.

I. **Classification.** Although phenotypic variability does not allow all diseases to be placed unambiguously into one category, it is still conceptually helpful to divide inborn errors of metabolism into the following 3 groups based on the time of presentation.

A. **Neonatal onset.** Diseases of neonatal onset are discussed in this chapter (Table 61–1). Five cardinal points to remember are:

1. Although these diseases are rare individually, collectively they contribute significantly to neonatal mortality and morbidity.

2. Many of these diseases are likely to be fatal if untreated and may cause permanent and severe sequelae (eg, central nervous system) if recognized and treated late.

3. Rapid laboratory diagnosis and effective therapy are available for many of these disorders.

4. Early diagnosis and treatment are essential for normal long-term neurologic development.

5. **Early diagnosis requires that the possibility of metabolic disease be considered in every sick neonate.**

B. **Insidious onset during infancy or childhood.** Although some metabolic diseases are fatal and have no treatment (eg, Tay-Sachs disease), most are not. Illness may result unless the disorders are diagnosed and treated (eg, phenylketonuria, hypothyroidism, partial ornithine transcarbamylase deficiency in females). Most newborn screening tests detect diseases in this category.

C. **Onset of symptoms in late childhood, adolescence, or adulthood.** This category includes some of the hyperlipidemias.

II. **Incidence.** The cumulative incidence of all inborn errors of metabolism is probably close to 1:500 live births. It has been conservatively estimated that 10% of inborn errors present in the neonatal period (ie, with an incidence of 1:5000 live births). Equivalently, it has also been suggested that metabolic disorders account for approximately 20% of acute disease in full-term neonates born without obvious risk factors (eg, prolonged rupture of maternal membranes).

III. **Pathophysiology.** Symptoms of metabolic disease usually result from the **abnormal accumulation of one or more toxic metabolites** (eg, ammonium in urea cycle disorders, organic acids in the organic acidemias, galactose-1-phosphate and galactitol in galactosemia). Less frequently, symptoms occur secondary to **underproduction of an essential metabolite** (eg, glucose in the glycogen storage diseases, adenosine triphosphate (ATP) in disorders of pyruvate metabolism and the respiratory electron transport chain). Occasionally, both mechanisms are operative; for example, in adrenogenital syndrome, hyponatremia, hyperkalemia, and vomiting arise

TABLE 61–1. LABORATORY SELECTED METABOLIC DISEASES PRESENTING IN THE NEWBORN PERIOD

Disorders of Carbohydrate Metabolism
Galactosemia
Fructose-1,6-diphosphatase deficiency
Glycogen storage diseases (types IA, IB, II, III)
Hereditary fructose intolerance

Disorders of Amino Acid Metabolism
Maple syrup urine disease (MSUD)
Nonketotic hyperglycinemia
Hereditary tyrosinemia
Pyroglutamic acidemia (5-oxoprolinuria)
Periodic hyperlysinemia
Hyperornithinemia-hyperammonemia-homocitrullinemia syndrome
Lysinuric protein intolerance

Disorders of Organic Acid Metabolism
Isovaleric acidemia
Propionic acidemia (ketotic hyperglycinemia)
Methylmalonic acidemia
Multiple carboxylase deficiency
Glutaric acidemia, type II (multiple acyl-CoA dehydrogenase deficiencies)
3-Methyl crotonyl-CoA carboxylase deficiency

Disorders of Pyruvate Metabolism and the Electron Transport Chain
Pyruvate carboxylase deficiency
Pyruvate dehydrogenase deficiency
Electron transport chain deficiencies

Disorders of Urea Synthesis
Carbamyl phosphate synthetase (CPS) deficiency
Ornithine transcarbamylase (OTC) deficiency
Argininosuccinate synthetase (AS) deficiency (citrullinemia)
Argininosuccinate lyase (AL) deficiency
Arginase deficiency
N-Acetylglutamate synthetase (NAGS) deficiency
Transient hyperammonemia of the newborn (THAN)

Lysosomal Storage Disorders
GM_1 gangliosidosis, type I (beta-galactosidase deficiency)
Gaucher's disease (glucocerebrosidase deficiency)
Niemann-Pick disease, types A and B (sphingomyelinase deficiency)
Wolman disease (acid lipase deficiency)
Mucopolysaccharidosis, type VII (beta-glucuronidase deficiency)
I-cell disease (mucolipidosis, type II)
Sialidosis, type II (neuraminidase deficiency)

Peroxisomal Disorders
Zellweger syndrome
Neonatal adrenoleukodystrophy

Miscellaneous Disorders
Adrenogenital syndrome (21-hydroxylase deficiency)
Pyridoxine-responsive seizures
Alpha$_1$-antitrypsin deficiency
Disorders of bilirubin metabolism (eg, Crigler-Najjar syndrome)
Fatty acyl-CoA dehydrogenase deficiencies (short chain, medium chain, and long chain)

---

from a deficiency of cortisol synthesis, while excessive production of adrenal androgens causes the characteristic physical stigmata (ambiguous genitalia) in the female infant. Finally, storage diseases, characterized by an inability to degrade some product(s) of cellular metabolism, may present diversely with hydrops fetalis (Niemann-Pick disease, Gaucher's disease), myocardial dysfunction (glycogen storage disease [type II] [Pompe's disease]), hepatosplenomegaly and ascites (sialadosis), or dysmorphic facies (gangliosidosis GM_1, the mucopolysaccharidoses, peroxisomal disorders).

TABLE 61-2. SIGNS AND SYMPTOMS OF NEONATAL METABOLIC DISEASE

Central nervous system
Lethargy, poor sucking
Irritability
Hypo- or hypertonicity
Seizures
Coma, encephalopathy

Gastrointestinal system
Poor feeding
Vomiting
Diarrhea

Cardiopulmonary system
Apnea
Tachypnea
Respiratory distress
Cardiomegaly
Nonimmune hydrops fetalis

Hepatic disorders
Jaundice
Coagulopathy
Hepatomegaly, hepatosplenomegaly

Miscellaneous signs
Abnormal odor of skin or urine
Coarse or dysmorphic facies
Cataracts, retinopathy
Macroglossia
Abnormal hair

IV. Clinical presentation

A. High-risk infant. An inborn error of metabolism should be strongly suspected under the following circumstances.

1. Presence of any of the signs and symptoms listed in Table 61-2. A high index of suspicion for metabolic disease is necessary because of the relative nonspecificity of these symptoms. Metabolic disease should be at the top of the differential diagnosis if family history reveals:
   a. Unexplained or suspicious neonatal deaths (eg, previous siblings, males from the maternal side of the family).
   b. Consanguinity.
2. Entertainment of any of the diagnoses in Table 61-3, especially when the available evidence does not support the presumed diagnosis. A diagnosis of sepsis supported by positive cultures does not exclude metabolic disease; for instance, *E coli* sepsis frequently complicates galactosemia.
3. Failure of the infant to improve with the usual therapy, or worsening neurologic status of unknown cause.
4. Presence of any of the laboratory findings listed in Table 61-4.

B. Symptoms and signs (Table 61-2)

TABLE 61-3. MISDIAGNOSIS OF METABOLIC DISEASE IN THE NEWBORN INFANT

Sepsis (bacterial or viral)
Asphyxia
Gastrointestinal tract obstruction
Hepatic failure, hepatitis
Central nervous system catastrophe
Persistent pulmonary hypertension
Myocardiopathy

TABLE 61—4. LABORATORY FINDINGS SUGGESTIVE OF METABOLIC DISEASE

	Galactosemia	Fructose-1,6-diphosphatase Deficiency	Glycogen storage Disease[a]	Maple Syrup Urine Disease	Nonketotic Hyperglycinemia[b]	Glutaric Acidemia, Type II[c]	Pyroglutamic Acidemia	Organic Acidemias	Disorders of Pyruvate[c] Metabolism	Disorders of Urea Synthesis	Transient Hyperammonemia of the Newborn
Hypoglycemia	+	+	+	±	−	±	−	±	±	−	−
Metabolic acidosis with or without elevated anion gap	+	+	+	+	−	±	+	+	+	−	±
Respiratory alkalosis	−	−	−	−	−	±	−	−	−	+	±
Hyperammonemia	−	−	−	N−1+	−	N−1+	−	N−3+	N−1+	1−3+	2−4+
Hyperlactatemia	−	−	±	−	−	±	−	N−1+	1−2+	−	±
Direct hyperbilirubinemia	↑	−	−	−	−	−	−	−	−	−	−
Urine											
Clinitest: +	+	+	+	−	−	−	−	−	±	−	−
Acetest + or Ketostix +	−	±	±	+	−	−	−	+	±	−	−
DNPH	−	−	−	+	−	−	−	±	−	−	−
Abnormal odor or color	−	−	−	+[d]	−	+[e]	−	+[e,f]	−	−	−
Neutropenia or thrombocytopenia	−	−	−	−	−	−	−	±	−	−	−

N = Normal
[a] Hypercholesterolemia. Hypertriglyceridemia. hyperuricemia.
[b] Elevated plasma glycine only metabolic abnormality.
[c] Dysmorphic features.
[d] Maple syrup or burnt sugar.
[e] Sweaty feet (isovaleric acidemia).
[f] Cat urine (3 methyl crotonyl CoA carboxylase deficiency).

1. **Time of onset.** Inborn errors of metabolism usually present in the newborn infant after a symptom-free period of 1 to several days after delivery. The onset of symptoms and their progression often correlate with introduction and advancement of enteral feedings. Disorders of pyruvate metabolism and the electron transport chain and the poorly understood transient hyperammonemia of the newborn (THAN) may present at delivery or shortly afterward with respiratory distress and metabolic (lactic) acidosis; certain storage disorders may present in utero or at birth with ascites or hydrops fetalis.

2. **Misdiagnosis.** Metabolic disease can masquerade as any of the neonatal emergencies listed in Table 61–3. Unfortunately, the correct diagnosis is often made only after a second sibling presents with an identical clinical picture. Undoubtedly, incorrect diagnosis has led to underestimation of the true incidence of some metabolic errors.

3. **Term vs preterm infants.** When present, metabolic disease is more likely to be found in term infants (THAN is only exception). More important, however, a sick term infant is much more likely than an ill preterm infant to have metabolic disease, because preterm infants are at greater risk for a wide variety of other diseases.

V. **Diagnosis**

A. **Prenatal studies (if known proband exists).** Prenatal diagnosis is possible for an increasing number of inborn errors of metabolism. For certain metabolic diseases, prenatal identification will ensure appropriate treatment from the time of birth and thereby optimize outcome. For disorders for which no effective treatment exists, parents are thus enabled to make an informed decision regarding continuation of pregnancy.

1. **Amniocentesis.** Amniocentesis has been used to obtain amniotic fluid or amniocytes for chemical or enzyme activity analysis, respectively. Not all disorders can be diagnosed this easily, however. In ornithine transcarbamylase (OTC) deficiency, for instance, there are no abnormal metabolites in the amniotic fluid and the OTC enzyme is not expressed by amniocytes. Diagnosis has been made by analysis of OTC activity in fetal liver biopsy specimens.

2. **Chorionic villus biopsy and DNA analysis.** More recently, biopsy of chorionic villi with linkage analysis of restriction fragment length polymorphisms has made prenatal diagnosis of OTC deficiency possible when DNA of the mother and a known proband can be similarly analyzed. Application of new genetic techniques is rapidly increasing the number of disorders for which prenatal diagnosis is possible.

B. **Sign and symptom complexes that suggest classes of metabolic disease**

1. **Neurologic signs and symptoms predominate.** A clinical presentation characterized by the insidious onset of lethargy, hypotonia, poor feeding and vomiting after the first day of life with progression to frank coma (with or without seizures) suggests disorders of urea synthesis, the organic acidemias, disorders of amino-acid metabolism, and fructose-1,6-diphosphatase deficiency. Seizures without abnormalities of tone may be a clue to nonketotic hyperglycinemia, pyridoxine-responsive seizures, fatty acyl CoA dehydrogenase deficiencies, and some of the rarer disorders of amino-acid metabolism (periodic hyperlysinemia, lysinuric protein intolerance, and the hyperornithinemia-hyperammonemia-homocitrullinemia [HHH] syndrome). Peroxisomal disorders may present with seizures accompanied by significant tone abnormalities (usu-

ally hypotonia); a degenerative retinopathy may be present as well. Respiratory alkalosis in conjunction with altered consciousness is often found in disorders of urea synthesis. Structural brain abnormalities (cortical cysts, agenesis of the corpus callosum) have been reported in pyruvate dehydrogenase deficiency.

2. **Liver disease (direct hyperbilirubinemia, coagulopathy, and/or hepatitis)** is prominent in galactosemia, hereditary fructose intolerance, alpha$_1$-antitrypsin deficiency, hereditary tyrosinemia.

3. **Nonimmune hydrops fetalis.** Storage disorders account for as many as 10% of cases of nonimmune hydrops. Leading candidates are Niemann-Pick disease and Gaucher's disease.

4. **Cardiomegaly.** Consider glycogen storage disease type II (Pompe's disease), long-chain fatty acyl CoA dehydrogenase deficiency.

5. **Coarse facial features and hepatosplenomegaly.** Consider GM$_1$-gangliosidosis (beta-galactosidase deficiency), mucopolysaccharidosis type VII (beta-glucuronidase deficiency), I-cell disease (mucolipidosis, type II), and sialidosis, type II. (**Note:** more familiar storage disorders [eg, Hurler's syndrome] generally present later than the neonatal period with some combination of coarse features, hepatosplenomegaly, failure to thrive, loss of developmental milestones, or bone and/or joint abnormalities.)

6. **Dysmorphology (eg, epicanthal folds, Brushfield's spots, large fontanelles, simian creases, renal cysts).** Relatively recent insights have blurred the traditional distinction between inborn errors of metabolism and genetic dysmorphology syndromes. Examples are glutaric acidemia (type II) and peroxisomal disorders such as Zellweger's syndrome (cerebrohepatorenal syndrome) and neonatal adrenoleukodystrophy.

7. **Abnormal odor.** An odor of maple syrup or burnt sugar suggests maple syrup urine disease. An odor of sweaty feet is found in isovaleric acidemia and glutaric acidemia, type II. A cat urine odor is associated with multiple carboxylase deficiency and 3-methylcrotonyl CoA carboxylase deficiency.

8. **Hypoglycemia and metabolic acidosis** *without* **ketonuria** should suggest the medium- and long-chain fatty acyl-CoA dehydrogenase deficiencies and HMG CoA lyase deficiency (an organic acidemia).

C. **Laboratory testing**
1. **Prenatal suspicion of disease.** Occasionally, a high-risk mother may decline prenatal diagnosis, in which case the neonate should be treated prophylactically (see below). Some disorders can be ruled in or out by appropriate tests on cord blood or neonatal serum, or both, collected during the first 24 hours of life. Diagnosis of other disorders may require specific enzymatic analyses using red cells or cultured fibroblasts or hepatocytes.

2. **If signs and symptoms suggest metabolic disease.** At a minimum, the following **metabolic battery of tests** should be performed (Table 61–5).
   a. Urine nonglucose-reducing substances (Clinitest).
   b. Plasma ammonium level.
   c. Urine ketones (Acetest, Ketostix).
   d. Serum electrolytes and pH.
   e. Serum glucose level.
   f. Urine dinitrophenyldrazine (DNPH).
   g. Complete blood count and smear.
   h. Serum lactate and pyruvate levels if metabolic acidosis and elevated anion gap are not explained by ketonuria or ketonemia.

D. **Diagnostic algorithms** (Figs 61–1 and 61–2). If metabolic disease is strongly suspected but none of the simple screening tests listed

TABLE 61-5. PROCEDURES FOR URINE TESTS HELPFUL IN THE DIAGNOSIS OF METABOLIC DISEASE

Clinitest (Ames)
1. Mix 5 drops of urine and 10 drops of water in a clean test tube. Add 1 tablet. Fifteen seconds after the end of the reaction, gently shake the test tube.
2. Compare the color after the reaction with the chart supplied. A negative test gives a blue color. Tests that produce green, brown, yellow, or red solutions may indicate the presence of carbohydrate reducing substances (eg, glucose, galactose), amino acids, or a variety of exogenous drugs.

Acetest (Ames)
1. Place 1 tablet on a clean white filter paper. Apply 1 drop of urine; wait 30 seconds.
2. Test is positive only if the tablet turns purple. Result is coded as small, moderate, or large amount of ketones by comparison to a color chart.

Ketostix (Ames)
1. Dip the reagent strip into urine.
2. Compare the color to the chart on the bottle.

Dinitrophenylhydrazine (DNPH)
1. Mix 10 drops of reagent (refrigerated solution of 100 mg 2,4-dinitrophenylhydrazine in 100 mL of 2-N HCl) with 1 mL of urine.
2. Yellow-white precipitates indicate the presence of ketoacids. This test is usually highly positive with maple syrup urine disease, though it may be positive with glycogen storage disease, fructose-1,6-diphosphatase deficiency, organic acidemias, phenylketonuria, or tyrosinemia.

above in **C.2** are abnormal, detailed analyses of plasma and urine for amino acids, organic acids, carnitine, and/or very long-chain fatty acids should be performed (guided by the class of metabolic disease suspected), using quantitative column chromatography or gas chromatography–mass spectrometry as appropriate (Table 61-6). These tests are available at special regional metabolic or genetic centers. It is important to be aware that in some disorders, metabolic abnormalities resolve if supportive care eliminates offending compounds or precursors, or both, from the diet. Tests drawn during such a period of metabolic normalcy will be falsely reassuring. For example, urine-reducing substances will become negative within hours of withholding enteral feeds and instituting intravenous dextrose.

E. **Postmortem studies**
1. **Indications.** Two situations can prompt immediate postmortem harvesting of skin fibroblasts and hepatocytes for enzyme and DNA analysis.
   a. **Rapid progression of disease,** that is, the fulminant nature of the disease did not allow an unambiguous antemortem diagnosis.
   b. **Metabolic disease was strongly suspected,** but available antemortem testing could not define a specific defect (common in disorders of pyruvate metabolism and the electron transport chain or in suspected storage diseases).
2. **Specific steps to take if death occurs or is likely to occur before diagnosis**
   a. Collect 30 mL urine and freeze at $-20\,°C$ in 5-10-mL aliquots.
   b. Collect 20–25 mL whole blood. Separate plasma from cells by centrifugation. Freeze plasma in 2 mL aliquots at $-20\,°C$. Refrigerate red cell fraction at $4\,°C$ for possible enzyme analysis.
   c. Obtain sample of cerebrospinal fluid. Freeze at $-20\,°C$.
   d. Obtain skin biopsy specimen (prepare with alcohol only, not iodine) and transport immediately at $25-37\,°C$ to tissue culture laboratory, preferably in tissue culture medium (but D5NS will suffice), for fibroblast culture and subsequent enzyme/DNA analysis.
   e. Obtain liver sample as soon as possible after death (by percuta-

FIGURE 61-1. Algorithm for initial diagnosis of metabolic disease with acute neonatal onset.

FIGURE 61-2. Algorithm for differential diagnosis of hyperammonemia.

AL = Argininosuccinate lyase deficiency
AS = Argininosuccinate synthetase deficiency (citrullinemia)
CPS = Carbamyl phosphate synthetase deficiency
HHH = Hyperornithemia, hyperammonemia, homocitrullinemia
        syndrome
LPI = Lysinuric protein intolerance
NAGS = N-Acetylglutamate synthetase deficiency
OTC = Ornithine transcarbamylase deficiency

TABLE 61-6. ANALYSIS OF AMINO AND ORGANIC ACIDS IN PLASMA AND URINE

	Organic Acids	Amino Acids
Isovaleric acidemia	Isovalerylglycine 3-Hydroxyisovalerate	Normal
Propionic acidemia	3-Hydroxypropionate Methylcitrate	Elevated glycine
Methylmalonic acidemia	Methylmalonate	Elevated glycine
Multiple carboxylase deficiency	3-Methylcrotonyl 3-Hydroxyisovalerate 3-Hydroxypropionate	
Glutaric acidemia, type II	Glutaric acid 2-Hydroxyglutarate Ethylmalonate 2-Hydroxyisovalerate	Elevated lysine
5-Oxoprolinuria (pyroglutamic acidemia)	Pyroglutamate	Normal or elevated oxoproline
Nonketotic hyperglycinemia	Normal	Elevated glycine

neous biopsy if autopsy is delayed) and freeze the unfixed specimen at −20 °C for later enzyme/DNA analysis and light/electron microscopy.

   f. Obtain biopsy samples of other organs if clinically indicated (eg, heart, skeletal muscle, brain) and freeze at −20 °C.

   g. Complete autopsy.

VI. Management. For optimal outcome in disorders for which treatment is available, **early consideration of the diagnosis of metabolic disease is critical.**

  A. General supportive care. Take appropriate measures to correct dehydration and restore normal electrolytes and acid-base balance. Assisted ventilation and aggressive therapy with antibiotics are often necessary. (***Note:*** Galactosemia is associated with an increased risk of *E coli* sepsis.)

  B. Elimination of toxic metabolites. Hemodialysis and peritoneal dialysis will remove compounds distributed throughout the total body water compartment. **Hemodialysis** is the more effective method and clears metabolites such as ammonium, amino acids, and ketoacids up to 10 times more rapidly than peritoneal dialysis. If hemodialysis is not immediately available, **peritoneal dialysis** should be initiated. **Exchange transfusion** is much less effective. Optimal therapy may require transport of the infant to a center with appropriate facilities.

  C. Nutritional therapy

    1. Restrict offending compounds and metabolic precursors.

      a. Protein restriction. In some disorders, protein must be severely restricted because it causes accumulation of toxic products (ammonium in disorders of ureagenesis; branched-chain amino acids in maple syrup urine disease; organic acids in disorders of organic acid metabolism).

      b. Carbohydrate modification. In galactosemia, elimination of lactose (a glucose-galactose disaccharide) is essential; in hereditary fructose intolerance, sources of fructose must be eliminated (eg, certain soy formulas, fruits, juices).

    2. Provide adequate calories.

      a. Start parenteral nutrition. In these disorders, intravenous glucose and lipid should provide sufficient calories (120 kcal/kg/d) to shut down tissue catabolism.

      b. Use specialized enteral formula. Dietary therapy should continue after metabolic and neurologic stabilization with the appropriate formula (eg, a nongalactose preparation such as

Isomil, ProSobee, or Nutramigen for galactosemia; MSUD diet powder for maple syrup urine disease; other special formulas for the organic acidemias)

3. **Add minimal essential amounts of offending compound or precursor after symptoms have resolved and metabolic profile has normalized.** For example, this measure would entail providing no more than 75–150 mg leucine/kg/d to an infant with isovaleric acidemia.

4. **High-dose vitamin therapy.** Some disorders have multiple phenotypes. Occasionally, the pathophysiology results from an inability to bind or utilize vitamin cofactors in enzymatic reactions. In these cases, high-dose therapy may normalize metabolism by a mass action effect.

   a. **Thiamine,** 10 mg/d intramuscularly, for maple syrup urine disease.

   b. **Biotin,** 10 mg/d intramuscularly, for isovaleric acidemia, propionic acidemia or multiple carboxylase deficiency.

   c. **Hydroxycobalamin,** 2 mg/d intramuscularly, for methylmalonic acidemia.

   d. **Combination therapy.** Disorders of pyruvate metabolism require combination therapy: thiamine, 10 mg/d intramuscularly; biotin, 10 mg/d intramuscularly; riboflavin, 50 mg/d intramuscularly; and lipoamide, 20 mg/d intramuscularly.

5. L-**Carnitine supplementation** may be useful in the organic acidemias and in the acyl-CoA dehydrogenase disorders that are characterized by a secondary carnitine deficiency.

D. **Metabolic therapies.** New therapies have sought to activate alternative excretory pathways and provide missing compounds for normal metabolism. For example, treatment of argininosuccinic acid synthetase deficiency (a disorder of ureagenesis) has included administration of sodium benzoate, sodium phenylacetate, or both, to activate alternative routes of nitrogen elimination, as well as supplementation with arginine (a missing metabolic product). It is best to contact a regional metabolic specialist for up-to-the-moment advice in this rapidly changing area.

E. **Long-term management.** Sustaining normal long-term nutrition and growth is a challenge to the clinical skills of the physician. Patients with metabolic diseases characterized by protein intolerance tend to become symptomatic during intercurrent illnesses despite maintenance therapy. Continued strict dietary therapy may be difficult. Family counseling and support should be provided early and continued on a long-term basis.

REFERENCES

Arn PH, Valle DL, Brusilow SW: Inborn errors of metabolism: Not rare, not hopeless. *Contemp Pediatr* 1988;**5**:47.

Batshaw ML: Hyperammonemia. *Curr Probl Pediatr* 1984;**14**:1.

Brusilow SW, Valle DL: Symptomatic inborn errors of metabolism in the neonate. In: *Current Therapy in Neonatal-Perinatal Medicine 1985–1986.* Nelson NM (editor). Decker, 1985.

Burton BK: Inborn errors of metabolism: Clinical diagnosis in early infancy. *Pediatrics* 1987;**79**:359.

Hudak ML, Jones MD, Brusilow SW: Differentiation of transient hyperammonemia of the newborn and urea cycle enzyme defects by clinical presentation. *J Pediatr* 1985;**107**:712.

Komrower GM: Inborn errors of metabolism. *Pediatr Rev* 1980;**2**:175.

Matsui SM, Mahoney MJ, Rosenberg LE: Natural history of the inherited methylmalonic acidemias. *N Engl J Med* 1983;**308**:857.

Waber L: Inborn errors of metabolism. *Pediatr Ann* 1990;**19**:105.

Ward JC: Inborn errors of metabolism of acute onset in infancy. *Pediatr Rev* 1990;**11**:205.

Wolf B et al: Propionic acidemia: Clinical update. *J Pediatr* 1981;**99**:835.

62 Infant of Diabetic Mother

Good control of maternal diabetes is the key factor in determining fetal outcome. Recent data indicate that perinatal morbidity and mortality rates in the offspring of women with diabetes mellitus have improved with dietary management and insulin therapy. However, when adequate control of diabetes has not been accomplished, the physician must be aware of possible complications in the infant, including hypoglycemia, hypocalcemia, hypomagnesemia, perinatal asphyxia, respiratory distress syndrome, other respiratory illnesses, hyperbilirubinemia, polycythemia, renal vein thrombosis, macrosomia, birth injuries, and congenital malformations. Because of better current understanding of the pathophysiology of diabetic pregnancies, these complications can be recognized and treated.

I. **Classification**
   A. **White's classification.** In earlier descriptions of diabetic pregnancies, physicians relied on White's classification (Table 62–1). This nomenclature is based on the age at onset, the duration of the disorder, and the complications. It is used today chiefly to compare groups of infants delivered.
   B. **National Diabetes Data Group classification.** Table 62–2 presents the nomenclature of the National Diabetes Data Group. It replaces the older White classification and is a simpler method for characterizing diabetic pregnancies.

II. **Incidence.** Insulin-dependent diabetes occurs in 0.5% of all pregnancies. In addition, 1–3% of women exhibit biochemical abnormalities during pregnancy consistent with gestational diabetes.

III. **Pathophysiology**
   A. **Macrosomia.** Macrosomia is the classic presentation of the infant of a diabetic mother (IDM). It is the result of biochemical events along the maternal hyperglycemia—fetal hyperinsulinemia pathway as described by Pedersen (1971). Infants born to mothers described by

TABLE 62-1. WHITE'S CLASSIFICATION OF DIABETES

Class	Description
A	Chemical diabetes with positive glucose tolerance test before or during pregnancy
B	Onset after age 20; less than 10 years' duration
C	Onset at age 10–19
D1	Onset before age 10
D2	Duration longer than 20 years
D3	Calcification of vessels of the leg
D4	Benign retinopathy
D5	Hypertension
E	Calcification of pelvic vessels (not used)
F	Nephropathy
G	Pregnancy failures
H	Vascular lesions developing in childbearing years; includes patients with cardiopathy
R	Malignant retinopathy

Adapted, with permission, from White P: Diabetes mellitus in pregnancy. *Clin Perinatol* 1974:**1**:331.

TABLE 62-2. NOMENCLATURE OF NATIONAL DIABETES DATA GROUP

Class	Description
Type I: Insulin-dependent diabetes mellitus (IDDM)	Ketosis-prone, insulin-deficient owing to islet cell loss. Often associated with specific HLA types, with predisposition to viral insulitis or diabetes autoimmune phenomena. Occurs at any age. Common in youth.
Type II: Non-insulin-dependent diabetes mellitus (NIDDM)	Ketosis-resistant. More common in adults but occurs at any age. Many patients are overweight. May be seen in family aggregates as an autosomal dominant genetic trait. May require insulin for hyperglycemia during stress. Invariably requires insulin during pregnancy.
Gestational diabetes mellitus (GDM)	Diabetes begins (or is recognized) during pregnancy. Above normal risk of perinatal complications. Glucose intolerance may be transitory but frequently recurs. Diagnosis requires at least 2 abnormal plasma glucose values on a 3-hour oral glucose tolerance test (100 g glucose). Fasting: 105 mg/dL or more 1 hour: 190 mg/dL or more 2 hours: 160 mg/dL or more 3 hours: 145 mg/dL or more

Adapted, with permission, from National Diabetes Data Group: Classification and diagnosis of diabetes mellitus and other categories of glucose intolerance. *Diabetes* 1979;**28:**1039.

White's classification as having class A (insulin-dependent), B, C, or D diabetes are typically macrosomic. Complications are minimal in gestational diabetes and in class A diabetes controlled by diet.

B. Small for gestational age (SGA). Mothers with renal, retinal, or cardiac diseases are more likely to have SGA or premature infants, poor fetal outcome, fetal distress, or fetal death.

C. Specific disorders frequently encountered in IDMs

1. Metabolic disorders

a. Hypoglycemia is defined as a blood glucose level less than 45 mg/dL in a pre-term or term infant. It is present in up to 40% of IDMs, most commonly in macrosomic infants. It usually presents within 1-2 hours after delivery. According to Pedersen, at birth, the transplacental glucose supply is terminated, and, because of high concentrations of plasma insulin, blood glucose levels fall. Mothers with well-controlled blood glucose levels have fewer infants with hypoglycemia. Hypoglycemia in the SGA infants born to mothers with diabetic vascular disease is due to decreased glycogen stores; it appears 6-12 hours after delivery.

b. Hypocalcemia. Serum calcium levels less than 7 mg/dL associated with symptoms or less than 6 mg/dL without symptoms— or an ionized calcium level less than 3 mg/dL—is considered hypocalcemic. The incidence is up to 50% of IDMs (Tsang, 1979). The severity of hypocalcemia is related to the severity of maternal diabetes and involves decreased function of the parathyroid glands (Tsang, 1975). Serum calcium levels are lowest at 24-72 hours of age.

c. Hypomagnesemia. A serum magnesium level less than 1.52 mg/dL in any infant is an indication of hypomagnesemia. It is related to maternal hypomagnesemia and the severity of maternal diabetes.

2. Cardiorespiratory disorders

a. Perinatal asphyxia. Perinatal asphyxia occurs in up to 25% of IDMs. It may be due to prematurity, cesarean delivery, intrauterine hypoxia caused by maternal vascular disease, or macrosomia.

b. **Hyaline membrane disease or respiratory distress syndrome (RDS)**

   (1) **Incidence.** The incidence has decreased to only 3% of IDM owing to better management of diabetes during pregnancy (Frantz, 1979). Most cases are due to premature delivery, delayed maturation of pulmonary surfactant production, or delivery be elective cesarean section.

   (2) **Fetal lung maturity.** Pulmonary surfactant production in the IDM is deficient or delayed principally in class A, B, and C diabetics. Fetal hyperinsulinism may adversely affect the lung maturation process in the IDM by antagonizing the action of cortisol (Smith, 1975).

   (3) **Cesarean section.** Infants delivered by elective cesarean section are at risk for RDS because of decreased prostaglandin production and increased pulmonary vascular resistance (Csaba, 1978).

c. **Other causes of respiratory distress**

   (1) **Transient tachypnea of the newborn (TTN)** occurs especially after elective cesarean section. This disorder may or may not require oxygen therapy and usually responds by 72 hours of age.

   (2) **Cardiomyopathy** occurs in up to 20% of IDMs (Way, 1979). It occurs secondary to increased fat and glycogen deposition in the myocardium and may lead to congestive heart failure.

3. **Hematologic disorders**

a. **Hyperbilirubinemia.** Bilirubin production is apparently increased in the IDM secondary to prematurity, macrosomia, hypoglycemia, and polycythemia.

b. **Polycythemia and hyperviscosity.** The cause of polycythemia is unclear but may be related to increased levels of erythropoietin in the IDM, increased red blood cell production secondary to chronic intrauterine hypoxia in mothers with vascular disease, and intrauterine placental transfusion due to acute hypoxia during labor and delivery.

c. **Renal vein thrombosis** is a rare complication most likely due to hyperviscosity, hypotension, or disseminated intravascular coagulation. It is usually diagnosed by ultrasonography and may present with hematuria and an abdominal mass.

4. **Morphologic and functional problems**

a. **Macrosomia and birth injury**

   (1) **Macrosomia** is due to fetal hyperglycemia, resulting in increased glucose uptake in insulin-sensitive tissues. It is seen in the offspring of gestational and class A, B, and C diabetics. Macrosomia is rarely seen in the other classes because of maternal vascular disease.

   (2) **Birth injury.** Macrosomia may lead to shoulder dystocia, which may cause birth asphyxia. Birth injuries include fractures of the clavicle or humerus, Erb's palsy, phrenic nerve palsy, and, rarely, central nervous system injury.

b. **Congenital malformations.** Congenital malformations occur in 4.1% of IDMs (Molsted-Pedersen, 1980)—a much higher incidence than in the general population. It is suspected that poor diabetic control in the first trimester is associated with a higher percentage of congenital malformations. Congenital malformations now account for up to 50% of perinatal deaths and include cardiac defects (transposition of the great vessels, ventricular septal defect, atrial septal defect), renal defects (agenesis), gastrointestinal tract defects (small left colon syndrome, situs inversus), neurologic defects (anencephaly, meningocele syndrome), skeletal defects (hemivertebrae, caudal regression syndrome), unusual facies and microophthalmia.

IV. **Risk factors.** The following factors or conditions may be associated with an increased risk for problems in IDMs.

A. **Maternal class of diabetes**
1. **In gestational diabetes and class A diabetes** controlled by diet alone, infants have few complications.
2. **Women with class A diabetes controlled with insulin and class B, C, and D diabetes** are prone to deliver macrosomic infants if diabetes is inadequately controlled.
3. **Diabetic women with renal, retinal, cardiac, and vascular disease** have the most severe fetal problems.

B. **Hemoglobin A$_{1c}$.** To decrease perinatal morbidity and mortality rates, the diabetic woman should attempt to achieve good metabolic control before conception. Elevated hemoglobin A$_{1c}$ levels during the first trimester appear to be associated with a higher incidence of congenital malformations (Miller, 1979).

C. **Diabetic ketoacidosis.** Pregnant women with insulin-dependent diabetes are apt to develop diabetic ketoacidosis. The onset of this complication may be life-threatening for the mother and fetus or may lead to preterm delivery.

D. **Preterm labor.** Premature onset of labor in a diabetic woman is a serious problem because of the increased likelihood of respiratory distress syndrome in the fetus. Furthermore, beta-sympathomimetic agents used to prevent preterm delivery may be associated with maternal hyperglycemia, hyperinsulinemia, and acidosis.

E. **Immature fetal lung profile.** Diabetic women who present at 36 weeks' gestation or later should undergo amniocentesis to evaluate fetal lung maturity. A mature lecithin:sphingomyelin ratio may not ensure normal respiratory function in the IDM. However, the presence of phosphatidylglycerol in the amniotic fluid is more apt to be associated with normal neonatal respiratory function (see also Chap 1).

V. **Clinical presentation**
A. **At birth,** the infant may be large for gestational age, or if the mother has vascular disease, small for gestational age. The size of most infants is appropriate for gestational age; however, if macrosomia is present, birth trauma may occur.

B. **After birth,** hypoglycemia can present as lethargy, poor feeding, apnea, or jitteriness in the first 6–12 hours after birth. Jitteriness that occurs after 24 hours of age may be due to hypocalcemia or hypomagnesemia. Signs of respiratory distress due to immature lungs can be noted on examination. Cardiac disease may be present as an enlarged cardiothymic shadow on a chest x-ray film or by physical evidence of heart failure. Gross congenital anomalies may be noted on physical examination.

VI. **Diagnosis**
A. **Laboratory studies.** The following tests *must* be closely monitored in the IDM.
1. **Serum glucose levels** should be checked at delivery and at $\frac{1}{2}$, 1, $1\frac{1}{2}$, 2, 4, 8, 12, 24, 36, and 48 hours of age. Glucose levels should be checked with Chemstrip-bG or Dextrostix. Readings below 40 mg/dL on Chemstrip-bG or below 45 mg/dL on Dextrostix should be verified by serum glucose measurements.
2. **Serum calcium levels** should be obtained at 6, 24, and 48 hours of

age. If serum calcium levels are low, **serum magnesium levels** should be obtained as they may also be low.

3. **The hematocrit** should be checked at birth and at 4 and 24 hours of age.
4. **Serum bilirubin levels** should be checked as indicated by physical examination.
5. **Other tests.** Arterial blood gas levels, complete blood counts, cultures, and Gram stains should be obtained as clinically indicated.

B. **Radiologic studies** are not necessary unless there is evidence of cardiac, respiratory, or skeletal problems.
C. **Electrocardiography and echocardiography** should be performed if hypertrophic cardiomyopathy or a cardiac malformation is suspected.

VII. **Management**

A. **Initial evaluation.** Upon delivery, the infant should be evaluated in the usual manner. In the transitional nursery, blood glucose levels and the hematocrit should be obtained. The infant should be observed for jitteriness, tremors, convulsions, apnea, weak cry, and poor sucking. A physical examination should be performed, paying particular attention to the heart, kidneys, lungs, and extremities.

B. **Continuing evaluation.** Over the first several hours after delivery, the infant should be assessed for signs of respiratory distress. During the first 48 hours, observe for signs of jaundice and for renal, cardiac, neurologic, and gastrointestinal tract abnormalities.

C. **Metabolic management**
   1. **Hypoglycemia.** See Chapter 41.
   2. **Hypocalcemia**
      a. **Calcium therapy.** Symptomatic infants should receive 10% calcium gluconate intravenously. The infusion should be given slowly to prevent cardiac arrhythmias, and the infant should be monitored for signs of extravasation. Following the initial dose, a maintenance dose is given by continuous intravenous infusion. The hypocalcemia should respond in 3-4 days, but until then, serum calcium levels should be monitored every 12 hours.
      b. **Magnesium maintenance therapy.** Magnesium is usually added to intravenous fluids or given orally as magnesium sulfate 50%, 0.2 mL/kg/d (4 meq/mL).

D. **Management of cardiorespiratory problems**
   1. **Perinatal asphyxia.** Close observation for fetal distress should continue (see Chap 68).
   2. **Hyaline membrane disease.** Obtaining amniotic fluid for a fetal lung maturity profile can decrease the incidence of hyaline membrane disease. However, some infants must be delivered even if the lung profile is immature.
   3. **Cardiomyopathy.** The treatment of choice is with propranolol. See Chapter 75 for dosage information. Digoxin is contraindicated due to possible ventricular outflow obstruction.

E. **Hematologic therapy**
   1. **Hyperbilirubinemia.** Frequent monitoring of serum bilirubin levels may be necessary. Phototherapy and exchange transfusion for infants with hyperbilirubinemia is discussed in Chapter 60.
   2. **Polycythemia.** See Chapter 56.
   3. **Renal vein thrombosis.** Treatment consists in fluid restriction and close monitoring of electrolytes and renal status. Supportive therapy is indicated to insure adequate blood circulation. Nephrectomy is usually only a last resort in unilateral disease.

F. **Management of morphologic and functional problems**
   1. **Macrosomia and birth injury**

    a. Fractures of the extremities should be treated with immobilization.

    b. Erb's palsy can be treated with range-of-motion exercises.

  2. Congenital malformations. If a gross malformation is discovered, a specialist should be consulted.

VIII. Prognosis. Less morbidity and mortality occur with adequate control during the diabetic pregnancy. Preconceptual counseling is used as an adjunct to preventive health care of the diabetic patient. The known pregnant diabetic is currently receiving better health care than before, but the challenge is early identification of women with biochemical abnormalities of gestational diabetes. The risk of subsequent diabetes in the infants of these women is at least 10 times greater than in the normal population.

REFERENCES

Csaba IF, Sulyok E, Ertl T: Relationship of maternal treatment with indomethacin to persistence of fetal circulation syndrome. *J Pediatr* 1978;**92**:484.

Cummins M, Norrish M: Follow-up of children of diabetic mothers. *Arch Dis Child* 1980;**55**:259.

Frantz IO III, Epstein MF: Fetal lung development in pregnancies complicated by diabetes. In: *The Diabetic Pregnancy: A Perinatal Perspective*. Merkatz IR, Adam PAJ (editors). Grune & Stratton, 1979.

Hollingsworth DR: Diabetes. In: *Medical Counseling Before Pregnancy*. Hollingsworth DR, Resnik R (editors). Churchill, 1988.

Kitzmiller JL, Cloherty JP, Graham CA: Management of diabetes and pregnancy. In: *Clinical Diabetes Mellitus*. Kozak GP (editor). Saunders, 1982.

Kulovich MV, Gluck L: The lung profile. 2. Complicated pregnancy. *Am J Obstet Gynecol* 1979;**135**:64.

Miller JM, Crenshaw MC Jr, Welt SI: Hemoglobin A$_{1c}$ in normal and diabetic pregnancy. *JAMA* 1979;**242**:2785.

Molsted-Pedersen L: Pregnancy and diabetes: A survey. *Acta Endocrinol [Suppl]* 1980;**238**:13.

Pedersen J: *The Pregnant Diabetic and Her Newborn,* 2nd ed. Williams & Wilkins, 1971.

Smith BT et al: Insulin antagonism of cortisol action on lecithin synthesis by cultured fetal lung cells. *J Pediatr* 1975;**87**:953.

Tsang RC, Brown DR, Steichen JJ: Diabetes and calcium: Calcium disturbances in infants of diabetic mothers. In: *The Diabetic Pregnancy: A Perinatal Perspective*. Merkatz IR, Adam PAJ (editors). Grune & Stratton, 1979.

Way GL et al: The natural history of hypertrophic cardiomyopathy in infants of diabetic mothers. *J Pediatr* 1979;**95**:1020.

White P: Diabetes mellitus in pregnancy. *Clin Perinatol* 1974;**1**:331.

63 Infectious Diseases

Isolation precautions for all infectious diseases, including maternal and neonatal precautions, breast-feeding, and visiting issues, can be found in Appendix H.

NEONATAL SEPSIS

I. **Definition.** Neonatal sepsis is a clinical syndrome of systemic illness accompanied by bacteremia occurring in the first month of life.

II. **Incidence.** The incidence of primary sepsis is 1–10 per 1000 live births. The mortality rate is high (13–50%), with the higher rates seen in premature infants and in those with early fulminant disease.

III. **Pathophysiology.** In considering the pathogenesis of neonatal sepsis, 3 different clinical situations may be defined: early onset, late onset, and nosocomial disease.

  A. **Early-onset disease** presents in the first 5–7 days of life and is usually a multisystem fulminant illness with prominent respiratory symptoms. In this situation, the infant is colonized with the pathogen in the perinatal period. Several infectious agents, notably treponemes, viruses, *Listeria,* and probably *Candida,* can be acquired transplacentally via hematogenous routes. Acquisition of other organisms is associated with the birth process. With rupture of the membranes, vaginal flora may ascend to reach the amniotic fluid and fetus. Chorioamnionitis develops, leading to fetal colonization and infection. Aspiration of infected amniotic fluid by the fetus or neonate may play a role in resultant respiratory symptoms. The presence of vernix or meconium impairs the natural bacteriostatic properties of amniotic fluid. Finally, the infant may be exposed to vaginal flora as it passes through the birth canal. The primary sites of colonization tend to be the skin, nasopharynx, oropharynx, conjunctiva, and umbilical cord. Trauma to these mucosal surfaces may lead to infection.

  B. **Late-onset disease** may occur as early as at 5 days of age; however, it is more common after the first week of life. Although these infants may have a history of obstetric complications, these complications are associated less frequently with late-onset than with early-onset disease. These babies usually have an identifiable focus, most often meningitis in addition to sepsis. Bacteria responsible for late-onset sepsis and meningitis include those acquired after birth from the maternal genital tract as well as organisms acquired after birth from human contact or from contaminated equipment. Therefore, horizontal transmission appears to play a significant role in late-onset disease. The reasons for delay in development in clinical illness, the predilection for central nervous system disease, and the less severe systemic and cardiorespiratory symptoms are unclear. Transfer of maternal antibodies to the mother's own vaginal flora may play a role in determining which exposed infants become infected, especially in the case of group B streptococcal infections.

  C. **Nosocomial sepsis.** This form of sepsis occurs in high-risk newborn infants. Its pathogenesis is related to the underlying illness and debilitation of the infant, the flora in the NICU environment, and invasive monitoring and other techniques used in neonatal intensive care. Infants, especially premature infants, have an increased susceptibility to infection because of immature immune defenses that are less efficient at localizing and clearing bacterial invasion.

D. **Causative organisms.** The principal pathogens involved in neonatal sepsis have tended to change with time. Primary sepsis must be contrasted with nosocomial sepsis. The agents associated with primary sepsis are usually the vaginal flora. Most centers report **group B streptococci** as the most common, followed by **gram-negative enteric organisms, especially *E coli.*** Other pathogens include ***Listeria monocytogenes, Staphylococcus,* other streptococci (including the enterococci), anaerobes, and *Haemophilus influenzae.*** In addition, many unusual organisms are documented in primary neonatal sepsis, especially in premature infants. The flora causing nosocomial sepsis varies in each nursery. ***Staphylococci* (especially *Staphylococcus epidermidis*), gram-negative rods (including *Pseudomonas, Klebsiella, Serratia,* and *Proteus*), and fungal organisms** predominate.

IV. **Risk factors**

A. **Prematurity and low birth weight.** Prematurity is the single most significant factor correlated with sepsis. The risk increases in proportion to the decrease in birth weight.

B. **Rupture of membranes.** Premature or prolonged rupture of the membranes is a risk factor for neonatal sepsis.

C. **Maternal peripartum fever or infection.** Chorioamnionitis, urinary tract infection (UTI), and other obstetric complications.

D. **Amniotic fluid problems.** Meconium-stained or foul-smelling, cloudy amniotic fluid.

E. **Resuscitation at birth.** Infants who had fetal distress, who were born by traumatic delivery, or who were severely depressed at birth and required intubation and resuscitation.

F. **Multiple gestation.**

G. **Invasive procedures.** Invasive monitoring and respiratory or metabolic support.

H. **Infants with galactosemia** (predisposition to *E coli* sepsis), immune defects, or asplenia.

I. **Iron therapy.** Iron added to serum in vitro enhances the growth of many organisms.

J. **Other factors.** Males are more commonly affected than females. Variations in immune function may play a role. Sepsis is more common in black than in white infants and may be explained by a higher incidence of premature rupture of membranes, maternal fever, and low birth weight. Low socioeconomic status is often reported as an additional risk factor, but again this may be explained by low birth weight.

V. **Clinical presentation.** The initial diagnosis of sepsis is by necessity a clinical one, because it is imperative to begin treatment before results of culture are available. Clinical signs and symptoms of sepsis are nonspecific, and the differential diagnosis is broad, including respiratory distress syndrome (RDS), metabolic diseases, hematologic disease, central nervous system disease, cardiac disease, and other infectious processes (ie, TORCH infections). Clinical signs and symptoms most often mentioned include the following.

A. **Temperature irregularity.** Hypo- or hyperthermia (greater heat output required by incubator or radiant warmer to maintain neutral thermal environment or frequent adjustments of infant servocontrol probe).

B. **Change in behavior.** Lethargy, irritability, or change in tone.

C. **Skin.** Poor peripheral perfusion, cyanosis, mottling, pallor, petechiae, rashes, sclerema, jaundice.

D. Feeding problems. Feeding intolerance, vomiting, diarrhea (water loss stool), abdominal distention with or without visible bowel loops.

E. Cardiopulmonary. Tachypnea, respiratory distress (grunting, flaring, retractions), apnea especially within the first 24 hours or new onset, especially after 1 week of age, tachycardia, hypotension (tends to be a late sign).

F. Metabolic. Hypo- or hyperglycemia, metabolic acidosis.

VI. Diagnosis

A. Laboratory studies

1. **Cultures.** Blood and other normally sterile body fluids should be obtained for culture. (In neonates less than 24 hours of age, a sterile urine specimen is not necessary, since the occurrence of UTIs is exceedingly rare in this age group.) Positive bacterial cultures will confirm the diagnosis of sepsis. Results may vary because of a number of factors, including maternal antibiotics administered before birth, organisms that are difficult to grow and isolate (ie, anaerobes), and sampling errors with small sample volumes. Therefore, in many clinical situations, infants are treated for presumed sepsis despite negative cultures, with apparent clinical benefit. Some controversy currently exists about whether lumbar puncture and CSF culture should be performed on asymptomatic newborns who are being evaluated for presumptive sepsis. Many institutions perform lumbar punctures only on babies who are clinically ill or who have documented positive blood cultures.

2. **Antigen detection tests.** Tests are available for **group B streptococci, Neisseria meningitidis, H influenzae,** and **Streptococcal pneumoniae.** Urine and cerebrospinal fluid are generally the specimens that can be tested. As an adjunct to making a definitive diagnosis, these tests can be especially helpful because of their rapid turn-around time. They can also be valuable if the mother or baby have received antibiotics prior to cultures being obtained. However, it is important to become familiar with the techniques used in a particular laboratory and their rates of false-positive or false-negative results.

3. **Gram's staining of various fluids.** Gram's staining is especially helpful for the study of cerebrospinal fluid. Gram's staining of the buffy coat has been helpful in several series of proved sepsis in infants. Gram's-stained smears and cultures of amniotic fluid or of material obtained by gastric aspiration is often performed. White cells in the samples are maternal in origin, and their presence along with bacteria indicates exposure and possible colonization but not necessarily actual infection.

4. **Adjunctive laboratory tests**

   a. **White blood count and differential.** These values alone are very nonspecific. There are references for total white blood count and absolute neutrophil count (probably a better measure) as a function of postnatal age in hours (see Appendix M). Neutropenia may be a significant finding; it carries an ominous prognosis when associated with sepsis. The presence of immature forms of white cells is more specific but is still rather insensitive. Ratios of bands to segmented forms greater than 0.3 and of bands to total PMNs greater than 0.1 have good predictive value if present. Serial white counts followed several hours apart may be helpful in establishing a trend.

   b. **Platelet count.** A decreased platelet count is usually a late sign and is very nonspecific.

   c. **Acute-phase reactants**

(1) **C-reactive protein** greater than 2 mg/dL may be helpful as a nonspecific marker of inflammation.

(2) **The standard erythrocyte sedimentation rate (ESR)** may be elevated but usually not until well into the course of the illness; it therefore is used infrequently in the initial workup.

(3) Changes in fibrinogen, haptoglobin, and IgM levels and leukocyte enzyme activity have not been shown to be diagnostically useful in neonates.

d. **Miscellaneous tests.** Abnormal values for bilirubin, glucose, and sodium may, in the proper clinical situation, provide supportive evidence for sepsis.

B. **Radiologic studies**
  1. **A chest x-ray study** may be helpful in cases accompanied by pneumonia, although it is often impossible to distinguish group B streptococcal or *Listeria* pneumonia from uncomplicated respiratory distress syndrome (RDS). (Group B streptococcal pneumonia will often have associated pleural effusions present.)
  2. **Urinary tract imaging (renal ultrasonography, intravenous pyelography, and voiding cystourethrography)** should be part of the evaluation if urinary tract infection accompanies sepsis. Sterile urine for culture must be obtained by either suprapubic collection (p 138) or bladder catheterization (p 140). Bag-urine samples should not be used to diagnose urinary tract infection.

C. **Other studies.** Examination of the placenta and fetal membranes may disclose evidence of chorioamnionitis and thus an increased potential for neonatal infection.

VII. **Management**
  A. **Initial therapy.** Treatment is most often begun before a definite causative agent is identified. It consists of a **penicillin, usually ampicillin** (the drug of choice for *Listeria* and enterococci, although some resistance has recently been reported), plus an **aminoglycoside such as gentamicin.** In nosocomial sepsis, the flora of the NICU must be considered; however, staphylococcal coverage with **vancomycin plus either an aminoglycoside or a third-generation cephalosporin** is usually begun. Dosages and other pharmacologic information are given in Chapter 76.
  B. **Continuing therapy** is of course based on culture and sensitivity results. Monitoring for antibiotic toxicity and following levels of aminoglycosides and vancomycin are important. When group B streptococci is documented as the causative agent, a **penicillin** is the drug of choice; however, often an **aminoglycoside** is also given because of documented synergism in vitro. See Chap 76 for specific drugs, dosages, and other pharmacologic information.
  C. **Complications and supportive therapy**
    1. **Respiratory.** Assure adequate oxygenation with blood gas monitoring and, if needed, initiate oxygen therapy or ventilator support.
    2. **Cardiovascular.** Support blood pressure and perfusion to prevent shock. Use volume expanders (normal saline, albumin, or blood), 10–20 mL/kg, and follow intake of fluids and output of urine. Pressor agents such as dopamine or dobutamine may be needed (see Chap 75).
    3. **Hematologic**
      a. **Disseminated intravascular coagulation (DIC).** With DIC, generalized bleeding may occur at puncture sites, in the GI tract, or at CNS sites. In the skin, large vessel thrombosis may cause gangrene. Laboratory parameters consistent with DIC include thrombocytopenia, increased prothrombin time (PT), and increased partial thromboplastin time (PTT). There is an increase

in fibrin split products (FSP). Measures include treating the underlying disease, fresh-frozen plasma (FFP) 10 mL/kg, vitamin K (see p 486), platelet infusion and, possibly, exchange transfusion (see Chap 21).

b. **Neutropenia.** Granulocyte transfusion in extremely ill infants has been successful in some studies. Intravenous gamma globulin (p 467) or exchange transfusion may also be used.

4. **Central nervous system.** For seizure control, use phenobarbital, 20 mg/kg as the loading dose, and monitor for syndrome of inappropriate secretion of antidiuretic hormone (SIADH), which is characterized by decreased urine output, hyponatremia, decreased serum osmolarity, and increased urine specific gravity and osmolality.

5. **Metabolic.** Monitor for and treat hypo- and hyperglycemia. Metabolic acidosis may accompany sepsis and is treated with bicarbonate and fluid replacement.

MENINGITIS

I. **Definition.** Neonatal meningitis is infection of the meninges and central nervous system in the first month of life. This period is the most common time of life for meningitis to occur.

II. **Incidence.** The incidence is about 1:2500 live births. The **mortality rate** is 30–60%, and there is a high incidence (up to 50% or more) of neurodevelopmental sequelae in survivors.

III. **Pathophysiology.** In most cases, infection occurs because of hematogenous seeding of the meninges and central nervous system. In patients with central nervous system or skeletal anomalies (eg, myelomeningocele) there may be direct inoculation of the central nervous system by flora on the skin or in the environment. Neonatal meningitis is often accompanied by **ventriculitis,** which makes resolution of infection more difficult. There is also a predilection for vasculitis, which may lead to hemorrhage, thrombosis, and infarction. Subdural effusions and brain abscess may also complicate the course.

Most organisms implicated in neonatal sepsis also cause neonatal meningitis. Some have a definite predilection for central nervous system infection. **Group B streptococcus** (especially type III) and the gram-negative rods (especially *E coli* with K1 antigen) are the **most common causative agents.** Other organisms with central nervous system predilection are *Listeria monocytogenes* and *Flavobacterium meningosepticum.*

With central nervous system anomalies involving open defects or indwelling devices (such as ventriculoperitoneal shunts), staphylococcal disease (*Staphylococcus aureus* and *Staphylococcus epidermidis*) is more common, as is disease caused by other skin flora, including streptococci and diphtheroids. Many unusual organisms, including fungi and anaerobes, are described in case reports of neonatal meningitis in debilitated and normal neonates.

IV. **Risk factors.** Premature infants with sepsis have a much higher incidence (up to threefold that of term infants) of central nervous system infection. Infants with central nervous system defects necessitating ventriculoperitoneal shunt procedures are also at increased risk.

V. **Clinical presentation.** The clinical presentation of meningitis is usually nonspecific, and it must be excluded in any infant being evaluated for sepsis or infection. Signs and symptoms of meningitis generally are similar to those reported for sepsis. A full or bulging fontanelle is often a late finding in patients with meningitis. The syndrome of inappropriate secretion of antidiuretic hormone (SIADH) may accompany meningitis.

VI. **Diagnosis**
   A. **Laboratory studies.** Cerebrospinal fluid (CSF) examination is critical

in the investigation of possible meningitis. The technique for obtaining fluid is discussed in Chapter 24. Normal CSF values are found in Appendix D.

1. **CSF culture** may be positive in association with normal (clear) or minimally abnormal CSF on inspection.
2. **A gram-stained CSF smear** is helpful. One study showed it to be positive in 78% of cases of meningitis caused by rods and 83% of cases caused by group B streptococci.
3. **Cerebrospinal glucose levels** must be compared with **serum glucose levels.** Normally, CSF values are one-half to two-thirds of serum values.
4. **CSF protein** is usually elevated, although normal values for infants, especially prematures, may be much higher (up to 150 mg/dL) than in later life and the test may be confounded by the presence of blood in the specimen.
5. **CSF pleocytosis** is variable. There are usually more cells with gram-negative rods than with group B streptococcal disease. Normal values allow up to 25 white cells in premature infants, some of which may be PMNs. Pleocytosis (with neutrophils early in the disease course) may also be an irritant reaction to central nervous system hemorrhage.
6. **Rapid antigen tests** are available for several organisms and should be done on a CSF specimen.
7. **Ventricular tap,** with culture and microscopic examination of the CSF, is indicated in cases not responding to treatment.

B. **Radiologic studies**
1. **Cranial ultrasonography** has been useful in the diagnosis of ventriculitis. (Ectogenic strands can be seen in the ventricles.)
2. **CT scan of the head** may be indicated to rule out abscess, subdural effusion, or an area of thrombosis, hemorrhage, or infarction.

VII. **Management**
A. **Drug therapy.** (See Chap 76 for drug dosages and other pharmacologic information.)
1. **Empiric antibiotic therapy.** Optimal antibiotic selection depends on culture and sensitivity testing of causative organisms. **Ampicillin and gentamicin** are usually started as empirical therapy for suspected sepsis or meningitis.
2. **Gram-positive meningitis (group B streptococci and *Listeria*). Penicillin or ampicillin** is the drug of choice. These infections usually respond well to treatment. Administration for 14–21 days is indicated.
3. **Staphylococcal disease.** This type of meningitis is seen mainly in infants with neurosurgical disorders. **Nafcillin, methicillin, or vancomycin** should be substituted for penicillin or ampicillin as initial coverage.
4. **Gram-negative meningitis.** *The optimal treatment for this type of meningitis is still under investigation.* Many organisms may be ampicillin-resistant, and penetration of CSF (even in the inflamed neonatal meninges) may be inadequate with aminoglycosides. Studies have shown no advantage to using intrathecal or intraventricular aminoglycosides. A better choice may be third-generation cephalosporins (eg, cefotaxime, cefuroxime).
   a. Currently, most clinicians use **ampicillin plus cefotaxime** as initial therapy. This infection may be difficult to eradicate, and 5–7 days of drug therapy may be needed to sterilize the CSF, even with adequate therapy. Treatment should continue until 14 days after cultures are negative or for 21 days, whichever is longer. Follow-up examination of the CSF is recommended until steril-

ity is documented. Screening for relapse of infection should continue for at least 48–72 hours after therapy is discontinued.
   b. **External ventricular drainage** may be indicated in certain cases complicated by ventriculitis.
B. **Supportive measures and monitoring for complications.** Measurement of head circumference, transillumination of the head, and neurologic examination should be performed daily.

TORCH INFECTIONS

TORCH is an acronym (**T**oxoplasma, **O**thers such as syphilis, hepatitis B, coxsackie virus, Epstein-Barr virus, varicella-zoster, and human parvovirus, **R**ubella virus, **C**ytomegalovirus, **H**erpes simples virus) that denotes chronic nonbacterial perinatal infection. Herpetic disease in the neonate does not fit the pattern of chronic intrauterine infection but is traditionally grouped with the others. TORCH infections may present in the neonate with similar clinical and laboratory findings (ie, SGA, hepatosplenomegaly, rash, central nervous system manifestations, early jaundice, low platelet count)—hence the usefulness of the TORCH concept.

TOXOPLASMOSIS

I. **Definition.** *Toxoplasma gondii* is a parasite capable of causing intrauterine infection.
II. **Incidence.** The incidence of congenital infection is 1:1000 live births.
III. **Pathophysiology.** *T gondii* is a coccidian parasite ubiquitous in nature. The primary natural host is the cat family. The organism exists in 3 forms: oocyst, tachyzoite, and tissue cyst. The **oocysts** are excreted in cat feces. Ingestion of oocysts is followed by penetration of gastrointestinal mucosa by sporazoites, and circulation of tachyzoites, the ovoid unicellular organism characteristic of acute infections. Most maternal organs, including the placenta, are "seeded" by the protozoan. Actual transmission to the fetus is by the transplacental-fetal hematogenous route. In the chronic form of the disease, organisms invade certain body tissues, especially those of the brain, eye, and striated muscle, forming **tissue cysts.**

Acute infection in the adult is often subclinical. If symptoms are present, they are generally nonspecific: mononucleosis-like illness with fever, lymphadenopathy, fatigue, malaise, myalgia, fever, skin rash, and splenomegaly. Infection is believed to occur solely in fetuses of nonimmune mothers experiencing primary acute infection. Placental infection occurs and persists throughout gestation. The infection may or may not be transmitted to the fetus. The later in pregnancy that infection is acquired, the more likely is transmission to the fetus (first trimester, 14%; second trimester, 29%; and third trimester, 59% transmission). Infections transmitted earlier in gestation are likely to cause more severe fetal effects (abortion-stillbirth, severe disease with teratogenesis). Infections transmitted later are more likely to be subclinical. Rarely, a parasite may be transmitted during parturition via an infected placenta. Infection in the fetus or neonate usually involves disease in one of 2 forms: infection of the central nervous system or the eyes (or both) or infection of the central nervous system and the eyes with disseminated infection.
IV. **Risk factors.** *T gondii* may be ingested during contact with soil or litter boxes contaminated with cat feces. It may also be transmitted in unpasteurized milk, in raw or undercooked meats (especially pork), and through transfusion of blood products. Premature infants have a higher incidence of congenital toxoplasmosis than term infants (25–50% of cases in some series).

V. Clinical presentation. Congenital toxoplasmosis may be manifested as clinical neonatal disease, disease in the first few months of life, late sequelae or relapsed infection, or subclinical disease.

   A. Clinical disease. Infants who present with evident clinical disease may have disseminated illness or isolated central nervous system (CNS) or ocular disease. Late sequelae are primarily related to ocular or central nervous system disease. Obstructive hydrocephalus, chorioretinitis, and intracranial calcifications form the **classic triad** of toxoplasmosis.

   B. Prominent signs and symptoms in infants with congenital toxoplasmosis include chorioretinitis, abnormalities of cerebrospinal fluid (high protein value), anemia, seizures, intracranial calcifications, direct hyperbilirubinemia, fever, hepatosplenomegaly, lymphadenopathy, vomiting, microcephaly or hydrocephaly, diarrhea, cataracts, eosinophilia, bleeding diathesis, hypothermia, glaucoma, optic atrophy, microphthalmia, rash, and pneumonitis.

   C. Associated findings. Toxoplasmosis has been associated with congenital nephrosis, various endocrinopathies (due to hypothalamic or pituitary effects), myocarditis, erythroblastosis with hydrops fetalis, and isolated mental retardation.

   D. Subclinical disease. Subclinical infection is believed to be the most common. Studies of infants in whom infection is identified by serologic testing or documented maternal infection indicate that a large percentage may have minor cerebrospinal fluid abnormalities at birth and later develop visual or neurologic sequelae or learning disabilities.

VI. Diagnosis

   A. Laboratory studies. The diagnosis of congenital toxoplasmosis is most often based on clinical suspicion plus serologic tests, which may be complex and difficult to interpret.

      1. Direct isolation of the organism from body fluids or tissues requires inoculating blood, body fluids, or placental tissue into mice or tissue culture, and the technique is not readily available. Isolation of the organism from placental tissue correlates strongly with fetal infection.

      2. Cerobrospinal fluid examination should be performed in suspected cases. The most characteristic abnormalities are xanthochromia, mononuclear pleocytosis, and a very high protein level. Tests for cerebrospinal fluid IgM to toxoplasmosis may also be performed.

      3. Serologic tests include maternal skin tests (a positive test indicates chronic or latent infection and little risk of transmission to the fetus). Because it is relatively easy to perform, the **indirect fluorescent antibody (IFA)** test has largely replaced the **Sabin-Feldman dye test.** It measures antibodies to surface antigen. A mother with a high IFA (1 to 512 or greater) and a positive IGM-IFA is highly suspect for recently acquired infection. The absence of a placental leak and a positive (1 to 2 or more) IGM-IFA in the newborn are firm evidence of congenital toxoplasmosis. A negative test does not rule out congenital toxoplasmosis, as most neonates with congenital disease do not have detectable IGM yet, and they must be followed by subsequent serologic testing.

   B. Radiologic studies

      1. A skull x-ray study or CT scan of the head may demonstrate characteristic intracranial calcifications (speckled throughout the central nervous system), including the meninges.

      2. Long-bone x-ray studies may show abnormalities; specifically, metaphyseal lucency and irregularity of the line of calcification at the epiphyseal plates without periosteal reaction.

   C. Other studies. Ophthalmologic examination characteristically shows chorioretinitis. Other ocular features are often present at some stages.

VII. Management. The efficacy of treatment of pregnant women and infants with congenital infection is unclear. Treatment of acute maternal toxoplasmosis appears to reduce the risk of fetal wastage and decrease the likelihood of congenital infection. In most cases, maternal infection is not suspected.

   A. Specific treatment. Treatment is with **pyrimethamine,** 1 mg/kg/d orally, plus **sulfadiazine,** 50–100 mg/kg/d in 2 divided doses, for a total of 21 days. For overt and subclinical infection, therapy with these drugs should be continued for the first year as 3–4 courses of 21 days each. These medications are potentially teratogenic and should be used only after the first trimester. Pyrimethamine is a folic acid antagonist and can cause marrow suppression that may be ameliorated by the concurrent administration of leucovorin. A third agent, **spiramycin** (available in Canada and Europe), is a macrolide antibiotic related to erythromycin. In Europe and Canada, it has been used throughout pregnancy without adverse effects on mother or fetus; it can be obtained from the CDC in Atlanta. Corticosteroids may alleviate some of the inflammatory processes (eg, chorioretinitis).

   B. Prevention. Pregnant women should avoid eating raw meat or raw eggs and exposure to cat litter boxes or cat feces.

RUBELLA

   I. Definition. Rubella is a viral infection capable of causing chronic intrauterine infection and damage to the developing fetus.

  II. Incidence. The incidence varies from 0.1 to 2.0% of births, with the higher incidence after rubella epidemics.

 III. Pathophysiology. Rubella virus is an RNA virus that typically has an epidemic seasonal pattern of increased frequency in the spring. Epidemics have occurred at 6- to 9-year intervals; major pandemics occur every 10 to 30 years. Humans are the only known hosts, with an incubation period of approximately 18 days following contact. The virus is spread by respiratory secretions and from stool, urine, and cervical secretions. A live virus vaccine has been available since 1969. Five to 20% of women of childbearing age are susceptible to rubella. The incidence of subclinical infections is high. Maternal viremia is a prerequisite for placental infection, which may or may not spread to the fetus. Most cases occur following primary disease. Maternal antibody to previous infection is protective for the fetus.

    The fetal infection rate varies, depending on the time of maternal infection during pregnancy. If infection occurs at 1–12 weeks, there is an 81% risk of fetal infection; at 13–16 weeks, 54% risk; at 17–22 weeks, 36% risk; at 23–30 weeks, 30% risk; a rise to 60% at 31–36 weeks; and 100% in the last month of pregnancy. No correlation exists between the severity of maternal rubella and teratogenicity. However, the incidence of fetal effects is greater the earlier in gestation infection occurs, especially at 1–8 weeks, when 85% of infected fetuses will be damaged. Rarely are rubella defects noted in those infected after the 16th week. The virus sets up chronic infection in the placenta and fetus. Placental or fetal infection may lead to resorption of the fetus, spontaneous abortion, stillbirth, fetal infection from multisystem disease, congenital anomalies, or inapparent infection.

    The pathology involves angiopathy as well as cytolytic changes. Other viral effects include chromosome breakage, decreased cell multiplication time, and mitotic arrest in certain cell types. There is little inflammatory reaction.

 IV. Risk factors. Women in the childbearing age group who are rubella nonimmune are at risk for rubella.

V. **Clinical presentation.** Congenital rubella has a wide spectrum of presentations, ranging from acute disseminated infection to deficits and defects not evident at birth.
   A. **Teratogenic effects** include intrauterine growth retardation, congenital heart disease (patent ductus arteriosus, pulmonary artery stenosis), sensorineural hearing loss, cataracts or glaucoma, neonatal purpura, dermatoglyphic abnormalities.
   B. **Systemic involvement** can be manifested by adenitis, hepatitis, hepatosplenomegaly, jaundice, anemia, decreased platelets with or without petechiae, bony lesions, encephalitis, meningitis, myocarditis, eye lesions (iridocyclitis, retinopathy), or pneumonia.
   C. **Later presenting defects.** More than one-half of all newborns with congenital rubella are normal at birth; however, the majority of these newborns later develop one or more signs and symptoms of the disease. Later presenting defects include immunologic dyscrasias, hearing deficit, psychomotor retardation, autism, brain syndromes such as subacute sclerosing panencephalitis, diabetes mellitus, and thyroid disease.

VI. **Diagnosis**
   A. **Laboratory studies**
      1. **Open cultures.** The virus can be cultured for up to 1 year despite a measurable antibody titer. The best specimens for viral recovery are from nasal pharyngeal swabs, conjunctival scrapings, urine, and cerebrospinal fluid (in decreasing order of usefulness).
      2. **Cerebrospinal fluid examination** may reveal encephalitis, with an increased protein:cellular ratio in some cases.
      3. **Serologic studies** may be helpful, but the disease itself may cause immunologic aberrations and delay the infant's ability to mount an IgM or IgG response. An IgM hemagglutination inhibition antibody test and an IgG hemagglutination inhibition titer are available.
   B. **Radiologic studies.** Long-bone x-ray studies may show metaphyseal radiolucencies that correlate with metaphyseal osteoporosis, caused by virus-induced inhibition of mitosis of bone-forming cells.

VII. **Management.** There is no specific treatment for rubella. Long-term follow-up is needed to detect late-onset symptoms. Prevention consists in vaccination of the susceptible population (especially young children). Vaccinations should not be given to pregnant women. Passive immunization does not prevent fetal infection when maternal infection occurs.

CYTOMEGALOVIRUS

I. **Definition.** Cytomegalovirus (CMV) is a DNA virus and a member of the herpesvirus group. It is an important cause of intrauterine infection in infants.

II. **Incidence.** In the United States, the incidence of congenital CMV infection is 1–2%.

III. **Pathophysiology.** CMV is a ubiquitous virus that may be transmitted in secretions, blood (white cells), and urine, and perhaps by sexual contact. More than 90% of primary CMV infections are asymptomatic. Infants with symptoms usually have a mononucleosis-like illness. Seroconversion and initial infection often occur around the time of puberty; shedding of the virus may continue for a long time. CMV can also become latent and reactivate periodically. Ten to 30% of pregnant women have cervical colonization with CMV. This virus is capable of penetrating the placental barrier as well as the blood-brain barrier. Both primary and recurrent maternal CMV can lead to transmission of the virus to the fetus. Infants with symptomatic disease usually are born to women with primary CMV infection. One to 2% of all newborns in the United States are infected with CMV and, of these, 10% are symptomatic and 90% have subclinical infection. **Symptomatic infants have a mortality rate of 20-30%.** Maternal virus-infected leukocytes are the proposed vehicle of transplacental transmission to the fetus. Fetal viremia is spread by the hematogenous route. The primary target organs are CNS, eye, liver, lung, and kidney. Characteristic histopathologic features of CMV include focal necrosis, inflammatory response, the formation of enlarged cells with intranuclear inclusions (cytomegalic cells), and the production of multinucleated giant cells. CMV may also be transmitted to the infant at delivery (if the mother has cervical colonization), via breast milk, and via transfusion of seropositive blood to an infant whose mother is seronegative.

IV. **Risk factors.** CMV infection in neonates has been associated with lower socioeconomic status, drug abuse, and sexual promiscuity of the mother. Premature infants are more often affected than full-term infants. Transfusion of unscreened blood is an additional risk factor for neonatal disease.

V. **Clinical presentation**

A. **Subclinical infection** is 10 times more common than clinical illness.

B. **Low birth weight.** Maternal CMV infection is associated with low birth weight and small-for-gestational-age (SGA) infants even when the infant is not infected.

C. **Classic cytomegalovirus inclusion disease** is rarely seen. It consists of intrauterine growth retardation, hepatosplenomegaly with jaundice, abnormal liver function tests, thrombocytopenia with or without purpura, and severe central nervous system disease including microcephaly, intracerebral calcifications (most characteristically in the subependymal area), chorioretinitis, and progressive sensorineural hearing loss (10-20% of cases). Other symptoms include hemolytic anemia and pneumonitis. By 2 years of age, 5-15% of infants who are asymptomatic at birth develop serious sequelae such as hearing loss or ocular abnormalities.

D. **Late sequelae.** With subclinical infection, late sequelae such as mental retardation, learning disability, and sensorineural hearing loss may be attributable to CMV infection.

VI. **Diagnosis**

A. **Laboratory studies**

1. **Urine culture for demonstration of the virus.** The "gold standard" for the diagnosis of CMV is urine culture. Most urine specimens from infants with congenital CMV are positive within 48-72 hours. Many laboratories now use a shell-vial tissue culture technique involving detection of CMV-induced antigens by monoclonal antibodies, allowing for identification of virus within 18 hours.

2. **Serologic tests** are available, but results may be hampered by the antigenic heterogeneity of the virus. A positive rheumatoid factor test is fairly specific but is positive in only 35-45% of cases. A complement fixation test that measures IgG will detect more than 75% of positive cases but also has a significant false-positive rate.

B. **Radiologic studies.** Skull x-ray films or CT scans of the head may demonstrate characteristic intracranial calcifications.

VII. **Management**

A. **Antiviral agents.** Treatment trials with available antivirals have only transiently altered viral excretion and have had little or no effect on the clinical course of the disease. Because of their appreciable side effects, antivirals should not be used. Limited clinical trials have begun with 2-candidate live attenuated vaccines.

B. **Prevention.** Affected infants may excrete the virus for months to years and are often a concern to personnel caring for them. In the nursery, they should be isolated, and people caring for these infants should use hand-washing, gowns, and gloves as protective measures. Sero-negative pregnant women should not have contact with these infants.

HERPES SIMPLEX

I. **Definition.** Herpes simplex virus (HSV) is a DNA virus related to cytomegalovirus, Epstein-Barr virus, and varicella virus. It is among the most prevalent of all viral infections encountered by humans.

II. **Incidence.** The estimated rate of occurrence of neonatal HSV is 1:1000 to 1:5000 deliveries per year.

III. **Pathophysiology.** Two serologic subtypes can be distinguished by antigenic and serologic tests: HSV-1 (orolabial) and HSV-2 (genital). Three-fourths of neonatal herpes infections are due to HSV-2; the remainder are caused by HSV-1. HSV-1, however, is the cause of 7–50% of primary genital herpes infections. HSV infection of the neonate can be acquired during one of 3 periods: intrauterine, intrapartum, or postnatal. Most infections are acquired in the intrapartum (80%) period as ascending infections with ruptured membranes (4–6 hours is considered a critical period for it to occur) or by delivery through an infected cervix or vagina. The usual portals of entry for the virus are the skin, eyes, mouth, and respiratory tract. Once colonization occurs, the virus may spread by contiguity or via a hematogenous route. The incubation period is from 2 to 20 days. The 3 general patterns of neonatal HSV infection are (1) disease localized to the skin, eyes, oral cavity, or central nervous system; (2) disseminated disease with or without central nervous system involvement; and (3) asymptomatic infection (less than 1%). Of infants born vaginally to mothers with a primary infection, 50% have HSV compared with only 4% of those born to mothers with recurrent infection. Maternal antibody is not necessarily protective in the fetus.

IV. **Risk factors.** The risk of genital herpes infection may vary with socioeconomic status and the number of sexual partners. Only approximately 40% of cases have signs or symptoms of genital herpes at labor and delivery despite having active infection. The primary infection may be active for as long as 2 months.

V. **Clinical presentation.** Subclinical HSV infections are very rare. The disease may be localized or disseminated. Humoral and cellular immune mechanisms appear important in preventing initial HSV infections or limiting its spread.

   A. **Localized infections** involving the skin, eyes, or oral cavity usually manifest at 10–11 days of age and account for approximately 20% of neonatal herpes. **Skin lesions** vary from discrete vesicles to large bullous lesions and occasionally denude the skin. Assertive **mouth lesions,** with or without cutaneous involvement, may be seen. **Ocular findings** include keratoconjunctivitis and chorioretinitis. About 25% of this group will subsequently develop neurologic abnormalities even though there is no evidence of CNS involvement in the neonatal period. A second group has localized **CNS involvement** with or without skin, eye, or mouth lesions. Clinical manifestations of encephalitis include seizures (focal and generalized), lethargy, irritability, tremors, poor feeding, temperature instability, bulging fontanelle, and pyramidal tract signs. These infants usually present at 15–17 days of age (one-third will have no herpetic skin lesions) and the mortality rate is about 17%; however, it may be as high as 50% in untreated patients. Of survivors, 40% have long-term neurologic sequelae, such as psychomotor retardation.

   B. **Disseminated disease** involves the **liver** and **adrenal glands** as well as virtually any other organ. Approximately one-half of these patients also have localized disease, as described above. Infants with disseminated HSV infection account for at least one-half of all neonatal herpes patients. Usually they present at 9–11 days of age. Presentation may include the signs and symptoms of localized disease as well as anorexia, vomiting, lethargy, fever, jaundice (with abnormal liver function tests), rash or purpura, apnea, respiratory distress, bleeding, and shock. Presentation with bleeding and cardiovascular collapse may be sudden and rapidly fatal. CNS involvement is present in two-thirds of these patients. Without antiviral therapy, 80% or more die, and most have serious neurologic sequelae. With appropriate treatment, the mortality rate decreases to 15–20%, and 40–55% of survivors suffer long-term neurologic impairment.

VI. Diagnosis
A. Laboratory studies
1. **Viral cultures.** The virus grows readily; preliminary results of culture are available in 24–72 hours. Cultures are usually obtained from the infant's conjunctiva, throat, feces, urine, nasal pharynx, and CSF.
2. **Tzanck smear.** Cytologic examination of the base of skin vesicles with a Giemsa or Wright stain looking for characteristic but nonspecific giant cells and eosinophilic intranuclear inclusions.
3. **Fluorescent antibody test** is becoming more readily available; however, it has a low sensitivity and perhaps increased false-positive results.
4. **Serologic tests** are virtually useless in the diagnosis of neonatal infection until a test for HSV IgM is available.
5. **Lumbar puncture** and CSF examination should be performed in all suspected cases. Evidence of hemorrhagic central nervous system infection (increased white and red cells and protein) is found.

B. Radiologic studies. CT scan of the head may be useful in the diagnosis of central nervous system disease, but MRI and electroencephalography (the EEG shows multiple independent foci of periodic slow and sharp wave discharge) are probably better for detecting earlier disease. In the neonate, central nervous system involvement is more diffuse than in older patients.

C. Other tests
1. **Brain biopsy** may be needed in certain cases to confirm the diagnosis; however, most clinicians currently recommend a trial of treatment before considering brain biopsy.
2. **Examination of parents.** The most valuable aid may be examination of the parents for lesions and questioning for a history of herpetic disease.

VII. Management
A. Antepartum and intrapartum treatments. The American College of Obstetrics and Gynecology (ACOG) has revoked previous guidelines of weekly antenatal surveillance cultures of the lower genital tract beginning at 36 weeks' gestation, because findings have little correlation with spreading of the virus at the time of delivery. Most infants with neonatal herpes are delivered to women with no history of infection and no lesions at delivery. Their current guidelines for management of genital herpes infection during pregnancy and at delivery recommend that a history of genital herpes in a pregnant woman or in her partner(s) be solicited and recorded in the prenatal record. If a positive history is obtained:
1. Weekly surveillance cultures during pregnancy are not necessary if there are no visible lesions.
2. To confirm the diagnosis, cultures should be done when there are active lesions during pregnancy. If there are no visible lesions at the onset of labor, vaginal delivery is acceptable.
3. In women with herpetic lesions of the genital tract when either labor

or membrane rupture occurs, cesarean section should be performed. Cesarean section should preferably be done within 4–6
hours of membrane rupture, but it may be beneficial in preventing
neonatal herpes regardless of the time that has passed since the
membranes ruptured. However, for patients with active HSV infection and extremely premature rupture of membranes (ie, at a remote
time from term), the risk of morbidity due to extreme immaturity
must be weighed against the risk of morbidity due to neonatal HSV
infection in deciding whether or not to perform cesarean section.

4. To identify potentially exposed neonates at the time of delivery, culture specimens should be obtained from the mother and the neonate. Neonatal cultures should be done at more than 24–48 hours
after delivery; earlier cultures may be surface contaminants.

B. Neonatal treatment

1. **Isolation.** Some controversy exists over strict isolation vs secretion
precautions. (Herpesvirus is coated with a lipid layer and is easily
killed with detergent soaps and water.)

2. **Pharmacologic therapy.** The drug of choice is **acyclovir,** with the
second choice being **vidarabine,** which requires 12-hour infusion
with a large volume of fluid. (See Chap 76 for dosages and other
pharmacologic information.)

3. **Feedings.** The infant may be breast-fed as long as no breast lesions
are present on the mother; the mother should be instructed in good
hand-washing technique.

VIRAL HEPATITIS

Hepatitis may be produced by many infectious and noninfectious agents. Typically, viral hepatitis refers to several clinically similar diseases of different
causes and epidemiology. These include hepatitis A, B, non-A, non-B, and D
(delta). All may be transmitted to the infant. The differential diagnosis of newborn liver disease includes neonatal hepatitis (giant cell), biliary atresia, other
infectious agents that cause hepatocellular injury, for example, cytomegalovirus (CMV), rubella, varicella, toxoplasmosis, *Listeria,* syphilis, and tuberculosis, as well as bacterial sepsis, which can cause nonspecific hepatic dysfunction. Table 63–1 outlines various hepatitis panel tests useful in the diagnosis
and management of this disease.

HEPATITIS A

I. **Definition.** Hepatitis A **(infectious hepatitis)** is caused by RNA virus transmitted by the fecal-oral route. A high concentration of virus is found in the
stools of infected persons; it has not been found in urine or other body
fluids. It causes the short-incubation form of viral hepatitis (15–50 days).
There is no chronic carrier state.

II. **Pathophysiology.** Pregnant women with hepatitis A usually do not transmit
the infection to their offspring. The risk of transmission is limited because
the period of viremia is short and fecal contamination does not occur at
delivery.

III. **Clinical presentation.** Most infants are asymptomatic and have only mild
abnormalities of liver function.

IV. **Diagnosis**

A. **IgM antibody to hepatitis A virus (HAV)** is present during the acute or
early convalescent phase of disease. IgG (anti-HAV) appears in the convalescent phase and remains detectable.

B. **Liver function tests.** Characteristically, the transaminases (AST [SGOT],

TABLE 63-1. HEPATITIS PANEL TESTS

Test	Comments
Hepatitis A virus (HAV)	Etiologic agent of "infectious" hepatitis.
Antibody to HAV (Anti-HAV)	Detectable at onset of symptoms; lifetime persistence.
IgM class antibody to HAV (IgM Anti-HAV)	Indicates recent infection. HAV positive up to 4 to 6 months after infection.
Hepatitis B virus (HBV)	Etiologic agent of "serum" hepatitis.
Hepatitis B surface antigen (HBsAg)	Detectable in serum; earliest indicator of acute infection or indicative of chronic infection; several subtypes identified.
Antibody to HBsAg (Anti-HBs)	Indicates past infection with (and immunity to) HBV, passive antibody from HBIG, or immune response from HBV vaccine.
Hepatitis Be antigen (HBeAG)	Correlates with HBV replication, high titer HBV in serum, and infectivity of serum.
Antibody to HBeAg (Anti-HBe)	Presence in carrier of HBsAg suggests lower titer of HBV and resolution of infection.
Hepatitis B core antigen (HBcAg)	No commercial test available.
Antibody to HBcAg (Anti-HBc)	Indicates past infection with HBV at undefined time.
IgM class antibody to HBcAg (IgM anti-HBc)	Indicates recent infection with HBV; positive for 4 to 6 months after infection.

ALT [SGPT]) and serum bilirubin levels (total and direct) are elevated, whereas the alkaline phosphatase level is normal.

V. Management

A. Maternal infection in the last trimester. If the mother had acute hepatitis A infection in the last trimester, the infant should be treated with **immune serum globulin (ISG),** 0.02 mL/kg intramuscularly, at birth. Development of a live attenuated HAV vaccine is an area of current research.

B. Isolation. The infant should be isolated, and enteric precautions should be taken.

NON-A, NON-B HEPATITIS

I. Definition. The majority of cases of non-A, non-B hepatitis have now been linked to hepatitis C virus. A small percentage of cases may be caused by other currently unidentified pathogens.

II. Pathophysiology. Primary infection in the infant is acquired by transfusion of infected blood or blood products. There is indirect evidence that maternal-to-infant transmission occurs during pregnancy or at delivery. Infection of the mother during the last trimester or at delivery is believed to carry the highest risk of transmission of infection to the infant.

III. Clinical presentation. At birth infants are asymptomatic, with elevation of liver-function tests. The incubation period is usually approximately 45 days but may range from 14–115 days. A chronic carrier state frequently develops and may cause significant chronic liver disease.

IV. Diagnosis. Recently, an anti-HCV antibody has been developed to screen for hepatitis C. Anti-HCV antibodies seem to be a reliable marker for non-A, non-B hepatitis. Liver function tests may be elevated and fluctuate widely with time.

V. Management. At birth the infant should be treated with **immune serum globulin (ISG),** 0.02 mL/kg intramuscularly; however, the efficacy of this treatment is unknown. The infant should be followed by means of routine serum alanine aminotransferase (ALT [SGPT]) levels.

HEPATITIS D

Hepatitis D, also known as *delta hepatitis,* is a defective RNA virus that cannot survive independently and requires the helper function of the DNA virus hepatitis B. Therefore hepatitis D occurs either as co-infection with hepatitis B or superinfection of a hepatitis B carrier. It has reportedly been transmitted from mother to infant. **Prevention** of hepatitis B infection will prevent hepatitis D. However, no treatments to prevent it in hepatitis B surface-antigen carriers before or after exposure are available. **Management** is similar to that for hepatitis B infection (see below).

HEPATITIS B

I. **Definition.** Hepatitis B **(serum hepatitis)** is caused by a double-shelled DNA virus. It has a long incubation period (45–160 days) after exposure.

II. **Pathophysiology.** If the mother is a chronic carrier, there is a substantial risk to the infant. HBeAg positivity in the mother is associated with an 80–90% chance of transmission to the infant. More than 85% of these infants will be chronic carriers. If the mother has antibody to HBeAg or no detectable HBe markers, the risk of transmission is only 25%. In the fetus and neonate, transmission has been suggested by the following mechanisms.

A. **Transplacental transmission** either during pregnancy or at delivery secondary to placental leaks.

B. **Natal transmission** by exposure to HBsAg in amniotic fluid, vaginal secretions, or maternal blood.

C. **Postnatal transmission** by fecal oral spread, blood transfusion, or other mechanisms.

III. **Risk factors**

A. **Factors associated with higher rates of HBV transmission to neonates** include:

1. Presence of HBe antigen and absence of anti-HBe in maternal serum (transmission rates of 80–95% [rate decreases 25% if anti-HBe antigen is present], with more than 85% of these infants being chronic carriers).

2. Asian racial origin, particularly Chinese (incidence of 40–70%).

3. Maternal acute hepatitis in third trimester or immediately postpartum (70% transmission rate).

4. Higher titer HBsAg in maternal serum (transmission rates parallel the titer).

5. Antigenemia present in older siblings.

B. **Factors not related to transmission** include:

1. The particular HBV subtype in mother.

2. Presence or absence of HB surface antigen in amniotic fluid.

3. Presence or titer or anti-HBc in cord blood.

IV. **Clinical presentation.** Maternal hepatitis B infection has not been associated with abortion, stillbirth, congenital malformations, or intrauterine growth retardation (IUGR). Prematurity has occurred, especially with acute hepatitis during pregnancy. Fetuses or newborns exposed to HBV present a wide spectrum of disease; the infants are rarely ill and usually are asymptomatic, with jaundice appearing less than 3% of the time. The various clinical presentations include:

A. Mild transient acute infection.

B. Chronic active hepatitis with or without cirrhosis.

C. Chronic persistent hepatitis.

D. Chronic asymptomatic HBsAg carrier state.

E. Fatal fulminant hepatitis B (rare).

V. **Diagnosis**

A. **Differential diagnosis.** Major diseases to consider include biliary atresia and acute hepatitis due to other viruses (hepatitis A, CMV, rubella, and HSV).

B. **Serum transaminases.** Serum AST (SGOT) and ALT (SGPT) levels may be markedly increased before the rise in serum bilirubin levels.

C. **Serum bilirubin (direct and indirect) levels** may be elevated. (The rise in the direct bilirubin level will occur later.)

D. **Liver biopsy** is occasionally indicated to differentiate biliary atresia from neonatal hepatitis.

E. **Hepatitis panel testing** (Table 63–1)
  1. **Mother.** Test for HBsAg, HBeAg, anti-HBe, and anti-HBc.
  2. **Infant.** Tests for HBsAg and anti-HBc. Most infants demonstrate antigenemia by 6 months of age, with peak acquisition at 3–4 months. Cord blood is not a reliable indicator of neonatal infection (a) because contamination could have occurred with antigen-positive maternal blood or vaginal secretions and (b) because of possible transmission of noninfectious antigenemia from the mother.

VI. **Management**

A. **HBsAg-positive mother.** If the mother is HBsAg-positive, regardless of the status of her HBe antigen or antibody, the **infant should be given hepatitis B immune globulin (H-BIG),** 0.5 mL intramuscularly, within 12 hours after delivery. **Additionally, hepatitis B vaccine** (plasma-derived or recombinant), 0.5 mL intramuscularly (anterolateral thigh), is given within 7 days and at 1 month and 6 months of age. If the first dose of hepatitis B vaccine is given simultaneously with HBIG, it should be administered at a separate site, preferably the opposite leg. HBIG and HB vaccinations do not interfere with routine childhood immunizations.

B. **Isolation.** Precautions are necessary in handling blood and secretions.

C. **Breast-feeding.** HBsAg has been detected in breast milk of HBsAg-positive mothers by means of special concentrating techniques. One study in Taiwan showed no difference in infection rates between bottle- and breast-fed infants. Because of the efficacy of HBV vaccine in combination with HBIG, even a theoretical risk of transmission through breast-feeding is of less concern.

D. **Follow-up.** At 12–15 months of age, the infant should be screened for HBsAg and anti-HBs antibody to confirm immunity. If HBsAg is not detectable and anti-HBs is present, the child can be considered protected. Long-term effects in infants who become carriers of the virus may include cirrhosis, hepatocellular carcinoma, or chronic hepatitis.

VARICELLA-ZOSTER INFECTIONS

Varicella-zoster (VZ) virus is a member of the herpesvirus family. There are 3 forms of varicella-zoster infections that may occur in the neonate: teratogenic, congenital, and postnatal. In the mother, infection is usually manifested as typical chickenpox or, occasionally, as herpes zoster, or shingles (intrauterine infection less common than with maternal varicella).

TERATOGENIC VARICELLA-ZOSTER INFECTION

I. **Definition.** This form occurs when the mother has her first exposure to VZ virus during pregnancy. Viremia occurs prior to the onset of rash, with fetal infection likely occurring during this time.

II. **Incidence.** Fortunately, this form is rare, since more than 95% of women in the USA are immune to varicella (only 30 reported cases as of 1987).

III. **Pathophysiology.** Transmission of the virus to the pregnant woman probably occurs via respiratory droplets. The virus replicates in the oropharynx, resulting in maternal viremia, with transplacental passage to the fetus. Almost all reported cases have involved exposure between the 8th and 20th weeks of pregnancy, except for one case at 28 weeks. Neonatal defects are the result of viral replication and destruction of developing fetal ectodermal tissue.

IV. **Clinical presentation.** Clinical examination of the neonate may disclose defects in a number of organ systems, as outlined below.
  A. **Limbs.** Hypoplasia or atrophy of an extremity, paralysis with muscular atrophy, and hypoplastic or missing fingers are frequent findings. These defects are caused by invasion of the brachial and lumbar plexus.
  B. **Eyes.** Microphthalmos, chorioretinitis, cataracts, optic atrophy, and Horner's syndrome (ptosis, miosis, enophthalmos) may all be seen.
  C. **Skin.** Findings are cicatricial skin lesions and the residua of infected bullous skin lesions.
  D. **Central nervous system.** Microcephaly, seizures, encephalitis, cortical atrophy, and mental retardation may be seen.
V. **Diagnosis**
  A. **Fluorescent antibody to membrane antigen (FAMA) test.** This test measures immune status only.
  B. **Serum VZ-specific IgM antibody test.** This test confirms VZ infection in the infant. It is performed at birth in any infant with suspected VZ infection.
VI. **Management**
  A. **Mother.** If the mother is exposed to VZ infection in the first or second trimester, some clinicians recommend treatment with **varicella-zoster immune globulin (VZIG)** if the history of varicella infection is negative or uncertain. It helps to reduce complications in the mother but not in the fetus. (See Chap 75 for dosage and other pharmacologic information.)
  B. **Infant.** Because there is usually profound neurologic impairment, supportive care of the infant is required. The infant often dies as a result of secondary infections. Survivors usually suffer profound mental retardation and major neurologic handicaps.
  Note: Isolation is not necessary.

CONGENITAL VARICELLA-ZOSTER INFECTION

I. **Definition.** This form of varicella-zoster infection occurs when a pregnant women suffers chickenpox during the last 14 to 21 days of pregnancy or within the first few days postpartum. Onset of disease in the neonate is within the first 10 days of life.
II. **Incidence.** Although the congenital form is more common than the teratogenic form, it is still rare—only 0.7 per thousand pregnant women develop chickenpox.
III. **Pathophysiology.** One of 4 newborns will become infected when maternal varicella occurs during the last 3 weeks of pregnancy. If the infant is born within 5 days of the onset of rash in the mother, the disease will be more severe, since there is insufficient time for maternal antibody formation; the resulting death rate is 30% in affected infants. If the onset of maternal disease is more than 5 days before delivery or onset of neonatal disease is within the first 4 days, transplacental antibody transmission occurs and fetal deaths are infrequent.
IV. **Clinical presentation.** There may be only mild involvement of the infant, with vesicles on the skin, or the following presentations may be seen.
  A. **Skin.** A centripetal rash (initially on the trunk and spreading to the face and scalp, sparing the extremities) begins as red macules and progresses to vesicles and encrustation. Lesions are more common in the diaper area and skin folds. There may be 2 or 3 lesions or thousands of them. The main complication is secondary staphylococcal or streptococcal skin infection, or both. (Septicemia was seen in fewer than 0.5% of patients in one study.)
  B. **Lungs.** Lung involvement is seen in all fatal cases. It usually appears

2–4 days after the onset of the rash but may be seen up to 10 days after. Signs include fever, cyanosis, rales, and hemoptysis. A chest x-ray film shows a diffuse nodular-miliary pattern, especially in the perihilar region.

C. **Other organs.** Focal necrosis may be seen in the liver, adrenals, intestines, kidneys, and thymus. Glomerulonephritis, myocarditis, encephalitis, and cerebellar ataxia are sometimes seen.

V. **Diagnosis.** Diagnosis of VZ is usually based on clinical findings only; laboratory confirmation is seldom needed. However, if the diagnosis is in question, the following studies may be performed.

A. **Tzanck smear** will demonstrate **multinucleated giant cells with intracellular inclusions** consistent with herpesvirus infection.

B. **Cultures.** VZ virus can be isolated from cultures of vesicular lesions during the first 3 days of the rash.

VI. **Management**

A. **Varicella-zoster immune globulin (VZIG)**

1. **Perinatal infection.** Infants of mothers who develop VZ infection within 5 days before or 48 hours after delivery should receive 125 units VZIG as soon as possible and not later than 96 hours after delivery (see Chap 75). These infants should be placed in strict respiratory isolation for 28 days after receiving VZIG, since treatment will prolong the incubation period. VZIG does not reduce the clinical attack rate in treated newborns; however, treated newborns tend to develop milder infections than untreated neonates.

2. **Maternal rash occurring more than 5 days before delivery.** Infants of mothers who develop a rash more than 5 days before delivery or more than 48 hours after delivery do not need VZIG. It is felt that these infants will have received antibodies via the placenta.

B. **Vidarabine and acyclovir** may be used in severely affected infants to decrease the chance of dissemination and shorten the duration of skin lesions. Dosages and other pharmacologic information are in Chapter 76.

C. **Use of antibiotics** is indicated if secondary bacterial skin infections occur.

D. **Serum test for varicella-zoster antibodies.** Performance of this test during the acute and convalescent periods documents resolution of the infection.

POSTNATAL VARICELLA-ZOSTER INFECTION

I. **Definition.** This form of the disease presents on days 10–28 of life. It does not represent transplacental infection from the mother.

II. **Pathophysiology.** Postnatal VZ infection occurs by droplet transmission. It is more common than congenital chickenpox. Postnatal varicella-zoster is usually mild because of passive protection from maternal antibodies.

III. **Clinical presentation.** The typical chickenpox rash is seen with centripetal spread, beginning on the trunk, spreading to the face and scalp, and sparing the extremities. All stages of the rash may appear at the same time, from red macules to clear vesicles to crusting lesions. Complications of this form of the disease are rare but may include secondary infections and varicella pneumonia.

IV. **Diagnosis.** Diagnosis is the same as that for congenital varicella-zoster (see p 351, **V**).

V. **Management.** This form of the disease is usually mild; death is extremely rare.

A. **VZIG** is recommended for infants less than 28 weeks' gestational age or weighing 1000 g or less, regardless of the maternal history. It is also recommended in premature infants whose mothers do not have a history of chickenpox. (See Chap 75 for dosage and other pharmacologic information.)

B. Infants of greater than 28 weeks' gestation should have sufficient transplacental antibodies if the mother is immune to protect them from the risk of complications.

C. Isolation. Exposed infants should be placed in strict isolation for 10–21 days after the onset of the rash in the index case. Exposed infants who receive VZIG should be in strict respiratory isolation for 28 days.

SYPHILIS

I. **Definition.** Syphilis is a sexually transmitted disease caused by *Treponema pallidum*. **Early congenital syphilis** is when clinical manifestations occur before 2 years of age; **late congenital syphilis** is when manifestations occur at greater than 2 years of age.

II. **Pathophysiology.** Treponemas appear able to cross the placenta at any time during pregnancy, thereby infecting the fetus. Syphilis can cause preterm delivery, stillbirth, congenital infection, or neonatal death, depending on the stage of maternal infection and duration of fetal infection prior to delivery. Untreated infection in the first and second trimester often leads to significant fetal morbidity, whereas with third-trimester infection, many infants are asymptomatic. Infection can also be acquired by the neonate via contact of infectious lesions during passage through the birth canal. Virtually all infants born to untreated women with primary and secondary syphilis will have congenital infection, with 50% clinically symptomatic. Infection rate is only 40% with early latent disease and 6–14% with late latent stages. Mortality may be as high as 54% in infected infants.

III. **Clinical presentation.** Generally neonates do not have signs of primary syphilis from infection acquired in utero. Their manifestations are systemic—similar to those of adults with secondary syphilis. There is an additional 40–60% chance of CNS involvement. Most common findings in the neonatal period include hepatosplenomegaly, jaundice, and osteochondritis. Other signs include generalized lymphadenopathy, pneumonitis, myocarditis, nephrosis, pseudoparalysis (atypical Erbs palsy), rash (vesicobullous, especially palms and soles), hemolytic anemia (normocytic, normochromic), leukemoid reaction, hemorrhagic rhinitis (snuffles). Late congenital syphilis is manifested as Hutchinson's teeth, healed retinitis, eighth-nerve deafness, saddle nose, mental retardation, arrested hydrocephalus, saber shins. Other clues to the diagnosis of congenital syphilis include placentomegaly or congenital hydrops.

IV. **Diagnosis**

A. **Laboratory studies.** Patients with congenital or acquired syphilis produce several different antibodies that are classified as nonspecific, nontreponemal antibody (NTA) or specific antitreponemal antibody (STA). NTA tests are inexpensive, rapid, and convenient screening tests that may indicate disease activity. They test the patient's serum or cerebrospinal fluid (CSF) for its ability to flocculate a suspension of a cardiolipin-cholesterol lecithin antigen. They are used as initial screening tests and quantitatively to follow the patient's response to treatment. False-positive reactions can be secondary to autoimmune disease, intravenous drug addiction, aging, pregnancy, and many infections such as hepatitis, mononucleosis, and endocarditis.

1. **Nonspecific reagin antibody tests.** The 2 most used of these nonspecific reagin antibody tests are:

a. **Venereal Disease Research Laboratory (VDRL) slide test.** A VDRL titer at least 2 dilutions (fourfold) higher in the infant than in the mother signifies probable active infection. Titers should be followed and repeated. If titers decrease in the first 8 months of life, the infant is probably not infected.

    b. Rapid plasma reagin (RPR) test. This nontreponemal test detects cardiolipid antibodies and is a screening test for syphilis. It should not be used on spinal fluid. Any positive test should be followed up with an FTA-ABS test. Titers can also be reported, as for VDRL.

2. Specific treponemal tests. Specific STA tests verify current or past infection. These tests should be performed if nontreponemal tests are positive.

    a. Fluorescent treponemal antibody absorption test (FTA-ABS test) may be positive in the infant if transfer of IgG from the mother to the neonate has occurred. If positivity persists after 6–12 months, the infant is probably infected.

    b. Microhemagglutination test for *T pallidum* (MHATP) uses less serum and is easier than FTA to perform; however, it may be less sensitive in early disease. It should be quantitative, as it can include IgG antibodies that crossed the placenta.

    c. IgM FTA-ABS test measures antibody to the treponeme developed in the infant. It is not as specific as initially thought; false-positive results may occur. The test must be done at the Centers for Disease Control.

3. Microscopic darkfield examination should be performed on appropriate lesions for spirochetes.

4. Complete blood count and differential. Monocytosis is typically seen; look for hemolytic anemia or leukemoid reaction.

5. Lumbar puncture. Central nervous system disease may be detected by positive serologic tests, darkfield examination positive for spirochetes, elevated monocyte count, or elevated CSF protein levels. A finding of fluorescent treponemal antibodies on CSF examination is not reliable.

B. Radiologic studies. X-ray studies of the long bones may show sclerotic changes of the metaphysis and diaphysis, with widespread osteitis and periosteitis.

V. Management

A. Treated mother. Infants born to mothers who received adequate penicillin treatment for syphilis during pregnancy are at minimal risk. An infant should be treated if maternal treatment was inadequate, unknown, or given during the last 4 weeks of pregnancy or if a drug other than penicillin was used. In a pregnant woman who has been treated for syphilis, quantitative NTA tests should be done monthly for the rest of her pregnancy.

B. VDRL-positive infant. Infants with positive VDRL tests, even if the results are only an indication of maternal transfer of IgG, should be treated if adequate follow-up is not possible.

C. Definitive treatment. See Chapter 76 for drug dosages and other pharmacologic information.

    1. CSF studies normal. A single dose of penicillin G benzathine, 50,000 units/kg intramuscularly, is given.

    2. CSF studies abnormal. Penicillin G procaine, 50,000 units/kg intramuscularly daily, is given for at least 10 days.

D. Isolation procedures. Precautions regarding drainage, secretions, and blood and body fluids are indicated for all infants with suspected or proven congenital syphilis until therapy has been given for 24 hours.

E. Follow-up care. The infant should have repeated quantitative NTA tests at 3, 6, and 12 months. Most infants will develop a negative titer with adequate treatment. A rising titer requires further investigation and re-treatment.

GONORRHEA

I. **Definition.** Infection with **Neisseria gonorrhoeae,** a gram-negative diplo-coccus, is the most commonly reported communicable disease. Infection in pregnancy is important because of transmission to the fetus.

II. **Incidence.** Prevalence of gonococcal infection among pregnant women varies from 0.6% or less to 7.6% or greater, depending on the population. Approximately 30–35% of neonates acquire infection during vaginal deliv-ery from infected mothers.

III. **Pathophysiology.** N gonorrhoeae primarily affects the endocervical canal. The infant may become infected during passage through an infected cervi-cal canal or by contact with contaminated amniotic fluid if rupture of the membranes has occurred.

IV. **Clinical presentations**

A. **Ophthalmia neonatorum.** The most common clinical manifestation is gonococcal ophthalmia neonatorum. If appropriate eye prophylaxis is given, this disorder occurs in fewer than 2% of cases of positive mater-nal gonococcal infection. For a description of this disease, see p 188.

B. **Gonococcal arthritis.** The onset of gonococcal arthritis can be at any time from 1 to 4 weeks after delivery. It is secondary to gonococcemia. The source of bacteremia has been attributed to infection of the mouth, nares, and umbilicus. The most common sites are the knees and ankles, but any joint may be affected. The infant may present with mild or moderate symptoms. Drainage and antibiotics are necessary.

C. **Amniotic infection syndrome** occurs when there is premature rupture of the membranes, with inflammation of the placenta and umbilical cord. The infant may develop clinical evidence of sepsis. Fluid obtained by gastric aspiration is usually positive for gonococci. This infection is associated with a high infant mortality rate.

D. **Meningitis.**

E. **Scalp abscess** is usually secondary to intrauterine fetal monitoring.

F. **Stomatitis.**

V. **Diagnosis**

A. **Mother.** Endocervical scrapings should be obtained for culture.

B. **Infant**

1. **Gram's stain** of any exudate, if present, should be obtained.

2. **Culture.** Material may be obtained by swabbing the eye or nasophar-ynx or the orogastric or anorectal areas. Blood should be obtained for culture.

3. **Cerebrospinal fluid studies.** Cell count and differential, Gram's stain, protein, glucose, and culture should be ordered.

VI. **Management**

A. **Antibiotic therapy.** (See also Chap 76.)

1. **Maternal infection.** Infection does not develop in most infants born to mothers with gonococcal infection. However, some cases have been reported and it is recommended that full-term infants receive a single injection of penicillin G, 50,000 units intramuscularly, and that premature infants receive 20,000 units intramuscularly.

2. **Ophthalmia.** Give penicillin G, 50,000 units/kg intravenously every 12 hours for 7–10 days, plus saline irrigations. For penicillin-resistant strains, give ceftriaxone, 50 mg/kg/d intramuscularly once daily for 7 days.

3. **Arthritis and septicemia.** Give penicillin G, 75,000–100,000 units/kg/d intravenously in 4 doses for 7 days. (Alternatively, give ceftriaxone, 50 mg/kg/d intravenously or intramuscularly once a day for 7–10 days.)
4. **Meningitis.** Give penicillin G, 100,000–150,000 units/kg/d in 4 divided doses for at least 10 days.

B. **Isolation.** All infants with gonococcal infection should be placed in contact isolation until effective parenteral antimicrobial therapy has been given for 24 hours.

CHLAMYDIAL INFECTION

I. **Definition.** *Chlamydia trachomatis* is a highly specialized gram-negative bacterium that possesses a cell wall, contains DNA and RNA, and can be inactivated by several antimicrobial agents. Due to its inability to generate adenosine triphosphate, however, it is an obligate intracellular parasite. It may cause urethritis, cervicitis, urethral symptoms, and salpingitis in the mother. In the infant, it may cause conjunctivitis and pneumonia.

II. **Incidence.** Chlamydial infection is currently the most common sexually transmitted disease. The risk of infection in infants born to infected mothers is 50–75%; conjunctivitis occurs in 20–50%, and pneumonia in about 30%. Cervical chlamydial infection varies widely, depending on the population, with a significantly increased incidence in young, low socioeconomic, and nonwhite populations (2–37%).

III. **Pathophysiology.** *C trachomatis* subtypes B–K cause the sexually transmitted form of the disease and the associated neonatal infection. These subtypes frequently cause a benign subclinical infection. The infant acquires infection during vaginal delivery through an infected cervix. Infection after cesarean section is rare and usually occurs only with early rupture of amniotic membranes.

IV. **Clinical presentation**
A. **Conjunctivitis.** See Chapter 33.
B. **Pneumonia.** *C trachomatis* is one of the most common causes of pneumonia in the first 3 months of life. The respiratory tract may be directly infected during delivery. Approximately half of infants presenting with pneumonia will have concurrent or previous conjunctivitis. Pneumonia usually presents at 3–11 weeks of life. A gradual increase in symptoms occurs over several weeks. Initially, there is often 1–2 weeks of mucoid rhinorrhea, followed by cough and increasing respiratory rate. More than 95% of infants are afebrile. The cough is characteristic—paroxysmal and staccato; it interferes with sleeping and eating. These infants may also have pulmonary congestion, and apnea may be present; however, the congestion tends to be associated with secondary infection.
C. **Otitis media** occurs in about one-third of infants with chlamydial infection.

V. **Diagnosis**
A. **Laboratory studies**
1. **Rapid screening tests.** Two rapid screening tests for *Chlamydia trachomatis* utilize direct smears of the conjunctiva or nasopharynx.
  a. **Fluorescent monoclonal antibody test (Microtrak)** takes only 30 minutes.
  b. **Enzyme immunoassay technique (Chlamydiazyme)** takes approximately 3 hours.
2. **Culture of respiratory tract.** Material should be obtained for culture by nasopharyngeal aspiration or deep suctioning of the trachea.
3. **IgM antibody to C trachomatis (pneumonia).** Either a significant rise in or high levels of the titer (1:64) indicate infection.

    4. Gram's stain of eye discharge. (See p 189, B.1.)
    5. Other tests. In pneumonia, the **white blood count** is normal, but there is eosinophilia in 70% of cases. **Blood gas measurements** show mild to moderate hypoxia.
  B. Radiologic studies. In cases of pneumonia, a **chest x-ray film** may reveal hyperexpansion of the lungs, with bilateral symmetric interstitial or alveolar infiltrates.
VI. Management
  A. Prevention. For high-risk mothers, a **cervical culture for** *Chlamydia* should be obtained and treatment of the mother should begin before delivery. After birth, use of **erythromycin eye drops** instead of silver nitrate drops will prevent conjunctivitis in the infant.
  B. Conjunctivitis. See Chapter 33.
  C. Pneumonia. Give **erythromycin,** 50 mg/kg/d in 3 divided doses for 14 days. This regimen will not only shorten the clinical course but will decrease the duration of nasopharyngeal shedding. No isolation measures are necessary. (See also Chap 76 for pharmacologic information about erythromycin.)

ACQUIRED IMMUNODEFICIENCY SYNDROME (AIDS)

  I. Definition. AIDS was originally recognized as a clinical entity in 1981 and was later found to be the end-stage of infection with human immunodeficiency virus (HIV), formerly known as HTLV-III, lymphadenopathy AIDS virus (LAV), and AIDS-associated retrovirus (ARV). HIV is a member of the lentivirus, or slow virus, a subgroup of retroviruses. Terminology has been confusing; *HIV infection* covers the entire spectrum of stages of the infection, ranging from apparently nonsymptomatic to critically ill, with *AIDS* being the most severe syndrome caused by HIV infection. As of April 1991, 171,865 cases of HIV infection in adults and adolescents and 3028 cases in children under 13 years of age have been reported.

  II. Incidence. Some authorities project that as many as 10,000 to 20,000 cases of AIDS will occur in the next several years. Currently, approximately 78% of HIV-infected children have acquired the infection perinatally: 13% received contaminated blood products; 5% were infected during treatment of hemophilia or other coagulation disorder. With improved control of the blood supply, the perinatal route will probably constitute the sole route of acquisition of pediatric AIDS in the future.

  III. Pathophysiology. HIV infects T_4 (helper) lymphocytes. The virus selectively inhibits the growth of T_4 lymphocytes and eventually destroys these inducer and helper T cells, although it probably remains latent in a few cells. In children, the loss of T_4 lymphocytes leads initially to lack of direction to B cells, which produce large amounts of nonspecific and ineffective immunoglobulins. Profound defects and cell-mediated immunity occur as well, allowing a predisposition to opportunistic infections such as fungal and *Pneumocystis carinii* infections. The virus can also invade the central nervous system and produce psychosis and brain atrophy.

  IV. Risk factors
    A. High-risk mother. Any infant born to a high-risk mother is at risk. High-risk mothers include intravenous drug users, hemophiliacs, spouses of bisexual males, women from areas where the disease is more prevalent in heterosexuals, and spouses of hemophiliacs. The rate of transmission is between 0% and 65%, although the timing of mother-to-child transmission is unknown. Transplacental infection is possible; the virus has been identified in 13- to 20-week abortae as well as in the thymus of a 20-day-old infant who had been born at 28 weeks' gestation.

B. **Blood transfusion.** Approximately 15–18% of pediatric AIDS cases have been attributed to blood transfusion. Screening of blood donors has reduced but not totally eliminated the risk, because some newly infected persons are viremic but seronegative for 2–4 months and because some infected persons (5–15%) are seronegative.

C. **Breast milk.** The HIV virus has been isolated in breast milk. In one case, the mother received a blood transfusion after delivery from a person who later developed AIDS. The mother breast-fed her infant, and both were seropositive for AIDS. Although transmission to infants through breast milk is believed to be rare, it is recommended that in developed countries with safe alternative nutrition, the infected mother not breast-feed.

V. **Clinical presentation.** The clinical presentation depends on the severity of the disease.

A. **Age.** Symptoms of HIV disease are generally evident between 4 and 6 months of age, but their onset has been delayed up to 7 years. The interval between HIV infection and the onset of symptoms and of AIDS is shorter in children infected congenitally than in those infected by transfusion and is shorter in children than in adults.

B. **Symptoms and signs.** The infant may be asymptomatic or may have low birth weight, weight loss, failure to thrive, recurrent infections or episodes of otitis media, diarrhea, persistent candidiasis, hepatosplenomegaly, lymphadenopathy, neutropenia, thrombocytopenia, interstitial pneumonitis, chronic eczematoid dermatitis, or fever. The course of the disease is variable, and long asymptomatic periods sometimes occur. In general, the course is ultimately characterized by progressive immune dysfunction and clinical deterioration.

C. **AIDS-related complex (ARC).** AIDS-related complex is associated with generalized lymphadenopathy, recurrent fevers, and mild immune dysfunction. Infants with ARC do not have opportunistic infections.

D. **Characteristic craniofacial appearance.** A characteristic craniofacial pattern has been described in infants infected with HIV (Marion, 1987). Specificity has not been confirmed. Craniofacial features include the following.
1. Microcephaly.
2. Prominent boxlike forehead.
3. Flattened nasal bridge that appears scooped-out in profile.
4. Mild upward or downward obliquity of the eyes.
5. Prominent palpebral fissures, with blue scleras.
6. Ocular hypertelorism.
7. Short nose with flattened columella.
8. Well-formed triangular philtrum with patulous lips.

VI. **Diagnosis.** Diagnosis is based on (1) suspicion of infection because of epidemiologic risk or clinical presentation and (2) confirmation by serologic tests.

A. **All other causes of immunodeficiency must be excluded.** These causes include both primary and secondary immunodeficiency states. Primary immunodeficiency diseases include DiGeorge's syndrome, Wiskott-Aldrich syndrome, ataxia-telangiectasia, agammaglobulinemia, severe combined immunodeficiency, and neutrophil function abnormality. Secondary immunodeficiency states include those caused by immunosuppresive therapy, starvation, and lymphoreticular cancer.

B. **Laboratory findings**
1. **Positive test for HIV antibody.** The **enzyme-linked immunoassay (ELISA) test** is most commonly used. If it is positive, it should be confirmed by a **Western blot antibody test** after a repeat ELISA is performed. Seropositivity may be secondary to maternal transfer of

IgG. It is estimated that 15 months are required before demonstration of antibody against HIV indicates infant infection. Some infected infants show a delayed or absent anti-HIV antibody. The status of the infant is indeterminate until follow-up tests are performed. No IgM-specific antibody test is used commercially as yet.

2. Abnormal B-lymphocyte activity.
3. High immunoglobulin levels of IgG and IgA (also IgD and IgM) may be an early finding.
4. Circulating immune complexes.
5. Absolute lymphopenia less than 1500 (more common in adults).
6. Thrombocytopenia with normal platelet size.
7. Other test results that may be helpful in diagnosis, usually later in the clinical course, are the following.
   a. Decreased numbers of T cells or T helper (T_4) cells.
   b. A reversed T helper to T suppressor (T_4:T_8) ratio. (Decline in helper T cells and an increase in suppressor T cells—ratio less than 1.)
   c. A decreased proliferative response to mitogens.
   d. Cutaneous anergy to delayed hypersensitivity antigens.

C. **Presence of a "marker" disease** that indicates cellular immunodeficiency. Marker diseases include candidiasis, cryptococcisis, *Mycobacterium avium* infection, Epstein-Barr virus infection, *Pneumocystis carinii* pneumonia, strongyloidiasis, and Kaposi's sarcoma. Cytomegalovirus infection is considered a marker disease if it occurs more than 6 months after birth, and toxoplasmosis if it occurs more than 1 month after birth.

VII. Management

A. **Prevention.** Currently, there is no highly effective treatment for AIDS; thus, prevention is paramount. An infected woman should avoid pregnancy. Testing of blood donors will help decrease the risk associated with transfusion. Transfusions should be avoided unless clinically indicated. Plasma protein fraction (Plasmanate) should be used instead of fresh-frozen plasma unless there is a documented clotting deficiency.

B. **General supportive care**
   1. Treat recurrent secondary infections aggressively.
   2. The efficacy of monthly administrations of parenteral gamma globulin, interferon, or interleukin 2 for the primary infection is under study.
   3. Irradiate blood or blood products to prevent graft-vs-host disease.

C. **Management during delivery.** The following procedures are recommended for delivery of an infant born to a mother with proven infection or one who is a member of a high-risk group.
   1. Wear gown and gloves.
   2. If meconium aspiration occurs, perform intubation and suction with suction equipment or a DeLee apparatus.
   3. Items soiled by blood or amniotic fluid should be handled and disposed of according to routine procedures for contaminated material.

D. **Postdelivery management**
   1. Thoroughly clean off amniotic fluid and blood from the infant.
   2. Isolate the infant with the same precautions as for hepatitis B (precautions against transmission through blood and secretions).
   3. Send serum for HIV antibody testing (State laws vary on requirements of consent for testing as well as on confidentiality required.)
   4. Make certain the infant has the best possible follow-up care.
   5. Perform and repeat HIV antibody testing at 6 months and 12 months

after birth. A positive test at birth may result from passive transfer of antibody from the mother; if the test is negative at 6 and 12 months, it confirms passive transfer. If the test is positive at birth and continues to be positive at 6 and 12 months, the infant has a primary infection and requires close follow-up.

E. **Antiretroviral treatment.** Azidothymidine (AZT), now known as **zidovudine,** first used in pediatrics in 1986, was administered via continuous intravenous infusion. Children with neurodevelopmental abnormalities improved on this therapy, and most patients also had increased appetite and weight gain. In some children a discordant response, that is, improved neurodevelopment but progression at other organ sites, occurred. The pharmacokinetics of zidovudine in children are similar to those in adults. Because of the short half-life of the drug, development of a sustained release formulation will be necessary for oral use to be possible. The question of when to begin treatment in children remains. It is currently being studied in newborns, especially the possibility of chemoprophylaxis, although determination of the exact time of transmission to the fetus or neonate will be important. Prolonged use of zidovudine is limited because of bone marrow toxicity (decreased red blood cells and white blood cells). Current studies on 2'3' dideoxycytidine, with and without alternating its use with zidovudine, may help diminish toxicity and increase effectiveness of both agents. Further studies of zidovudine in children will be needed to define the optimal route of administration, dosage, and efficacy in various clinical settings.

LYME DISEASE

Lyme disease is caused by the spirochete *Borrelia burgdorfi* and is transmitted by the bite of a deer tick. Over 90% of cases have been reported in the Northeast coastal states. Diagnosis in the adult is made on the basis of clinical findings (flulike symptoms, skin lesions of erythema chronicum migrans, joint pain and swelling), because many diagnostic tests are often negative during active disease.

Transplacental transmission to neonates has been reported; however, the Centers for Disease Control has concluded that none of the adverse outcomes in these newborns could be definitively linked to Lyme disease. In the few reported cases of maternal-fetal transmission, problems in the infants have included stillbirths, heart diseases, and respiratory distress syndrome. Although prevention of maternal exposure is paramount, many obstetricians prescribe prophylactic antibiotics (amoxicillin, penicillin, erythromycin) for tick bites during pregnancy (see Chap 76 for dosages and other pharmocologic information). If there is concern that an infant has been born with Lyme disease, the CDC recommends treatment with the same regimen as that for congenital syphilis (p 352).

REFERENCES

Andiman WA: Virologic and serologic aspect of human immunodeficiency virus infection in infants and children. *Semin Perinatol* 1989;**13**:16.

Arvin AM et al: Consensus: Management of the patient with herpes simplex encephalitis. *J Pediatr Inf Dis* 1987;**6**:2.

Baley JE: Neonatal sepsis: The potential for immunotherapy. *Clin Perinatol* 1988;**15**:755.

Balfour HH et al: Antiviral drugs in pediatrics. *Am J Dis Child* 1989;**143**:1307.

Balis FM et al: Pharmacokinetics of zidovudine administered intravenously and orally in children with immunodeficiency virus infection. *J Pediatr* 1989;**114**:880.

Balisteri W: Viral hepatitis. *Pediatr Clin North Am* 1988;**35**:375.

Blanche S et al: A prospective study of infants born to women seropositive for human immunodeficiency virus type I. *N Engl J Med* 1989;**320**:1643.

Bradley JS: Neonatal infections. *J Pediatr Inf Dis* 1985;**4**:315.

Chirico G et al: Intravenous gammaglobulin therapy for prophylaxis of infection in high-risk neonates. *J Pediatr* 1987;**110**:437.

Christensen RD et al: Granulocyte transfusions in neonates with bacterial infection, neutropenia, and depletion of mature marrow neutrophils. *Pediatrics* 1987;**70**:1.

Dillon HC: Group B streptococcal carriage and disease: A 6-year prospective study. *J Pediatr* 1987;**110**:31.

Donowitz LG: Practical infection control for human immunodeficiency virus infection in children. *J Pediatr Inf Dis* 1989;**8**:133.

Falloon J et al: Human immunodeficiency virus infection in children. *J Pediatr* 1989;**114**:1.

Feinkind L et al: HIV in Pregnancy. *Clin Perinatol* 1988;**15**:189.

First 100,000 cases of acquired immunodeficiency syndrome—United States. *MMWR* (Aug) 1989:561.

Freij BJ: Herpesvirus infections in pregnancy: Risks to embryo, fetus, and neonate. *Clin Perinatol* 1988;**15**:203.

Freij BJ et al: Maternal rubella and the congenital rubella syndrome. *Clin Perinatol* 1988;**15**:247.

Grossman M: Human immunodeficiency virus infections in children: Public health and public policy issues. *J Pediatr Inf Dis* 1987;**6**:113.

Hall RT et al: Characteristics of coagulase-negative staphylococci from infants with bacteremia. *J Pediatr Inf Dis* 1987;**6**:377.

Hammerschlag MR: Chlamydial infections. *J Pediatr* 1989;**114**:727.

Hodgman JE: Sepsis in the neonate. *Perinatol Neonatal* 1981;**5**:45.

Johnson JP: Natural history of serologic diagnosis of infants born to human immunodeficiency virus–infected women. *Am J Dis Child* 1989;**143**:1147.

Kinney JS et al: Should we expand the TORCH complex? *Clin Perinatol* 1988;**15**:727.

Koskiniemi M et al: Neonatal herpes simplex virus infection: Report of 43 patients. *J Pediatr Inf Dis* 1989;**8**:30.

Lee RV: Parasites and pregnancy: Problems of malaria and toxoplasmosis. *Clin Perinatol* 1988;**15**:351.

Manroe BL et al: Neonatal blood count in health and disease. Reference values for neutrophilic cells. *J Pediatr* 1979;**95**:85.

Marion RW et al: Fetal AIDS syndrome score. *Am J Dis Child* 1987;**14**:429.

McDonald LK et al: Lack of toxicity in two cases of neonatal acyclovir overdose. *J Pediatr Inf Dis* 1989;**8**:529.

Nelson SN et al: Early onset group B streptococcal disease: Is it underdiagnosed? *J Perinatol* 1986;**6**:234.

Oxtoby MJ: Human immunodeficiency virus and other viruses in human milk: Placing the issues in broader perspective. *J Pediatr Inf Dis* 1988;**7**:825.

Perinatal herpes simplex virus infections. *ACOG Technical Bulletin;* No. 122, Nov, 1988.

Pickering LK: Management of the infant of a mother with viral hepatitis. *Pediatr Rev* 1988;**9**:315.

Pizzo PA: Emerging concepts in the treatment of HIV infection in Children. *JAMA* 1989;**262**:14.

Pizzo PA et al: Effect of continuous intravenous infusion of zidovudine (AZT) in children with symptomatic HIV infection. *N Engl J Med* 1988;**319**:889.

Recommendations of the Immunization Practices Advisory Committee: Prevention of perinatal transmission of hepatitis B virus: Prenatal screening of all pregnant women for hepatitis B surface antigen. MMWR 1988;**37**:22.

Remington JS, Klein JO: Bacterial sepsis and meningitis. Chap 18, p 601 in: *Infectious Diseases of Fetus and Newborn Infant,* 3rd ed. Saunders; 1990.

Remington JS, Klein JO: Gonococcal infection. Chap 26, p 848 in: *Infectious Diseases of the Fetus and Newborn Infant,* 3rd ed. Saunders; 1990.

Rettig PJ: Infections due to chlamydia trachomatis from infancy to adolescence. *J Pediatr Inf Dis* 1986;**5**:449.

Rettig PJ: Perinatal infections with chlamydia trachomatis. *Clin Perinatol* 1988;**15**:321.

Rodriguez EM et al: Diagnostic methods for chlamydia trachomatis disease in neonates. *J Perinatol* 1987;**11**:232.

Sarff LD et al: Cerebrospinal fluid evaluation in neonates: Comparison of high-risk infants with and without meningitis. *J Pediatr* 1976;**88**:473.

Scutchfield FD et al: AIDS update. *Postgrad Med* 1989;**85**:289.

Teberg AJ: Clinical manifestations of epidemic neonatal listeriosis. *J Pediatr Inf Dis* 1987;**6**:817.

Wasserman RL: Intravenous gamma globulin prophylaxis for newborn infants. *J Pediatr Inf Dis* 1986;**5**:62.

Wendel GD: Gestational and congenital syphilis. *Clin Perinatol* 1988;**15**:287.

Whitley RJ: Neonatal herpes simplex virus infections. *Clin Perinatol* 1988;**15**:903.

Williams CL, Strobino BA: Lyme disease transmission during pregnancy. *Contemp OB/GYN* 1990;**35**:48.

64 Intrauterine Growth Retardation (Small-for-Gestational-Age Infant)

I. **Definition.** The terms **intrauterine growth retardation (IUGR)** and **small for gestational age (SGA)** are used more or less interchangeably. There is considerable variability in the definition of what constitutes a growth-retarded infant. The term *IUGR* signifies an abnormality of the fetus itself or means that some insult to the fetus has interfered with normal growth. IUGR may also be defined as birth weight **below the 10th percentile** for gestational age or more than **2 standard deviations below the mean** for gestational age. The **ponderal index,** arrived at by the following formula,

$$\text{Ponderal index} = \frac{\text{Birth weight} \times 100}{\text{Crown-heel length}}$$

can be used to identify infants whose soft tissue mass is below normal for the stage of skeletal development (Battaglia, 1967). Thus, a ponderal index of below the 10th percentile may be used to identify IUGR infants.

   A. **Term IUGR** infants are those born at 37 weeks or later who are small for gestational age.

   B. **Preterm IUGR** infants are those who are delivered prematurely (before 37 weeks) who are small for gestational age.

II. **Incidence.** About 3–10% of all pregnancies are associated with IUGR, and 20% of stillborn infants are growth retarded. The perinatal mortality rate is 4–8 times higher for growth-retarded fetuses, and serious short- or long-term morbidity is noted in half of the affected surviving infants. It is estimated that one-third of infants with birth weights under 2800 g are in fact growth-retarded and not premature. In the USA, uteroplacental insufficiency is the leading cause of IUGR. An estimated 10% of cases are secondary to congenital infection. Chromosomal and other genetic disorders are reported in 5–15% of IUGR infants.

III. **Pathophysiology.** Fetal growth is influenced by fetal, maternal, and placental factors.

   A. **Fetal factors** (Table 64–1)

   1. **Genetic factors.** Potential for fetal growth is ultimately determined by genetic endowment. Racial and ethnic backgrounds influence size at birth irrespective of socioeconomic status. Males weigh an average of 150–200 G more than females at birth. This weight in-

TABLE 64–1. FETAL FACTORS IN IUGR

Genetic factors
  Racial, ethnic, and population differences
  Genetic disorders
  Chromosomal disorder
  Female sex
  Congenital anomalies
Congenital infections
Inborn errors of metabolism

crease occurs late in gestation. Genetic disorders such as achondroplasia, Russell-Silver syndrome, and leprechaunism also present with IUGR.

2. **Chromosomal anomalies.** Growth retardation is observed as a major feature of trisomies 13, 18, and 21.

3. **Congenital malformations.** Anencephaly, gastrointestinal atresia, Potter's syndrome, and pancreatic agenesis are examples of congenital anomalies associated with IUGR.

4. **Fetal cardiovascular anomalies** (with the possible exception of transposition of the great vessels and tetralogy of Fallot). Abnormal hemodynamics are thought to be the basis of IUGR.

5. **Congenital infection.** TORCH infections are often associated with IUGR (see p 339). The clinical findings in different congenital infections are nonspecific and overlap considerably. IUGR with rubella causes damage during organogenesis and results in a decreased number of cells, whereas cytomegalovirus infection results in cytolysis and localized necrosis within the fetus.

6. **Inborn errors of metabolism.** Transient neonatal diabetes, galactosemia, and phenylketonuria are other disorders associated with IUGR.

B. **Maternal factors** (Table 64–2)

1. **Reduced uteroplacental blood flow.** Maternal disorders such as preeclampsia-eclampsia, chronic renovascular disease, and chronic hypertensive vascular disease often result in decreased uteroplacental blood flow and associated IUGR. Impaired delivery of oxygen and other essential nutrients is thought to limit organ growth and musculoskeletal maturation.

2. **Maternal malnutrition.** Maternal malnutrition leads to deficient substrate supply to the fetus. Total caloric consumption rather than protein or fat consumption appears to be the principal nutritional influence on birth weight. Famine causes a modest decline in birth weight, and in third-world countries, severe maternal malnutrition is the leading cause of IUGR. Negative effects on birth weight are most pronounced when starvation occurs in the last trimester.

3. **Multiple pregnancy.** Impaired growth results from failure to provide optimal nutrition for more than one fetus in utero. There is a progressive decrease in weight of singletons, twins, and triplets. In parabiotic twins, the smaller twin has decreased nutrient delivery

TABLE 64–2. MATERNAL FACTORS IN IUGR

Pregnancy-induced hypertension (> 140/90 mm Hg)
Weight gain (< 0.9 kg/every 4 weeks)
Fundal lag (< 4 cm for gestational age)
Cyanotic heart disease
Heavy smoking
Residing at high altitude
Substance abuse and drugs
Short stature
Low socioeconomic class
Anemia (Hct < 30%)
Prepregnancy weight (< 50 kg)
Prior history of IUGR
Chronic hypertension
Renal disease
Severe maternal malnutrition
Multiple pregnancy
Low maternal age

secondary to abnormal placental blood flow resulting from arterio-venous communication in the chorionic plate.

4. **Drugs**
   a. **Cigarettes and alcohol.** Chronic abuse of cigarettes or alcohol is demonstrably associated with IUGR. The effects of alcohol and tobacco seem to be dose-dependent, with IUGR becoming more serious and predictable with heavy abuse.
   b. **Heroin.** Maternal heroin addiction is also often associated with IUGR.
   c. **Cocaine.** Cocaine use in pregnancy is associated with increased rates of IUGR (Orro, Dixon, 1987). The cause of IUGR may be mediated by placental insufficiency or direct toxic effect on the fetus.
   d. **Others.** Other drugs and chemical agents causing IUGR include known teratogens, antimetabolites, and therapeutic agents such as trimethadione, warfarin, and phenytoin. Each of these agents causes characteristic malformation syndromes.
5. **Maternal hypoxemia.** Mothers with hemoglobinopathies, especially sickle cell disease, often have IUGR infants. Infants born at high altitudes tend to have lower mean birth weights for gestational age.
6. **Other maternal factors.** Maternal short stature, young maternal age, low socioeconomic class, primiparity, grand multiparity, and low prepregnancy weight are associated with subnormal birth weight.

C. **Placental factors** (Table 64–3)
1. **Placental insufficiency.** In the first and second trimesters, fetal growth is determined mostly by inherent fetal growth potential. By the third trimester, placental factors—ie, an adequate supply of nutrients—assume major importance for fetal growth. When the duration of pregnancy exceeds the capacity of the placenta to nurture, placental insufficiency results, with subsequent impaired fetal growth. This phenomenon occurs mostly in postterm gestations but may occur at any time during gestation.
2. **Anatomic problems.** Various anatomic factors such as multiple infarcts, aberrant cord insertions, umbilical vascular thrombosis, and hemangiomas are described in IUGR placentas. Premature placental separation may reduce the surface area exchange, resulting in impaired fetal growth. An adverse intrauterine environment is apt to affect both placental and fetal development; hence IUGR infants usually have small placentas.

IV. **Classification**
A. **Symmetric IUGR.** (HC = Ht = Wt, all < 10%.) The head circumference, length, and weight are all proportionately reduced for gestational age. Symmetric IUGR is due either to decreased growth potential of the fetus (congenital infection, genetic disorder) or to extrinsic conditions that are active early in pregnancy.
B. **Asymmetric IUGR.** (Hc = Ht > Wt, all < 10%.) Fetal weight is reduced out of proportion to length and head circumference. The head circum-

TABLE 64–3. PLACENTAL FACTORS IN IUGR

Abruptio placentae
Hemangioma
Single umbilical artery
Infarction
Aberrant cord insertion
Umbilical vessel thrombosis

ference and length are closer to the expected percentiles for gestational age than is the weight. In these infants, brain growth is usually spared. The usual causes are uteroplacental insufficiency, maternal malnutrition, or extrinsic conditions appearing late in pregnancy.

V. Diagnosis

A. Establishing gestational age.
Determining the correct gestational age is imperative. The last menstrual period, size of the uterus, time of quickening (fluttering movements in the abdomen caused by fetal activity, appreciated by the mother for the first time), and early ultrasound measurements are used to determine gestational age.

B. Fetal assessment

1. **Clinical diagnosis.** The patient's history will raise the index of suspicion regarding suboptimal growth. Manual estimations of weight, serial fundal height measurements, and maternal estimates of fetal activity are simple clinical measures. Imprecision and inconsistency have prevented widespread confidence in these clinical methods.

2. **Hormonal evaluation.** Hormonal assays were at one time popular for assessment of IUGR but are rarely used today. Maternal urinary estriol and human placental lactogen levels tend to be low or falling in pregnancies with IUGR, though there is marked individual variation.

3. **Ultrasonography.** Currently, diagnostic ultrasound offers the greatest promise for diagnosis of IUGR. The following parameters used in combination will usually predict growth impairment with a high degree of accuracy:

   a. **Biparietal diameter (BPD).** When serial measurements of BPD are less than optimal, 50–80% of infants will have subnormal birth weights.

   b. **Abdominal circumference.** The liver is the first organ to suffer the effects of growth retardation. Reduced abdominal circumference is the earliest sign of asymmetric growth retardation and diminished glycogen storage.

   c. **Ratio of head circumference to abdominal circumference.** The ratio normally changes as pregnancy progresses. In the second trimester the head circumference is greater than the abdominal circumference. At about 32–36 weeks' gestation, the ratio is 1:1, and after 36 weeks the abdominal measurements become larger. Persistence of a head:abdomen ratio greater than 1 late in gestation is predictive of asymmetric IUGR.

   d. **Femur length.** Femur length appears to correlate well with crown-heel length and provides an early and reproducible measurement of length. Serial measurements of femur length are as effective as head measurements for detecting symmetric IUGR.

   e. **Placental morphology and amniotic fluid assessment** may help in distinguishing a constitutionally small fetus from a growth-retarded fetus. For example, placental aging with oligohydramnios suggests IUGR and fetal jeopardy, whereas normal placental morphology with a normal amount of amniotic fluid suggests a constitutionally small fetus.

C. Neonatal assessment. (See also Chap 3.)

1. **Reduced birth weight** for gestational age is the simplest method of diagnosis.

2. **Lubchenco charts** (see Fig 3–2) may underestimate IUGR because they are based on observations made well above sea level.

3. **The ponderal index** can help identify neonates with IUGR whose birth weight is over 2500 g.

4. **Ballard score.** Gestational age can also be assessed by means of

the Ballard scoring system. This examination has a predictive value of 2 weeks in infants weighing more than 999 g at birth and is most accurate at 30–42 hours of age. IUGR infants have a higher rating on this scale than premature infants with similar weights. See p 20 for Ballard examination and scoring.

VI. Complications (Table 64–4)

A. Hypoxia

1. **Perinatal asphyxia.** IUGR infants frequently have birth asphyxia, because they tolerate the stress of labor poorly.

2. **Persistent pulmonary hypertension (persistent fetal circulation).** Many IUGR infants are subjected to chronic intrauterine hypoxia, which results in abnormal thickening of the smooth muscles of the small pulmonary arterioles, which in turn reduces pulmonary blood flow and results in varying degrees of pulmonary artery hypertension. Because of this, IUGR infants are at risk of developing persistent fetal circulation. Hyaline membrane disease is less frequently seen in IUGR, since these infants tend to manifest advanced pulmonary maturity secondary to chronic intrauterine stress.

3. **Meconium aspiration.** Postterm IUGR infants are at risk for meconium aspiration.

B. Hypothermia.
Thermoregulation is compromised in IUGR infants because of diminished subcutaneous fat insulation. Infants with IUGR secondary to fetal malnutrition late in gestation tend to be scrawny as a result of loss of subcutaneous fat. They tend to be more alert than their premature counterparts.

C. Metabolic

1. **Hypoglycemia.** Carbohydrate metabolism is seriously disturbed, and IUGR infants are highly susceptible to hypoglycemia as a consequence of diminished glycogen reserves and decreased capacity for gluconeogenesis. Hypothermia may potentiate the problem of hypoglycemia.

2. **Hypocalcemia.** Idiopathic hypocalcemia may also occur in IUGR infants.

D. Hematologic disorders.
Hyperviscosity and polycythemia may result from increased erythropoietin levels secondary to fetal hypoxia associated with IUGR. Polycythemia may also contribute to hypoglycemia and lead to cerebral injury.

VII. Management.
Antenatal diagnosis is the key to proper management of IUGR.

A. History of risk factors.
The presence of maternal risk factors should alert the obstetrician to the likelihood of fetal growth retardation. Ultrasonography confirms the diagnosis. Correctable causes of impaired fetal growth warrant immediate attention.

B. Delivery and resuscitation.
Appropriate timing of delivery is important. Delivery is usually undertaken when the lungs are mature or when biophysical data obtained by monitoring reveal fetal distress. Labor is particularly stressful to IUGR fetuses. Skilled resuscitation should be available, as birth asphyxia is common.

TABLE 64–4. NEONATAL COMPLICATIONS OF IUGR

Metabolic disorders: hypoglycemia, hypocalcemia
Hypothermia
Hematologic disorders: polycythemia
Hypoxia: birth asphyxia, meconium aspiration, persistent fetal circulation
Congenital malformation

    C. **Prevention of heat loss.** Meticulous care should be taken to prevent heat loss (see Chap 5).

    D. **Hypoglycemia.** Close monitoring of blood glucose levels is essential for all IUGR infants. Hypoglycemia should be treated promptly with parenteral dextrose and early feeding, as outlined in Chapter 41.

    E. **Hematologic disorders.** A central hematocrit reading should be obtained to detect polycythemia.

    F. **Congenital infection.** IUGR infants should be examined for congenital malformations or signs of congenital infections. Many intrauterine infections are clinically silent, and screening for these should be done routinely in IUGR infants. (See TORCH infections, p 339.)

    G. **Genetic anomalies.** Screening for genetic anomalies should be done as indicated by the physical examination.

VIII. Outcome. The neurodevelopmental outcome depends mostly on the cause of the IUGR.

    A. **Symmetric versus asymmetric IUGR.** Infants with symmetric IUGR caused by decreased growth potential generally have a poor outcome, whereas infants with asymmetric IUGR in which brain growth is spared usually have a good outcome.

    B. **Preterm IUGR** infants have a higher incidence of abnormalities than the general population, as these infants are subjected to the risks of prematurity in addition to the risks of IUGR.

    C. **Chromosomal disorders.** IUGR infants with major chromosomal disorders have a 100% incidence of handicap.

    D. **Congenital infections.** Infants with congenital rubella or CMV infection with microcephaly have a poor outcome, with a handicap rate exceeding 50%.

    F. **Learning ability.** The school performance of IUGR infants is significantly influenced by social class, with children from higher social classes scoring better on achievement tests.

REFERENCES

Allen MC: Developmental outcome and follow-up of the small for gestational age infant. *Semin Perinatol* 1984;**8**:123.

Ballard JL, Kazmaier K, Driver M: A simplified assessment of gestational age. *Pediatr Res* 1977;**11**:374.

Battaglia FC, Lubchenco LO: A practical classification of newborn infants by weight and gestational age. *J Pediatr* 1967;**17**:159.

Cassady G: The small for date infant. *Pathophysiol Manage Newborn* 1981;**15**:262.

Lockwood CJ, Weiner S: Assessment of fetal growth. *Clin Perinatology* 1986;**13**:3.

Lubchenco LO et al: Intrauterine growth and estimated from live born birthweight data. *Pediatrics* 1963;**32**:793.

Orro AS, Dixon SD: Perinatal cocaine and methamphetamine exposure. *J Pediatr* 1987;**111**:571.

Queenan JT: How to diagnose intrauterine growth retardation. *Contemp Obstet Gynecol* 1982;**19**:195.

Seeds JW: Impaired fetal growth: Definition and clinical diagnosis. *Obstet Gynecol* 1984:**64**:303.

Warshaw JB: Intrauterine growth retardation. *Pediatr Rev* 1986;**8**:107.

Williams RL et al: Fetal growth and perinatal viability in California. *Obstet Gynecol* 1982;**52**:624.

65 Multiple Gestation

I. **Incidence.** The incidence of multiple gestation is probably underestimated. Fewer than half of twin pregnancies diagnosed with ultrasonography during the first trimester are finally delivered as twins, a phenomenon that has been termed *vanishing twin.* Twins occur in 1–2% of deliveries after 20 weeks, and the triplet rate is about 0.1%. Two gestational sacs can be identified with ultrasonography by 6 weeks' gestation. In addition, routine screening for maternal alpha-fetoprotein (AFP) will identify about half of the pregnancies with multiple gestations at an early gestational age. About 12–20% of twins are identified after the onset of labor.

The incidence of monozygotic twinning is remarkably constant at 3–5 per 1000 pregnancies, while the rate for dizygotic twinning varies from 4 to 50 per 1000 pregnancies. About one-third of twins in the USA are monozygotic. The rate of monozygotic twinning is considered a chance phenomenon, whereas dizygotic twinning is believed to be due to multiple ovulation and may have a familial tendency.

II. **Risk factors.** The incidence of dizygotic twinning increases with a family history of twins, maternal age (peak at 35–39 years), previous twin gestation, increasing parity, maternal height, fecundity, social class, frequency of coitus, and exposure to exogenous gonadotropins (20–40% incidence) and clomiphene (6–8% incidence).

The risk of twinning decreases with undernourishment. Ethnic background (Black > Caucasian > Oriental) is a preconception risk factor for multiple gestation.

III. **Placentation**
   A. **Classification.** Placental examination affords a unique opportunity to identify two-thirds to three-fourths of monozygotic twins at birth. Twin placentation is classified according to the placental disc (single, fused, or separate), number of chorions (monochorionic, dichorionic), and number of amnions (monoamniotic, diamniotic). Heterosexual (assuredly dizygotic) twins always have a dichorionic placenta, and monochorionic twins are always of the same sex. All monochorionic twins are believed to be monozygotic. In 70% of monozygotic twin pregnancies, the placentas are monochorionic, and the possibility exists for commingling of the fetal circulations. Fewer than 1% of twin pregnancies are monoamniotic.
   B. **Complications.** Twin gestations are associated with an increased frequency of anomalies of the placenta and adnexa—eg, single umbilical artery or velamentous or marginal cord insertion (6–9 times more common with twin gestation). The cord is more susceptible to trauma from twisting. The vessels near the insertion are often unprotected by Wharton's jelly and are especially prone to thrombosis when compression or twisting occurs. Intrapartum fetal distress from cord compression and fetal hemorrhage from associated vasa previa are potential problems with velamentous insertion of the cord.
   C. **Determination of zygosity.** The most efficient way to identify zygosity is as follows.
      1. **Gender examination.** Male-female pairs are dizygotic. The dichorionic placenta may be separate or fused.
      2. **Placental examination.** Twins with a monochorionic placenta (mo-

noamniotic or diamniotic) are monozygotic. Care should be taken not to confuse apposed fused placentas for a single chorion. If doubt exists upon gross inspection of the dividing membranes, a transverse section should be studied. The zygosity of twins of the same sex with dichorionic membranes cannot be immediately known. Genetic studies are needed (eg, blood typing, HLA typing, chromosome marking) to determine zygosity.

IV. **Mortality rates.** Although perinatal mortality rates for singleton pregnancies have continued to fall during the last decade, there has been little change in mortality rates for multiple pregnancies.

   A. **Twins.** For twin gestations, the fetal mortality rate is 4%, the neonatal mortality rate is 7.6% (1.2% for singletons), and the perinatal mortality rate is 11.6% (2.2% for singletons). The perinatal death rate for twins is 9 times the rate for first-born singletons, and 11 times the rate for second-born singletons.

      1. **Monoamniotic twins.** The mortality rate for monoamniotic twins is highest (50–60%), largely because of cord entanglement.

      2. **Monozygotic twins.** Monozygotic twins have a perinatal mortality and morbidity rate that is 2–3 times that of dizygotic twins. Diamnionic monochorionic twins have a mortality rate of 25% and dichorionic twins a mortality rate of 8.9%.

      3. **Prematurity in twins.** Approximately 10% of preterm deliveries are twin gestations, and they account for 25% of perinatal deaths in preterm deliveries.

      4. **Fetal death.** Death of one fetus may affect the outcome of the survivor profoundly or minimally (Dudley, 1986). When the cause of death is intrinsic to one dichorionic fetus and does not threaten the other fetus, complications are rare. Hazardous intrauterine environments threaten both twins, whether monochorionic or dichorionic. With monochorionic placentas, the incidence of major complications or death in the surviving twin is approximately 50%.

   B. **Triplets.** The neonatal mortality rate for triplets is 18.8%, and the perinatal mortality rate is 25.5%.

V. **Morbidity**

   A. **Prematurity.** Prematurity and uteroplacental insufficiency are the major contributors to perinatal complications. The average twin delivery occurs at 37 weeks, and multiple gestation is complicated by preterm delivery (< 35 weeks) in 21.5% of patients.

   B. **Intrauterine growth retardation.** The incidence of low birth weight in twins is approximately 50–60%, a figure that is 5–7 times higher than the incidence of low birth weight in singletons. In general, the more fetuses in a gestation, the smaller their weight for gestational age. Twins tend to grow at normal rates up to about 30–34 weeks' gestation, when they reach a combined weight of 4 kg. Thereafter, they grow more slowly. Two-thirds of twins show some signs of growth retardation at birth.

   C. **Uteroplacental insufficiency.** The incidence of acute and chronic uteroplacental insufficiency is increased in multiple gestations. Five-minute Apgar scores of 0–3 are reported for 5–10% of twin gestations. These low scores may relate to acute stresses of labor, cord prolapse (1–5%), or trauma during delivery superimposed on chronic uteroplacental insufficiency.

VI. **Congenital anomalies.** Congenital malformations are more common in twins than in singletons. In twin gestations, the incidence of major malformations is 2.12% and of minor malformations 4.13% (Wenstrom, Stanley 1988). It is now generally agreed that the increased incidence of anomalies is confined to monozygotic twins. The anomalies are usually discordant.

A. **Anomalies unique to multiple pregnancies.** Certain anomalies, such as conjoined twins and acardia, are unique to multiple pregnancies.

B. **Other anomalies.** Neural tube defects, hydrocephalus, congenital heart disease, orofacial clefts, chromosomal abnormalities, and anomalies of the urogenital system are suspected but not proved to be more common in multiple gestations. Twins are more likely to suffer positional defects due to intrauterine crowding and restriction of movement (MacLennan, 1984).

VII. **Twin-twin transfusion syndrome**

A. **Vascular anastomoses.** The chorionic vascular bed of monozygotic (and usually monochorionic) twins seem to have limitless variations. However, almost all monochorionic placentas demonstrate vascular anastomoses, whereas dichorionic placentas rarely do. Vascular anastomoses may be superficial direct communications easily visible upon inspection between arteries (most common) or veins (uncommon); deep connections from arteries to veins via villi; or combinations of superficial and deep connections. This commonality of chorionic vasculature sets the stage for twin-twin transfusion syndrome.

B. **Incidence.** Despite the high frequency of vascular anastomosis in monochorionic placentation, the twin-twin transfusion syndrome is relatively uncommon (about 15% of monochorionic gestations).

C. **Clinical manifestations.** Clinically, the twin-twin transfusion syndrome is diagnosed when twins have a hemoglobin difference of more than 5 g/dL.

  1. The **donor twin** tends to be pale and have a low birth weight, oligohydramnios, anemia, hypoglycemia, decreased organ mass, hypovolemia, and amnion nodosum. Donor twins often require volume expansion or red cell transfusion, or both.

  2. The **recipient twin** is frequently plethoric and has a high birth weight, polyhydramnios, polycythemia/hyperviscosity, increased organ mass, hypervolemia, and hyperbilirubinemia. Recipient twins often require partial exchange transfusion with fresh-frozen plasma.

  3. Rarely, either or both of the twins involved in a fetofetal transfusion may present with hydrops fetalis.

VIII. **Neonatal implications and management**

A. **Site of delivery.** When a complicated twin gestation has been identified, delivery should ideally be conducted at a high-risk perinatal center with 2 experienced pediatric delivery teams in attendance.

B. **Placental examination.** Examination of placenta(s) in the delivery room provides an early opportunity to determine zygosity and anticipate certain problems.

C. **Physical examination.** Infants should be examined for evidence of IUGR, congenital anomalies, and twin-twin transfusion syndrome. Central hematocrits should be obtained in both infants to look for anemia or polycythemia.

D. **Complications in newborn period.** The second-born twin is 2–4 times as likely to develop respiratory distress syndrome (Rokos, 1968), probably secondary to perinatal stress; however, the first-born twin may be at risk for developing necrotizing enterocolitis (Samm, 1986).

IX. **Risks beyond the neonatal period**

A. **Catch-up growth.** In monozygotic twins, birth weight differences may be as much as 20%, but the lighter twin has a remarkable ability to make up intrauterine growth deficits. However, if the birth weight of the lighter twin is less than the tenth percentile, the prognosis is guarded. With such marked discordance, the undersized twin often continues to be inferior in growth and intelligence into adult life.

B. **Acquired illnesses.** Illness in one twin increases the risk of illness in the other (Seigle, 1982). Epilepsy has an 85% concordance rate in identical twins. With acute lymphocytic leukemia or juvenile diabetes mellitus of one twin, the incidence in the other twin is 20% and 50%, respectively.

C. **Social problems.** Inadequate nurturing and child abuse are more likely with twins. Counseling for parents of twins may be invaluable (Seigel, 1982).

REFERENCES

Babson SG, Phillips DS: Growth and development of twins dissimilar in size at birth. *N Engl J Med* 1973;**289**:937.

Benirschke K: Multiple gestation: Incidence, etiology, and inheritance. Pages 511–526 in: *Maternal-Fetal Medicine.* Creasy RK, Resnik R (editors). Saunders, 1984.

Dudley DKL, Dalton ME: Single fetal death in twin gestation. *Semin Perinatol* 1986;**10**:65.

Hecht F, Hecht BK: Genetic and related biomedical aspects of twinning. *Pediatr Rev* 1983;**5**:179.

Johnson SF, Driscoll SG: Twin placentation and its complications. *Semin Perinatol* 1986;**10**:9.

Keet MP, Jaroszewica AM, Lombard CJ: Follow-up study of physical growth of monozygous twins with discordant within-pair birth weights. *Pediatrics* 1986;**77**:336.

Little J, Bryan E: Congenital anomalies in twins. *Semin Perinatol* 1986;**10**:50.

Macgillivray I: Epidemiology of twin pregnancy. *Semin Perinatol* 1986;**10**:4.

MacLennan AH: Multiple gestation: Clinical characteristics and management. Pages 527–538 in: *Maternal-Fetal Medicine.* Creasy RK, Resnik R (editors). Saunders, 1984.

Newton ER: Antepartum care in multiple gestation. *Semin Perinatol* 1986;**10**:19.

Rokos J et al: Hyaline membrane disease in twins. *Pediatrics* 1986;**42**:204.

Samm M et al: Necrotizing enterocolitis in infants of multiple gestation. *Am J Dis Child* 1986;**140**:937.

Seigle SJ, Seigle MM: Practical aspects of pediatric management of families of twins. *Pediatr Rev* 1982;**4**:8.

Smith DW: *Recognizable Patterns of Human Malformation,* 3rd ed. Saunders, 1982.

Wenstrom KD, Stanley SA: Incidence, morbidity and mortality, and diagnosis of twin gestations. *Clin Perinatol* 1988;**15(1)**:1.

66 Necrotizing Enterocolitis

I. **Definition.** Necrotizing enterocolitis (NEC) is an acquired neonatal disorder representing an end-expression of serious intestinal injury following a combination of vascular, mucosal, and toxic (and yet unidentified) insults to a relatively immature gut.

II. **Incidence**

A. **NEC is predominantly a disorder of preterm infants,** with an incidence of 8–12% in infants under 1–5 kg. The incidence increases with decreasing gestational age. **Sixty to 80% of cases occur in high-risk premature infants,** while 10–25% occur in low-risk and full-term newborns. Infants with NEC represent 2–5% of NICU admissions.

B. **NEC occurs sporadically or in epidemic clusters.**

III. **Pathophysiology.** Currently there is no single unifying theory for the pathogenesis of NEC that satisfactorily explains all of the clinical observations associated with this disorder. The generally accepted pathophysiologic sequence of events resulting in overt clinical disease is thought to involve an initial ischemic or toxic mucosal damage resulting in a loss of mucosal integrity. Then, with the availability of suitable substrate provided by enteral feedings, there is bacterial proliferation followed by invasion of the damaged intestinal mucosa by gas (hydrogen), producing organisms causing intramural bowel gas (pneumatosis intestinalis). This sequence of events may then progress to transmural necrosis or gangrene of the bowel and finally to perforation and peritonitis.

IV. **Risk factors**

A. **Prematurity.** There is an inverse relationship between risk and gestational age. The lower the gestational age, the greater the risk, owing to the immaturity of the circulatory, gastrointestinal, and immune systems.

B. **Asphyxia and acute cardiopulmonary distress** lead to low output states, resulting in redistribution of cardiac output away from the mesenteric circulation and causing episodic intestinal ischemia.

C. **Enteral feedings.** NEC is rare in unfed infants. About 90–95% of infants with NEC have received at least one oral feeding.

1. Enteral feeding provides necessary substrate for proliferation of enteric pathogens.

2. Hyperosmolar formula or medications cause direct mucosal damage.

3. There is a loss or lack of immunoprotective factors in enteral formula or breast milk.

D. **Polycythemia and hyperviscosity syndromes.** These have been shown to be definite risk factors both clinically and experimentally.

E. **Exchange transfusions.** There has been a clinically observed association between NEC and exchange transfusions, which is probably due to intestinal ischemia secondary to wide variations in venous and/or arterial perfusion pressures.

F. **Feeding volume and rapid increase in enteral feedings.** These probably play a minor role, but clinical evidence is *controversial* and inconclusive.

G. **Enteric pathogenic microorganisms.** Bacterial and viral pathogenesis, including *E coli, Klebsiella, Enterobacter, Pseudomonas, Salmonella,*

Clostridia sp, coronaviruses, rotaviruses, and enteroviruses, have all been implicated.

V. Clinical presentation. NEC usually presents within the first week of life and 3-7 days after initiating enteral feedings. The presentation may vary from a benign gastrointestinal abnormality such as abdominal distention (the most frequent early sign, noted in 70% of cases), ileus, and increased volume of gastric aspirate (two-thirds of cases) to frank signs of shock, blood per rectum, peritonitis, and perforation. It can also present with nonspecific signs such as labile temperature, apnea, bradycardia, or other signs that would make one suspect sepsis.

The clinical syndrome has been classified into stages by Bell et al (1978) and modified by Walsh and Kliegman (1986) to include systemic, intestinal, and radiographic findings.

A. Stage I: Suspected of pre-NEC
1. **Systemic** findings are nonspecific, including apnea, bradycardia, lethargy, and temperature instability.
2. **Intestinal** findings include gastric residuals and guiac positive stools.
3. **Radiographic** findings are normal or nonspecific.

B. Stage IIA: Mild NEC
1. **Systemic** findings are similar to stage I.
2. **Intestinal** findings include prominent abdominal distention with or without tenderness, absent bowel sounds, and gross blood in the stools.
3. **Radiographic** findings include ileus, with dilated loops with focal areas of pneumatosis intestinalis.

C. Stage IIB: Moderate NEC
1. **Systemic** findings include mild acidosis and thrombocytopenia.
2. **Intestinal** findings include abdominal wall edema, tenderness with or without a palpable mass.
3. **Radiographic** findings include extensive pneumatosis and early ascites. Intrahepatic portal venous gas may be present.

D. Stage IIIA: Advanced NEC
1. **Systemic** findings include respiratory and metabolic acidosis, assisted ventilation for apnea, decreasing blood pressure and urine output, neutropenia, and disseminated intravascular coagulation (DIC).
2. **Intestinal** findings include spreading edema, erythema, and induration of the abdomen.
3. **Radiographic** findings include prominent ascites and possibly persistent sentinel loop with no perforation.

E. Stage IIIB: Advanced NEC
1. **Systemic** findings reveal deteriorating vital signs and laboratory indices, shock syndrome, and electrolyte imbalance.
2. **Intestinal and radiographic** findings reveal evidence of perforation.

VI. Diagnosis. A high index of suspicion should be entertained for any infant with a history of a combination of the risk factors enumerated under **IV,** above.

A. Clinical diagnosis. NEC is a tentative diagnosis in any infant presenting with the triad of feeding intolerance, abdominal distention, and grossly bloody stools (hematochezia) or acute change in stool character. Alternatively, the earliest signs may be identical to neonatal sepsis, that is, apnea, bradycardia, lethargy and abnormal white blood count indices, and thrombocytopenia.

B. Laboratory studies. The following should be performed as baseline studies. If there is clinical progression of disease or if these laboratory tests are abnormal, the tests should be repeated every 8-12 hours.

1. **Complete blood count and differential.** The white count may be normal but is more frequently either elevated, with a shift to the left, or low (leukopenia).
2. **Platelet count.** Thrombocytopenia is seen. Fifty percent of patients with proven NEC have platelet counts less than 50,000/mL.
3. **Blood culture** for aerobic and anaerobes.
4. **Stool screening** for occult blood. Even though a clinical study has found that routine testing of stools for occult blood does not identify a population at greater risk for NEC, testing still continues on suspected patients so that changes in the stool can be followed.
5. **Stool screening** for reducing substances > 1% sugar or +2/+3 for reducing substances.
6. **Arterial blood gas measurements.** Metabolic acidosis or hypoxia may be seen.
7. **Serum potassium level.** The serum potassium level may be high, secondary to hemolysis of red blood cells.
8. **Stool cultures for rotaviruses and enteroviruses** should be obtained if diarrhea is an epidemic in the nursery.
   C. **Radiologic studies**
1. **Flat-plate x-ray studies of the abdomen**
   a. **Supportive for NEC.** Look for abnormal bowel gas patterns, ileus, or areas suspicious for pneumatosis intestinalis.
   b. **Confirmatory of NEC.** Look for (1) the presence of intramural bowel gas (pneumatosis intestinalis) and (2) the presence of intrahepatic portal venous gas (in the absence of an umbilical venous catheter).
2. **Lateral decubitus, cross-table lateral, or upright x-ray studies of the abdomen.** These studies may show free air with perforation.
   Note: In the presence of pneumatosis intestinalis or portal venous gas, flat-plate and lateral decubitus or cross-table lateral x-ray studies of the abdomen should be obtained every 6–8 hours to check for the development of pneumoperitoneum signaling intestinal perforation. Serial x-ray studies may be discontinued with clinical improvement, usually after 48–72 hours.

VII. **Management.** The main principle of management for confirmed NEC is to treat it as an acute abdomen with impending or septic peritonitis. The goal is to prevent progression of disease, intestinal perforation, and shock. If NEC occurs in epidemic clusters, cohort isolation has been shown to limit transmission.
   A. **Basic NEC protocol.** Any infant with suspected NEC should be managed according to the following protocol.
1. **Nothing by mouth (NPO)** to allow gastrointestinal rest.
2. **Use of a nasogastric tube** (on low suction) to keep the bowel decompressed.
3. **Frequent monitoring of vital signs** (every 2–4 hours) and **abdominal circumference.**
4. **Removal of umbilical catheter and placement of peripheral venous (and possibly arterial) catheter,** depending on severity of illness.
5. **Antibiotics.** Start ampicillin and gentamicin or cefotaxime intravenously. Add anaerobic coverage (clindamycin or metronidazole [Flagyl]) if peritonitis or perforation is suspected (*controversial*). (See Chap 76 for dosages and other pharmacologic information.)
6. **Monitoring for gastrointestinal bleeding.** Check all gastric aspirates and stools for blood.
7. **Strict monitoring of fluid intake and output.** Try to maintain urine output of 1–3 mL/kg/h.
8. **Removal of potassium from intravenous fluids.**

9. **Laboratory monitoring.** Check CBC, platelet count, potassium level, and blood gas levels frequently.
10. **Septic workup.** Culture blood, urine, and sputum. Some institutions routinely perform lumbar puncture for culture of cerebrospinal fluid prior to starting antibiotics (*controversial*).
11. **Radiologic studies.** Perform abdominal flat-plate x-ray studies every 6–8 hours.

B. **Management of stage 1.** Start the basic NEC protocol described above in **A.** If all cultures are negative and the infant has improved clinically, antibiotics can be stopped after 3 days. The infant can also be fed after 3 days if clinically improved.

C. **Management of stage IIA + B**
1. **Basic NEC protocol,** including antibiotics for 10 days (see **A.5,** above).
2. **NPO for 2 weeks.** Oral feedings may be started 7–10 days after radiographic demonstration of clearing of pneumatosis.
3. **Total parenteral nutrition (TPN)** should be initiated. A caloric intake of at least 90–110 cal/kg/d should be attempted. TPN should be continued until full enteral feedings have been well established.
4. **Supplemental oxygen.** Place infant under a 25% oxygen hood. (With further understanding of reperfusion syndromes, supplemental oxygen therapy has become *controversial* unless blood gas levels reveal hypoxia.)
5. **Thrombocytopenia,** if severe, can be treated with platelets.
6. **Acidosis,** if progressive, can be treated with tromethamine (THAM) or sodium bicarbonate and mechanical ventilation.
7. **Surgical consultation** is required.

D. **Management of stage IIIA + B**
1. **Basic NEC protocol,** as described in **A,** above.
2. **Stage II management,** as described in **C,** above.
3. **Respiratory support,** as indicated by blood gas levels and clinical status.
4. **Blood pressure support.** Declining blood pressure and urine output, increasing nasogastric output, and increasing abdominal circumference suggest increasing third-space losses, perforation, or septic shock. Treatment includes replacement of ongoing fluid losses, volume expansion with colloids (see p 220) and vasopressors such as dopamine (see Chap 75 for dosage and other pharmacologic information). The goal is to maintain adequate mean blood pressure (see Appendix C, Fig C–1) and urine output (1–3 mL/kg/h).
5. **Progressive leukopenia, granulocytopenia, and thrombocytopenia** usually parallel a deteriorating clinical status. Granulocyte transfusions are usually not indicated. Blood and platelet transfusion are frequently needed.

E. **Surgical management.** Surgical intervention is indicated if there is evidence of intestinal perforation. Perforations usually occur within 24–48 hours following the appearance of pneumatosis. Other indications (relative and not absolute) for surgical intervention in the absence of free intraperitoneal air include:
1. **Deteriorating clinical condition** with failure to respond to appropriate medical management.
2. **Evidence of a persistent, fixed sentinel loop over 24 hours** suggesting a segment of gangrenous bowel. In these instances, paracentesis and peritoneal lavage to obtain peritoneal fluid for visual examination, Gram's staining, white blood cell count, and culture are helpful. The presence of of brown-colored or particulate peritoneal fluid and bacteria on Gram's stain, a white count of more than 300/mm^3, and positive culture results are strongly suggestive of gangre-

nous bowel. Introduction of air may confound later diagnosis of perforation.

    3. Right lower quadrant mass.

VIII. **Prognosis**

    A. **NEC with perforation** is associated with a mortality of 20–40%.

    B. **Recurrent NEC** is a rare complication.

    C. **Subacute or intermittent symptoms of bowel obstruction** due to stenosis or strictures of the colon and, less frequently, of the small bowel are seen in about 10–20%. A barium enema is usually confirmatory.

    D. **Infants undergoing extensive surgical resection** require long-term parenteral nutrition, enterostomy care, and management of short gut syndrome. Chronic electrolyte imbalance and failure to thrive are common.

    E. **In the absence of short gut syndrome,** growth, nutrition, and gastrointestinal function appear to catch up and are normal by the end of the first year.

REFERENCES

Abrams TJ et al: Occult blood in stools and necrotizing enterocolitis: Is there a relationship? *Am J Dis Child* 1988:**142(4):**451.

Bell MJ et al: Necrotizing enterocolitis: Therapeutic decisions based on clinical staging. *Ann Surg* 1978;**187:**1.

Kliegman RM, Faranoff AA: Necrotizing enterocolitis. *N Engl J Med* 1984;**310:**1093.

Kosloski AM: Pathogenesis and prevention of NEC: Hypothesis based on personal observation and review of the literature. *Pediatrics* 1984;**74:**1086.

Kosloski AM, Goldthorn J: Paracentesis as an aid to the diagnosis of intestinal gangrene. *Arch Surg* 1982;**117:**571.

Walsh MC, Kliegman RM: Necrotizing enterocolitis: Treatment based on staging criteria. *Pediatr Clin North Am* 1986;**33(1):**179.

67 Neurologic Diseases

HYDROCEPHALUS

I. **Definition**. Hydrocephalus is defined as dilatation of the cerebral ventricular system. It is usually associated with large head circumference, but ventricular dilatation usually precedes head growth, so that head circumference may be normal. **Macrocephaly** is defined as a head circumference 2 or more standard deviations greater than the mean. Macrocephaly is not always associated with hydrocephalus.

II. **Pathophysiology and etiology**
   A. **Obstruction of cerebrospinal fluid flow.** Hydrocephalus is usually due to obstruction of cerebrospinal fluid flow.
      1. It is usually associated with increased intracranial pressure.
      2. It is termed *noncommunicating hydrocephalus* if obstruction occurs at the foramen of Monro, along the cerebral aqueduct (aqueduct of Sylvius), or at the base of the brain at the foramina of Magendie and Luschka. It is termed *communicating hydrocephalus* if cerebrospinal fluid passes through the foramen at the base of the brain but is improperly drained by the cerebral and cerebellar subarachnoid spaces.
   B. **Destructive process.** Less commonly, hydrocephalus is due to a destructive or atrophic process. This type is termed *hydrocephalus ex vacuo* and is *not* associated with increased pressure.
   C. **Increased cerebrospinal fluid production.** Rarely, hydrocephalus results from excessive production of cerebrospinal fluid, eg, due to papilloma of the choroid plexus.
   D. **Common causes**
      1. Congenital aqueductal stenosis. This disorder may be an X-linked recessive trait.
      2. Neural tube defects with Arnold-Chiari malformation.
      3. Posthemorrhagic obstruction (see Intraventricular Hemorrhage, p 379).
   E. **Less common causes**
      1. Postinfectious.
      2. Dandy-Walker malformation.
      3. Aneurysm of vein of Galen.
      4. Tumors.
      5. Achondroplasia.
      6. Osteopetrosis.
   F. **Macrocephaly without hydrocephalus** is usually familial and benign, but it may be associated with neurocutaneous diseases (eg, neurofibromatosis, Sturge-Weber syndrome), metabolic storage diseases (eg, Hunter's or Hurler's syndrome), Beckwith-Wiedemann syndrome, or achondroplasia.
   G. **Multifactorial inheritance.** Most cases result from an interaction between genetic and environmental factors.

III. **Risk factor.** The risk factor depends upon the underlying cause.

IV. **Clinical presentation**
   A. **Prenatal diagnosis**

      1. **Ultrasonographic** diagnosis in utero is becoming more common.
      2. **Polyhydramnios** is present in 10% of cases.
      3. **Breech presentation** is reported in 30% of cases.
  B. Associated conditions include an increased incidence of prematurity, postmaturity, and stillbirths.
  C. With neural tube defects
      1. Eighty percent of infants with neural tube defects have hydrocephalus.
      2. The head circumference may be normal or nearly normal at birth.
  D. Due to posthemorrhagic obstruction
      1. This form is usually detected by screening ultrasonography or CT scan of the head in asymptomatic high-risk infants.
      2. Ventriculomegaly may be detected 2–3 weeks prior to onset of rapid head growth.
      3. With this form of hydrocephalus, the ventricles either return to normal size, arrest with mild hydrocephalus, or develop progressive hydrocephalus with signs of increased intracranial pressure.
  E. Signs of hydrocephalus include apnea, bradycardia, lethargy, vomiting, tense fontanelle, widely split sutures, dilated scalp veins, rapid head growth, and scleras visible above the irises **(setting-sun sign)**. Papilledema is rarely observed in neonates.

V. Diagnosis
  A. Intrauterine ultrasonographic screening may detect hydrocephalus as early as 15–18 weeks' gestation. It is indicated when there is a family history of neural tube defect or congenital aqueductal stenosis.
  B. Physical examination. The occipitofrontal head circumference should be carefully determined for all infants. The head circumference of the parents may be increased in up to 50% of cases when infants have macrocephaly. (Normal [± 2 SD] is 54 ± 3 cm for women and 55 ± 3 cm for men.) No further evaluation is required unless there are signs of increased intracranial pressure.
  C. CT scan or MRI of the head is indicated if increased intracranial pressure is suspected or if the cause of macrocephaly is still uncertain.
  D. Neonatal screening
      1. **Neural tube defects** are screened by CT scan or MRI of the head.
      2. **Premature infants** are screened with CT scan or ultrasonography.
         a. Indications
            (1) Birth weight of less than 1500 g.
            (2) Larger, sick premature infants.
            (3) Rapidly enlarging head circumference.
            (4) Signs of increased intracranial pressure.
         b. Yield. Screening at 2 weeks of age will detect 98% of cases of posthemorrhagic hydrocephalus.
         c. Follow-up. Weekly follow-up examinations are indicated to observe for progression until there is definite stabilization or regression of the hydrocephalus.

VI. Management
  A. Prenatal diagnosis established
      1. **With pulmonary maturity,** based on L:S ratio (see p 3), proceed to prompt delivery.
      2. **If the lungs are immature,** there are 3 options.
         a. Immediate delivery (with the risks of prematurity).
         b. Delayed delivery (with the risks of persistent increased intracranial pressure).
         c. In utero placement of a ventriculoamniotic shunt.
      3. **Consultation.** Ideal management calls for consultation with the obstetrician, neonatologist, neurosurgeon, ultrasonographer, geneticist, ethicist, and family members.

B. **Congenital aqueductal stenosis or neural tube defects.** Therapy for neonates with hydrocephalus associated with congenital aqueductal stenosis or neural tube defects is **decompression** by prompt placement of a ventricular bypass shunt into an intracranial or extracranial compartment. **Ventriculoperitoneal shunts** are considered the method of choice. **Long-term complications of shunts** include infection (usually staphylococcal), occlusion, and organ perforation (due to intraperitoneal contact of a catheter with a hollow viscus).

C. **Posthemorrhagic hydrocephalus**
   1. **Mild hydrocephalus** usually arrests or returns to normal size within the first few months of life.
   2. **Severe, rapidly progressive hydrocephalus**
      a. **Temporary measures** (unproved in randomized controlled trials)
         (1) Perform serial lumbar punctures.
         (2) Administer drugs to decrease cerebrospinal fluid production (eg, acetazolamide; see Chap 75).
         (3) Perform cranial compression with head-wrapping techniques.
         (4) Insert external ventricular drain.
      b. **Permanent management.** Perform a ventricular shunt procedure.

VII. Prognosis

A. Previously the prognosis for infants with congenital hydrocephalus was poor, but with modern neurosurgical techniques, it has improved. **Long-term survival approaches 90%,** and **approximately two-thirds of infants who survive have normal or near-normal intellectual capabilities.**

B. Once an infant has a ventricular bypass shunt placed, the infant will probably need a shunt for the rest of his life. Complications associated with shunts (see **VI.B,** above), are very common.

C. The long-term outcome for preterm infants with posthemorrhagic hydrocephalus is strongly correlated with the severity of the hemorrhage and the degree of prematurity.

INTRAVENTRICULAR HEMORRHAGE

I. **Definition.** Intraventricular hemorrhage (IVH) is an intracranial hemorrhage usually arising in the germinal matrix and periventricular regions of the brain. It is predominantly a disorder of preterm infants.

II. **Incidence.** IVH occurs in 40% of infants weighing less than 1500 g at birth and in 60% of infants weighing less than 1000 g at birth. Although cases of prenatal IVH have been reported, the disorder usually occurs shortly after delivery: 60% in the first 24 hours, 85% in the first 72 hours, and 95% in the first week.

III. **Pathophysiology**
   A. **Subependymal germinal matrix.** The germinal matrix is present in premature infants but dissipates by 40 weeks' gestation. It is a weakly supported, highly vascularized area and is the site of production of neurons and glial cells of the cerebral cortex and basal ganglia.
   B. **Blood pressure changes.** Sudden elevations of arterial or venous pressure cause hemorrhage into the germinal matrix.
   C. **Rupture** through the ependyma causes IVH in 80% of infants with germinal matrix hemorrhage.
   D. **Hydrocephalus.** Acute hydrocephalus may develop as a result of obstruction at the cerebral aqueduct or, less commonly, at the foramen of Monro. A more slowly progressive hydrocephalus sometimes develops as a result of obliterative arachnoiditis in the posterior fossa.
   E. **Periventricular hemorrhagic infarction.** Twenty percent of infants with

IVH have associated intraparenchymal hemorrhage into an area of cortical ischemia and infarction.

IV. **Risk factors**
  A. **Strong risk factors**
    1. Extreme prematurity.
    2. Birth asphyxia.
    3. Hypoxia.
    4. Hypercapnia.
    5. Acidosis.
    6. Respiratory distress syndrome.
    7. Pneumothorax.
    8. Sudden rise in arterial blood pressure.
  B. **Other risk factors** include administration of sodium bicarbonate, rapid blood volume expansion, patent ductus arteriosus, elevated central venous pressure, and disturbances of hemostasis.

V. **Classification.** Any method of classifying IVH must describe the location of the hemorrhage and the size of the ventricles. Numerous systems have been proposed, but the one developed by **Papile** is most often used. Although it was developed for CT scanning, it has also been applied to ultrasonography.

  Grade I. Subependymal, germinal matrix hemorrhage.
  Grade II. Intraventricular extension without ventricular dilatation.
  Grade III. Intraventricular extension with ventricular dilatation.
  Grade IV. Intraventricular and intraparenchymal hemorrhage.

VI. **Clinical presentation.** The clinical presentation is extremely diverse. IVH may be totally asymptomatic, or there may be subtle symptoms, eg, bulging fontanelle, sudden drop in hematocrit, apnea, bradycardia, acidosis, seizures, and changes in muscle tone or level of consciousness. A catastrophic syndrome is characterized by rapid onset of stupor or coma, respiratory abnormalities, tonic seizures, decerebrate posturing, pupils fixed to light, eyes fixed to vestibular stimulation, and flaccid quadriparesis.
  A. **Symptoms and signs may mimic those of other common neonatal disorders** such as metabolic disturbances, asphyxia, sepsis, or meningitis.
  B. **A diagnosis based upon clinical symptoms is inadequate.**
    1. Of infants with IVH confirmed by CT scan, only 60% of cases were predicted on the basis of clinical criteria.
    2. Of infants with no IVH documented by CT scan, 25% had been judged to have hemorrhage by clinical criteria.

VII. **Diagnosis**
  A. **Laboratory studies**
    1. Examination of cerebrospinal fluid is normal in up to 20% of infants with IVH.
    2. The cerebrospinal fluid usually shows elevated red and white cells, with elevated protein concentration.
    3. It is frequently difficult to distinguish IVH from a "traumatic tap."
    4. Within a few days after hemorrhage, the cerebrospinal fluid becomes xanthochromic, with a decreased glucose concentration.
    5. Diagnosis by analysis of cerebrospinal fluid is often unreliable, and confirmatory imaging techniques are required.
    6. Often the cerebrospinal fluid shows a persistent increase in white cells and protein and a decreased glucose level, therefore making it difficult to rule out meningitis except by negative cultures.
  B. **Radiologic studies.** CT scanning and ultrasonography of the head are both useful. MRI is an acceptable alternative, although it is usually more expensive and more complex; also, motion of the patient interferes with the study and therefore makes it difficult to perform in neonates.

VIII. Management
    A. Prevention
        1. Avoidance of premature delivery and perinatal asphyxia will prevent many cases of IVH.
        2. General supportive care of premature infants should be given to maintain a stable acid-base status and avoid fluctuation of arterial and venous blood pressures.
        3. Pharmacologic prevention may be considered. None of the following regimens have been definitely proved safe and effective. All are considered experimental and *controversial.*
            a. Phenobarbital
                (1) **Mother.** Give 500 mg by slow intravenous infusion and then 100 mg orally every 24 hours until delivery or until labor ceases.
                (2) **Infant.** Give 2 doses of 10 mg/kg intravenously 12 hours apart and then 2.5 mg/kg every 12 hours intravenously, intramuscularly, or orally for 6 days.
            b. Pancuronium, 0.1 mg/kg intravenously as needed for paralysis for the first 72 hours of life.
            c. Indomethacin, 0.1 mg/kg intravenously every 12 hours for a total of 5 doses.
            d. Ethamsylate (125 mg/mL), 0.1 mL/kg intravenously within 2 hours of birth, then every 6 hours for 4 days. (Currently not available in USA.)
            e. Vitamin E. Dosage and route are *controversial.*
            f. Vitamin K, 10 mg intramuscularly, given to the mother every 5 days until delivery if still in labor.
    B. Screening ultrasonography or CT scanning of head
        1. All infants weighing less than 1500 g at birth should be screened.
        2. Larger infants should be screened if risk factors are present or if there is evidence of increased intracranial pressure or hydrocephalus.
        3. The optimal age for diagnosis of IVH is 4–7 days, with follow-up at 14 days.
        4. The optimal age for diagnosis of hydrocephalus is 14 days, with follow-up at 3 months.
        5. The advantages of ultrasonography are that it provides acceptable resolution with portable equipment and no radiation exposure. IVH may be isodense 7–14 days after hemorrhage on CT scanning.
    C. Acute hemorrhage
        1. General stabilization and supportive measures
            a. Maintain cerebral perfusion pressure by maintaining an adequate arterial blood pressure.
            b. Maintain normal blood volume and acid-base status.
        2. Follow-up serial imaging (ultrasonography or CT scanning) should be done to detect progressive hydrocephalus.
    Note: A randomized controlled trial of **lumbar punctures** to prevent hydrocephalus following IVH demonstrated no difference between a group of infants undergoing lumbar puncture with supportive care and a control group receiving supportive care only.
    D. Hydrocephalus
        1. With mild hydrocephalus, ventricular enlargement will usually cease without additional therapy.
        2. For treatment of moderate or severe posthemorrhagic hydrocephalus, see p 379, **C.2.**
  IX. Prognosis. The prognosis depends on the grade of hemorrhage.
    Grade I or II. There is no increase in morbidity or mortality rates compared to those in infants with no IVH at 2 years of age.

Grade III. Up to 80% of patients have severe developmental delays.
Grade IV. Almost all (90%) die or suffer severe developmental delays.

NEONATAL SEIZURES

I. **Definition.** A seizure is defined clinically as a paroxysmal alteration in neurologic function, ie, behavioral, motor, or autonomic function, or all three (Volpe, 1989).
II. **Incidence.** Neonatal seizures are not uncommon. The incidence ranges from 1.5:1000 to 14:1000 live births.
III. **Pathophysiology.** The neurons within the central nervous system undergo depolarization as a result of inward migration of sodium. Repolarization occurs via efflux of potassium. A seizure occurs when there is excessive depolarization, resulting in excessive synchronous electrical discharge. Volpe has proposed the following 3 possible reasons for excessive depolarization: (1) failure of the sodium-potassium pump owing to a disturbance in energy production; (2) alteration in the neuronal membrane, causing a change in sodium permeability; and (3) a relative excess of excitatory versus inhibitory neurotransmitters. The basic mechanisms of neonatal seizures, however, are unknown.

There are numerous causes of neonatal seizures but relatively few account for most cases (Table 67–1). Therefore, only common causes of seizures are discussed below.
A. **Perinatal asphyxia** is the most common cause of neonatal seizures. These occur within the first 24 hours of life in most cases and may progress to overt status epilepticus. In premature infants, seizures are of the generalized tonic type, while in full-term infants they are of the multifocal clonic type. Accompanying subtle seizures are usually present in both types.
B. **Intracranial hemorrhage** whether subarachnoid, periventricular, or intraventricular, may occur as a result of hypoxic insults that can lead to neonatal seizures. Subdural hemorrhage, usually a result of trauma, can cause seizures.
   1. **Subarachnoid hemorrhage.** In primary subarachnoid hemorrhage,

---

TABLE 67–1. CAUSES OF NEONATAL SEIZURES

Perinatal asphyxia
Intracranial hemorrhage
   Subarachnoid hemorrhage
   Periventricular or intraventricular hemorrhage
   Subdural hemorrhage
Metabolic abnormalities
   Hypoglycemia
   Hypocalcemia
   Electrolyte disturbances: hypo- and hypernatremia
Amino acid disorders
Infections
   Meningitis
   Encephalitis
   Syphilis, cytomegalovirus infections, toxoplasmosis
   Cerebral abscess
Drug withdrawal
Toxin exposure (particular local anesthetics)
Inherited seizure disorders
   Benign familial epilepsy
   Tuberous sclerosis
   Zellweger's syndrome
Pyridoxine dependency

convulsions often occur on the second postnatal day, and the infant appears quite well during the interictal period.

2. **Periventricular or intraventricular hemorrhage** arising from the subependymal germinal matrix is accompanied by subtle seizures, decerebrate posturing, or generalized tonic seizures, depending on the severity of the hemorrhage.

3. **Subdural hemorrhage** over the cerebral convexities leads to focal seizures and focal cerebral signs.

C. **Metabolic disturbances**

1. **Hypoglycemia** is frequently seen in infants with intrauterine growth retardation (IUGR) and in infants of diabetic mothers (IDMs). The duration of hypoglycemia and the time lapse before initiation of treatment determine the occurrence of seizures. Seizures are less frequent in IDMs, perhaps because of the short duration of hypoglycemia.

2. **Hypocalcemia** has been noted in low birth weight infants, IDMs, asphyxiated infants, infants with DiGeorge's syndrome, and infants born to mothers with hyperparathyroidism. Hypomagnesemia is a frequent accompanying problem.

3. **Hyponatremia** occurs because of improper fluid management or as a result of syndrome of inappropriate secretion of antidiuretic hormone (SIADH).

4. **Hypernatremia** is seen with dehydration or excessive use of sodium bicarbonate.

5. **Other metabolic disorders**
   a. **Pyridoxine dependency** leads to seizures resistant to anticonvulsants. Infants with this disorder experience intrauterine convulsions and are born with meconium staining. They resemble asphyxiated infants.
   b. **Amino acid disorders.** Seizures in infants with amino acid disturbances are invariably accompanied by other neurologic disorders. Hyperammonemia and acidosis are commonly present in amino acid disorders.

D. **Infections.** Intracranial infection due to bacterial or nonbacterial agents may be acquired by the neonate in utero, during delivery, or in the immediate perinatal period.

1. **Bacterial infection.** Meningitis due to **group B streptococcus,** *Escherichia coli,* or *Listeria monocytogenes* infection is accompanied by seizures during the first week of life.

2. **Nonbacterial infection.** Nonbacterial causes such as toxoplasmosis and infection with herpes simplex, cytomegalovirus, rubella, and coxsackie B viruses lead to intracranial infection and seizures.

E. **Drug withdrawal.** Three categories of drugs used by the mother lead to passive addiction and drug withdrawal (sometimes accompanied by seizures) in the infant. These are **analgesics** such as heroin, methadone, and propoxyphene (Darvon); **sedative-hypnotics** such as secobarbital; and **alcohol.**

F. **Toxins.** Inadvertent injection of local anesthetics into the fetus at the time of delivery (paracervical, pudendal, or saddle block anesthesia) may cause generalized tonic-clonic seizures. Mothers often notice the absence of pain relief during delivery.

IV. **Clinical presentation.** It is important to understand that **seizures in the neonate are different from those seen in older children.** The differences are perhaps due to the neuroanatomic and neurophysiologic developmental status of the newborn infant. In the neonatal brain, glial proliferation, neuronal migration, establishment of axonal and dendritic contacts, and myelin deposition are incomplete. **Four types of seizures,** based on clinical presentation, are recognized: subtle, clonic, tonic, and myoclonic.

1. **Subtle seizures.** These seizures are not clearly clonic, tonic, or myoclonic and are more common in premature than in full-term infants. Subtle seizures are more commonly associated with an electroencephalographic seizure in premature infants than in full-term infants. They consist of tonic horizontal deviation of the eyes with or without jerking; eyelid blinking or fluttering; sucking, smacking, or drooling; "swimming," "rowing," or "pedaling" movements; and apneic spells. Apnea accompanied by electroencephalographic abnormalities has been called **convulsive apnea.** It is differentiated from nonconvulsive apnea, which is due to sepsis, lung disease, or metabolic abnormalities, by the absence of electroencephalographic abnormalities. Furthermore, during nonconvulsive apnea of 20 seconds' duration or longer, the heart rate decreases by 40% or more within 8 seconds, whereas in convulsive apnea, the heart rate does not change even when apnea lasts longer than 20 seconds. Apnea as a manifestation of seizures is usually accompanied or preceded by other subtle manifestations. In premature infants, apnea is unlikely to be a manifestation of seizures.

2. **Clonic seizures** are more common in full-term infants than in premature infants and are commonly associated with an electroencephalographic seizure. There are 2 types of clonic seizures.
   a. **Focal seizures.** Well-localized, rhythmic, slow jerking movements involving the face and upper or lower extremities on one side of the body or the neck or trunk on one side of the body. Infants are usually unconscious during or after the seizures.
   b. **Multifocal seizures.** Several body parts seize in a sequential, non-Jacksonian fashion (eg, left arm jerking followed by right leg jerking).

3. **Tonic seizures** occur primarily in premature infants. Two types of tonic seizures are seen.
   a. **Focal seizures.** Sustained posturing of a limb or asymmetric posturing of the trunk or neck, or both. Commonly associated with an electroencephalographic seizure.
   b. **Generalized seizures.** Most commonly, a tonic extension of both upper and lower extremities (as in decerebrate posturing) but may also present with tonic flexion of upper extremities with extension of the lower extremities (as in decorticate posturing). Uncommon to see electroencephalographic seizure disorders.

4. **Myoclonic seizures** are seen in both full-term and premature infants and are characterized by single or multiple synchronous jerks. Three types of myoclonic seizures are seen.
   a. **Focal seizures.** Typically involve the flexor muscles of an upper extremity and not commonly associated with electroencephalographic seizure activity.
   b. **Multifocal seizures.** Asynchronous twitching of several parts of the body and not commonly associated with electroencephalographic seizure activity.
   c. **Generalized seizures.** Bilateral jerks of flexion of the upper and sometimes the lower extremities. More commonly associated with electroencephalographic seizure activity.

   Note: It is important to distinguish **jitteriness** from seizures. Jitteriness is not accompanied by abnormal eye movements, and movements cease on application of passive flexion. In jitteriness, movements are stimulus-sensitive and are not jerky.

V. **Diagnosis**
   A. **History.** While it is often difficult to obtain a thorough history in infants transported to tertiary care facilities from other hospitals, the physician must make a concerted effort to elicit pertinent historical data.

1. **Family history.** A positive family history of neonatal seizures is usually obtained in cases of metabolic errors and benign familial neonatal convulsions.
2. **Maternal drug history** is critical in cases of narcotic withdrawal syndrome.
3. **Delivery.** Details of the delivery provide information regarding maternal analgesia, the mode and nature of delivery, the fetal intrapartum status, and the resuscitative measures employed. Information regarding maternal infections during pregnancy point toward an infectious basis for seizures in an infant.

B. **Physical examination**
1. A thorough general physical examination should precede a well-planned neurologic examination. Determine the following:
   a. Gestational age.
   b. Blood pressure.
   c. Presence of skin lesions.
   d. Presence of hepatosplenomegaly.
2. **Neurologic evaluation.** Neurologic evaluation should include assessment of the level of alertness, cranial nerves, motor function, primary neonatal reflexes, and sensory function. Some of the specific features to look for are the site and "feel" of the fontanelle, retinal hemorrhages, chorioretinitis, pupillary size and reaction to light, extraocular movements, changes in muscle tone, and the status of primary reflexes.
3. **Notation of seizure pattern.** When seizures are noted, they should be described in detail, including size of onset, spread, nature, duration, and level of consciousness. Recognition of subtle seizures requires special attention.

C. **Laboratory studies.** In selecting and prioritizing laboratory tests, one must utilize the information obtained by history taking and physical examination and look for common and treatable causes.
1. **Serum chemistries.** Estimations of serum glucose, calcium, sodium, blood urea nitrogen and magnesium and blood gas levels must be performed. They may reveal the abnormality causing the seizures.
2. **Spinal fluid examination.** Evaluation of the cerebrospinal fluid is essential, since the consequences of delayed treatment or nontreatment of bacterial meningitis are grave.
3. **Metabolic disorders.** (See also Chap 61.) With a family history of neonatal convulsions, a peculiar odor about the infant, milk intolerance, acidosis, alkalosis, or seizures not responsive to anticonvulsants, other metabolic causes should be investigated.
   a. **Blood ammonia levels** should be checked.
   b. **Amino acids** should be measured in urine and plasma. The urine should be tested for reducing substances.
      (1) **Urea cycle disorders.** Respiratory alkalosis is seen as a result of direct stimulation of the respiratory center by ammonia.
      (2) **Maple syrup urine disease.** With 2,4-dinitrophenylhydrazine (2,4-DNPH) testing of urine, a fluffy yellow precipitate will be seen in cases of maple syrup urine disease (see Table 61-5).

D. **Radiologic studies**
1. **Ultrasonography of the head** is performed to rule out intraventricular or periventricular hemorrhage.
2. **CT scanning of the head** provides detailed information regarding intracranial disease. CT scanning is helpful in looking for evidence of infarction, hemorrhage, calcification, and cerebral malformations. Recent experience with this technique suggests that valuable

information is obtained in term infants with seizures, especially when seizures are asymmetric.

E. Other studies

  1. Electroencephalography. EEGs obtained during a seizure will be abnormal. Interictal EEGs may be normal. However, an order to obtain an ictal EEG should not delay other diagnostic and therapeutic steps. The diagnostic value of EEG is greater when it is obtained in the first few days, since diagnostic patterns indicative of unfavorable prognosis disappear thereafter. Electroencephalography is valuable in confirming the presence of seizures when manifestations are subtle or when neuromuscular paralyzing agents have been given. EEGs are of prognostic significance in full-term infants with recognized seizures. For proper interpretation of EEGs, it is important to know the clinical status of the infant (including the sleep state) and any medications given.

VI. Management. Since repeated seizures may lead to brain injury, **urgent treatment is indicated. The method of treatment depends on the cause.**

A. Hypoglycemia. Hypoglycemic infants with seizures should receive 10% dextrose in water, 2–4 mL/kg intravenously, followed by 6–8 mg/kg/min by continuous intravenous infusion.

B. Hypocalcemia is treated with slow intravenous infusion of calcium gluconate (see dosage and other pharmacologic information in Chap 75). If serum magnesium levels are low (< 1.52 meq/L), magnesium should be given.

C. Anticonvulsant therapy. Conventional anticonvulsant treatment is employed when no underlying metabolic cause is found. Loading doses of phenobarbital and phenytoin control 70% of neonatal seizures.

  1. Phenobarbital is usually given first (see Chap 75 for dosage and other pharmacologic information). Neither gestational age nor birth weight seems to influence the loading or maintenance dose of phenobarbital. When phenobarbital alone fails to control seizures, another agent is employed. Gilman and associates (1989) found that sequentially administered phenobarbital controlled seizures in term and preterm newborns in 77% of cases. If seizures are not controlled at a serum phenobarbital level of 40 μg/mL, they recommend administering a second agent (eg, phenytoin [Dilantin]).

  2. Phenytoin (Dilantin) is employed next by many practitioners (see dosage and other pharmacologic information in Chap 75).

  3. Diazepam (Valium) has not been used extensively in control of neonatal seizures, and when utilized as a third agent, it did not improve seizure control. However, when used as a continuous intravenous infusion, 0.3 mg/kg/h, it was quite effective in controlling seizures in 8 neonates, all of whom became somnolent but did not require artificial ventilation.

  4. Lorazepam (Ativan) given intravenously has been quite effective and safe, even when repeated 4–6 times in a 24-hour period (see dosage and other pharmacologic information in Chap 75).

  5. Paraldehyde, given rectally, has been used as an effective anticonvulsant (see Chap 75 for dosage and other pharmacologic information).

D. Duration of anticonvulsant therapy. The optimal duration of anticonvulsant therapy has not been established. While some recommend continuation of phenobarbital for a prolonged period, others recommend stopping it after seizures have been absent for 2 weeks.

VII. Prognosis. Since 1969, there has been some improvement in the neurologic outcome of infants experiencing seizures, but morbidity and mortality rates are still about 50%. As would be expected, the prognosis varies with the cause. Infants with hypocalcemic convulsions have an excellent prognosis, while those with seizures due to congenital malformations have a poor prognosis. Symptomatic hypoglycemia has a 50% risk of death or complications, while central nervous system infection carries a risk of 70%. Asphyxiated infants with seizures have a 60% chance of a poor outcome. Seventeen percent of patients with neonatal seizures have recurrent seizures later in life.

NEURAL TUBE DEFECTS

I. **Definition.** Neural tube defects (NTD) are any malformations of the developing brain and spinal cord, including:
   A. **Open lesions.** These defects arise during the process of neuralation, which is a well-defined period between the 17th and 30th day after ovulation. Open lesions include:
      1. Craniorachischosis (total dysraphism).
      2. Anencephaly.
      3. Meningomyelocele.
   B. **Closed lesions.** These lesions are postneuralation defects that arise after the 30th day postovulation. They include:
      1. Iniencephaly.
      2. Encephalocele.
      3. Hydrocephalus.
      4. Spina bifida occulta.
      5. Meningocele. **Clinically, the most frequently encountered lesion is myelomeningocele,** which will be discussed in detail here.
II. **Incidence**
   A. **Worldwide,** there is an average incidence of 1 case per 1000 births for both anencephaly and meningomyelocele.
   B. There is an east-west gradient. Even within the United States, there is a higher prevalence of open neural tube defects on the East Coast than on the West Coast.
   C. **In the United States,** approximately 6000 infants are born with neural tube defects each year.
III. **Pathophysiology of myelomeningocele.** Most myelomeningocele lesions occur in the lumbar region, but occasionally they extend upward to involve the thoracic spine. The more extensive the lesion, the more serious the long-term handicaps. Nearly 80% of myelomeningoceles are confined to the lumbar region and affect spinal cord segments L2–S1. Abnormalities associated with myelomeningocele include hydrocephalus, lower limb deformities, and urologic abnormalities.
   A. **Hydrocephalus** is often secondary to **Arnold-Chiari malformation** of the foramen magnum and upper cervical canal, with resultant downward displacement of the medulla, pons, and cerebellum. Obstructed cerebrospinal fluid flow and resulting hydrocephalus are probably due to partial blockage caused by deformities of the posterior fossa and fourth ventricle.
   B. **Urinary tract dysfunction.** The loss of normal bladder function (hypertonic of hypotonic dysfunction), ureteral reflux, and urinary incontinence reflect loss of development of the lower lumbar segments.
   C. **Neurologic abnormalities.** The lower extremities lack peripheral nervous system innervation, and there is loss of secondary muscle development.
   D. **Infections.** Patients with myelomeningocele are at increased risk for infections, especially *Staphlococcus epidermitis.*
IV. **Risk factors.** Environmental factors that have been considered related to open NTD include:
   A. **Ingestion of nitrate.** Cured meat, blighted potatoes, salicylates, and hard water.

    B. Antineoplastic drugs.

    C. Anticonvulsant drugs (ie, sodium valproate).

    D. Anesthetic agents.

    E. Infectious agents.

    F. Other factors. Accumulating data point toward nutritional and vitamin deficiencies as important contributing factors in the development of human open neural tube defects.

V. Clinical presentation. Meningomyelocele presents as a failure of closure of the caudal neural tube, with protrusion of a portion of the spinal cord and membrane through a defect in the vertebral column. The most commonly affected area is the lumbosacral region of the spine. Neurologic, musculoskeletal, urologic, and developmental abnormalities may accompany this condition.

VI. Diagnosis

  A. Antenatal diagnosis

    1. **Alpha-fetoprotein (AFP) levels.** Antenatal diagnosis of open neural tube defects is possible by measuring AFP levels in maternal serum or amniotic fluid. Exposure of fetal neural tissue causes large quantities of AFP to leak into the amniotic fluid and pass into the maternal circulation. Screening of pregnancies at high risk for dorsal neural defects is possible by sampling the maternal serum before 14 weeks' gestation.

    2. **Acetylcholinesterase.** Amniotic-fluid acetylcholinesterase determination is another test that is beneficial in diagnosing open NTDs. When amniotic-fluid AFP and acetylcholinesterase determinations are combined and both show elevated levels, it indicates open NTD, thus eliminating false-positive results of the AFP test alone.

    3. **Ultrasonography.** Both longitudinal examinations of fetal spine and serial transverse sections through the fetal spine are helpful in diagnosing neural tube defects.

    4. **Immunocytochemical staining of amniotic fluid cells** for macrophages.

  B. Postnatal diagnosis. Determine the extent of the myelomeningocele lesion and the associated neurosensory and neuromuscular deficits.

  C. Physical examination

    1. **Head measurements.** Initial measurements of head circumference and anterior fontanelle establish baseline information from which the rate of increasing hydrocephalus can be judged.

    2. **Level of defect.** If the uppermost part of the dorsal lesion extends into the thoracic spine, it supports an early suspicion of hydrocephalus.

    3. **Size and tone of the urinary bladder** offer indications of urinary tract involvement.

    4. **Anal sphincter tone and retention or involuntary passage of meconium** give an indication of the lower extent of involvement, namely, of the sacral spinal segments.

    5. **Scoliosis** may be seen, especially if the thoracic vertebrae are involved.

    6. **Extremity disorders.** The lower extremities may be flaccid, and muscle mass may be diminished in the most severe cases.

    7. **Deformities of the hips and ankles** may also be present (eg, dislocation of hips, equinovarus [club foot]).

VII. Management

  A. Supportive measures

    1. **A careful evaluation** of the infant must be conducted for associated defects or coincidental disorders.

    2. **Fluid management** must include assessment of insensible water loss and appropriate replacement.

3. **Heat loss** should be prevented (see Chap 5).
4. **Antibacterial prophylactic measures** include:
   a. **Blood and urine cultures.**
   b. **Dressings.** Wet sterile dressings are used to cover the lesion prior to surgery.
   c. **Antibiotics.** Intravenous antibiotics for broad-spectrum coverage are used at most institutions. **Ampicillin** and **gentamicin** are most frequently used, but some institutions prefer to use a penicillinase-resistant penicillin. (See Chap 76 for dosages and other pharmacologic information.)
B. **Surgical measures**
   1. **Surgical closure of the defect** should be performed expeditiously by a neurosurgeon. Some myelomeningocele defects are amenable to primary closure, but many require skin grafting.
   2. **Ventriculoperintoneal shunting.** Follow-up neurosurgical placement of a ventricular shunt at a later date is required for hydrocephalus.
C. **Follow-up**
   1. **Neurologic follow-up.** Reevaluation of neurologic sequelae by a pediatric neurologist will give the parents a developing picture of any physical handicaps.
   2. **Shunt infections.** Possible neurosurgical complications, especially shunt infections, must be anticipated and explained to the family.
   3. **Physical therapy.** Early muscle evaluation by physical therapists will familiarize the parents with plans for ongoing, long-term adaptive therapy.
   4. **Orthopedic and urologic follow-up.** Evaluations are necessary, depending on the individual case. Urologic complications are often encountered and may require routine procedures such as intermittent bladder catheterization for urinary retention.
D. **Counseling of parents.** Parents need patient, extended, repeated counseling regarding the lesion, long-term outcome, and short-term invasive medical procedures. A **team approach** to counseling is important. A social worker, genetic counselor, physicians, and primary care nurses with special interests in caring for handicapped children should combine their experience to support and help the family make a lifelong adjustment and commitment to the child.
VIII. **Prognosis.** The prognosis for infants with meningomyelocele is related to the site of the lesion. The risk of hydrocephalus is 96% for infants with thoracolumbar lesions and 60% for those with sacral lesions. Infants with thoracolumbar lesions have a 35% mortality rate; 44% have an IQ greater than 80, and 71% are able to walk with braces and other supports. Infants with sacral lesions have no mortality; 100% of them have an IQ greater than 80 and are able to walk with braces; 83% can walk without the use of devices.

REFERENCES

Bergman I, Painter MJ, Crumine PK: Neonatal seizures. *Semin Perinatol* 1982;**6**:54.
Brock DJH, Barron L, van Heyningen V: Prenatal diagnosis of neural tube defects with monoclonal antibody specific for acetylcholinesterase. *Lancet* 1985;**21**:5.
Donn SM, Goldstein GW, Roloff DW: Prevention of intraventricular hemorrhage with phenobarbital therapy: Now what? *Pediatrics* 1986;**77**:779.
Dykes FD et al: Posthemorrhagic hydrocephalus in high-risk preterm infants: Natural history, management and long-term outcome. *J Pediatr* 1989;**114**:611.
Dykes FD et al: Intraventricular hemorrhage: A prospective evaluation of etiopathogenesis. *Pediatrics* 1980;**66**:42.
Gilman JT et al: Rapid sequential phenobarbital treatment of neonatal seizures. *Pediatrics* 1989;**83**:674.
Glick PL et al: Management of ventriculomegaly in the fetus. *J Pediatr* 1984;**105**:97.

Hudgins RJ et al: Natural history of fetal ventriculomegaly. *Pediatrics* 1988;**82:**692.

Lazzara A et al: Clinical predictability of intraventricular hemorrhage in preterm infants. *Pediatrics* 1980;**65:**30.

Lemire RJ: Neural tube defects: Clinical correlations. *Clin Neurosurg* 1983;**30:**165.

Lemire RJ et al: Neural tube defects. *JAMA* 1988;**259(4):**558.

Main DM, Mennuti MT: Neural tube defects: Issues in prenatal diagnosis and counseling. *Obstet Gynecol* 1986;**67:**1.

McCullough DC, Balzer-Martin LA: Current prognosis in overt neonatal hydrocephalus. *J Neurosurg* 1982;**57:**378.

Michejda M, Queenan JT, McCullough D: Present status of intrauterine treatment of hydrocephalus and its future. *Am J Obstet Gynecol* 1986;**155:**873.

Myianthopoulos NC, Melnick M: Studies in neural tube defects: Epidemiologic and etiologic aspects. *Am J Med Genet* 1987;**26:**738.

Painter MJ, Berman I, Crumine PK: Neonatal seizures. *Pediatr Clin North Am* 1986;**63:**91.

Philip AGS et al: Intraventricular hemorrhage in preterm infants: Declining incidence in the 1980s. *Pediatric* 1989;**84:**797.

Poland RL: Vitamin E for prevention of perinatal intracranial hemorrhage. *Pediatrics* 1990;**85:**865.

Sandovnick AD et al: Use of genetic counseling services for neural tube defects. *Am J Med Genet* 1987;**26:**811.

Vintzileos AM, Ingardia CT, Nochinson DJ: Congenital hydrocephalus: Review and protocol for perinatal management. *Obstet Gynecol* 1983;**62:**539.

Volpe JJ: Intraventricular hemorrhage and brain injury in the premature infant. *Pediatr Clin North Am* 1989;**2:**361.

Volpe JJ: *Neurology of the Newborn.* Saunders, 1987.

Volpe JJ: Neonatal Seizures: Current concepts and revised classification. *Pediatrics* 1989;**84:**422.

Warkany J: Hydrocephalus. Chapter 25 in: *Congenital Malformations.* Year Book, 1971.

68 Perinatal Asphyxia

I. **Definition.** Perinatal asphyxia exists when an antepartum event, labor, or a birth process diminishes the oxygen supply to the fetus, causing decreased fetal or newborn heart rate, which results in impairment of exchange of respiratory gases, oxygen, and carbon dioxide, and inadequate perfusion of the tissues and major organs.

II. **Incidence.** Consensus on the incidence of perinatal asphyxia has been difficult to arrive at because of the non-uniform clinical criteria on which different institutions base their definitions. In a 1987 Finland study by Ranta-kallio, the overall incidence was 12.7% (diagnosis based on blood gas analysis and whether extra oxygen or assisted ventilation was needed, and including newborns with a low Apgar score alone), compared with the incidences of severe asphyxia of 3.2% and 2.6% in a Swedish series of the 1970s (diagnosis based on Apgar score of 3 or less at 5 minutes).

III. **Pathophysiology**

A. **Disorders associated with perinatal asphyxia**

1. **Antepartum period.** Maternal diabetes, preeclampsia, fetal malformation, postmaturity, prematurity, and intrauterine growth retardation.

2. **Intrapartum period.** Breech presentation (4.4:1000), meconium staining, cephalopelvic disproportion (6.6:1000), and cord compression (8.9:1000). Mann (1986) concluded that evidence for cord compression can be found in 30% of all deliveries.

3. **Less common causes** include uterine malformation, precipitous labor, abruptio placentae, maternal shock, cord prolapse, and infection. Infection is of special importance when coincident with prolonged rupture of membranes.

4. **Postnatal period.** Severe pulmonary disease, congenital heart disease, large patent ductus arteriosus, severe recurrent apneic spells, and sepsis with cardiovascular collapse.

B. **Pathophysiologic events** following perinatal asphyxia (Table 68–1).

TABLE 68–1. PATHOPHYSIOLOGIC EVENTS FOLLOWING PERINATAL ASPHYXIA

Event	Time from Birth		
	1 Minute	5 Minutes	10 Minutes
Respiratory effort	Increased	Returns briefly	Falls again, becomes agonal
Approximate blood pH	7.25	7.00	6.75
Heart rate	Increased	Plateau at about 50/min	< 50/min; becomes idio-ventricular
Cardiac output	Slightly increased	Falling	Minimal
Pulmonary blood flow	Decreases rapidly	Minimal	Negligible
Cerebral blood flow	Slightly increased	Rapidly falling	Ischemia resulting in brain damage
Renal perfusion	Unchanged	Rapidly declining	Ischemia, cortical necrosis

Modified and reproduced, with permission, from Cunningham MD, TePas KE: Newborn care in the delivery room. Page 501 in *High Risk Pregnancy: A Team Approach.* Knuppel RA, Drukker JE (editors), Saunders, 1986.

1. Altered carbohydrate and energy metabolism results in profound **disturbance of respiration and oxidative metabolism,** regional alterations in high energy compounds (eg, ATP), accumulation of extracellular potassium and intracellular calcium, intracellular **acidosis,** accumulation of hydrogen ions, steady decrease of pH to levels below 7.25, **decreasing heart rate and cardiac output,** and **altered neurotransmitters.** Dawes (1968) has suggested a timed sequence that establishes loss of major organ function and irreparable tissue damage after 10 minutes of complete asphyxia.

2. **Loss of vascular autoregulation.** Initial circulatory effects of perinatal asphyxia include redistribution of cardiac output so that a larger proportion enters the brain, increase in cerebral blood flow, and loss of cerebrovascular autoregulation. Later effects include diminution of cardiac output, hypotension, and decrease in cerebral blood flow.

3. **Toxic effect of synaptically released excitatory amino acids.** Synaptic release of glutamate, or failure of the glutamate re-uptake system in the face of ATP deficiency associated with oxygen deprivation, results in accumulation of extracellular glutamate, which causes either immediate or delayed neuronal death. **Immediate neuronal death (minutes)** is due to sodium, chloride, and water influx, which results in an osmolar load and eventual lysis of the cell membrane. **Delayed neuronal death (hours)** is due to calcium influx. High intracellular free calcium results in activation of undesirable second messengers and enzymes, generation of free radicals, and disturbance of oxidative phosphorylation.

C. **Clinical events**
  1. **The initial response** is hypertension and hyperpnea, followed by primary apnea, then gasping attempts to breathe.
  2. **Unresolved hypoxia** leads to secondary apnea, bradycardia, and shock. This latter phase sets the stage for central nervous system damage.
  3. **Diminished cerebral blood flow** and loss of oxygen supply results in vessel injury.
  4. **Cerebrovascular injury** leads to **cerebral edema.**
  5. **Cerebrovascular hemorrhage** occurs upon reperfusion of ischemic and damaged areas of the brain.

D. **Pathologic findings**
  1. **Cortical changes.** Cortical edema, with flattening of cerebral convolutions, is followed by cortical necrosis until finally a healing phase results in gradual cortical atrophy. Cortical atrophy, if severe, may result in **microcephaly.**
  2. **Other pathologic findings** common in term infants exposed to oxygen deprivation include selective neuronal necrosis (involving the Sommer's sector of the hippocampus and the Purkinje cells of the cerebellum), status marmoratus of the basal ganglia (the marbled appearance is due to the characteristic feature of hypermyelination), and parasagittal cerebral injury (bilateral and usually symmetrical, with the parietal-occipital regions affected more often than those regions anteriorly).
  3. **Periventricular leukomalacia (PVL)** is necrosis of periventricular white matter, which has a predilection for premature infants. The incidence increases with length of survival and severity of postnatal cardiorespiratory disturbances; 25% of cases of PLV are complicated by hemorrhage into the lesion. PVL involving the pyramidal tracts usually results in spastic diplegic or quadriplegic cerebral palsy.

4. **Porencephaly or hydrocephaly** may follow cortical necrosis, intra-ventricular hemorrhage, or intracerebral hemorrhage.
5. **Brain-stem damage** is seen in the most severe cases of hypoxic-ischemic brain injury and results in permanent respiratory impairment.

IV. **Clinical presentation**
  A. **Assessment at delivery.** Although the Apgar score is not an ideal measure of perinatal asphyxia because it does not correlate well with intrapartum indicators of asphyxia, it is still in wide use today because it is the only **standardized** method of clinical assessment available. According to the Internal Classification of Diseases (Annotated I.C.D.9 C.M., Clinical Modification, Volume I):
    1. **Mild to moderate asphyxia (blue asphyxia): Apgar score of 4–7 at 1 minute** is a cause for concern.
    2. **Severe asphyxia (pale asphyxia): Apgar score of 0–3 at 1 minute** (HR < 100 or falling, absent respiration or generalized pale color) is an indication for immediate intubation and resuscitation.
  B. **Syndrome of hypoxic-ischemic encephalopathy.** This occurs in asphyxiated infants with Apgar scores of 0–3 for more than 5 minutes, onset of seizures at 12–24 hours of life, and onset of motor abnormalities by the end of the first week. Weakness in the full-term infant can be either a hemiparesis or involve the proximal limbs, upper more than lower. Weakness in the premature infant involves the lower limbs.
    1. **Mild:** hyperalertness, uninhibited reflexes, sympathetic overactivity (duration of less than 24 hours).
    2. **Moderate:** lethargy or stupor, hypotonia, suppressed primitive reflexes, seizures.
    3. **Severe:** coma, flaccid tone, suppressed brain-stem function, seizures, increased intracranial pressure.
  C. **Birth injury.** A diagnosis of hypoxic-ischemic encephalopathy secondary to birth injury is made when there is clinical evidence of birth trauma (eg, subdural hematoma) coexistent with Apgar scores of 0–3 within the first 5 minutes of life.

V. **Diagnosis**
  A. **Antepartum diagnosis**
    1. **Fetal heart rate (FHR) monitoring.** Fetal bradycardia and late decelerations indicate a lack of oxygen supply to the fetus and suppression of the fetal myocardium.
    2. **"Chronic fetal distress" pattern of FHR**
      a. Stable baseline heart rate between 120–160 beats/min.
      b. Persistently absent short-term variability.
      c. Intermittent, usually small, variable decelerations with overshoot, with amplitude less than 20 beats/min and duration less than 20 seconds.
      d. Absence of reactivity. Shields and Schifrin (1988) showed that almost all infants with this pattern had 1-minute Apgar scores of less than 7 and that almost 80% of the 5-minute Apgar scores were low.
    3. **Real-time ultrasonography** shows decreased frequency of fetal activity, fetal breathing movements, decreased muscle tone (biophysical profile), pupillary dilatation in response to light, and abnormal fetal movement in response to external acoustic or vibrotactile stimuli.
    4. **Aminiotic fluid volume.** An aminiotic fluid index (AFI) of 5 or less is associated with an increased incidence of meconium, fetal distress in labor, and a low 5-minute Apgar score.
    5. **Assessment of fetoplacental blood flow using Doppler ultrasonography** shows that changes in the aortic blood flow velocity waveform

may precede the development of pathologic fetal heart rate patterns and may provide an early warning of impending asphyxia.

B. **Intrapartum diagnosis**
   1. **Fetal heart rate monitoring.**
   2. **Sampling of fetal scalp capillary blood** to determine pH and Pao_2.
   3. **Sampling of umbilical cord blood** for acid-base status.
   4. **Observation of early passage of "heavy" meconium** (ie, at the time of rupture of membranes during active labor).

C. **Newborn asphyxia (asphyxia neonatorum).** There is no ideal measure of perinatal asphyxia in clinical practice.
   1. **Apgar scores** have been shown to be not specific for hypoxia and do not appear to closely correlate with intrapartum indicators of asphyxia. Most infants with low Apgar scores do not show evidence of biochemical asphyxia. Other factors that can account for low Apgar scores include gestational age, maternal medications, type of anesthetic administered, and the person who assigned the score. Fetal heart rate may diminish because of vagal influences unrelated to fetal hypoxia such as endotracheal, orogastric, or nasogastric suctioning. The sensitivity and positive predictive values of a low 5-minute Apgar score (< 7) are 12% and 19% respectively (Ruth, 1988). Regardless, the Apgar scoring system continues to be the most commonly used method to define birth asphyxia.
   2. **Acid-base analysis of umbilical cord blood** provides objective information about the acute and chronic respiratory and metabolic condition of the fetus at birth. However, its value as a true predictor of fetal condition is best judged when maternal acid-base analysis is normal. Cord arterial pH correlates best with 1-minute Apgar score and has a sensitivity and positive predictive value for adverse neurologic outcome of 21% and 8% respectively (Ruth, 1988). Conversely, a normal cord arterial pH may be useful in ruling out the diagnosis of birth asphyxia in the newborn with respiratory depression (Thorp, 1989).
   3. **Base deficit calculation** is used as an index of severity of metabolic acidosis and the degree of compensation achieved by resuscitative efforts. A base deficit of 4 or more warrants further evaluation and correction.
   4. Numerous abnormal **metabolites in blood and CSF** have been identified, possibly reflecting metabolic derangement associated with hypoxic-ischemic encephalopathy. Such research "markers" (not refined for use in clinical practice) include creatine kinase, hypoxanthine, lactate, lactate dehydrogenase, cord erythropoietin, and cord arginine vasopressin.

D. **Other organ systems requiring assessment.** Approximately 60% of "asphyxiated" newborn infants exhibit single- or multiple-organ injury.
   1. **Cardiovascular system.** Hypotension, tachycardia, poor perfusion, and congestive heart failure may follow severe asphyxia.
      a. **Chest x-ray** may reveal an **enlarged heart.**
      b. **Electrocardiography may show myocardial ischemia** with ST segment depression and T wave inversion.
      c. **Two-dimensional echocardiography with Doppler interrogation** shows both **right and left ventricular dysfunction** in 25% of severely asphyxiated infants. Left ventricular dilatation or dysfunction alone is infrequent (10%). Right ventricular dysfunction is more common (30%) and is manifested by a dilated right ventricle with high-velocity tricuspid regurgitation and atrial shunting. It is most frequently observed in infants with meconium-stained amniotic fluid.
      d. **Serum creatinine phosphokinase levels** for myocardial damage

(CPK-MB) have not been as diagnostically useful as previously reported.

2. **Renal function** may be depressed or transiently abolished following asphyxia, resulting in acute tubular or cortical necrosis or renal failure. **Oliguria** may be transient (present in the first 24 hours) or persistent (present for at least 36 hours). Poor outcome in term infants is associated with persistent oliguria, and in preterm infants, with both transient and persistent oliguria (Perlman, Tack, 1988).

   a. **Serum urea nitrogen and creatinine studies** for baseline levels are suggested. Careful documentation of urine output and specific gravity is needed to evaluate possible onset of syndrome of inappropriate antidiuretic hormone secretion (SIADH).

   b. **Elevated urinary B-2-microglobulin** in the first void and normal urine output suggest mild to moderate CNS insult resulting in proximal tubular injury but not enough to cause cerebral injury. However, if accompanied by persistent oliguria, it is likely that the brain has suffered ischemic injury (Perlman, Tack, 1988).

   c. **Catheter drainage of the bladder** may be required, as some asphyxiated infants may have acute urinary retention.

3. **Liver function.** Liver enzymes, especially gamma-glutamyl transpeptidase activity, clotting factors, serum ammonia, serum indirect bilirubin and total bile acid concentration are useful studies at 3–4 days' postnatal age in moderate to severe asphyxia.

4. **Gastrointestinal tract.** The GI tract may be compromised, and necrotizing enterocolitis is an associated delayed (5–7 days) complication. Caution with the first feeding is advised: isotonic or hypotonic feedings, small volumes, and close observation of gut tolerance to feedings are recommended.

5. **Lungs.** Observe for **respiratory distress syndrome** (see p 413) and **persistent pulmonary hypertension,** especially in infants with a history of meconium-stained amniotic fluid (see p 284).

6. **Hematologic system. Thrombocytopenia** due to shortened platelet survival time when exposed to hypoxia may be present.

7. **Brain.** The neurologic examination provides **critical** information concerning the presence, site, extent of hypoxic-ischemic injury, and the prognosis.

   a. Infants are usually **obtunded** if not comatose.

   b. **Depressed reflexes,** loss of auditory and cranial reflexes, and cranial nerve palsies are the most common findings.

   c. **Muscle tone is poor or flaccid.** Generalized hypotonia and paucity of spontaneous movements are common clinical features of severe hypoxic-ischemic encephalopathy.

   d. **Hypoxic-ischemic spinal cord injury.** Ischemic injury to anterior horn cells within spinal cord gray matter is relatively common among hypotonic-hyporeflexic neonates following severe perinatal hypoxia-ischemia. Electromyographic examinations show injury to the lower motor neuron above the level of the dorsal root ganglion (Clancy, Sladky, Rorke, 1989).

   e. **Serum osmolality and electrolytes** should be monitored for possible onset of SIADH.

   f. **Traumatic deliveries** may cause skull fracture, subdural hematoma, or subarachnoid hemorrhage.

   g. Onset of **seizures** in 12–72 hours is not unusual. Serial EEG may be used to document severity and to follow progression of damage. Watch for seizures due to **low serum glucose levels.**

   h. **Evoked electrical potentials** (auditory, cortical auditory, middle latency responses, visual, or somatosensory) may help to document levels of CNS damage.

i. **Intracranial pressure** (ICP) should be monitored in the severely asphyxiated term newborn. It is not a recognized feature in the preterm infant in the absence of hydrocephalus. ICP is normal initially and rises to a maximum at 24–72 hours of age; the cerebral perfusion pressures remain normal throughout this time period. The typical temporal profile of changes in ICP suggests that clinically recognizable brain swelling is a *consequence* of extensive cerebral necrosis rather than a cause of ischemic cerebral injury.

j. **Ultrasonography** is the **technique of choice for routine assessment of the brain in the premature newborn.** Although of major value for identification of IVH, major limitations in the first weeks of life exist for diagnosis of ischemic injury because of the inability of ultrasonography to reliably identify mild injury and to visualize lesions that are peripherally located and because of the poor specificity of increased echogenicity for distinguishing between hemorrhagic and ischemic injury in cerebral parenchyma.

k. **Doppler ultrasonography.** Higher cerebral blood flow velocity is found in asphyxiated infants during the first 4 days of life, coincidental with cerebral edema and neurologic abnormalities, thus suggesting that the changes in the cerebral circulation are at least partly caused by cerebral edema-induced increase of intracranial pressure following severe perinatal asphyxia (van Bel et al, 1987).

l. **CT scan.** Currently, CT scanning is the **technique of choice for evaluation of hypoxic-ischemic cerebral injury in the term newborn.** The value of CT in the assessment of diffuse cortical neuronal injury is most apparent several weeks after severe asphyxial insults. During the first week after insult, the striking bilateral diffuse hypodensity reflects marked cortical neuronal injury, with associated edema corresponding closely to the occurrence of maximum intracranial pressure.

m. **Magnetic resonance imaging** (MRI) demonstrates better anatomic definition of the hypoxic-ischemic cerebral lesions. However, the application of MRI in the newborn is fraught with practical difficulties related to the prolonged scanning time, inability to use ferromagnetic life-support equipment in proximity to the scanner, and difficulties in differentiating white and gray matter.

n. **Other potentially useful imaging techniques** include technetium scan (detects areas with disturbances of the blood-brain barrier), positron emission tomography (detects decreased parasagittal cerebral blood flow), cerebral hemodynamics using xenon-133 inhalation and single-photon emission computer tomography (Taudorf, Vorstrup, 1989), magnetic resonance spectroscopy (a measure of oxidative phosphorylation), and near infrared spectroscopy (Wyatt et al, 1989).

VI. Management

A. **Optimal management is prevention** using the antepartum and intrapartum diagnostic modalities (see pp 393, 394).

B. **Immediate resuscitation**

1. **Maintenance of adequate ventilation and perfusion**

a. **Maintain tidal volumes between 4 and 6 mL/kg.**

b. **During the initial period of resuscitation, $Paco_2$ should be maintained between 25 and 30 mm Hg** to minimize cerebral edema. $Paco_2$ can then be normalized to 35–45 mm Hg after initial resuscitation.

c. **Maintain a pH of more than 7.35** with hyperventilation, sodium bicarbonate, or tromethamine (THAM), as acidic pH can potentiate pulmonary vasoconstriction.

    d. Avoid hypoxemia (Pao_2 < 40 in premature infants and Pao_2 < 50 in term infants) **and hypercarbia** ($Paco_2$ > 50). Overcorrection of hypoxemia with resultant hyperoxemia may contribute to brain injury.

    e. Avoid hypovolemia. Central venous pressure monitoring can be very helpful. Capillary refill time of 5 seconds or greater is consistent with poor perfusion.

    f. Inotropic support may be required to maintain the systemic mean blood pressure in the normal range appropriate for gestational age and birth weight. Do not treat just a low blood pressure value; evaluate the "whole" patient (ie, perfusion, renal output, oxygenation). Attempts should be made to maintain the systemic mean blood pressure above the pulmonary artery pressure to reverse the right-to-left shunt seen in asphyxia.

    g. Conversely, **avoid systemic hypertension** to prevent hemorrhagic injury.

    h. Observe minimal handling of infant. Hypoxemia may result even from routine handling of the infant.

    i. Give partial exchange transfusion for significant polycythemia.

2. Control of seizures. Seizures associated with severe hypoxic-ischemic cerebral injury commonly occur on the first day of life and may be prolonged and refractory to anticonvulsant medication.

    a. Phenobarbital is the **drug of choice** for the treatment of seizures in neonatal hypoxic-ischemic encephalopathy. Some centers start it before the onset of clinical seizures, based on the clinical impression that prophylaxis treatment reduces the likelihood of subsequent uncontrolled seizures by reducing catecholamines and cerebral edema and lowering overall metabolic activity at a time of great stress. Phenobarbital is discontinued after 7 days if no clinical seizures occur; otherwise, it is continued until the EEG and clinical observation show no seizure activity for at least 2 months.

    b. Further anticonvulsant therapy must be considered if seizures occur despite adequate phenobarbital doses. Other agents that may be tried include diazepam, lorazepam, and phenytoin (see Chap 75 for dosages and other pharmacologic information).

3. Prevention of cerebral edema

    a. Monitor intracranial pressures, if possible, in severely asphyxiated infants.

    b. Avoid excessive volume expansion or rapid infusion of colloid solutions or sodium bicarbonate.

    c. Maintain adequate oxygenation. Avoid aminophylline, as it may decrease cerebral blood flow and potentiate cerebral anoxia.

    d. Maintain a normal range of $Paco_2$ (35–45 mm Hg). Hyperventilation to decrease Pco_2 to the range of 20–30 mm Hg may lower cerebral blood flow and is one way to minimize cerebral edema acutely, although further hyperventilation to Pco_2 less than 20 mm Hg may result in cerebral ischemia. Conversely, increased carbon dioxide levels may increase cerebral blood flow, cause vasodilatation, and risk new or extended intracranial hemorrhage.

    e. Maintain a normal serum glucose level to provide adequate substrate for brain metabolism. Avoid hyperglycemia to prevent hyperosmolality or increased brain lactate levels.

    f. Fluid and electrolyte management

        (1) Maintain moderate to slight fluid restriction (eg, 60 mL/kg). If cerebral edema is severe, further restriction of fluid intake to 50 mL/kg is imposed.

   (2) **Monitor serum sodium** and maintain normal levels.

   (3) **Monitor urine output and specific gravity.** A urine output of 2.0–2.5 mL/kg/h and a urine specific gravity of 1.012–1.015 reflect adequate fluid management in the face of early cerebral edema.

   (4) **Observe the infant for syndrome of inappropriate secretion of antidiuretic hormone (SIADH),** which is treated by stringent fluid restriction.

   g. Glucocorticoids, mannitol, and phenobarbital are not proven therapeutic approaches to cerebral edema secondary to perinatal asphyxia.

VII. Prognosis

A. Useful prognostic factors

1. Data from electronic fetal monitoring, blood gas sampling, imaging studies, and biochemical markers.

2. Normalization of tone by 15 minutes of life is a good prognostic sign.

3. Apgar scores, especially extended scores, may be helpful (Table 68–2). However, Thomson and co-workers (1977) reported that as many as 29 out of 31 infants with 1-minute Apgar scores of 0–1 survived without mental or physical handicap when given prompt and effective resuscitation.

4. Neonatal neurologic syndrome.

   a. Severity.

   b. Seizures

      (1) Early onset and difficult to control.

      (2) Duration of more than 1–2 weeks.

   c. Increased intracranial pressure.

   d. Specific patterns of motor weakness may be predictive of the type of later cerebral palsy.

   e. Persistent abnormalities of brain-stem function (generally incompatible with long-term survival).

B. Hypoxic-ischemic injury is a much more common cause of neurodevelopmental impairments seen at follow-up in sick or preterm infants than hemorrhage.

C. Environmental, psychosocial, behavioral, and developmental variables are more predictive of 36-month outcome than are maternal, prenatal and perinatal variables.

D. Rantakallio and coworkers (1987) reported that perinatal brain damage accounted for 57.5% of all neonatal deaths, 30% of admissions to a special nursery and 12.5% of mental retardation (IQ < 71), epilepsy, and cerebral palsy at the age of 14.

TABLE 68–2. HYPOXIC-ISCHEMIC ENCEPHALOPATHY FOLLOWING APGAR SCORES OF 0–3 FOR 1 MINUTE OR MORE

Time (min)	Death by 1 Year of Age	
	Birth Weight < 2.5 kg (%)*	Birth Weight > 2.5 kg (%)*
1	25 (1.9)	3 (0.7)
5	55 (7.1)	8 (9)
10	67 (6.7)	18 (4.7)
20	96	59 (57)

* Numbers in parentheses are percentages of survivors with cerebral palsy.

Modified and reproduced, with permission, from Nelson KB, Ellenberg JH: Apgar scores: Predictors of chronic neurologic disability. *Pediatrics* 1981;**68**:36.

E. The outcome of severe asphyxia neonatorum is always ominous, but efforts to resuscitate must always be undertaken as quickly as possible, with the expectation that every infant has the potential to respond and recover fully.

REFERENCES

Castle V et al: The effect of hypoxia on platelet survival and site of sequestration in the newborn rabbit. *Thromb Haemos* 1988;**59**:45.

Clancy RR, Sladky JT, Rorke LB: Hypoxic-ischemic spinal cord injury following perinatal asphyxia. *Ann Neurol* 1989;**26**:185.

Clark GD: Role of excitatory amino acids in brain injury caused by hypoxia-ischemia, status epilepticus, and hypoglycemia. *Clin Perinatol* 1989;**16**:459.

Dawes GS: *Foetal and Neonatal Physiology.* Year Book, 1968.

Gilstrap III LC et al: Diagnosis of birth asphyxia on the basis of fetal pH, Apgar score, and newborn cerebral dysfunction. *Am J Obstet Gynecol* 1989;**161**:825.

Hill A: Assessment of the fetus: Relevance to brain injury. *Clin Perinatol* 1989;**16**:413.

Lou HC: The "lost autoregulation hypothesis" and brain lesions in the newborn—an update. *Brain Devel* 1988;**10**:143.

Mann LI: Pregnancy events and brain damage. *Am J Obstet Gynecol* 1986;**155**:6.

Manning FA, Platt LD, Sipos L: Antepartum fetal evaluation: Development of a fetal biophysical profile. *Am J Obstet Gynecol* 1980;**136**:787.

Nelson KB, Ellenberg JH: Apgar scores: Predictors of chronic neurologic disability. *Pediatrics* 1981;**68**:36.

Painter MJ: Fetal heart rate patterns, perinatal asphyxia, and brain injury. *Pediatr Neurol* 1989;**5**:137.

Perlman JM, Tack ED: Renal injury in the asphyxiated newborn infant: Relationship to neurologic outcome. *J Pediatr* 1988;**113**:875.

Rantakallio P, von Wendt L, Koivu M: Prognosis of perinatal brain damage: Prospective study of a one-year birth cohort of 12,000 children. *Early Hum Develop* 1987;**15**:75.

Ruth VJ, Raivio KO: Perinatal brain damage: Predictive value of metabolic acidosis and the Apgar score. *Br Med J Clin Res* 1988;**297**:24.

Ruth VJ et al: Prediction of perinatal brain damage by cord plasma vasopressin, erythropoietin, and hypoxanthine values. *J Pediatr* 1988;**113**:880.

Shields JR, Schifrin BS: Perinatal antecedents of cerebral palsy. *Obstet Gynecol* 1988;**71**:899.

Standards and guidelines for cardiopulmonary resuscitation (CPR) and emergency cardiac care (ECC). 6. Neonatal advanced life support. *JAMA* 1986;**255**:2969.

Taudorf K, Vorstrup S: Cerebral blood flow abnormalities in cerebral palsied children with a normal CT scan. *Neuropediatrics* 1989;**20**:33.

Thomson AJ, Searle M, Russell G: Quality of survival after severe birth asphyxia. *Arch Dis Child* 1977;**52**:620.

Thorp JA et al: Routine umbilical cord blood gas determinations? *Am J Obstet Gynecol* 1989;**161**:600.

van Bel F et al: Cerebral blood flow velocity pattern in healthy and asphyxiated newborns: Controlled study. *Eur J Pediatr* 1987;**146**:461.

Volpe JJ: Hypoxic-ischemic encephalopoathy: Biochemical and physiological aspects. In: *Neurology of the Newborn*, 2nd ed. Saunders, 1987.

Wyatt JS et al.: Magnetic resonance and near infrared spectroscopy for investigation of perinatal hypoxic-ischemic brain injury. *Arch Dis Child* 1989;**64**:953.

69 Pulmonary Diseases

AIR LEAK SYNDROMES

I. **Definition.** The air leak syndromes (pneumomediastinum, pneumothorax, pulmonary interstitial emphysema [PIE], and pneumopericardium) comprise a spectrum of disease with the same underlying pathophysiology. Overdistention of alveolar sacs or terminal airways leads to disruption of airway integrity, resulting in dissection of air into surrounding spaces.

II. **Incidence.** Although the exact incidence of the air leak syndromes is hard to determine, they are most commonly seen in infants with lung disease who are on ventilatory support in the NICU. In general, the more severe the lung disease, the higher the incidence of pulmonary air leak. Whereas air leak syndromes are seen most commonly in infants on ventilatory support, they all have been reported to occur spontaneously.

III. **Pathophysiology.** Overdistention of terminal air spaces or airways—the common denominator in all the pulmonary air leaks—can result from uneven alveolar ventilation; air trapping, or injudicious use of alveolar distending pressure in infants on ventilatory support. As lung volume exceeds physiologic limits, mechanical stresses occur in all planes of the alveolar or respiratory bronchial wall, with eventual tissue rupture.

   A. **Barotrauma.** The common denominator of the air leak syndromes is overdistention of the lung; the most common cause of overdistention is barotrauma. Barotrauma results whenever positive pressure is applied to the lung; it cannot be avoided in the ill newborn infant needing ventilatory support, but its effects should be minimized.

   1. **Peak inspiratory pressure (PIP), positive end-expiratory pressure (PEEP), inspiratory time (IT), respiratory rate, and the inspiratory waveform** all play an important role in the development of barotrauma. It is difficult to determine which of these parameters is the most damaging and which plays the largest role in the development of the air leaks. Frequent and large oscillating pressures associated with intermittent positive-pressure ventilation (IPPV) may be more important than distending pressure (PIP) or PEEP by themselves; the duration of positive pressure (IT) may be more important than the positive end-expiratory pressure (PEEP); distending pressure may be more important than either of the above.

   2. **Inadvertent PEEP** secondary to a very rapid rate and a short expiratory time may also be important.

   B. **Other causes of lung overdistention.** Barotrauma is not the only cause of lung overdistention. Gas trapping secondary to a ball-valve effect may occur with meconium aspiration or with the presence of other material such as mucous plugs in the airway. Other events, such as inappropriate intubation of the right main-stem bronchus, failure to wean following surfactant replacement therapy, or the development of high opening pressures with the onset of air breathing, can also lead to overdistention, with rupture of airway integrity at birth.

IV. **Risk factors**

   A. **Ventilatory support.** The infant on ventilatory support has an increased risk of developing one of the air leak syndromes. Some investigators report an incidence as high as 12% in infants on any type of ventilatory support.

B. **Meconium staining.** Other infants at risk include those who are meconium stained at birth. In these infants meconium may be plugging the airways, with resultant air trapping. During inspiration the airway expands, allowing air to enter, but during exhalation there is airway collapse, with resultant trapping of air behind meconium plugs.

C. **Surfactant therapy.** Infants receiving surfactant replacement therapy may be at increased risk for the development of air leaks. With the return of pulmonary compliance, appropriate weaning must occur and may be necessary immediately following therapy. The clinician must watch for improvement in the infant's arterial blood gas levels and must wean ventilatory support as required.

V. **Clinical presentation.** A high index of suspicion is necessary for the diagnosis of air leak syndromes. On clinical grounds, respiratory distress or a deteriorating clinical course strongly suggests air leak. See specific syndromes in **IX**, below.

VI. **Diagnosis.** The definitive diagnosis of all of these syndromes is made radiographically. An anteroposterior chest x-ray film along with a cross-table lateral film is essential in diagnosing an air leak.

VII. **Prevention.** The best mode of treatment for all of the air leak syndromes is prevention—judicious use of ventilatory support, with close attention to distending pressure, PEEP inspiratory time, and appropriate weaning of ventilatory support as the clinical condition improves. Despite excellent ventilatory management, however, air leak syndromes will continue to be a problem in neonatal intensive care. Despite major advancement in ventilatory support and respiratory monitoring, barotrauma remains a prominent disadvantage to ventilatory support. The judicious use of ventilatory pressures and the adjustment of ventilator settings to provide a minimum of barotrauma is extremely important in the NICU.

VIII. **Prognosis.** The prognosis for the infant in whom an air leak develops depends on the underlying condition. In general, if the air leak is treated rapidly and effectively, the long-term outcome should not change. However, it must be remembered that early onset (PIE) (prior to 24 hours of age) is associated with a high mortality rate. Chronic lung disease of the newborn, or bronchopulmonary dysplasia (BPD), is also associated with severe pulmonary air leak syndromes.

IX. **Specific air leak syndromes**

A. **Pneumomediastinum**

1. **Definition.** Pneumomediastinum is air in the mediastinum from ruptured alveolar air that has traversed fascial planes.

2. **Incidence.** The incidence of pneumomediastinum prior to the era of neonatal intensive care was approximately 2:1000 live births. The exact incidence is related to the degree of ventilatory support and is clearly higher today.

3. **Pathophysiology.** Pneumomediastinum is preceded by PIE in almost every case. Following alveolar rupture, air traverses fascial planes and passes into the mediastinum.

4. **Risk factors.** See p 400.

5. **Clinical presentation.** Unless accompanied by pneumothorax, pneumomediastinum may be totally asymptomatic. Spontaneous pneumomediastinum may develop in term infants not on ventilatory support and may be accompanied by mild respiratory distress. Physical findings in addition to respiratory distress may include an increase in anteroposterior diameter of the chest, and heart sounds may be difficult to auscultate.

6. **Diagnosis.** On radiograph, pneumomediastinum may present in several different ways. The classic description is that of a "wind-

blown spinnaker sail" (a lobe or lobes of the thymus being elevated off the heart). In other cases a halo may be seen around the heart in the anteroposterior projection, or evidence on this projection may be completely absent. Again, the cross-table lateral projection will show an anterior collection of air that may be difficult to distinguish from a pneumothorax.

7. **Management.** There is no definitive treatment for pneumomediastinum. The temptation to insert a drain into the mediastinum should be resisted, as it will not be beneficial and may cause more problems than it will solve. An oxygen-rich environment can be used in the term infant to attempt nitrogen washout if the pneumomediastinum is felt to be clinically significant.

8. **Prognosis.** See p 400.

B. **Pneumothorax**

1. **Definition.** Pneumothorax is air between the visceral and parietal pleural surfaces.

2. **Incidence.** Before the modern era of neonatal intensive care, the incidence of pneumothorax was 1–2%. With the advent of neonatal ventilator care, however, the incidence has risen dramatically. While the exact incidence is difficult to determine, it is directly related to the degree of ventilatory support delivered.

3. **Pathophysiology**

   a. **The term infant not on ventilatory support.** Pneumothorax may develop spontaneously. It usually happens at the time of delivery, when a large opening pressure is initially necessary to inflate collapsed alveolar sacs.

   b. **The infant on ventilatory support** will have alveolar overdistention secondary to either injudicious use of distending pressure or failure to wean ventilatory pressure when compliance begins to return. Pneumothorax is usually preceded by rupture of the alveoli, with the interstitial air then traversing via fascial planes to the mediastinum. The pneumomediastinum breaks through the mediastinal pleura to form a pneumothorax.

4. **Risk factors.** See p 400.

5. **Clinical presentation.** The clinical presentation of the neonate with pneumothorax depends on the setting in which it develops.

   a. **The term infant with a spontaneous pneumothorax** may be asymptomatic or only mildly symptomatic. These infants usually present with tachypnea and mild oxygen needs but may have the classic signs of respiratory distress (grunting, flaring, retractions, and tachypnea).

   b. **The infant on ventilatory support** will generally have a sudden, rapid clinical deterioration characterized by cyanosis, hypoxemia, hypercarbia, and respiratory acidosis. The most common time for the development of this complication is either immediately following the initiation of ventilatory support or when the infant begins to improve and compliance returns (for example, following surfactant therapy). In either case, other clinical signs may include decreased breath sounds on the involved side, shifted heart sounds, and asynchrony of the chest.

6. **Diagnosis.** A high index of suspicion is necessary for the diagnosis of pneumothorax.

   a. **Transillumination of the chest.** With the aid of transillumination, the diagnosis of pneumothorax may be made without a chest x-ray study. A **fiberoptic light probe** placed on the infant's chest wall will illuminate the involved hemithorax. While this technique is beneficial in an emergency, it should not replace a chest x-ray study as the means of diagnosis.

   b. Chest x-ray study. Radiographically, pneumothorax is diagnosed on the basis of the following characteristics.
      (1) Presence of air in the pleural cavity separating the parietal and visceral pleura.
      (2) Collapse of the ipsilateral lobes.
      (3) Displacement of the mediastinum to the contralateral side.
      (4) Downward displacement of the diaphragm.
      In infants with respiratory distress syndrome (RDS), the compliance may be so poor that the lung may not collapse, with only minimal shift of the mediastinal structures. The anteroposterior x-ray film may not demonstrate the classic radiographic appearance if a large amount of the intrapleural air is situated just anterior to the sternum. In these situations, the cross-table lateral x-ray film will show a large lucent area immediately below the sternum, or the lateral decubitus x-ray film (with the suspected side up) will show free air.
7. Management. Treatment of pneumothorax depends on the clinical status of the infant.
   a. Oxygen supplementation. In the term infant who is mildly symptomatic, an oxygen-rich environment is often all that is necessary. The inspired oxygen facilitates nitrogen washout of the blood and tissues and thus establishes a difference in the gas tensions between the loculated gases in the chest and those in the blood. This diffusion gradient results in rapid resorption of the loculated gas, with resolution of the pneumothorax. This mode of therapy is not appropriate in the preterm infant because of the risk of retinopathy of prematurity.
   b. Decompression. In the symptomatic neonate or the neonate on mechanical ventilatory support, immediate evacuation of air is necessary. The technique is described on p 231, **V.A.** Placement of a chest tube of appropriate size will eventually be necessary (see p 142).
C. Pulmonary interstitial emphysema (PIE)
   1. Definition. PIE is dissection of air into the perivascular tissues of the lung from alveolar overdistention or overdistention of the smaller airways.
   2. Incidence. This disorder arises almost exclusively in the very low birth weight infant on ventilatory support. If seen within the first 24 hours of life, it generally is associated with a poor prognosis. As time passes, its occurrence is less common, but it may be seen at any time during ventilatory management.
   3. Pathophysiology. PIE may be the precursor of all the other types of pulmonary air leaks. With alveolar overdistention or overdistention of the conducting airways, or both, rupture may occur and there may be dissection of the air into the perivascular tissue of the lung. The interstitial air moves in the connective tissue planes and around the vascular axis, particularly the venous ones. Once in the interstitial space, the air moves along bronchioles, lymphatics, vascular sheaths, or directly through the lung interstitium to the pleural surface. The extrapulmonary air is trapped in the interstitium (PIE), or it may extend and cause pneumomediastinum, pneumopericardium, or pneumothorax.
   4. Risk factors. See p 400.
   5. Clinical presentation. The patient in whom PIE develops may have sudden deterioration, but more commonly, the onset of PIE will be heralded by a slow, progressive deterioration of arterial blood gas levels and the apparent need for increasing ventilatory support. Invariably a diffusion block develops in these patients, with the al-

veolar membrane becoming separated from the capillary bed by the interstitial air. The response to increased ventilatory support in the face of poor arterial blood gas levels may lead to worsening of PIE and sudden clinical deterioration. Infants with severe PIE may have sudden and rapid deterioration or may actually improve if the PIE progresses to pneumothorax.

6. **Diagnosis.** In infants with PIE, the chest x-ray film will generally reveal radiolucencies that are either linear or cystlike in nature. The linear radiolucencies vary in length and do not branch; they are seen in the periphery of the lung as well as medially and may be mistaken for air bronchograms. The cystlike lucencies vary from 1.0 to 4.0 mm in diameter and can be lobulated.

7. **Management**
   a. **Lessening barotrauma.** In general, once PIE is diagnosed, an attempt should be made to decrease ventilatory support and lessen barotrauma. Decreasing the peak inspiratory pressure, decreasing the PEEP, or shortening the inspiratory time may be required. All of these maneuvers will decrease barotrauma and possibly lessen PIE. During this time, some degree of hypercarbia and hypoxia may have to be accepted.
   b. **Splinting of the affected side** has also proved beneficial in some cases of unilateral PIE.
   c. **Other treatments.** More invasive measures include selective collapse of the involved lung on the side with the worse involvement, with selective intubation or even the insertion of chest tubes prior to the development of pneumothorax.
   d. **High-frequency jet ventilation** (HFJV) (see p 122) has proved useful in infants with severe PIE. While this treatment modality may improve survival of the infant with PIE, the long-term pulmonary outcome of these infants remains uncertain. However, randomized controlled trials have been completed and have revealed good results. The earlier HFJV is begun following the onset of PIE, the greater the chance for survival.

8. **Prognosis.** See p 401.

D. **Pneumopericardium**
   1. **Definition.** Pneumopericardium is air in the pericardial sac, which is usually secondary to passage of air along vascular sheaths. It is always a complication of mechanical ventilatory support.
   2. **Incidence.** Pneumopericardium is a rare occurrence.
   3. **Pathophysiology.** It is often said that pneumopericardium is always preceded by pneumomediastinum, but this is not universally true. The mechanism by which pneumopericardium develops is not well understood, but it is probably due to passage of air along vascular sheaths.
   4. **Risk factors.** See p 400.
   5. **Clinical presentation.** The clinical signs of pneumopericardium range from asymptomatic to the full picture of cardiac tamponade. The first sign of pneumopericardium may be a decrease in blood pressure or a decrease in pulse pressure. There may also be an increase in heart rate with distant heart sounds.
   6. **Diagnosis.** Pneumopericardium has the **most classic radiographic appearance** of all the air leaks. A **broad radiolucent halo completely surrounds the heart, including the diaphragmatic surface.** This picture is easily distinguished from all the other air leaks by its extension completely around the heart in all projections.
   7. **Treatment.** Treatment of pneumopericardium is essential and requires the placement of a **pericardial drain or repeated pericardial taps.** The procedure is described on p 159.

APNEA AND PERIODIC BREATHING

I. **Definitions.** Simply defined, apnea is the absence of respiratory gas flow for a period of 20 seconds, with or without a decrease in heart rate. There are several types.
   A. **Central apnea** is of central nervous system origin and is characterized by the absence of gas flow with no respiratory effort.
   B. **Obstructive apnea** is continued respiratory effort not resulting in gas flow.
   C. **Mixed apnea** is a combination of the above and is usually initiated by a central event.
   D. **Periodic breathing,** defined as 3 or more periods of apnea lasting 3 seconds or more within a 20-second period of otherwise normal respiration, is also common in the newborn period. Currently it is not known whether or not there is an association between apnea and periodic breathing.
II. **Incidence.** The incidence of apnea and periodic breathing in the term infant has not been adequately determined. Approximately 50–60% of preterm infants have evidence of apnea: 35% present with central apnea, 5–10% with obstructive apnea, and 15–20% with mixed apnea. Another 30% will have periodic breathing.
III. **Pathophysiology.** Apnea and periodic breathing probably have a common pathophysiologic origin, apnea being a step further along the continuum than periodic breathing. While the exact pathophysiology of these events has not yet been elucidated, there are many theories.
   A. **Immaturity of respiratory control.** Since apnea is seen most commonly in the premature infant, some type of immaturity of the respiratory control mechanism is thought to play a role in most cases of apnea.
      1. **Hypoxic response.** The preterm infant is known to have an abnormal biphasic response to hypoxia: a brief period of tachypnea followed by apnea. This response is unlike that seen in the adult or older child in whom hypoxia produces a state of prolonged tachypnea.
      2. **Carbon dioxide response.** The carbon dioxide response curve is shifted in the preterm infant, with higher levels of carbon dioxide required before respiration is stimulated.
   B. **Sleep-related responses.** Sleep states may also play an important role in the development of apnea in the preterm infant. A shift from one sleep state to another is often characterized by instability of respiratory activity in the adult. The preterm infant spends about 80% of the time in sleep and has a difficult time making the transition between sleeping and waking states, which could lead to an increased risk for the development of apnea in these infants.
   C. **Protective reflexes** such as the apneic response to noxious substances in the airway may also play a role in the apneic episodes seen in the newborn infant.
   D. **Muscle weakness.** Overall muscle weakness (of both the muscles of respiration and the muscles that maintain airway patency), also plays an important role in pathophysiology.
   E. All of the above point to an **immature respiratory control mechanism** in the preterm infant. Whether the immaturity is operational at the level of the brain stem, the peripheral chemoreceptors, or the central receptors has yet to be determined. What is likely is that apnea results from a combination of immature afferent impulses to the respiratory control centers along with immature efferents from these same centers, giving rise to the poor ventilatory control.
   F. **Pathologic states** can also lead to apnea in the infant. The following disorders have all been associated with apnea in the neonatal period.

1. **Hypothermia.**
2. **Metabolic disturbances** such as hypoglycemia and hyponatremia.
3. **Sepsis.**
4. **Anemia.**
5. **Hypoxemia.**
6. **Central nervous system abnormalities** such as intraventricular hemorrhage.
7. **Necrotizing entercolitis.**

IV. **Risk factors**
  A. **Preterm infants.** The preterm infant is at the greatest risk for the development of apnea. Since apnea is believed to develop secondary to an immature or poorly developed respiratory control mechanism, this association should be obvious.
  B. **SIDS sibling.** The sibling of an infant who died from sudden infant death syndrome (SIDS) is also at great risk for having periods of apnea. Again, a poorly developed respiratory control mechanism is believed to be involved.
  C. **Neurologic disorders.** Since respiration depends on the integration of numerous central nervous system functions, the child with certain neurologic diseases may be at increased risk for the development of apnea.

V. **Clinical presentation**
  A. **Apnea within 24 hours after delivery.** Although apnea may present at any time during the neonatal period, if it presents within the first 24 hours of life, it is usually not simple apnea of prematurity. Apnea during this time period is **strongly associated with sepsis.**
  B. **Apnea after the first 3 days of life.** When apnea occurs after the first 3 days of life and is not associated with any other pathologic condition, it may be classified as **apnea of prematurity.** Apnea may also occur following weaning from ventilatory support and may be associated with intermittent hypoxia.

VI. **Diagnosis.** A high incidence of suspicion is necessary to diagnose apnea. If significant apnea is detected, an extensive workup is required in order to make an accurate diagnosis and develop a logical treatment plan.
  A. **Monitoring of infants at risk.** All preterm infants should be closely monitored for the development of this often life-threatening condition. Close attention should be paid to the type of monitoring that is given to infants in intensive care units. Preterm infants are commonly on heart rate monitors only, and they will be identified as having apnea only if the heart rate drops below the monitor alarm limit (usually set at 80 beats/min). In this case, these infants may suffer profound hypoxia before bradycardia develops, or they may have apnea with significant hypoxemia but without a drop in heart rate. In order to detect apnea, these infants should have continuous monitoring of respiratory activity or monitoring of oxygenation, or both, using either transcutaneous oximetry or pulse oximetry.
  B. **Physical examination.** Specific attention should be paid to physical findings such as lethargy, hypothermia, cyanosis, and respiratory effort. A good neurologic examination should also be performed.
  C. **Laboratory studies**
    1. **Complete blood count with differential and platelet count** will help to rule out sepsis.
    2. **Arterial blood gas determinations** will screen for hypoxia.
    3. **Serum glucose, electrolyte, and calcium levels** will aid in the diagnosis of metabolic disturbances.
  D. **Radiographic studies**
    1. **Chest x-ray study** to detect evidence of pathologic lung changes (eg, atelectasis, pneumonia, air leak).

    2. Abdominal x-ray study to detect signs of necrotizing entercolitis (see Chap 66).

    3. Ultrasonography of the head to detect intraventricular hemorrhage or other central nervous system abnormality.

    4. CT scan of the head may also be appropriate in infants with definite signs of neurologic disease.

E. Other studies

    1. Electroencephalography. An EEG may be necessary to complete the workup if there is any question about the neurologic status of the infant.

    2. Pneumography. A pneumogram is another essential tool in the diagnosis of apnea. Chest leads provide a tracing that gives a continuous recording of both heart rate and chest wall movement and can detect periods of central apnea and periodic breathing.

        a. Abnormal pneumogram. An abnormal pneumogram is defined as one in which one of the following patterns is demonstrated.

            (1) Periods of prolonged apnea (cessation of respiratory movement of > 20 seconds).

            (2) Short apnea (cessation of respiratory movement of < 20 seconds) if accompanied by bradycardia.

            (3) Episodes of periodic breathing lasting more than 5% of the total quiet or sleep time.

        b. Three-channel pneumogram. A more accurate instrument for the diagnosis of apnea is a 3-channel pneumogram, in which a nasal thermistor to detect air flow is added to the standard heart-rate and chest-wall channels. With the addition of the thermistor, central apnea can easily be distinguished from obstructive apnea. This distinction carries more than academic interest, since treatment of the disorder should be directed specifically to the type of apnea that is detected.

        c. Polysomnography. In research-oriented centers, a polysomnogram (a study that monitors specific EEG leads and muscle movement) can be used for a more thorough workup of apnea. This study will not only determine the type of apnea that occurs but can also relate it to the sleep stage of the infant. While polysomnography is certainly not indicated in all infants with apnea, its use may be beneficial in determining the exact pathogenesis of this enigmatic condition. Only after a thorough diagnostic evaluation, can adequate therapy for apnea be instituted.

VII. Management. Treatment for apnea must be individualized.

    A. Specific therapy. If an identifiable cause of apnea is determined, it should be treated accordingly. For example: sepsis should be treated with antibiotics (see Chap 76); hypoglycemia with glucose infusion (see p 210); electrolyte abnormalities (see specific abnormality in On-Call Problems) and anemia (see p 256) should be corrected.

    B. General therapy. If a cause cannot be identified or if one can be identified but is not amenable to treatment (eg, intraventricular hemorrhage), there are several approaches to treatment.

        1. Supplemental oxygen. Merely increasing the ambient oxygen concentration will often alleviate apneic spells. The mechanism of action is probably secondary to decreasing the number of unidentified hypoxic spells.

        2. Continuous positive airway pressure (CPAP) is used with some success, probably acting by the same mechanism as supplemental oxygen. This method is an invasive therapeutic modality and should be used only when other methods have failed.

        3. Oscillating water bed. Placing the infant on an oscillating water bed has been used with some success. This procedure is felt to increase the tactile stimulation the infant is receiving and thereby increase output from efferent nerves in the respiratory centers. Randomized, controlled trials have shown that it may not be effective therapy, but some centers may use it in selected cases.

4. **Pharmacologic therapy.** If the above methods fail, the next line of approach is to begin administration of respiratory stimulants.

   a. **Theophylline** is the drug used most commonly in the treatment of apnea. The exact mechanism of action is open to debate, but it probably works through direct stimulation of the respiratory centers as well as by lowering the threshold to carbon dioxide. Some clinicians think it may act by direct stimulation of the diaphragm. (See Chap 75 for dosage and other pharmacologic information.)

   b. **Caffeine** can also be used in the treatment of apnea, and since it has a longer half-life than theophylline, it may be a better drug. If caffeine is used, it is imperative that caffeine levels be monitored. (See Chap 75 for dosage and other pharmacologic information.)

   c. **Doxapram.** Doxapram, a potent respiratory stimulant, has recently been shown to be effective when theophylline and caffeine have failed. The duration of treatment with doxapram has been limited to 5 days, but the drug may be used longer if indicated. Benzyl alcohol is the preservative used in doxapram. Duration of therapy depends upon the cumulative dose of benzyl alcohol.

5. **Mechanical ventilation.** Some infants continue to have apneic spells despite adequate treatment. If the apnea is severe and is associated with hypoxia or significant bradycardia, intubation and mechanical ventilation may be indicated.

C. **Discharge planning and follow-up.** A major issue in the management of infants with apnea is deciding when to stop administration of theophylline and whether or not the infant needs to be discharged on theophylline, a home monitor, or both.

1. **Discontinuing medications.** Consider stopping theophylline therapy when the apnea has resolved and the infant weighs between 1800 and 2000 g. If the infant remains asymptomatic following the discontinuation of theophylline therapy, the child may be discharged without further therapy.

2. **Reinstituting medications.** If symptomatic apnea recurs after discontinuing therapy, theophylline therapy should be reinstituted and a decision made to discharge the infant on this medication or to keep the infant hospitalized longer. The use of home monitors in addition to theophylline therapy is *controversial.* Therapeutic theophylline levels are maintained until the child reaches 52 weeks of postconceptual age; then theophylline therapy is discontinued and pneumography is performed. If the pneumogram is normal, therapy can be stopped. If the pneumogram is abnormal, the infant needs to be restarted on theophylline and monitoring continued. Another attempt can be made to discontinue theophylline in 4 weeks.

3. **Home apnea monitoring.** Even though home monitoring has not been proved to prevent morbidity and mortality associated with apnea and remains controversial, most neonatologists and pediatricians feel that until a better understanding of this condition is reached, home monitoring is the best approach available. The use of home monitors with theophylline remains *controversial.* If an infant is discharged on theophylline and a monitor, the guidelines are the same as in **C.2,** above.

VIII. Prognosis. In most infants, apnea resolves without the occurrence of long-term deficiencies. Once the child is weaned from medication or a monitor, or both, outcome is no different from gestational age–matched counterparts.

BRONCHOPULMONARY DYSPLASIA

I. **Definition.** Bronchopulmonary dysplasia (BPD) has become a general term for various forms of chronic lung disease that develop in premature infants treated with mechanical ventilation for respiratory distress syndrome (RDS). The term *bronchopulmonary dysplasia* was coined by Northway in 1967 to denote a chronic pulmonary syndrome associated with the use of mechanical ventilation in premature infants with RDS. He noted an orderly progression of clinical, pathologic, and radiologic changes from the early findings of severe RDS (stage 1) to severe, chronic pulmonary insufficiency (stage 4). However, these infants with RDS were more mature and larger at birth than are many survivors of RDS today. Two more recent definitions of BPD have been suggested. In the first, the diagnosis of BPD is made in the infant who requires positive-pressure ventilation in the first week of life and has clinical signs of chronic respiratory disease, an oxygen requirement, and an abnormal chest x-ray film at 28 days of age. More recently, it has been shown that an abnormal pulmonary outcome is better predicted by a requirement for oxygen at 36 weeks' postconceptional age. The terms *BPD* and *chronic lung disease* are often used interchangeably to refer to a variety of chronic respiratory disorders.

II. **Incidence.** The reported incidence of BPD is variable, depending on how BPD is defined and on the patient population under study. In babies with birth weights under 1000 g, the incidence of BPD has been reported to be as low as 3–4% when defined as Northway stage 3 or 4 disease or as high as 70% when defined as the need for supplemental oxygen at 28 days of age. Exogenous surfactant replacement therapy has not yet been shown to consistently decrease the incidence of BPD.

III. **Pathophysiology.** BPD is a multifactorial disorder. It begins with acute lung injury in a susceptible host. Continued lung injury and abnormal repair lead to structural changes and chronic pulmonary dysfunction.

A. **Lung injury** can occur as a result of:

1. **Surfactant deficiency.** Collapse of saccules, with distention of distal alveolar ducts and further maldistribution of ventilation, may lead to injury.

2. **Pulmonary edema.** RDS is almost always accompanied by pulmonary edema, which may be worsened by hypoproteinemia and increased pulmonary blood flow (as occurs in infants with patent ductus arteriosus).

3. **Oxygen exposure.** Prolonged exposure to high concentrations of oxygen can have multiple adverse effects, including epithelial and endothelial cell damage and/or death, ciliary dysfunction, decreased lung lymph flow, alteration of surfactant synthesis, and inhibition of lung growth.

4. **Mechanical ventilation.** Positive distending pressure, the presence of an endotracheal tube, tracheal suctioning, and improperly warmed or humidified inspired gases may all lead to lung injury.

5. **Inflammation.** Neutrophils are capable of releasing a variety of toxic substances including proteases, oxygen free radicals, and a host of mediators of inflammation. The presence of neutrophils in the tracheal aspirates of infants with RDS who subsequently develop BPD, suggests that they may contribute to the pathogenesis of BPD.

    B. **Pathologic changes.** The pathology of BPD varies with the stage of the disease. Early pathologic lung changes include areas of atelectasis filled with proteinaceous fluid alternating with areas of overexpansion. Airway injury is seen as loss of epithelium and cilia or, in a more severe form, as necrotizing tracheobronchitis. Late findings may include interstitial fibrosis, cystic dilatation, atelectasis, interstitial edema, and lymphatic distention.

IV. **Risk factors.** The risk of developing BPD increases with decreasing gestational age and birth weight. Prematurity, white race, male sex, and a family history of reactive airway disease have all been associated with an increased risk of BPD.

V. **Clinical presentation**

    A. **General presentation.** Typically, BPD occurs in infants weighing less than 2000 g and of less than 34 weeks' gestation at birth who have required supplemental oxygen and mechanical ventilation for RDS. Infants who develop BPD often fail to demonstrate the rapid improvement in the first week of life that is common in uncomplicated RDS. Instead, they frequently have a prolonged course of ventilator and oxygen dependency. This course may be accompanied by poor growth, intermittent pulmonary edema, or airway reactivity, or all three.

    B. **Physical examination**

        1. **General signs.** Tachypnea, tachycardia, retractions, and nasal flaring are common. Upon breathing room air, these signs may worsen and cyanosis may occur.

        2. **Pulmonary examination.** Retractions and diffuse rales are also common. Wheezing or prolongation of expiration may also be noted. The presence of digital clubbing indicates long-standing hypoxemia.

        3. **Cardiovascular examination.** A right ventricular heave, single S_2, or prominent P_2 may accompany cor pulmonale.

        4. **Abdominal examination.** The liver may be enlarged secondary to right heart failure or may be displaced downward into the abdomen secondary to pulmonary hyperinflation.

VI. **Diagnosis**

    A. **Laboratory studies.** Laboratory studies reflect the chronic nature of the disease.

        1. **Arterial blood gas levels** frequently reveal carbon dioxide retention. However, if the respiratory difficulties are chronic and stable, the pH is usually normal.

        2. **Electrolytes.** Abnormalities of electrolytes may result from chronic carbon dioxide retention (elevated serum bicarbonate), diuretic therapy (hyponatremia, hypokalemia, hypochloremia), or fluid restriction (elevated urea nitrogen and creatinine), or all three.

    B. **Radiologic studies**

        1. **Chest x-ray study.** Radiographic findings may be quite variable. They may appear only as diffuse haziness and hypoinflation in infants who were very immature at birth and have persistent oxygen requirements, while in other infants, they may be more similar to those originally described by Northway—streaky interstitial markings, atelectasis, cysts, and hyperinflation. It is often difficult to distinguish new x-ray findings from chronic changes without the benefit of comparison to previous x-ray films.

        2. **Abdominal ultrasonography or x-ray study.** Radiologic studies of the abdomen may demonstrate the presence of renal or, less commonly, biliary tract stones secondary to long-term use of diuretics (eg, furosemide).

    C. **Other studies. Electrocardiography** and **echocardiography** may show right ventricular hypertrophy and elevation of pulmonary artery pressure with right axis deviation, increased right systolic time intervals, thickening of the right ventricular wall, and abnormal right ventricular geometry.

VII. Management

A. Prevention. Much recent attention has been focused on the development of ways to prevent the occurrence of both RDS and BPD.

1. **Prevention of prematurity.** Therapies directed toward decreasing the risk of prematurity and the incidence of RDS include improving prenatal care and the use of tocolytic agents, antenatal corticosteroids, and exogenous surfactants.

2. **Prevention of BPD.** Management of the infant with RDS is directed toward reducing the risk of subsequent BPD.

   a. **Established modalities** include minimizing exposure to oxygen and barotrauma, restricting fluids, and aggressively treating patent ductus arteriosus.

   b. **Other modalities**

   (1) **Antioxidant therapy.** Treatment with the dietary antioxidant, **vitamin E,** has been attempted, with variable results. However, there was an unacceptably high incidence of side effects in infants receiving parenteral vitamin E. Extensive therapeutic trials of other antioxidants have not been performed.

   (2) **Dexamethasone.** There is evidence that dexamethasone may be effective in preventing or ameliorating BPD when started early in the course and tapered very gradually. Little work has been done to either identify optimal dosing regimens or compare corticosteroid preparations.

   (3) **Vitamin A.** Vitamin A is known to be important in epithelial cell differentiation and repair. When administered intramuscularly, it has been shown to decrease the incidence of BPD in very low birth weight infants. Although this study was small, the results are promising and await confirmation in a larger trial.

B. Treatment of BPD. The management of infants with BPD is often complex and time-consuming. It requires recognition of the gradual transition from RDS to BPD and corresponding changes in the therapeutic approach. Once BPD is present, the goal of management is to prevent further injury, augment pulmonary function, prevent cor pulmonale, and aid growth and development.

1. **Respiratory management**

   a. **Supplemental oxygen.** In contrast to RDS—for which the emphasis is on minimizing exposure to oxygen—maintaining adequate oxygenation is important in the infant with BPD in order to prevent complications such as cor pulmonale and growth failure. Supplemental oxygen is required. Monitoring of oxygenation is most easily accomplished with a pulse oximeter that measures arterial oxygen saturation (Sao_2), although transcutaneous oxygen monitoring is also useful. The infant should be studied during its various activities, including rest, sleep, and feeding. Blood gas measurements are important for the assessment of pH and $Paco_2$ but are of limited use in monitoring oxygenation, since they provide information about only one point in time. For infants with fully vascularized retinas (usually about 40 weeks' postconceptional age), it is probably optimal to maintain $Sao_2 > 95\%$ or $Pao_2 \geq 70$ torr. For less mature infants, Sao_2 should probably be maintained in the 90–94% range.

   b. **Positive-pressure ventilation.** Prolonged mechanical ventilation is frequently required. Problems with air trapping can be significant and may be reduced by decreasing ventilator rate and increasing the time for exhalation. Weaning is a gradual process that can be facilitated by tolerating $Paco_2$ in excess of 50 torr. Nasal continuous positive airway pressure (CPAP) can be useful as an adjunctive therapy following extubation.

c. **Bronchodilators.** A response to bronchodilators has been demonstrated in very young and very immature infants. A variety of agents are available for the treatment of airway reactivity. (See also Chap 75 for detailed pharmacologic information.)

   (1) **Beta-2 agonists.** Several beta-2 agonists have been shown to produce measurable improvements in lung mechanics and gas exchange in infants. Among those available as inhaled agents are **metaproterenol** (0.25–0.5 mg/kg, every 2–8 hours), **albuterol** (0.05–0.15 mg/kg every 2–8 hours), **isoetharine** (0.1–0.2 mg/kg every 2–8 hours) and **terbutaline** (0.1–0.3 mg/kg every 2–8 hours).

   (2) **Theophylline.** Theophylline has potentially beneficial actions, including smooth muscle dilation, improvement of diaphragmatic contractility, central respiratory stimulation, and mild diuretic effects. It appears to improve lung function in BPD when levels are maintained at more than 10 μg/mL. Side effects are fairly common and may include CNS irritability, gastroesophageal reflux, and GI irritation.

   (3) **Cromolyn sodium.** The precise mechanism of action is unknown, but this drug is believed to reduce the mediators of inflammation released into the airways following both antigenic and nonspecific stimuli. There is some evidence to suggest that it may be of benefit in infants with BPD when given as an aerosol in doses of 20 mg every 6–8 hours.

   (4) **Anticholinergic agents. Aerosolized atropine** (0.08 mg/kg) has been shown to improve lung function, similarly to metaproterenol, in infants with BPD. Systemic absorption occurs, and side effects, including flushing, urinary retention, tachycardia, dryness of the skin and mouth, and mental status changes, may occur with repeated doses.

   (5) **Corticosteroids.** The benefits of inhaled corticosteroids and short courses of oral or parenteral corticosteroids in the treatment of asthma in pediatric and adult patients are well established. However, their use for treatment of reactive airway disease in BPD has not been studied.

2. **Management of pulmonary edema**

   a. **Fluid restriction.** Restricting fluid to 150 mL/kg/d or less is often required. It can be accomplished by concentrating proprietary formulas to 24 cal/oz. Increasing the caloric density further, to 27–30 cal/oz, requires the addition of fat (eg, MCT oil, corn oil) and carbohydrate (eg, Polycose) to avoid excessive protein intake.

   b. **Diuretic therapy**

   (1) **Chlorothiazide and spironolactone.** This combination is ideal for chronic management. It has been shown to improve lung function and has relatively few side effects. When used in doses of 20 mg/kg/d (chlorothiazide) and 2 mg/kg/d (spironolactone), a good diuretic response can often be obtained without the need for electrolyte supplementation.

   (2) **Furosemide.** Furosemide is a more potent diuretic than chlorothiazide and spironolactone and is particularly useful acutely for rapid diuresis. It is associated with side effects such as electrolyte abnormalities, calciuria with bone de-

mineralization and renal stone formation, and ototoxicity, thereby limiting its usefulness as a chronic medication.

3. **Corticosteroids.** The use of corticosteroids in established BPD remains *controversial*. Long courses of dexamethasone in gradually tapering doses appear to benefit some patients. Possible side effects include infection, hypertension, gastric ulcer, and hyperglycemia. Alternate delivery methods (eg, aerosols) and dosing strategies have not been thoroughly studied.

4. **Nutrition.** Because growth is essential for recovery from BPD, adequate nutritional intake is crucial. Infants with BPD frequently have high caloric needs (120–150 kcal/kg/d or more) due to increased metabolic expenditures. Concentrated formula is often necessary to provide sufficient calories and prevent pulmonary edema.

5. **Discharge planning.** Oxygen can often be discontinued prior to NICU discharge. However, home oxygen therapy can be a safe alternative to long-term hospitalization. The need for home apnea and bradycardia monitoring must be decided on an individual basis but is generally recommended for infants discharged home on oxygen. All parents should be instructed in CPR.

6. **General care.** Care plans for older infants with BPD should include adapting their routine for home life and involving the parents in their care. Immunizations should be given at the appropriate chronologic age. Periodic screening for chemical evidence of rickets and echocardiographic evidence of right ventricular hypertrophy is recommended. Assessment by a developmentalist and occupational or physical therapist, or both, can be useful for prognostic and therapeutic purposes.

VIII. **Prognosis.** The prognosis for infants with BPD depends on the degree of pulmonary dysfunction and the presence of other medical conditions. Most deaths occur in the first year of life as a result of cardiorespiratory failure, sepsis or respiratory infection or as sudden, unexplained death.

A. **Pulmonary outcome.** The short-term outcome of infants with BPD, including those requiring oxygen at home, is surprisingly good. Weaning from oxygen is usually possible prior to their first birthday, and they demonstrate catch-up growth as their pulmonary status improves. However, in the first year of life, rehospitalization is necessary for about 30% of patients for treatment of wheezing or respiratory infections, or both. Although upper respiratory infections are probably no more common in infants with BPD than in normal infants, they are more likely to be associated with significant respiratory symptoms. The 10-year outcome, assessed in children who were more mature and larger at birth than many infants today, is characterized by increased airway resistance and reactivity.

B. **Neurodevelopmental outcome.** Children with BPD appear to be at increased risk for adverse neurodevelopmental outcome compared to comparable infants without BPD. Neuromotor and cognitive dysfunction appear to be more common. In addition, children with BPD may be at higher risk for significant hearing impairment and retinopathy of prematurity. They are also at risk for later problems, including learning disabilities, attention deficits, and behavior problems.

HYALINE MEMBRANE DISEASE (RESPIRATORY DISTRESS SYNDROME)

I. **Definition.** Hyaline membrane disease (HMD) is also called *respiratory distress syndrome (RDS)*. This clinical diagnosis is warranted in a preterm newborn with respiratory difficulty—including tachypnea (60/min), chest retractions, and cyanosis on room air—that persists or progresses over the first 48–96 hours of life and with a characteristic chest x-ray film (uniform reticulogranular pattern and air bronchograms). The clinical course of the disease varies with the size of the infant, the severity of the disease, the presence of infection, the degree of shunting of blood through a patent ductus arteriosus, and whether or not assisted ventilation was initiated (Stark, 1986).

II. **Incidence.** HMD severe enough to require assisted ventilation occurs in about 25% of infants born at 30 weeks' gestation. The incidence increases with increasing prematurity. In the United States, 40,000 newborns are affected annually. Although survival is over 90%, RDS accounts for 20% of all neonatal deaths.

III. **Pathophysiology.** The infant with HMD exhibits dependency on supplemental oxygen and increased work of breathing. Both are due to progressive atelectasis from lack of surfactant and an overly compliant chest wall. Surfactant is a surface-active material produced by airway epithelial cells called **type II pneumocytes.** This cell line differentiates, and surfactant synthesis begins at 24–28 weeks' gestation. Type II cells are sensitive to and decreased by asphyxial insults in the perinatal period. The maturation of this cell line is delayed in the presence of fetal hyperinsulinemia. The maturity of type II cells is enhanced by chronic intrauterine stress such as pregnancy-induced hypertension, intrauterine growth retardation (IUGR), and twin gestation. Surfactant, composed chiefly of phospholipid (75%) and protein (10%), is produced and stored in the characteristic **lamellar bodies** of type II pneumocytes. This lipoprotein is released into the airways, where it functions to decrease surface tension and maintain alveolar expansion at physiologic pressures.

   A. **Lack of surfactant.** In the absence of surfactant, the small air spaces collapse, with each expiration resulting in progressive atelectasis. Exudative proteinaceous material and epithelial debris, resulting from progressive cellular damage, collect in the airway and directly decrease total lung capacity. In pathologic specimens, this material stains typically as **eosinophilic hyaline membranes**—thus the pathologic diagnosis of hyaline membrane disease.

   B. **Presence of an overly compliant chest wall.** In the presence of a chest wall with weak structural support owing to prematurity, the large negative pressures generated to open the collapsed airways cause retraction and deformation of the chest wall instead of inflation of the poorly compliant lungs.

   C. **Shunting.** The presence or absence of a cardiovascular shunt through a patent ductus arteriosus or foramen ovale, or both, may change the presentation or course of the disease process. The course of HMD results in acidosis and hypoxia, which can increase pulmonary vascular resistance. When pulmonary (right) pressure exceeds systemic (left) pressure, right-to-left shunting results. The clinical course is often complicated by cardiomegaly and pulmonary edema, owing to a large left-to-right shunt through the patent ductus or foramen ovale.

   D. **Decreased intrapulmonary pressure.** The infant with HMD who is less than 30 weeks' gestational age often presents with immediate respiratory failure due to inability to generate the intrapulmonary pressure necessary to inflate the lungs without surfactant.

IV. **Risk factors.** Factors that increase or decrease the risk of HMD are listed in Table 69–1.

V. **Clinical presentation**

   A. **History.** The infant is **preterm,** either by dates or by gestational examination, *or* has a **history of asphyxia in the perinatal period.** It presents with some **respiratory difficulty at birth that becomes progressively more severe.** The classic worsening of the atelectasis, as seen on chest x-ray film, and increasing oxygen requirement for 48–72 hours

TABLE 69-1. RISK FACTORS THAT INCREASE OR DECREASE THE RISK OF HYALINE MEMBRANE DISEASE

Increased Risk	Decreased Risk
Prematurity	Chronic intrauterine stress
Male sex	Prolonged ruptured membranes
Familial predisposition	Maternal hypertension
Cesarean without labor	Narcotic/cocaine use
Perinatal asphyxia	IUGR or SGA
Chorioamnionitis	Corticosteroids
Hydrops	Thyroid hormone
	Tocolytic agents

with subsequent diuresis and improvement (or death), have been modified by the increased ability to provide respiratory support for these infants.

B. Physical examination. The infant exhibits **cyanosis on room air, nasal flaring, tachypnea, grunting on expiration,** and **retractions** of the chest wall. The infant grunts to prolong expiration, and this mechanism actually improves alveolar ventilation. The retractions occur and increase as the infant is forced to develop high transpulmonary pressure to reinflate atelectatic air spaces.

VI. Diagnosis

A. Laboratory studies

1. **Blood gas sampling** is essential in the management of HMD. Usually intermittent arterial sampling is performed. Although there is no consensus, most neonatologists agree that **arterial oxygen tensions of 50–70 mm Hg and arterial carbon dioxide tensions of 45–60 mm Hg are acceptable.** Most would maintain the pH at or above 7.25 and the arterial oxygen saturation at 88–95%. *Note:* In addition, continuous transcutaneous oxygen and carbon dioxide monitors or oxygen saturation monitors, or both, are proving invaluable in the minute-to-minute monitoring.

2. **Hemoglobin or hematocrit measurements** are needed early to guide the choice of plasma volume expanders if the infant has evidence of shock.

3. **Serum glucose levels** may be high or low initially and must be followed closely to assess the adequacy of dextrose infusion.

4. **Septic workup.** A partial septic workup, including complete blood count, platelet count, blood culture, amniotic fluid culture, urine culture, and latex agglutination test of the infant's urine for group B streptococcal antigen, should be considered for each infant with a diagnosis of HMD, since early-onset sepsis, eg, infection with group B streptococcus or *Haemophilus influenzae,* can be indistinguishable from HMD on clinical grounds alone.

5. **Serum electrolyte levels** should be followed very 12–24 hours for management of parenteral fluids.

6. **Serum calcium levels** should be followed daily, since hypocalcemia is common in sick, nonfed, preterm, or asphyxiated infants.

7. **Blood type, Rh, and Coombs' test determinations** are needed because:

   a. Transfusion may be indicated to correct hypotension, persistent poor perfusion, or falling blood hematocrit resulting from routine phlebotomy.

   b. The possibility of significant hyperbilirubinemia and the need for exchange blood transfusions exists in these infants, owing to prematurity, acidosis, and delayed feeding and stooling.

B. Chest x-ray study. An anteroposterior chest x-ray film should be obtained for all infants with respiratory distress of any duration. If the infant is close to term, a cross-table lateral view may be considered to search for evidence of free air between the chest wall and lung parenchyma. The typical radiographic finding is a **uniform reticulogranular pattern, referred to as a "ground glass" appearance accompanied by air bronchograms.** During the clinical course, sequential x-ray films may reveal air leaks secondary to ventilatory intervention as well as the onset of changes compatible with bronchopulmonary dysplasia.

C. **Echocardiography** is a valuable diagnostic tool in the evaluation of an infant with hypoxemia and respiratory distress. Significant congenital heart disease can be excluded by this technique. Vascular shunts either away from or toward the lungs may be demonstrated and appropriate therapy instituted.

VII. **Management**
A. **Prevention.** The following preventive measures have resulted in improved survival of infants at risk for RDS.
  1. **Antenatal ultrasonography** for more accurate assessment of gestational age and fetal well-being.
  2. **Continuous fetal monitoring** to document fetal well-being during labor or to signal the need for intervention when fetal distress is discovered.
  3. **Prevention and intervention of premature labor,** using both tocolytic agents and corticosteroids to induce lung maturation.
  4. **Assessment of fetal lung maturity** prior to delivery (lecithin:sphingomyelin ratio and phosphatidyl glycerol). (See p 3.)
B. **Respiratory support**
  1. **Endotracheal intubation and mechanical ventilation** are the mainstays of therapy for infants with respiratory distress syndrome in whom apnea or hypoxemia with respiratory acidosis develops. Mechanical ventilation usually begins with rates of 30–60 breaths/min and inspiratory:expiratory ratios of 1:2. An initial peak inspiratory pressure (PIP) of 18–30 cm water is used, depending on the size of the infant and the severity of the disease. A positive end-expiratory pressure (PEEP) of 4 cm water results in improved oxygenation probably due to increased airway pressure, which is kept as low as possible while still maintaining ventilation and oxygenation. The lowest possible pressures and inspired oxygen concentrations are maintained in an attempt to minimize damage to parenchymal tissue.
  2. **Continuous positive airway pressure (CPAP).** Nasal prong or nasopharyngeal CPAP (NPCPAP) may be used early to delay or prevent the need for endotracheal intubation. It works best on larger infants with mild to moderate disease and good respiratory effort. NPCPAP may be used upon extubation and it may decrease the chance of reintubation. Nasopharyngeal tubes plug frequently. Therefore, their use must be accompanied by routine replacement of the tube each 6–8 hours.
  3. **Complications.** Pulmonary air leaks, such as pneumothorax, pneumomediastinum, pneumopericardium, and pulmonary interstitial emphysema, may occur. Chronic complications include respiratory problems such as bronchopulmonary dysplasia and tracheal stenosis.
C. **Fluid and nutritional support.** In the very ill infant, it is now possible to maintain nutritional support with parenteral nutrition for an extended period. The specific needs of preterm and term infants are becoming better understood, and the nutrient preparations available reflect this understanding (see Chap 8).

TABLE 69-2. PROGNOSIS AND OUTCOMES IN PATIENTS WITH HYALINE MEMBRANE DISEASE BASED ON BIRTH WEIGHT

Birth Weight (g)	Survival Percentage	Risk of BPD[a]	Risk of Stage III/IV ROP[b]
501	5	All	Very high
501-750	40	Most	Moderate
751-1000	75	Half	Present
1001-1500	98	Few	Low

[a] Bronchopulmonary dysplasia, patients on oxygen at 28 days.
[b] Retinopathy of prematurity.

    D. Drug therapy. Sedation with **phenobarbitol, pentobarbitol,** and **chloral hydrate** is commonly used to control ventilation in these sick infants. Muscle relaxation with pancuronium in infants with RDS remains *controversial.* Sedation might be indicated for infants with respiratory patterns that increase the likelihood of an air leak. These infants "fight" the ventilator support and consistently exhale on the inspiratory part of the ventilator cycle. Sedation or muscle paralysis of infants with fluctuating cerebral blood flow velocity theoretically decreases the risk of intraventricular hemorrhage.

    E. Surfactant replacement. (See also Chap 13.) Surfactant replacement is the most exciting advance in the treatment of HMD. Double-blind randomized trials have proved that exogenous surfactant given either as a preventilatory dose or within 6 hours of birth in "rescue" studies dramatically reduces the number of cases of severe RDS (80% oxygen and mean airway pressures of more than 10 cm water). Two products (**Exosurf Pediatric** and **Survanta**) have been released by the FDA. It has granted new drug approval (NDA) to Exosurf Pediatric and approval for investigational use to Survanta. These products are available in all institutions that provide ventilatory support in neonatal intensive care settings. Strict protocols for enrollment and administration are required so that evaluation can continue. Surfactant replacement, although proved to be immediately effective in reducing the severity of RDS, has not clearly been shown to decrease the long-term oxygen requirements or the development of chronic lung changes. Currently, long-term follow-up studies have not shown significant differences between surfactant-treated patients and nontreated control groups with regard to PDA, IVH, ROP, NEC, BPD, and long-term mortality. In 2-4 year follow-up studies, no adverse effects attributable to surfactant therapy have been identified.

VIII. Prognosis. The prognosis for infants with HMD is highly dependent on birth weight (see Table 69-2).

MECONIUM ASPIRATION

    I. Definition. Normally, meconium is the first intestinal discharge of the newborn infant and is composed of epithelial cells, fetal hair, mucus, and bile. However, intrauterine stress may cause in utero passage of meconium into the amniotic fluid. Subsequent to passage, the meconium-stained amniotic fluid may be aspirated by the fetus in utero or by the newborn during labor and delivery. If meconium is aspirated, it can cause airway obstruction and an intense inflammatory reaction, resulting in severe respiratory distress. The presence of meconium in amniotic fluid is a **warning sign of fetal distress,** calling for careful supervision of labor and assessment of fetal well-being.

    II. Incidence. The incidence of meconium-stained amniotic fluid varies from 8% to 20% of all deliveries. The passage of meconium in an asphyxiated

infant under 34 weeks' gestation is unusual; thus, meconium aspiration affects chiefly **term and postmature infants.**
III. **Pathophysiology**
  A. **In utero passage of meconium.** Asphyxia and other forms of intrauterine stress may cause increased intestinal peristalsis, with relaxation of the external anal sphincter and passage of meconium. The effect of intrauterine hypoxia on peristalsis and sphincter tone seems to increase with gestational age, so that a premature infant with meconium-stained fluid at birth may have suffered a more severe insult than a postmature infant.
  B. **Aspiration of meconium.** After passage of meconium into the amniotic fluid, gasping respirations of the asphyxiated fetus, either in utero or during labor and delivery, can cause aspiration of the meconium-stained amniotic fluid into the large airways of the lung. (Normal fetal respiratory activity results in movement of lung secretions from the airways into the amniotic fluid.) The thick meconium causes airway obstruction, resulting in respiratory distress.
    1. **Airway obstruction.** With aspiration of meconium distally, total or partial airway obstruction may occur. In areas of total obstruction, atelectasis develops; but in areas of partial obstruction, a ball-valve phenomenon occurs, resulting in air trapping and hyperexpansion. Air trapping increases the risk of air leak to 21–50%.
    2. **Chemical pneumonitis.** Ultimately, interstitial and chemical pneumonitis develops, with resulting bronchiolar edema and narrowing of the small airways. Uneven ventilation due to areas of partial obstruction and superimposed pneumonitis causes severe carbon dioxide retention and hypoxemia. Pulmonary vascular resistance increases as a direct result of hypoxia, acidosis, and hyperinflation of the lungs. The increase in pulmonary vascular resistance may lead to atrial or ductal right-to-left shunting and further desaturation.
IV. **Risk factors.** The following factors have been associated with an increased risk of meconium passage and subsequent aspiration.
  A. Postterm pregnancy.
  B. Preeclampsia-eclampsia
  C. Maternal hypertension.
  D. Maternal diabetes mellitus.
  E. Abnormal fetal heart rate.
  F. Small-for-gestational-age infants.
  G. Biophysical profile ≤ 6.
  H. Maternal heavy smoking, chronic respiratory disease, or cardiovascular disease.
V. **Clinical presentation.** The presentation of an infant with meconium-stained amniotic fluid who has aspirated meconium in the trachea is variable. Symptoms depend on the severity of the hypoxic insult and the amount and viscosity of the meconium aspirated.
  A. **General features**
    1. **The infant.** Infants with meconium-stained amniotic fluid often exhibit signs of postmaturity: they are small for gestational age with long nails and peeling skin stained with yellow or green pigment. These infants may have respiratory depression at birth, with poor respiratory effort and decreased muscle tone if there has been significant perinatal asphyxia associated with the passage of meconium.
    2. **The amniotic fluid.** The meconium present in amniotic fluid varies in quantity, appearance, and viscosity, ranging from a small to a copious amount and from a thin green-stained fluid to a thick "pea soup" consistency. It appears that heavily stained fluid is more

clearly associated with severe respiratory distress and higher morbidity and mortality rates than lightly stained fluid.

B. Airway obstruction. If a large amount of thick meconium is aspirated, the infant presents with acute airway obstruction manifested by deep gasping respirations, cyanosis, and poor air exchange. The airway must be rapidly cleared by endotracheal suctioning.

C. Respiratory distress. The infant who has aspirated meconium into the distal airways but does not have total airway obstruction manifests signs of respiratory distress secondary to increased airway resistance and air trapping, ie, **tachypnea, nasal flaring, rib retraction, and cyanosis.** Some infants who do not experience acute airway obstruction **may have a delayed presentation,** with only mild initial respiratory distress, which becomes more severe hours after delivery as chemical pneumonitis develops.

Note: Although many infants with meconium-stained amniotic fluid appear normal at birth and exhibit no signs of respiratory distress, a short episode of asphyxia may well have induced passage of meconium.

D. Other pulmonary abnormalities. There may be a noticeable increase in the anteroposterior diameter of the chest if air trapping develops. With air trapping, auscultation reveals decreased air exchange, ie, variable rales, rhonchi, and wheezing.

VI. Diagnosis

A. Laboratory studies. Arterial blood gas levels characteristically reveal hypoxemia. Hyperventilation may result in respiratory alkalosis in mild cases, but infants with severe disease usually manifest respiratory acidosis with carbon dioxide retention due to airway obstruction and pneumonitis. If the patient has suffered severe perinatal asphyxia, combined respiratory and metabolic acidosis are present.

B. Radiologic studies. A **chest x-ray film** typically reveals hyperinflation of the lung fields and flattened diaphragms. There are coarse, irregular patchy infiltrates with increased lung fluid. Pneumothorax or pneumomediastinum may be present.

VII. Management

A. Prenatal management. The key to management of meconium aspiration lies in prevention during the prenatal period.

1. **Identification of high-risk pregnancies.** The approach to prevention begins with recognition of predisposing maternal factors that may cause uteroplacental insufficiency and subsequent fetal hypoxia during labor (see **IV,** p 418).

2. **Monitoring.** During labor, careful observation and fetal monitoring should be performed. Any signs of fetal distress (eg, appearance of meconium-stained fluid with membrane rupture, loss of beat-to-beat variability, deceleration patterns) warrant assessment of fetal well-being by scrutiny of fetal heart tracings and fetal scalp pH. If assessment indicates a compromised fetus, delivery by the most appropriate route should be accomplished as soon as possible.

B. Delivery room management. Delivery room management of the meconium-stained infant is discussed on p 15.

C. Management of the newborn with meconium aspiration. Infants who have meconium suctioned from the trachea are at risk for pneumonitis and air leak syndromes and must be observed closely for signs of respiratory distress. In addition, infants with meconium-stained fluid and low Apgar scores may have suffered asphyxial injury and should be examined for signs of end-organ damage.

1. **Respiratory management**

   a. **Pulmonary toilet.** If suctioning the trachea does not result in clearing of secretions, it may be advisable to leave an endotracheal tube in place for pulmonary toilet. Chest physiotherapy every 30 minutes to 1 hour, as tolerated, will aid in clearing the airway.

b. **Arterial blood gas levels.** On admission to the NICU, the infant requires arterial blood gas measurements to assess ventilatory compromise and supplemental oxygen needs. If the patient requires more than 40% FIO_2, an arterial line should be placed.

c. **Oxygen monitoring.** A transcutaneous oxygen monitor or pulse oximeter may provide information regarding the patient's ability to tolerate stress and will assist in preventing hypoxemia.

d. **Chest x-ray films** should be obtained after delivery if the infant is in distress. It may help determine which patients will develop respiratory distress.

e. **Antibiotic coverage.** Meconium promotes the growth of bacteria in vitro. Since it is impossible to differentiate meconium aspiration from pneumonia radiographically, infants with infiltrates on chest x-ray film should be started on broad-spectrum antibiotics (ampicillin and gentamicin; see Chap 76 for dosages and other pharmacologic information) after appropriate cultures have been obtained.

f. **Supplemental oxygen.** If oxygen requirements continue to increase and acceptable oxygenation cannot be maintained, a trial of continuous positive airway pressure (CPAP) may be considered. CPAP may help with oxygenation in certain patients, but it may also aggravate preexisting air trapping and increase the risk of air leak. If possible, arterial oxygen tension should be maintained in the range of 80–90 mm Hg to prevent hypoxic pulmonary vasoconstriction, which may result in development of persistent pulmonary hypertension (PPH).

g. **Mechanical ventilation.** Patients with severe disease who are in impending respiratory failure with hypercapnia and persistent hypoxemia require mechanical ventilation.

   (1) **Rate settings.** Ventilation must be tailored to the individual patient. These patients typically require higher inspiratory pressures than patients with hyaline membrane disease, and they do better with rates of 60 breaths/min or greater. Relatively short inspiratory times allow for adequate expiration in patients with preexisting air trapping.

   (2) **Complications.** The clinician must maintain a high index of suspicion for air leak. For any unexplained deterioration of clinical status, a chest x-ray study should be done to rule out air leak. With the development of edema, exudation, air trapping and the resulting decrease in lung compliance, high mean airway pressures may be required in a patient who is at risk for air leak. The approach to ventilation must be directed at preventing hypoxemia and providing adequate ventilation at the lowest mean airway pressure possible to reduce the risk of catastrophic air leak.

h. **Extracorporeal membrane oxygenation (ECMO).** Patients who cannot be ventilated by conventional means may be candidates for ECMO (see Chap 15).

i. **High-frequency jet ventilation.** Reports suggest that high-frequency jet ventilation may offer an alternative ventilatory mode for selected patients (see p 122).

2. **Cardiovascular management.** Persistent pulmonary hypertension is frequently associated with meconium aspiration. The development of pulmonary hypertension may be a result of hypoxic pulmonary vasoconstriction, abnormal muscularization of the pulmonary

microcirculation, or both. To minimize the risk of PPH, aggressive resuscitation and stabilization are essential (see p 284).

3. **General management.** Infants who have aspirated meconium and require resuscitation often develop metabolic abnormalities such as hypoxia, acidosis, hypoglycemia, hypocalcemia, and hypothermia. Because these patients may have suffered perinatal asphyxia, surveillance for any end-organ damage is essential (see Chap 68).

VIII. **Prognosis.** Complications are common, and the mortality rate may exceed 50%. In patients surviving severe meconium aspiration, bronchopulmonary dysplasia may result from oxygen toxicity and prolonged mechanical ventilation. Those with significant asphyxial insult may demonstrate neurologic sequelae.

TRANSIENT TACHYPNEA OF THE NEWBORN

I. **Definition.** Transient tachypnea of the newborn (TTN) is also known as *"wet lung"* and *type II respiratory distress syndrome.* It is usually a benign disease of near-term or term infants who have respiratory distress shortly after delivery that resolves within 3–5 days. It may be hard to differentiate TTN from HMD. However, infants with HMD are usually premature and have worse respiratory symptoms, and x-ray findings are completely different.

II. **Pathophysiology.** TTN is thought to occur because of delayed resorption of fetal lung fluid from the pulmonary lymphatic system. The increased fluid volume causes a reduction in lung compliance. Infants delivered by cesarean section are at risk because of lack of the normal vaginal thoracic squeeze, which forces lung fluid out. One study noted that a mild degree of pulmonary immaturity is a central factor in the cause of TTN. They found a mature L:S ratio but negative phosphatidylglycerol (the presence of phosphatidylglycerol means completed lung maturation), and infants who were closer to 36 weeks' gestation than 38 weeks had an increased risk of TTN.

III. **Risk factors**
   A. Cesarean delivery.
   B. Male sex.
   C. Macrosomia.
   D. Excessive maternal sedation.
   E. Prolonged labor.
   F. Negative amniotic fluid phophatidylglycerol.
   G. Low Apgar score (< 7 at 1 minute).

IV. **Clinical presentation.** The infant is usually near-term or term and shortly after delivery has tachypnea (> 80 breaths/min). The infant may also have grunting, nasal flaring, rib retraction, and varying degrees of cyanosis. There are usually no signs of sepsis. The disease usually does not last longer than 72 hours.

V. **Diagnosis**
   A. **Laboratory studies**
      1. **Prenatal testing.** A mature L:S ratio with presence of phosphatidylglycerol in the amniotic fluid may help to rule out hyaline membrane disease.
      2. **Postnatal testing**
         a. **Arterial blood gas** on room air will show some degree of hypoxia.
         b. **Complete blood count and differential** will help rule out any infectious process.
         c. **Urine Wellcogen test** may help rule out group B streptococcal pneumonia.
   B. **Radiologic studies**
      1. **Chest x-ray study.** The typical findings are:

     a. Prominent perihilar streaking (secondary to engorgement of peri-arterial lymphatics).
     b. Mild to moderately enlarged heart.
     c. Increased lung volume with depression of the diaphragm and hyperaeration.
     d. Fluid in the minor fissue, and perhaps fluid in the pleural space.

C. Other tests. Any infant who is hypoxic on room air must have a **100% oxygen test** to rule out heart disease. (This test is described on p 275.) If the infant has cyanotic heart disease, the oxygen content will not change.

VI. Management

A. General

1. **Oxygenation.** Initial management consists of providing adequate oxygenation. Start with hood oxygen. If 100% hood oxygenation does not work, change to nasal CPAP. If that does not work, intubate the infant and proceed with mechanical ventilation. The majority of infants with TTN require low to moderate levels of hood oxygen. If the infant requires 100% oxygen or endotracheal intubation with ventilator support, another disease process should be suspected.

2. **Feeding.** Because of the risk of aspiration, an infant should not be fed by mouth if the respiratory rate is over 60/min. If the respiratory rate is less than 60 breaths/min, oral feeding is permissible. If the rate is 60–80 breaths/min, feeding should be by nasogastric tube. If the rate is over 80/min, intravenous nutrition is indicated.

B. Confirm the diagnosis.
It is important to rule out other causes of tachypnea before assuming it is TTN. The usual causes are:

1. **Pneumonia.** If the infant has pneumonia, the prenatal history will usually suggest infection. There may be maternal chorioamnionitis, premature rupture of membranes, and fever. The blood count may show evidence of infection. It can either show neutropenia or leukocytosis with abnormal amount of immature cells. The urine Wellcogen test may be positive if the infant has group B streptococcal infection. Remember, it is better to give broad-spectrum antibiotics if there is any suspicion or evidence of infection. The antibiotics can always be discontinued if the cultures are negative in 3 days.

2. **Heart disease.** The 100% oxygen test should be done to rule out heart disease (see p 275). Cardiomegaly may be seen.

3. **Hyaline membrane disease.** The infant will normally be premature or have some reason for delayed lung maturation, such as maternal diabetes. The chest x-ray film is helpful because it shows the typical reticulogranular pattern with air bronchograms.

4. **Cerebral hyperventilation.** This disorder is also seen in term infants, but they have birth asphyxia. The infant has tachypnea with minimal x-ray changes. Arterial blood gas measurements show respiratory alkalosis.

VII. Prognosis.
The disease is self-limited, and there is no risk of recurrence or further pulmonary dysfunction.

REFERENCES

Allen RW, Jung AL, Lester PD: Effectiveness of chest tube evacuation of pneumothorax in neonates. *J Pediatr* 1981;**99**:629.

Alpan G et al: Doxapram in the treatment of idiopathic apnea on prematurity unresponsive to aminophylline. *J Pediatr* 1984;**104**:634.

Ballard J, Musial MJ, Myers MG: Hazards of delivery room resuscitation using oral methods of endotracheal suctioning. *Pediatr Infect Dis* 1986;**5**:198.

Bancalari E, Gerhardt T: Bronchopulmonary dysplasia. *Pediatr Clin North* 1986;**33**:1.

Bednarek FJ, Roloff DW: Treatment of apnea of prematurity with aminophylline. *Pediatrics* 1973;**55**:335.

Blanchard PW, Brown TM, Coates AL: Pharmacotherapy in bronchopulmonary dysplasia. *Clin Perinatol* 1987;**14**:881.

Brooks JG et al: Selective bronchial intubation for the treatment of severe localized pulmonary emphysema in newborn infants. *J Pediatr* 1977;**91**:648.

Carson BS: Prevention of meconium aspiration syndrome. *Neonatal Grand Rounds* 1986;**3**:3.

Creasy RK, Resnik R: *Maternal-Fetal Medicine: Principles and Practice.* Saunders, 1984.

Escobedo MB, Gonzales A: Bronchopulmonary dysplasia in the tiny infant. *Clin Perinatol* 1986;**13**:315.

Fanaroff AA, Martin RJ: *Neonatal-Perinatal Medicine: Diseases of the Fetus and Infant,* 4th ed. Mosby, 1987.

Fiascone JM et al: Bronchopulmonary dysplasia: Review for the pediatrician. *Curr Probl Pediatr* 1989;**19**:169.

Ficheux H et al: Simultaneous determination of hemoglobin and coproporphyrin by second derivative differential spectrophotometry: Application to the diagnosis of meconium aspiration. *Clin Chim Acta* 1989;**189(1)**:53.

Goetzman BW: Understanding bronchopulmonary dysplasia. *Am J Dis Child* 1986;**140**:332.

Goldsmith JP, Klarotkin EH. Pages 189–199 in: *Assisted Ventilation of the Neonate.* Saunders, 1981.

Jobe AH, Taeusch HW (editors): *Surfactant Treatment of Lung Disease.* Report of the Ninety-Sixth Ross Conference on Pediatric Research. Ross Laboratories, 1988.

Kattwinkel J: Neonatal apnea: Pathogenesis and therapy. *J Pediatr* 1977;**90**:342.

Kattwinkel J et al: Apnea of prematurity. *J Pediatr* 1985;**86**:588.

Keszler M et al: Combined high-frequency jet ventilation in a meconium aspiration model. *Crit Care Med* 1986;**14(1)**:34.

Linder N et al: Need for endotracheal intubation and suction in meconium-stained neonates. *J Pediatr* 1988;**112(4)**:613.

Mansfield PB et al: Pneumopericardium and pneumomediastinum in infants and children. *J Pediatr Surg* 1973;**8**:691.

Merritt TA et al: Immunologic consequences of exogenous surfactant administration. *Semin Perinatol* 1988;**12**:221.

Merritt TA, Northway WH Jr, Boynton BR: *Contemporary Issues in Fetal and Neonatal Medicine (4): Bronchopulmonary Dysplasia.* Blackwell Scientific, 1989.

Miller MJ, Carlo WA, Martin RJ: Continuous positive airway pressure selectively reduces obstructive apnea in preterm infants. *J Pediatr* 1985;**100**:91.

Murphy JD, Vawter GF, Reid LM: Pulmonary vascular disease in fatal meconium aspiration. *J Pediatr* 1984;**104**:758.

O'Brodovich HM, Mellins RB: Bronchopulmonary dysplasia: Unresolved neonatal acute lung injury. *Am Rev Respir Dis* 1986;**132**:694.

Perleman EJ, Moore GW, Hutchins GM: Pulmonary vasculature in meconium aspiration. *Hum Pathol* 1989;**20(7)**:701.

Philips III JB: Management of the meconium-stained infant. *Neonatal Grand Rounds* 1986;**3**:1.

Reynolds MS, Wallander KA: Use of surfactant in the prevention and treatment of neonatal RDS. *Clin Pharmacol* 1989;**8**:559.

Shapiro DL, Notter RH: Controversies regarding surfactant replacement therapy. *Clin Perinatol* 1988;**15**:891.

Spitzer AR, Fox WW: Infant apnea. *Pediatr Clin North Am* 1986;**33**:561.

Stark AE, Frantz III ID: Respiratory distress syndrome. *Pediatr Clin North Am* 1986;**33**:533.

Stevens JC, Eigen H, Wysomierski D: Extracorporeal membrane oxygenation as treatment of severe meconium aspiration syndrome. *South Med J* 1989;**82(6)**:696.

Taylor GA, Short BL, Kriesemer P: Extracorporeal membrane oxygenation: Radiographic appearance of the neonatal chest. *Am J Radiol* 1986;**146(6)**:1257.

Thibeault DW, Gregory GA: Pages 499–519 in: *Neonatal Pulmonary Care.* Appleton-Century-Crofts, 1986.

Trento A, Griffith BP, Hardesty RL: Extracorporeal membrane oxygenation experience at the University of Pittsburgh. *Am Thorac Surg* 1986;**42(1)**:56.

Trindade O et al: Conventional vs. high-frequency jet ventilation in a piglet model of meconium aspiration: Comparison of pulmonary and hemodynamic effects. *J Pediatr* 1985;**107(1)**:115.

Vance J: Antenatal and neonatal management of meconium staining. *MO Perinatal Prog* 1984;**7**:1.

Van Golde LMG et al: The pulmonary surfactant system: Biochemical aspects and functional significance. *Physiol Rev* 1988;**68**:374.

70 Renal Diseases

ACUTE RENAL FAILURE

I. **Definition.** In neonates, acute renal failure is defined as the absence of urinary output (anuria) or as urine output of less than 0.5 mL/kg/24 h (oliguria) with an associated increase in serum creatinine. Ninety-nine percent of infants void by 48 hours (see Table 40–1 for average times from birth to first voiding).

II. **Incidence.** In some studies, as many as 23% of neonates have some form of renal failure, with prerenal factors identified as the cause in 73%.

III. **Pathophysiology.** Normal urine output is about 1–3 mL/kg/h in newborns, and the normal newborn kidney has poor concentrating ability. Renal failure leads to problems with volume overload, hyperkalemia, acidosis, hyperphosphatemia, and hypocalcemia. Acute renal failure is traditionally divided into 3 categories, as follows.

  A. **Prerenal failure.** Prerenal failure is due to decreased renal perfusion. Causes include dehydration (poor feeding, increased insensible losses referable to radiant warmers), perinatal asphyxia, and hypotension (septic shock, hemorrhagic shock, cardiogenic shock due to congestive heart failure).

  B. **Intrinsic renal failure.** If poor renal perfusion persists, acute tubular necrosis with intrinsic renal failure may result. Other causes are nephrotoxins such as aminoglycosides and methoxyflurane anesthesia, congenital anomalies (eg, renal agenesis, polycystic kidney disease), disseminated intravascular coagulation (DIC), and renal vein or renal artery thrombosis.

  C. **Postrenal failure.** All the causes involve obstruction to urinary outflow. These include bilateral ureteropelvic obstruction, bilateral ureterovesical obstruction, posterior urethral valves, urethral diverticulum or stenosis, large ureterocele, neurogenic bladder, blocked urinary drainage tubes, and extrinsic tumor compression.

IV. **Risk factors.** Dehydration, sepsis, asphyxia, and administration of nephrotoxic drugs to the neonate are risk factors for acute renal failure. Maternal diabetes may increase the risk for renal vein thrombosis and subsequent renal insufficiency.

V. **Clinical presentation**

  A. **Decreased or absent urine output.** Low or absent urine output is usually the presenting problem. Ninety-nine percent of infants void by 48 hours (see Table 46–1).

  B. **Family history.** A history or urinary tract disease in other family members should be sought, a history of oligohydramnios, which frequently accompanies urinary outflow obstruction or severe renal dysplasia or agenesis.

  C. **Physical examination.** The following abnormalities on physical examination are significant.

    1. **Abdominal mass,** suggesting a distended bladder, polycystic kidneys, or hydronephrosis.

    2. **Potter's facies,** associated with renal agenesis.

    3. **Meningomyelocele,** associated with neurogenic bladder.

TABLE 70-1. RENAL FAILURE INDICES IN THE NEONATE

	Prerenal	Renal
Urine osmolality (mosm)	> 400	< 400
Urine Na (meq/L)	31 ± 19	63 ± 35
Urine/plasma Cr	29 ± 16	10 ± 4
Fractional excretion of Na	< 2.5	> 2.5
Renal failure index (RFI)	< 3.0	> 3.0

4. **Pulmonary hypoplasia,** due to severe oligohydramnios in utero secondary to inadequate urinary output.
5. **Urinary ascites,** which may be seen with posterior urethral valves.
6. **Prune belly** (hypoplasia of the abdominal wall musculature and cryptorchidism), associated with urinary abnormalities.

VI. Diagnosis

A. **Bladder catheterization.** Perform bladder catheterization, using a 5F or 8F feeding tube to confirm inadequate urine output (see Chap 18 for details of procedure). Immediate passage of large volumes of urine suggests obstruction (eg, posterior urethral valves) or a hypotonic (neurogenic) bladder.

B. **Laboratory studies**
   1. **Serum urea nitrogen and creatinine levels**
      a. **Urea nitrogen level** > 15–20 mg/dL suggests dehydration or renal insufficiency.
      b. **Creatinine level.** Normal serum creatinine values are 0.8–1.0 mg/dL at 1 day, 0.7–0.8 mg/dL at 3 days, and less than 0.6 mg/dL by 7 days of life. Higher values suggest renal disease except in low birth weight infants; a creatinine level of < 1.6 mg/dL is considered normal in them.
   2. **Urinary indices** of acute renal failure are listed in Table 70-1. Order a spot urine osmolality, a serum and spot urine sodium, and serum and urine creatinine and calculate the fractional excretion of sodium and the renal failure index. These indices are of limited value if measured while the effect of diuretics such as furosemide are present.

$$\text{Fractional excretion of sodium (FeNa)} = \frac{\text{Urine Na}}{\text{Urine Cr}} \times \frac{\text{Plasma Cr}}{\text{Plasma Na}} \times 100$$

$$\text{Renal failure index (RFI)} = \frac{\text{Urine Na}}{\text{Urine Cr}} \times \text{Plasma Cr}$$

   3. **Complete blood count and platelet count** may reveal thrombocytopenia, seen with sepsis or renal vein thrombosis.
   4. **Serum potassium levels** should be followed to rule out hyperkalemia.
   5. **Urinalysis** may reveal hematuria (associated with renal vein thrombosis, tumors, DIC; see Hematuria, p 426), or pyuria, suggesting urinary tract infection that is either the cause of renal insufficiency (sepsis) or the result of mechanical obstruction.

C. **Diagnostic fluid challenge.** If the patient does not have clinical volume overload or congestive failure, give a fluid challenge. Give normal saline or colloid solution, 5–10 mL/kg as IV bolus; repeat once PRN. If there is no response, give furosemide, 1 mg/kg. If there is still no increase in urine output, obstruction above the level of the bladder must be ruled out by ultrasound examination. If there is no evidence of obstruction and the patient does not respond to these maneuvers, the most likely cause of anuria or oliguria is intrinsic renal failure.

D. Radiologic studies

1. **Abdominal ultrasonography** can delineate hydronephrosis, dilated ureters, abdominal masses, a distended bladder, or renal vein thrombosis.

2. **Intravenous urography** has limited usefulness in the neonatal period, owing to the poor concentrating ability of the kidney, and is of limited value in the setting of renal failure.

3. **Abdominal x-ray studies** may show spina bifida or an absent sacrum, which can cause neurogenic bladder.

4. **Radionuclide scanning** can delineate functioning renal parenchyma (dimercaptosuccinic acid [DMSA]) and give some indication of renal flow and function (diethyltriamine pentaacetic acid [DTPA]).

VII. Management

A. General management

1. **Replace insensible fluid losses** (preterm, 50–70 mL/kg/d; term, 30 mL/kg/d) plus fluid output (urine, gastrointestinal tract).

2. **Keep strict intake and output and frequent weight records.**

3. **Follow serum sodium and potassium levels** frequently, and replace losses cautiously as needed. Infants with renal failure should never be given intravenous fluids containing potassium, since hyperkalemia, if it occurs, may be lethal. If hyperkalemia does occur, treat as outlined in Chapter 39.

4. **Restrict protein** to less than 2 g/kd/d and ensure adequate nonprotein caloric intake. Formulas such as SMA and PM 60/40 are frequently used for infants with renal failure.

5. **Hyperphosphatemia and hypocalcemia frequently coexist, and phosphate binders such as aluminum hydroxide,** 50-150 mg/kg/d orally, **should be used to normalize the phosphate.** Once the phosphate is normal, calcium with or without vitamin D supplements is usually needed.

6. **Metabolic acidosis may require chronic oral bicarbonate supplementation. Blood pressures should be followed serially,** because these infants are always at risk for developing chronic hypertension.

B. Definitive management

1. **Prerenal failure** is treated by correcting the specific cause (see section above).

2. **Postrenal failure.** Acute management involves bypassing the obstruction with a bladder catheter or by percutaneous nephrostomy drainage, depending on the level of the obstruction. Surgical correction is usually indicated at some point.

3. **Intrinsic renal disease.** If renal disease is caused by toxins or acute tubular necrosis, renal function may recover to some extent with time.

4. **Dialysis.** If recovery of renal function is expected or if renal transplantation is considered an option when the child is older, peritoneal dialysis is the treatment most commonly used in the neonate.

HEMATURIA

I. **Definition.** Hematuria is the presence of gross or microscopic blood in the urine. More than 3 red cells per high-power field is usually considered abnormal. A red-stained diaper usually signifies hematuria but may be due to bile pigments, porphyrins, or urates.

II. **Incidence.** Hematuria is not a common problem in newborns.

III. **Pathophysiology.** Hematuria in the newborn may be caused by perinatal asphyxia, cortical or medullary necrosis, infection, trauma (birth or iatrogenic, such as bladder aspiration), renal vein or renal artery thrombosis, hyperosmolar infusions into umbilical catheters, neoplasms (rhabdomyosarcoma, nephroblastoma), urinary tract obstruction or infection, coagulopathy, and neonatal glomerulonephritis (most commonly caused by syphilis).

IV. **Risk factors** include coagulopathy, urinary tract infection, obstruction, maternal diabetes (renal vein thrombosis), indwelling urinary catheters, and traumatic delivery.

V. **Clinical presentation**
   A. **History.** A maternal history of diabetes may arouse a suspicion of renal vein thrombosis. The birth history and Apgar scores may suggest perinatal asphyxia.
   B. **Physical examination.** Examination may reveal the presence of an abdominal mass (obstruction, neoplasm, renal vein thrombosis). The presence of an umbilical or bladder catheter should be noted.

VI. **Diagnosis**
   A. **Laboratory studies**
      1. **Urinalysis.** Microscopic examination and dipstick testing will confirm the presence of blood or other causes of "red urine." **Red cell casts** are seen with intrinsic renal disease such as glomerulonephritis. **Bacteria or white cells** suggest urinary tract infection.
      2. **Urine culture.** Collection of urine by bladder aspiration or catheterization is preferred and is outlined in Chapters 17 and 18.
      3. **Serum urea nitrogen and creatinine levels** may reveal renal insufficiency.
      4. **Coagulation studies.** PT, PTT, and thrombin time may provide clues to DIC or hemorrhagic disease of the newborn. Thrombocytopenia suggests renal vein thrombosis.
   B. **Radiologic studies**
      1. **Ultrasonography** will show neoplasms, renal vein thrombosis, or obstruction in the urinary tract.
      2. **Ancillary testing** such as intravenous urography, arteriography, and nuclear scans may be indicated.

VII. **Management.** Treatment is directed at the underlying cause.

URINARY TRACT INFECTION

I. **Definition.** Urinary tract infection (UTI) is the presence of pathogenic organisms in the urinary tract with or without symptoms of infection. A definitive diagnosis is made by culture of any organism in a urine specimen that has been properly collected by suprapubic bladder aspiration.

II. **Incidence.** Various series report an incidence of 0.5–1.0% in term infants weighing more than 2500 g and higher rates (3–5%) in premature infants or infants weighing less than 2500 g.

III. **Pathophysiology.** When urinary tract infection is present in an infant less than 1 year of age, an associated urinary tract abnormality is found in most males and in about one-third of females. Associated anomalies that may give rise to urinary tract infection include neurogenic bladder, urethral valves, vesicoureteral reflux, and ureteropelvic junction obstruction. The predominant organisms are gram-negative rods, with *E coli* the most common.

IV. **Risk factors** include indwelling urinary catheters, systemic sepsis with hematogenous seeding of the urinary tract, urinary tract obstruction, neurogenic bladder (myelodysplasia), and male newborns. Recent evidence suggests that uncircumsized males may be at higher risk for UTI.

V. **Clinical presentation**
   A. **Signs of sepsis.** The infant may present with frank signs of sepsis (respiratory distress, apnea, bradycardia, hypoglycemia, poor perfusion).

   B. **Nonspecific findings.** The signs are often subtle and may include poor
      feeding, vomiting, jaundice, or failure to thrive.
VI. **Diagnosis**
   A. **Laboratory studies**
      1. **Urine culture.** Suprapubic aspiration or catheterization is manda-
         tory for a good urine culture in a neonate. "Bag" urine is felt by
         some to be inadequate to achieve reliable culture results.
      2. **Blood cultures** should be obtained before starting antibiotic
         therapy.
      3. **Urinalysis.** Microscopic examination may show white blood cells,
         but the presence of bacteria is a more reliable sign of UTI in the
         neonate, especially when urine is collected by suprapubic aspira-
         tion.
      4. **Complete blood count** may show leukocytosis.
      5. **Serum bilirubin** may be elevated.
   B. No other studies are indicated.
VII. **Management**
   A. **Initial antibiotic treatment.** Initial antibiotic therapy usually consists
      of intravenous ampicillin and gentamicin until definitive urine and
      blood culture results are reported. (See Chap 76 for dosages and other
      pharmacologic information.)
   B. **Further investigations.** To rule out anatomic abnormalities in the neo-
      nate, abdominal ultrasonography, intravenous pyelography (IVP), and
      voiding cystourethrography (VCUG) may be indicated. Urologic con-
      sultation is usually indicated.
VIII. **Prognosis.** Up to one-fourth of infants can have recurrent UTI within the
      first year of life. Effective use of long-term suppressive antibiotics along
      with any indicated corrective surgery has dramatically reduced the long-
      term incidence of renal scarring and renal insufficiency.

REFERENCES

Ginsburg CM, McCracken GH: Urinary tract infections in young infants. *Pediatrics*
   1982;**69**:409.
Greenhill A, Gruskin AP: Laboratory evaluation of renal function. *Pediatr Clin North Am*
   1976;**23**:661.
Matthew OP et al: Neonatal renal failure: Usefulness of diagnostic indices. *Pediatrics*
   1980;**65**:57.
Norman ME, Asadi FK: A prospective study of acute renal failure in the newborn infant.
   Pediatrics 1979;**63**:475.

71 Retinopathy of Prematurity

I. Definitions

A. Retinopathy of prematurity (ROP) is ocular underdevelopment due to interruption of normal progression of newly forming retinal vessels. Vasoconstriction and obliteration of the advancing capillary bed is followed in succession by neovascularization extending into the vitreous, retinal edema, retinal hemorrhages, fibrosis, and traction on, and eventual detachment of, the retina. In most cases, the process is reversed before fibrosis occurs. **Advanced stages may lead to blindness.**

B. Retrolental fibroplasia. As originally described, the condition was seen only in its most advanced form, after extensive fibrosis and scarring had already occurred. It was therefore termed *retrolental fibroplasia*. It is now understood that several recognizable changes occur in the developing vasculature before end-stage fibrosis occurs. This condition is considered a true retinopathy; because it is found chiefly in prematures, it is now called *retinopathy of prematurity (ROP)*.

C. Cicatricial ROP. The term *cicatricial ROP*, referring to fibrotic disease, is essentially equivalent to the older term *retrolental fibroplasia*.

II. Incidence.
About 400–600 children per year may be blinded by ROP, representing 20% of blindness in preschool children. Of particular concern are the increasing numbers of survivors weighing less than 1000 g who have the highest incidence of ROP and who may account for much of the current epidemic. Of infants weighing 1000–1500 g, 2.2% have scarring and 0.3–1.1% are blinded; of those weighing less than 1000 g, 22–44% have scarring and 5–11% are blinded without treatment.

III. Pathophysiology

A. Historical perspective. Retrolental fibroplasia (RLF) was first described by Terry in the 1940s and was associated with the use of oxygen in newborn infants by Patz and associates (1984). The **first epidemic,** estimated to be responsible for 30% of cases of blindness in preschool children by the end of the 1940s, occurred during a period of relatively liberal oxygen administration. After this association was recognized, oxygen use in nurseries was curtailed. Although the incidence of RLF fell, infant mortality rates in newborn infants increased. In the 1960s, improved oxygen monitoring techniques made possible the cautious reintroduction of oxygen into the nursery. Despite improved oxygen monitoring, however, a **second epidemic** of retrolental fibroplasia (retinopathy of prematurity) appeared in the late 1970s and has continued into the 1990s.

B. Normal embryology of the eye. In the normally developing retina, there are no retinal vessels until about 16 weeks' gestation. Until then, oxygen diffuses from the underlying choroidal circulation. At 16 weeks, in response to an unknown stimulus (relative hypoxia as the retina thickens has been suggested), cells derived from mesenchyme traveling in the nerve fiber layer emanate from the optic nerve head. These cells, called *spindle cells* are the precursors of the retinal vascular system. A fine capillary network advances through the retina to the ora serrata, or retinal edge. More mature vessels form behind this advancing network. Vascularization on the nasal side of the ora serrata is complete at about 8 months' gestation, whereas that on the temporal side is ordi-

narily complete at term. Once completely vascularized, the retinal vasculature is no longer susceptible to insults of the type that lead to ROP.

C. Etiology
  1. There appear to be 2 phases in the development of ROP, as described by Patz.
      a. Early vasoconstriction and obliteration of the capillary network in response to high oxygen concentrations noted experimentally.
      b. Vasoproliferation, which follows the period of high oxygen exposure, perhaps in response to an **angiogenic factor** released by the hypoxic retina. Considerable evidence has been developed to support this hypothesis. Phelps and Rosenbaum (1984) studied kittens made hyperoxic and then allowed to recover in room air (21% oxygen) or 13% oxygen. Those recovering in the hypoxic environment had worse retinopathy than those recovering in room air, suggesting that retinal hypoxia may play a role.
  2. Alternatively, Kretzer et al (see McPherson [1986] reference) have proposed that the mesenchymal spindle cells form intercellular gap junctions in response to increased oxygen tensions. These increased gap junctions then form a barrier to ongoing mesenchymal migration into the retina, and the normal progression of vascularization ceases. These authors postulate further that the spindle cells produce an angiogenic substance that leads secondarily to abnormal vasoproliferation. They have reported experimental evidence that the administration of vitamin E decreases gap junction formation.

IV. Risk factors. The association of ROP with oxygen alone is now not so clear. There have been many recorded instances of ROP in premature infants not exposed to elevated oxygen concentrations. Many other factors such as extreme prematurity, maternal complications, apnea, sepsis, hyper- and hypocapnia, vitamin E deficiency, intraventricular hemorrhage, anemia, exchange transfusion, hypoxia, lactic acidosis, and bright light have been implicated. The pathophysiology of ROP is still unclear. Experimental studies have focused chiefly on the role of oxygen.

V. Clinical presentation. Several methods of classification of ROP have been used. With development of the **International Classification of ROP,** there is now general agreement on staging of active disease.
  Stage I. A thin **demarcation line** develops between the vascularized region of the retina and the avascular zone.
  Stage II. This line develops into a **ridge** protruding into the vitreous, in which there is histologic evidence for an arteriovenous shunt.
  Stage III. Extraretinal fibrovascular proliferation occurs with the ridge. Neovascular tufts may be found just posterior to the ridge (Fig 71–1).
  Stage IV. Fibrosis and scarring occur as the neovascularization extends into the vitreous. Traction occurs on the retina, resulting in **retinal detachment.**
  Plus disease (eg, stage III+) may occur when vessels posterior to the ridge become dilated and tortuous.

VI. Diagnosis. Ophthalmoscopic examination by an experienced examiner usually confirms the diagnosis. Various protocols are used, depending on the institution.
  A. The American Academy of Pediatrics recommends ophthalmoscopic examination at 6–8 weeks for all oxygen-exposed premature infants who weigh less than 2000 g.
  B. Screening criteria suggested by Brown et al (1987) and based on examinations of 2986 neonates, attempt to decrease unnecessary examinations by limiting them to those who weigh less than 1600 g, examining those over 1600 g only if they have been exposed to oxygen for more than 50 days.

FIGURE 71-1. Schematic drawing of moderate stage III retinopathy of prematurity. Optic nerve head is at the bottom of drawing, and periphery of the retina is at the top. (*Reproduced, with permission, from Garner A: International classification of retinopathy of prematurity. Pediatrics 1984;74:127.*)

C. In the recently completed trial of cryopexy for ROP, examinations for infants who weigh less than 1251 g were begun at 4-6 weeks of age and repeated every 2 weeks until maturity or until eyes were prethreshold, just prior to eligibility for treatment. Because rapid progression can occur, they were then examined every week until eligible for treatment at stage III+ or until regression occurred. Overall, an initial examination between 4-6 weeks in smaller infants is advised. In the absence of disease, examinations should be repeated every 3-4 weeks until the retina is mature.

VII. Management

A. **Circumferential cryopexy** is now the treatment of choice for progressive (stage III+) disease in an attempt to prevent further progression by destroying cells that may be releasing angiogenic factors. Results of the recent large collaborative NIH-sponsored trial indicate that cryopexy carried out at state III+ can reduce the incidence of severe visual impairment by 50% if performed within 72 hours of detecting threshold disease. If both eyes are involved, cryopexy is usually performed in one eye only as there are some risks with the procedure, such as vitreal hemorrhage. If there are enough risk factors for retinal detachment, however, cryopexy may be performed in both eyes. It is imperative that an ophthalmologist skilled in cryopexy perform the procedure.

B. **Vitamin E.** The administration of pharmacologic doses of vitamin E for ROP is *controversial;* currently there is no proof of clear benefit. Reported side effects include sepsis, necrotizing enterocolitis, and intraventricular hemorrhage. Even so, maintenance of normal serum vitamin E levels is a prudent management objective.

C. **Decreased lighting intensity.** Glass et al (1985) reported a decreased incidence of ROP in infants cared for in an area of reduced light intensity. A subsequent study (Ackerman et al, 1989) showed no effect. A collaborative study is now under way.

    D. **Retinal reattachment.** Stage IV disease has been treated by attempts at retinal reattachment without significant success to date. Reattachment of late retinal detachments in childhood has met with more success.

    E. **Vitrectomy** has not substantially improved the outcome in cicatricial disease.

    F. **Follow-up eye examinations** are advocated every 1–2 years for infants with fully regressed ROP and every 6–12 months for infants with cicatricial ROP.

VIII. Prognosis. Ninety percent of cases of stage I and stage II disease regress spontaneously. Current information suggests that 50% of cases of stage III + disease regress spontaneously. Of those that do progress to stage III +, the incidence of severe visual impairment can be reduced by approximately 50% if circumferential cryopexy is carried out by a skilled ophthalmologist. Sequelae of regressed disease such as myopia, strabismus, amblyopia, glaucoma, and late detachment require regular follow-up.

REFERENCES

Ackerman B, Sheruonit E, Williams J: Reduced incidental light exposure: Effect on the development of retinopathy of prematurity in low birth weight infants. *Pediatrics* 1989;**83**:958.

Committee Report: Vitamin E and the prevention of retinopathy of prematurity. *Pediatrics* 1985;**76**:315.

Cryotherapy for Retinopathy of Prematurity Cooperative Group. Multicenter trial of cryotherapy for retinopathy of prematurity: Preliminary results. *Pediatrics* 1988;**81**:697.

Flynn JT: Retinopathy of prematurity. *Pediatr Clin North Am* 1987;**34**:1847.

Garner A: International classification of retinopathy of prematurity. *Pediatrics* 1984;**74**:127.

Glass P et al: Effect of bright light in the hospital nursery on the incidence of retinopathy of prematurity. *N Engl J Med* 1985;**313**:401.

Lucey JF, Dangman BD: A reexamination of the role of oxygen in retrolental fibroplasia. *Pediatrics* 1984;**82**:73.

McPherson AR, Hittner HM, Kretzer FL: *Retinopathy of Prematurity: Current Concepts and Controversies.* Decker, 1986.

Patz A: Current concepts of the effect of oxygen on the developing retina. *Curr Eye Res* 1984;**3**:159.

Phelps DL: Retinopathy of prematurity: An estimate of vision loss in the United States—1979. *Pediatrics* 1981;**67**:924.

Phelps DL: Role of vitamin E therapy in high-risk neonates. *Clin Perinatol* 1988;**15**:955.

Phelps DL, Phelps CE: Cryotherapy in infants with retinopathy of prematurity. A decision model for treating one or both eyes. *JAMA* 1989;**261**:1751.

Phelps DL, Rosenbaum AL: Effects of marginal hypoxemia on recovery from oxygen-induced retinopathy in the kitten model. *Pediatrics* 1984;**73**:1.

72 Rickets and Disorders of Calcium and Magnesium Metabolism

RICKETS

I. **Definition.** Rickets is a chronic disorder of calcium metabolism characterized by x-ray evidence of bone demineralization and elevated serum alkaline phosphatase levels.

II. **Incidence.** The incidence of rickets in low birth weight infants is approximately 30%.

III. **Pathophysiology**

A. **Chronic diseases.** Infants with chronic debilitating diseases (notably **broncho-pulmonary dysplasia [BPD])** are at greatest risk for rickets. Typically, these infants require high caloric intake to sustain good weight gain. Bone demineralization can progress despite intakes of calcium, 50–60 mg/kg/d; phosphorus, 25 mg/kg/d; and vitamin D, 400 IU/d. These infants also have an increased incidence of rib fractures secondary to severe bone demineralization, with peak occurrence at about 2 months of age. Most infants with rickets also have received intermittent or routine doses of furosemide.

B. **Diuretics. Furosemide** has marked calciuric effect, and the increased calcium loss exacerbates calcium efflux from bones. **Thiazide diuretics** (eg, hydrochlorothiazide) tend to reduce urinary calcium losses and therefore can ameliorate bone demineralization.

IV. **Rick factors**

A. Chronic diseases, especially BPD.

B. Chronic stress.

C. Malnutrition.

D. Administration of inappropriate quantities of calcium, phosphorus, or vitamin D.

E. Diuretics.

V. **Clinical presentation**

A. **Poor weight gain** despite very high caloric intake is often seen in these infants.

B. **Rib and other bone fractures** may be seen in advanced stages of rickets.

C. **Respiratory distress** is occasionally seen.

VI. **Diagnosis**

A. **Laboratory studies**

1. **Alkaline phosphatase levels** are usually more than 280 IU/L and can be over 500 IU/L.

2. **Serum calcium levels** are usually normal.

3. **Serum phosphorus levels** may be low (< 3 mg/dL).

4. **Vitamin D levels.** Infants with rickets typically have increased levels of 1,25-hydroxyvitamin D, which reverts to normal when the disease resolves. 25-Hydroxyvitamin D levels may be depressed with active rickets, which resolves after treatment.

B. **Radiologic studies.** Sequential x-ray studies demonstrate gradual bone demineralization ("washed-out bones"). Some centers utilize the more sensitive bone mineral analyzer to follow smaller changes in bone density, but this instrument is not widely available. X-ray films provide evidence of progressive bone demineralization. Serial films may also show lucency at the metaphyses of long bones and loss of the normal opaque line at the metaphyseal end. In advanced stages, metaphyseal fraying and cupping can be seen—most markedly at the knees and wrists. Poor mineralization at the anterior aspects of the ribs (rachitic rosary) and rib fractures may also be seen.

VII. **Management and prognosis**
  A. **Nutrition.** In order to sustain adequate weight gain, infants with rickets usually have an increased need for calories and for additional calcium, vitamin D, and phosphate. A formula such as one of the special care formulas for premature infants (Similac Special Care, Enfamil Premature), which contain 1.2–1.4 g/L of calcium and have a calcium:phosphate ratio of 2:1 with 400–800 IU vitamin D per day, has been shown to stimulate bone mineralization and resolution of rickets. **Alkaline phosphatase levels** should be monitored every 1–2 weeks until normal levels are obtained.
  B. **Calcium supplementation.** Infants who are NPO should be given about 45 mg/kg/d of elemental calcium intravenously with a calcium:phosphate ratio of 2–3:1 and 400–800 IU vitamin D per day. Rarely, additional benefit can be achieved with higher doses of vitamin D.
  C. **Prognosis.** This condition is completely reversible with careful management. Depending on the severity of the disease, most infants should fully recover within weeks to months of detection and treatment.

HYPOCALCEMIA

  I. **Definition.** In infants in intensive care nurseries, disorders of calcium metabolism frequently develop; hypocalcemia is the most common. Hypocalcemia is defined as total serum calcium (tCa) levels less than 6 mg/dL, tCa levels of less than 7 mg/dL with symptoms, or ionized calcium (iCa) levels of less than 3 mg/dL (1.0 mM). Some authors have suggested that iCa levels greater than 2.5 mg/dL (0.8 mM) are adequate in some infants.
 II. **Pathophysiology.** Ionized calcium is the biologically important form of calcium. Total serum calcium levels have repeatedly been shown not to be predictive of serum ionized calcium levels. Therefore, tCA levels are unreliable as criteria for true hypocalcemia. In premature infants, it has been shown that tCa levels as low as 6 mg/dL or less correspond to iCa levels greater than 3 mg/dL.
  A. **Early-onset neonatal hypocalcemia (ENH).** During the third trimester of pregnancy, the human fetus receives at least 140 mg/kg/d of elemental calcium via the umbilical cord. Most of this calcium is readily incorporated into the newly forming bones. Following delivery, this massive supply of calcium is suddenly stopped, and calcium must be given enterally.
    1. **A full-term infant** receiving 100–120 mL of normal formula would be receiving 50–60 mg/kg/d of calcium orally. Despite this drop in supply, full-term infants tolerate the change well and do not become hypocalcemic.
    2. **Premature or sick infants** often become hypocalcemic during the first 3 days of life. Total serum calcium levels can drop to less than 7 mg/dL and occasionally fall below 6 mg/dL.
    3. **Calcium levels** (both iCa and tCa) usually return to normal within 48–72 hours whether or not supplemental calcium is given. It has also been shown that immunoreactive parathyroid hormone (iPTH) is often low at birth but rises to higher levels within 24–72 hours

after delivery. Intravenous calcium supplementation has been shown to suppress this increase in iPTH.

B. **Hypocalcemia secondary to prolonged poor enteral intake.** After 3 days of life, infants tolerating enteral feedings usually do not need calcium supplementation. Normal formula supplies adequate calcium for bone mineralization in full-term infants. Calcium-rich formula—formula with an elemental calcium concentration of 1.2–1.4 g/L and a calcium:phosphate ratio of 2:1—is usually sufficient for bone growth in premature infants. However, if feedings cannot be advanced rapidly or if the infant must be maintained NPO, parenteral calcium supplementation is needed to prevent bone demineralization. These infants often maintain normal iCa and tCa levels at the expense of bone calcium. Furthermore, magnesium deficiency secondary to malnutrition can suppress iPTH levels and thus cause hypocalcemia.

C. **Hypocalcemia secondary to maternal diabetes.** After infants of diabetic mothers are born, their serum glucose levels rapidly decline as a result of **hyperinsulinemia.** These infants also secrete higher amounts of **calcitonin,** which inhibits calcium mobilization from bone. iPTH may also be lower in these infants and may not increase as rapidly following delivery. Therefore, these infants can have a relative intolerance to phosphate and have an increased risk of developing hypocalcemia.

D. **Hypocalcemia secondary to perinatal stress.** Stressed neonates who have suffered from perinatal sepsis, asphyxia, TORCH infections, compromised placental blood flow, or meconium aspiration also have an increased risk of hypocalcemia. This is believed to be due to the effects of corticosteroids and catecholamines during stress.

E. **Hypocalcemia secondary to alkalosis.** The amount of tCa that is ionized is inversely proportionate to serum pH. Infants who are acidotic have higher than expected iCa levels, and alkalotic infants can likewise be clinically hypocalcemic even if their tCa level is greater than 7 mg/dL. This is a direct pH effect.

F. **Hypocalcemia secondary to blood transfusions.** Citrate, a normal component of stored blood, forms a neutral soluble complex with calcium and thus reduces the amount of calcium that is ionized. Citrate is metabolized to bicarbonate within a few hours after administration and may induce a mild metabolic alkalosis that will also tend to decrease the amount of iCa. The amount of citrate administered with periodic blood replacement usually does not lead to clinical hypocalcemia. However, the amount of citrate given as a result of exchange transfusion—especially repeated transfusions—is much higher and may reduce serum iCa.

G. **Hypocalcemia secondary to furosemide therapy.** Due to its action on the ascending loop of Henle and the proximal tubule, furosemide causes hypercalciuria, which can lead to hypocalcemia, bone demineralization, or both. This effect can be most severe with chronic use of this medication.

III. **Risk factors.** There is an increased incidence of hypocalcemia within the first 3 days of life in premature or sick neonates. The risk of hypocalcemia increases with the degree of prematurity. Infants who also have an increased risk of hypocalcemia are:

A. Infants with poor enteral intake.
B. Infants of diabetic mothers.
C. Infants stressed during the perinatal period.
D. Infants receiving blood transfusions.
E. Infants with alkalosis.
F. Infants receiving furosemide.
G. Infants receiving excessive phosphate intake.

H. Infants with insufficient magnesium intake.

I. Infants with congenital hypoparathyroidism (eg, DiGeorge's syndrome).

IV. Clinical presentation

A. Acute hypocalcemia. Infants who are acutely hypocalcemic may present with apnea, irritability, slight tremors of the extremities, profound tetany, or seizures. Cardiac dysfunction may also occur, characterized by prolonged QT intervals and arrhythmias.

B. Chronic hypocalcemia. Infants who are chronically hypocalcemic may develop rickets characterized by apnea, bone demineralization, elevated alkaline phosphatase levels, and rib and long bone fractures.

V. Diagnosis

A. Laboratory studies

1. **Total and ionized calcium.** Serum iCa levels of less than 3 mg/dL are diagnostic of hypocalcemia. In the absence of iCa levels, serum tCa levels of less than 6 mg/dL or tCa levels of less than 7 mg/dL with clinical symptoms can be considered diagnostic of hypocalcemia.

2. **Serum magnesium levels** of less than 1.5 mg/dL indicate hypomagnesemia, which can accompany hypocalcemia.

3. **Alkaline phosphatase levels** greater than 225 IU/L are elevated and can be an early sign of rickets.

4. **Urinary calcium losses** can be estimated either by **random spot or 24-hour urine collections.** Calcium:creatinine ratios (measured in spot urine specimens) greater than 0.21–0.25 are indicative of hypercalciuria. Twenty-four-hour urinary calcium levels greater than 4 mg/kg/24h also indicate hypercalciuria.

B. Radiologic studies. Bone demineralization can be grossly estimated by reviewing sequential x-ray films of ribs and long bones. Rickets can be suggested by metaphyseal lucency accompanied by metaphyseal fraying and cupping. These findings are best seen at the knees and anterior rib ends (rachitic rosary). Rib fractures can also be seen in severe cases.

C. Other studies. Electrocardiography may show prolonged QT intervals or arrhythmias as a result of hypocalcemia or hypomagnesemia.

VI. Management. Parental calcium therapy may be associated with significant untoward effects. These include nephrolithiasis, cardiac arrhythmias, subcutaneous calcium deposition endangering joint mobility, peripheral skin sloughs, and the recently recognized possibility of metastatic calcifications in the brains of very sick neonates. **Expectant nonintervention** is therefore suggested for early-onset neonatal hypocalcemia, reserving treatment with parenteral calcium therapy for cases in which profound or clinical (symptomatic) hypocalcemia exists.

A. Early-onset neonatal hypocalcemia (ENH). If treatment is necessary based on iCa or tCa levels or symptoms, intravenous **10% calcium gluconate** (containing 9 mg elemental calcium per mL) should be given (for dosage, see Chap 75). This is usually more than adequate to maintain normal ionized calcium levels. Excessive treatment can suppress iPTH levels and for that reason should be avoided. There is no real benefit to continuous drip infusion compared to bolus administration in the treatment of ENH. When calcium gluconate is given without phosphate, most of the calcium is rapidly excreted in the urine. But in the acute stage and during the first 3 days of life, calcium can be given every 6 hours because it is impractical to give phosphate at this time.

B. Hypocalcemia secondary to poor enteral intake. Parenteral nutrition is usually started on days 3–4 of life, and calcium and phosphate must be started both for maintenance and to support bone growth. The intrauterine dose of 140 mg/kg/d of elemental calcium cannot be achieved by the intravenous route because of precipitation with phosphate. **An intravenous dosage of 45 mg/kg/d of elemental calcium with a calcium:phosphate ratio of 1.3:1.0 or 2:1 has been shown to be optimal in promoting both calcium and phosphate retention.** Supplementation with intravenous calcium can cause hypercalciuria. If intravenous calcium is given without phospate, most of the calcium is released in the urine and thus is not utilized for bone formation. Although phospate is needed, excessive phosphate can lead to hypocalcemia. **Vitamin D supplements** of 400 IU/d should also be provided.

C. **Hypocalcemia secondary to maternal diabetes.** Since these infants are at greater risk for developing hypocalcemia, serum calcium levels must be closely monitored. The treatment criteria are the same as those outlined above for ENH.

D. **Hypocalcemia secondary to perinatal stress.** The treatment criteria are the same as those for ENH except when the infant is maintained alkalotic (see below).

E. **Hypocalcemia secondary to alkalosis.** Since alkalotic infants (eg, infants being treated for persistent pulmonary hypertension) can be clinically hypocalcemic with tCa levels greater than 7 mg/dL, maintenance calcium therapy should be started when blood pH levels reach 7.5.

F. **Hypocalcemia secondary to blood transfusions.** The amount of citrate administered with periodic blood replacement usually does not lead to clinical hypocalcemia. However, the rate of citrate given as a result of exchange transfusion is much higher and may reduce serum iCa. Hypocalcemia secondary to blood transfusion can be treated prophylactically (with calcium gluconate) or if symptoms of hypocalcemia are noted (see Chap 75 for dosages and other pharmacologic information). Low iCa levels and clinical symptoms of hypocalcemia are rarely encountered even when extra calcium is not given.

G. **Hypocalcemia secondary to furosemide therapy.** Infants receiving furosemide have an increased urinary loss of calcium. This loss can be demonstrated by measurement of calcium:creatinine ratios in spot urines or tCa in 24-hour urine collections. If hypercalciuria exists, an attempt should be made to **substitute a thiazide diuretic (most commonly chlorothiazide) for furosemide.** However, if furosemide is thought to be essential, a lower dose of furosemide in combination with a thiazide should be used (1 mg furosemide to 10 mg chlorothiazide 3 times daily). Thiazides tend to cause calcium retention and can overcome the hypercalciuric effect of furosemide. These efforts will reduce the risk of nephrocalcinosis, which is directly related to the amount of calcium excreted in the urine. However, this combination can cause significant diuresis and increase urinary potassium loss. Fluids and electrolytes must therefore be carefully monitored if combination therapy is chosen. If more than 5 meq/kg/d of potassium supplementation is required after diuretics are started, **spironolactone** therapy should also be started (see Chap 75). Spironolactone has little or no effect on urinary calcium loss but helps to reduce the severity of hypokalemia in infants receiving either furosemide or thiazide therapy.

VII. **Prognosis.** Hypocalcemia can be effectively controlled with close monitoring of calcium, phosphate, and vitamin D intake, and urinary calcium losses.

HYPERCALCEMIA

I. **Definition.** Hypercalcemia is defined as total serum calcium levels greater than 11 mg/dL and ionized calcium levels greater than 5 mg/dL (1.7 mM). tCa is not predictive of iCa levels and thus is not a reliable measure of hypercalcemia. Acidotic infants may have iCa levels greater than 5 mg/dL even though tCa levels are 10 mg/dL or less.

II. **Pathophysiology.** Hypercalcemia may be due to parathyroid-related causes or to mechanisms unrelated to the parathyroid.
   A. Congenital primary hyperparathyroidism (rare).
   B. Congenital secondary hyperparathyroidism due to maternal hypoparathyroidism (rare).
   C. Subcutaneous fat necrosis (if extensive, may lead to hypercalcemia when large amounts of calcium are released from subcutaneous fat).
   D. Fanconi's syndrome.
   E. Benign familial hypercalcemia.
   F. Iatrogenic hypercalcemia due to excessive calcium supplements.
   G. Hypervitaminiosis D.
   H. Hypoproteinemia.
   I. Excessive thiazide treatment.

III. **Risk factors**
   A. Excessive supplemental calcium.
   B. Rare congenital hypercalcemia.

IV. **Clinical presentation.** Clinical symptomatology is important in establishing significant hypercalcemia. Symptoms include poor feeding with poor weight gain, depressed tone, lethargy, polyuria, and shortening of the QT interval as evidenced by eletrocardiography. Seizures can also be seen in severe cases.

V. **Diagnosis**
   A. **Laboratory studies**
      1. **Total and ionized calcium.** Ideally, iCa levels greater than 5 mg/dL establish hypercalcemia. If iCa levels are not available, tCa levels greater than 11 mg/dL can be considered abnormal. Infants who are acidotic or hypoproteinemic may have iCa levels greater than 5 mg/dL even though tCa is 10 mg/dL or less. Therefore, clinical symptoms are important in establishing the diagnosis of hypercalcemia.
      2. **Intakes of calcium, phosphate, and vitamin D** should be checked. The calcium:phosphate ratio should be 2:1, and vitamin D dosage should be 400–800 IU/d.
      3. **Serum total protein** and the **albumin:globulin ratio** should also be obtained.
      4. **Tubular resorption of phosphate** is usually reduced when hyperparathyroidism exists.
      5. **Immunoreactive parathyroid hormone (iPTH)** can be measured to establish hyperparathyroidism.
      6. **Vitamin D levels.** Hypervitaminosis D can usually be determined by careful review of vitamin intake. However, if this is not clear, **25-hydroxyvitamin D** can be measured. This value would be elevated if excess vitamin D has been given.
   B. **Radiologic studies.** X-rays are helpful in establishing the cause of hypercalcemia. Bone demineralization is typical of hyperparathyroidism, and osteosclerotic lesions are seen with hypervitaminosis D. Hypercalciuria can be very severe with excessive calcium intake or with normal calcium intake plus inadequate phosphate intake.

VI. **Management**
   A. **General.** Treatment depends on the cause, but in general the calcium intake should be reduced and vitamin D supplements withheld. Some authors recommend avoidance of sunlight. After hypercalcemia has resolved, the actual calcium, phosphate, and vitamin D needs can be estimated based on normal bone mineralization without recurrence of hypercalcemia. If the infant is receiving a thiazide diuretic (which in-

creases calcium retention in the kidneys), the drug should be discontinued.

B. **Acute symptomatic hypercalcemia**

1. When acute symptomatic hypercalcemia exists, **furosemide** may be effective in reducing serum calcium due to its marked hypercalciuric effect (see dosage in Chap 75). Fluid and electrolyte intake must be monitored closely if furosemide is used.

2. In older children and adults, calcitonin has been used for hypercalcemia associated with immobilization (patients in traction) and for acute hypercalcemic states at a dosage of 5–8 units/kg/dose intravenously or intramuscularly every 12 hours. It is unlikely that calcitonin therapy would be needed in neonates.

C. **Surgical intervention.** Very rarely, when severe hyperparathyroidism exists, parathyroidectomy may be needed.

VII. **Prognosis.** Complete resolution of hypercalcemia occurs rapidly if it is treated promptly.

HYPOMAGNESEMIA

I. **Definition.** Hypomagnesemia is defined as a serum magnesium level less than 1.52 meq/L (0.75 mmol/L).

II. **Pathophysiology.** Magnesium is required as a catalyst for many intracellular enzymatic reactions. Calcium homeostasis cannot be maintained if serum calcium levels are low. The usual cause of low magnesium levels is inadequate intake following delivery.

III. **Risk factors**

A. Hypocalcemia.

B. Inadequate intake of magnesium.

IV. **Clinical presentation.** The most common manifestation of hypomagnesemia is hypocalcemia that fails to respond to calcium therapy.

V. **Diagnosis.** Serum magnesium levels should be checked in all severely stressed infants. If the level is adequate and there is normal magnesium intake, repeated checks are not necessary unless hypocalcemia occurs.

VI. **Management.** Acute hypomagnesemia should be treated with **magnesium sulfate** until the magnesium level is normalized or symptoms resolve. The route may be intramuscular or intravenous; however, with intravenous administration, careful electrocardiographic monitoring is indicated, owing to the risk for arrhythmias (see Chap 75 for dosage and other pharmacologic information). If feedings are started early, parenteral magnesium is unnecessary; however, if the infant has poor enteral intake, parenteral nutrition should include magnesium.

VII. **Prognosis.** This condition often goes unrecognized. However, when detected, complete resolution occurs with treatment.

HYPERMAGNESEMIA

I. **Definition.** Hypermagnesemia is defined as serum magnesium levels in excess of 2.3 meq/L (1.15 mmol/L).

II. **Pathophysiology.** Increased serum magnesium levels depress the central nervous system and decrease skeletal muscle contractility. These effects can be reversed by increased serum iCa levels. The most common cause of hypermagnesemia in neonates is treatment of the mother with magnesium sulfate. Less commonly, it can occur with administration of a magnesium-containing antacid, especially when urine output is decreased. Hypermagnesemia can also be caused by magnesium sulfate enemas, which are absolutely contraindicated in neonates.

III. **Risk factors**

A. Administration of magnesium sulfate to mother prior to delivery.

B. Administration of magnesium-containing antacids to neonate, especially when urinary output is decreased.

C. Magnesium sulfate enemas (absolutely contraindicated in neonates).

IV. Clinical presentation. The symptoms of hypermagnesemia are very similar to those of hypercalcemia. These include poor feeding, lethargy, depressed tone, hyporeflexia, apnea, and decreased gastrointestinal motility with abdominal distention.

V. Diagnosis

A. Laboratory studies. Elevated **serum magnesium levels** are diagnostic.

B. Electrocardiography. A shortened QT interval is seen on ECG.

VI. Management

A. Fluids and electrolytes. If enteral feedings are not tolerated, maintenance intravenous fluids should be provided, with careful monitoring of serum electrolytes and pH.

B. Respiratory care. In rare cases of severe apnea, intubation and mechanical ventilation are needed.

C. Exchange transfusion can effectively reduce serum magnesium levels; but this should be reserved for extreme cases.

VII. Prognosis. Hypermagnesemia usually resolves spontaneously, provided renal function is maintained.

REFERENCES

Brown DR, Steranka BH, Taylor FH: Treatment of early-onset neonatal hypocalcemia: Effects on serum calcium and ionized calcium. *Am J Dis Child* 1981:**135**:24.

Chesney RW: Requirements and upper limits of vitamin D intake in the term neonate, infant, and older child. *J Pediatr* 1990;**116**:159.

Cooper LJ, Anast CS: Circulating immunoreactive parathyroid hormone levels in premature infants and the response to calcium therapy. *Acta Paediatr Scand* 1985;**74**:669.

Greer FR, Steichen JJ, Tsang RC: Effects of increased calcium, phosphorus, and vitamin D intake on bone mineralization in very low-birth-weight infants fed formulas with Polycose and medium-chain triglycerides. *J Pediatr* 1982;**100**:951.

Knight P, Heer D, Abenour G: CaxP and Ca/P in the parenteral feeding of preterm infants. *JPEN* 1983;**7**:110.

Koo WWK: Calcium, phosphorus, and vitamin D requirements of infants receiving parenteral nutrition. *J Perinatol* 1989;**8**:263.

Rudloff S, Lonnerdal B: Calcium retention from milk-based infant formulas, whey-hydrolysate formula, and human milk in weanling rhesus monkeys. *Am J Dis Child* 1990;**144**:360.

Steichen JJ et al: Elevated serum 1,25-dihydroxyvitamin-D concentrations in rickets of very low-birth-weight infants. *J Pediatr* 1981;**99**:293.

Vileisis RA: Furosemide effect on mineral status of parenterally nourished neonates with chronic lung disease. *Pediatrics* 1990;**85**:316.

73 Surgical Diseases of the Newborn

ALIMENTARY TRACT OBSTRUCTION

VASCULAR RING

I. **Definition.** *Vascular ring* denotes a variety of anomalies of the aortic arch and its branches that result in a "ring" of vessels around the trachea and esophagus.

II. **Pathophysiology.** Partial obstruction of the trachea or the esophagus, or both, may result from extrinsic compression by the encircling ring of vessels.

III. **Clinical presentation.** Dysphagia or stridor (respiratory insufficiency), or both, are the 2 modes of presentation.

IV. **Diagnosis** is by **barium swallow,** which identifies extrinsic compression of the esophagus in the region of the aortic arch.

V. **Management** consists of surgical division of a portion of the constricting ring of vessels. The specific surgical plan must be tailored to the particular type of aortic arch anomaly present.

ESOPHAGEAL ATRESIA

I. **Definition.** The esophagus ends blindly about 10–12 cm from the nares. In 85% of cases, the distal esophagus communicates with the posterior trachea (distal tracheoesophageal fistula [TEF]).

II. **Pathophysiology.** Complete esophageal obstruction results in inability of the infant to handle his own secretions, producing "excess salivation" and aspiration of pharyngeal contents. More importantly, the direct communication between the stomach and the tracheobronchial tree via the distal TEF allows the crying newborn to greatly distend the stomach with air; embarrassment of diaphragmatic excursion promotes basilar atelectasis and subsequent pneumonia. Additionally, the distal TEF permits reflux of gastric secretion directly into the tracheobronchial tree, causing chemical pneumonitis, which may be complicated by bacterial pneumonia.

III. **Clinical presentation.** The pregnancy may have been complicated by polyhydramnios. After delivery, the infant typically is unable to swallow saliva, which drains from the corners of the mouth and requires frequent suctioning. Attempts at feeding will result in prompt regurgitation, coughing, choking, and cyanosis.

IV. **Diagnosis** is established by **attempting to pass a nasogastric tube and meeting resistance at 10–12 cm from the nares** followed by **chest x-ray** for confirmation. Chest x-ray will show the tube to end or coil in the region of the thoracic inlet. The x-ray film should also be examined for possible skeletal anomalies, pulmonary infiltrates, cardiac size and shape, and abdominal bowel gas patterns. The absence of gas in the gastrointestinal tract implies esophageal atresia without TEF, for which surgical management will probably differ from that for the more common esophageal atresia with TEF. Careful contrast x-ray study of the proximal esophageal pouch can also be performed to delineate the precise length of the proximal pouch and to rule out the rare proximal TEF.

V. **Management**
   A. **Preoperative treatment** should focus on protecting the lungs by evacuating the proximal esophageal pouch with an **indwelling Replogle tube or frequent suctioning,** and by **placing the baby in a relatively upright position (45 degrees)** to lessen the likelihood of reflux of gastric contents up the distal esophagus into the trachea. **Broad-spectrum antibiotics** should be administered.
   B. **Surgical therapy.** The steps and timing of surgical therapy must be individualized. Some surgeons perform preliminary gastrostomy to decompress the stomach and provide additional protection against reflux. Ligation of the tracheoesophageal fistula and esophageal anastomosis are the essential steps in total surgical correction.

DUODENAL OBSTRUCTION

I. **Definition.** Obstruction of the lumen of the duodenum may be either complete or partial, preampullary or postampullary, and may be caused by either intrinsic or extrinsic problems.

II. **Pathophysiology**
   A. **Duodenal atresia** results in complete obstruction of the lumen of the duodenum, whereas symptoms of partial obstruction will result from a stenotic lesion.
   B. **Annular pancreas** is a congenital anomaly of pancreatic development, which results in an encircling "napkin ring" of pancreatic tissue about the descending duodenum. It can result in either complete or, more commonly, partial duodenal obstruction.
   C. **Malrotation** may cause complete or partial duodenal obstruction in 1 of 2 ways. In uncomplicated malrotation, peritoneal attachments (Ladd's bands) may compress the duodenum, resulting in total or, more commonly, partial obstruction. Midgut volvulus may complicate nonrotation and nonfixation of the intestine. The entire midgut may twist on the pedicle of its blood supply, the superior mesenteric artery, resulting in duodenal obstruction and eventual nonviability of the midgut.

III. **Clinical presentation**
   A. **General.** Infants with duodenal obstruction typically present with **vomiting (often bilious).** Abdominal distention is not usually a prominent feature. Polyhydramnios may have been present.
   B. **Duodenal atresia.** The presence of **Down's syndrome, esophageal atresia,** or **imperforate anus** suggests duodenal atresia.
   C. **Midgut volvulus** typically presents with symptoms of **duodenal obstruction (bilious vomiting)** and evidence of **intestinal ischemia (mucoid bloody stools),** usually in an infant who for days or weeks has eaten and stooled normally.

IV. The **differential diagnosis** includes duodenal atresia (stenosis), annular pancreas, and malrotation with or without the complication of midgut volvulus.

V. **Diagnosis.** The exact cause of the obstruction may not be known until laparotomy.
   A. **Abdominal x-ray study.** In complete duodenal obstruction, the pathognomonic x-ray finding is a **"double-bubble."**
   B. **Radiologic contrast studies**
      1. **Partial obstructions** will probably require an **upper GI series** to identify the site of difficulty.
      2. **Malrotation.** It is important to eliminate malrotation as a possibility since its complication, midgut volvulus, is a true surgical emergency. This is best done by an **upper GI series,** identifying a trans-

verse portion of the duodenum leading to a fixed ligament of Treitz, or by **barium enema,** localizing the cecum to its normal, right lower quadrant position.

VI. **Management**
  A. **Duodenal atresia or annular pancreas.** In cases of atresia or annular pancreas, **gastric suction** will control vomiting and allow "elective" surgical correction.
  B. **Malrotation** mandates **immediate surgical intervention,** because the viability of the intestine from the duodenum to the transverse colon may be at risk from midgut volvulus.

PROXIMAL INTESTINAL OBSTRUCTION

  I. **Definition.** Proximal intestinal obstruction is obstruction of the jejunum.
 II. **Pathophysiology.** Jejunal obstruction typically results from atresia of that segment of the bowel, usually as a result of a vascular accident in utero.
III. **Clinical presentation.** Infants with jejunal obstruction usually present with **bilious vomiting associated with minimal abdominal distention** since few loops of intestine are involved in the obstructive process.
 IV. **Diagnosis.** A plain **abdominal x-ray study** reveals only a few dilated small bowel loops with no gas distally.
  V. **Management.** Surgical correction is required.

DISTAL INTESTINAL OBSTRUCTION

  I. **Definition.** The term *distal intestinal obstruction* denotes partial or complete obstruction of the distal portion of the gastrointestinal tract. It may be either small bowel (ileum) or large bowel obstruction. The list of causes includes:
  A. **Ileal atresia.**
  B. **Meconium ileus**
    1. **Uncomplicated (simple) obstruction of the terminal ileum** by pellets of inspissated meconium.
    2. **Complicated meconium ileus,** implying compromise of bowel viability either prenatally or postnatally.
  C. **Colonic atresia.**
  D. **Meconium plug–hypoplastic left colon syndrome.**
  E. **Hirschsprung's disease (congenital aganglionic megacolon).**
 II. **Clinical presentation.** Infants with obstructing lesions in the distal intestine all have similar signs and symptoms. They typically have **distended abdomens, fail to pass meconium,** and **vomit bilious material.**
III. **Diagnosis**
  A. **Abdominal x-ray studies** show multiple dilated loops of intestine; the site of obstruction (distal small bowel vs colon) cannot be determined on plain x-ray films.
  B. **Contrast radiologic studies.** The preferred diagnostic test is contrast enema. It may identify colonic atresia, outline microcolon (which may signify complete distal small bowel obstruction), or suggest a transition zone (which may signify Hirschsprung's disease). The procedure can identify and treat meconium plug–hypoplastic left colon syndrome. If the test is normal, ileal atresia, meconium ileus, and Hirschsprung's disease are possibilities.
  C. **Sweat test.** A sweat test may be needed to document cystic fibrosis in cases of meconium ileus (unlikely to be helpful in the first few weeks of life).
  D. **Mucosal rectal biopsy** for histologic detection of ganglion cells is the safest and most widely available screening test for Hirschsprung's disease. However, **laparotomy** is often necessary to determine the exact nature of the problem in infants with normal results of barium enema.

IV. **Management**
   A. **Nonoperative management** is "curative" in cases of meconium plug and hypoplastic left colon.
      1. Passage of time and **colonic stimulation by digital examination and rectal enemas** promote return of effective peristalsis.
      2. **In infants who achieve apparently normal bowel function,** one must rule out Hirschsprung's disease by **mucosal rectal biopsy;** a small percentage of patients with meconium plug will prove to have aganglionosis.
      3. Interestingly, **uncomplicated meconium ileus,** if identified, can often be treated by nonoperative means. **Repeated enemas with Hypaque or acetylcysteine (Mucomyst)** may disimpact the inspissated meconium in the terminal ileum and relieve the obstruction.
   B. **Surgical therapy.** Surgical intervention is required for atresia of the ileum or colon, for complicated meconium ileus, and when the diagnosis is in doubt. Hirschsprung's disease is treated in the neonatal period by colostomy through ganglionic bowel.

IMPERFORATE ANUS

   I. **Definition.** Imperforate anus is the lack of an anal opening of proper location or size. There are 2 types: high and low.
   A. **In high imperforate anus,** the rectum ends above the puborectalis sling, the main muscle responsible for maintaining fecal continence. There is never an associated fistula to the perineum. In males there may be a rectourinary fistula, and in females, a rectovaginal fistula.
   B. **In low imperforate anus,** the rectum has traversed the puborectalis sling in correct position. Variants include anal stenosis, imperforate anus with perineal fistula, and imperforate anus without fistula.
   II. **Diagnosis** is by **inspection and calibration of any perineal opening.** All patients with imperforate anus should have **x-ray studies of the lumbosacral spine and urinary tract,** because there is a high incidence of dysmorphism in these areas.
   III. **Management.** Surgical therapy in the neonate consists of colostomy for high anomalies and perineal anoplasty or dilation of fistula for low lesions. If the level is not known, colostomy is preferable to blind exploration of the perineum. If colostomy is done, a contrast x-ray study of the distal limb should be performed to ascertain the level at which the rectum ends and to determine the presence or absence of an associated fistula.

CAUSES OF RESPIRATORY DISTRESS

CHOANAL ATRESIA

   I. **Definition.** Choanal atresia is a congenital blockage of the posterior nares, caused by persistence of a bony septum (90%) or a soft tissue membrane (10%).
   II. **Pathophysiology.** Unilateral or bilateral obstruction at the posterior nares may be due to soft tissue or bone. Choanal atresia, which is complete and bilateral, is one of the causes of respiratory distress immediately following delivery. The effects of upper airway obstruction are compounded because neonates are obligate nose-breathers and will not "think" to breathe through the mouth.
   III. **Clinical presentation.** Respiratory distress due to partial or total upper airway obstruction is the mode of presentation.
   IV. **Diagnosis** is made by **inability to pass a catheter into the nasopharynx** via either side of the nose.

V. **Management.** Simply **making the infant cry and thereby breathe through its mouth** will temporarily improve breathing. Insertion of an **oral airway** will maintain the ability to breathe until surgical correction of the atresia is performed.

PIERRE-ROBIN SYNDROME

I. **Definition.** This anomaly consists of mandibular hypoplasia in association with cleft palate.
II. **Pathophysiology.** Airway obstruction is produced by posterior displacement of the tongue associated with the small size of the mandible.
III. **Clinical presentation.** Severity of symptoms varies, but most infants manifest a high degree of partial upper airway obstruction.
IV. **Management**
  A. **Infants with mild involvement** can be cared for in the **prone position** and fed through a special **Breck nipple.** Adjustment to the airway compromise will take place over days or weeks.
  B. **More severe cases** require **nasopharyngeal tubes or surgical procedures** to hold the tongue in an anterior position. **Tracheostomy** is generally a last resort.

VASCULAR RING

Airway compromise is rarely severe and is usually manifested by stridor (see p 441).

LARYNGOTRACHEAL CLEFT

I. **Definition.** Laryngotracheal cleft is a rare congenital anomaly in which there is incomplete separation of the larynx (and sometimes the trachea) from the esophagus, resulting in a common channel of esophagus and airway. This communication may be short or may extend almost the entire length of the trachea.
II. **Pathophysiology.** The persistent communication between the larynx (and occasionally a significant portion of the trachea) and the esophagus results in recurring symptoms of aspiration and respiratory distress with feeding.
III. **Clinical presentation.** Respiratory distress during feeding is the presenting symptom.
IV. **Diagnosis. Contrast swallow** may suggest the anomaly, but **endoscopy** is essential in firmly establishing the diagnosis and delineating the extent of the defect.
V. **Management.** Laryngotracheal cleft is treated by surgical correction, which is difficult and often unsuccessful.

H-TYPE TRACHEOESOPHAGEAL FISTULA

I. **Definition.** This anomaly is the third most common type of tracheoesophageal fistula (TEF), making up 5% of cases. Esophageal continuity is intact, but there is a fistulous communication between the posterior trachea and the anterior esophagus.
II. **Pathophysiology.** If the fistula is small, as is usually the case, "silent" aspiration takes place during feedings with resulting pneumonitis. If the fistula is unusually large, coughing and choking may accompany each feeding.
III. **Clinical presentation.** Symptoms, as noted above, depend on the size of the fistula.
IV. **Diagnosis. Barium swallow** is the initial diagnostic study and may identify the fistula. The most accurate procedure, however, is **bronchoscopy** (per-

haps combined with esophagoscopy); this should allow discovery and perhaps cannulation of the fistula.
V. **Management.** Surgical correction is required. The approach (neck or chest) is determined by location of the fistula.

INTRINSIC ABNORMALITIES OF THE AIRWAY

I. **Definition.** Abnormalities of, or within, the airway that cause partial obstruction fall into this category. Examples include laryngomalacia, paralyzed vocal cord, subglottic web, and hemangioma.
II. **Pathophysiology.** These lesions result in partial obstruction of the airway and cause stridor and respiratory distress of varying severity.
III. **Clinical presentation.** See **II**, above.
IV. **Diagnosis.** The diagnosis is established by **endoscopy** of the airway.
V. **Management** is individualized. Some problems, such as laryngomalacia, will be outgrown if the child can be supported through the period of acute symptoms. Other lesions, such as subglottic webs, may be amenable to endoscopic resection or laser therapy.

CONGENITAL LOBAR EMPHYSEMA

I. **Definition.** *Lobar emphysema* is a term used to denote hyperexpansion of the air spaces of a segment or lobe of the lung.
II. **Pathophysiology.** Inspired air is trapped in an enclosed space. As the cyst of entrapped air enlarges, normal lung is increasingly compressed. Cystic problems are more common in the upper lobes.
III. **Clinical presentation.** Small cysts may cause few or no symptoms and are readily seen on x-ray film. Giant cysts may cause significant respiratory distress, with mediastinal shift and compromise of the contralateral lung.
IV. **Diagnosis.** Usually the cysts are easily seen on plain **chest x-ray films.** However, the radiologic findings may be confused with that of tension pneumothorax.
V. **Management.** Therapeutic options include **observation** for small asymptomatic cysts, **repositioning of the endotracheal tube** to selectively ventilate uninvolved lung for 6–12 hours, **bronchoscopy** for endobronchial lavage, and operative resection of the cyst with or without the segment or lobe from which it arises.

CYSTIC ADENOMATOID MALFORMATION

I. **Definition.** The term *cystic adenomatoid malformation* encompasses a spectrum of congenital pulmonary malformation involving varying degrees of adenomatosis and cyst formation.
II. **Pathophysiology.** Severity of symptoms is related to the amount of lung involved and particularly to the degree to which normal ipsilateral and contralateral lung is compressed.
III. **Clinical presentation.** Signs of respiratory insufficiency such as **tachypnea** and **cyanosis** are modes of presentation.
IV. **Diagnosis.** The characteristic pattern on **chest x-ray film** is multiple discrete air bubbles, occasionally with air fluid levels, involving a region of the lung. The radiographic appearance can mimic that of congenital diaphragmatic hernia.
V. **Management.** Treatment is surgical resection of involved lung, allowing reexpansion of compressed normal pulmonary tissue.

CONGENITAL DIAPHRAGMATIC HERNIA

I. **Definition.** A patent pleuroperitoneal canal through the foramen of Bochdalek is the essential defect in congenital diaphragmatic hernia (CDH).

II. Pathophysiology

A. Prenatal. The abnormal communication between the peritoneal and pleural cavities allows herniation of intestine into the pleural space as the developing gastrointestinal tract returns from its extracoelomic phase at 10–12 weeks' gestation. Depending on the degree of pulmonary compression by herniated intestine, there may be marked diminution of bronchial branching, limited multiplication of alveoli, and persistence of muscular hypertrophy in pulmonary arterioles. These anatomic abnormalities are most notable on the side of the CDH (usually the left); they are also present to some degree in the contralateral lung.

B. Postnatal. After delivery, the anatomic anomaly may contribute to the development of one or both of the following pathologic conditions.

1. Pulmonary parenchymal insufficiency. Infants with CDH have a abnormally small functional lung mass. Some have so few conducting air passages and developed alveoli—a condition known as *pulmonary parenchymal insufficiency*—that survival is unlikely.

2. Pulmonary hypertension. Infants with CDH are predisposed anatomically to pulmonary hypertension, also known as *persistent fetal circulation (PFC)*. In this condition, blood is shunted around the lungs through the foramen ovale and patent ductus arteriosus. Shunting promotes acidosis and hypoxia, both of which are potent stimuli to additional pulmonary vasoconstriction. Thus, a vicious cycle of clinical deterioration is established.

III. Clinical presentation. Most infants with CDH exhibit significant respiratory distress within the first few hours of life.

IV. Diagnosis. Afflicted babies tend to have scaphoid abdomens since there is a paucity of the gastrointestinal tract located in the abdomen. **Auscultation** reveals diminished breath sounds on the affected side. Diagnosis is established by a **chest x-ray film** that reveals a bowel gas pattern in one hemithorax, with shift of mediastinal structures to the other side and compromise of the contralateral lung.

V. Management

A. Indwelling arterial catheter. Blood gas levels should be monitored by an indwelling arterial catheter.

B. Supportive care. Appropriate **respiratory and metabolic support** should be provided.

C. Nasogastric intubation should be done to lessen gaseous distention of the stomach and intestine. For the same reason, any positive-pressure ventilation must be delivered by endotracheal tube, never by mask.

D. Surgical correction is by reduction of intrathoracic intestine and closure of the diaphragmatic defect. Surgical intervention is obviously an essential element of treatment, but it is not the key to survival.

E. Extracorporeal membrane oxygenation (ECMO) is being employed at an increasing number of centers in the treatment of neonates with severe respiratory failure (see Chap 15).

VI. Prognosis. With conventional therapy, mortality rates for infants with CDH are still in the range of 50–80%. This high rate has prompted a search for other modes of treatment in addition to the expensive, labor-intensive modality ECMO.

A. Fetal surgery has been done successfully on a limited basis, with the idea that in utero intervention will lessen the risk for development of pulmonary hypoplasia, which may be incompatible with life after delivery.

B. Medications. Another major area of research is the attempt to develop a pharmacologic agent to selectively decrease pulmonary vascular resistance. Such an agent would help solve the problem of PFC.

ABDOMINAL MASSES

RENAL MASSES

In most clinical series, the majority of abdominal masses in neonates are renal in origin. They may be unilateral or bilateral, solid or cystic. After physical examination, evaluation begins with ultrasonography, which is simple and safe to perform. Ultrasonography should define the solid or cystic nature of the mass, the presence or absence of normal kidneys, and yield information on other intra-abdominal abnormalities. Intravenous pyelography (IVP) may be helpful but is not necessary in every case. In selected instances, more involved procedures such as renal scan, CT scan, retrograde pyelography, venography, and arteriography may be needed to define the problem and plan appropriate therapy.

I. **Multicystic kidney.** This is a form of renal dysplasia and the most common renal cystic disease of the newborn. Fortunately, it is usually unilateral. Ultrasonography can define the nature of the disorder, and IVP is useful in assessing the remainder of the urinary system. Nephrectomy is appropriate treatment.

II. **Hydronephrosis.** Urinary obstruction, depending on its location, can cause unilateral or bilateral flank and abdominal masses. Treatment is by correction of the obstructing lesion or decompression proximal to it. A kidney rendered nonfunctional by back pressure is usually best removed. Obstructive uropathy is one category of lesion suitable for in utero intervention. Surgery on the developing fetus to decompress the obstructed urinary system may improve the postnatal status and increase survival.

III. **Infantile polycystic kidney disease.** Inherited in an autosomal recessive fashion, this entity involves both kidneys and carries a grim prognosis.

IV. **Renal vein thrombosis.** The typical presentation is flank mass(es) and hematuria, usually within the first 3 days of life. Risk factors are maternal diabetes and dehydration. In general, conservative nonoperative management is recommended.

V. **Wilms' tumor.** See p 449.

OVARIAN MASSES

Simple ovarian cyst has been called the most frequently palpated abdominal mass in the female neonate. It presents as a relatively mobile smooth-walled abdominal mass. It is not associated with malignancy, and excision with preservation of any ovarian tissue is curative.

HEPATIC MASSES

The liver can be enlarged, often to grotesque proportions, by a variety of problems. When physical examination, ultrasonography, and IVP suggest hepatic origin, angiography should be performed. This study may be diagnostic and will aid in surgical planning. Lesions include:

I. **Hepatic cysts.**

II. **Solid, benign tumors.**

III. **Vascular tumors.**

    A. **Hemangiomas** of the liver may cause heart failure, thrombocytopenia, and anemia. Therapeutic options include digitalis, corticosteroid administration, embolization, hepatic artery ligation, and liver resection.

    B. **Hemangioendothelioma.**

IV. **Malignant tumors. Hepatoblastoma** is by far the most common liver cancer in the neonate. Serum alpha-fetoprotein may be elevated. While surgical resection remains the key to achieving cure, new chemotherapeutic protocols (cisplatin [Platinol] and doxorubicin [Adriamycin]) may significantly improve the formerly dismal prognosis for infants with this tumor.

GASTROINTESTINAL MASSES

Palpable abdominal masses that arise from the gastrointestinal tract are unusual and tend to be cystic, smooth-walled, and mobile (depending on size). Causes include intestinal duplication and mesenteric cyst.

RETROPERITONEAL TUMORS

NEUROBLASTOMA

I. **Definition.** Neuroblastoma is a primitive malignant neoplasm that arises from neural crest tissue. It is probably the most common congenital tumor and is usually located in the adrenal gland.

II. **Clinical presentation.** This tumor typically presents as a firm, fixed, irregular mass extending obliquely from the costal margin, occasionally across the midline and into the lower abdomen.

III. **Diagnosis**
   A. **Laboratory studies.** A **24-hour urine collection** should be analyzed for VMA and other metabolites.
   B. **Radiologic studies.** A plain **abdominal x-ray film** may reveal calcification within the tumor. **IVP** and **CT scan** typically show extrinsic compression and inferolateral displacement of the kidney. Search for possible metastatic deposits involves **bone marrow aspiration and biopsy, bone scan, chest x-ray study,** and **chest CT scan.**

IV. **Management.** Planned therapy should take into account the well-recognized but poorly understood fact that neuroblastoma is notably less aggressive in the young infant than in the older child.

WILMS' TUMOR (NEPHROBLASTOMA)

I. **Definition.** Wilms' tumor is an embryonal renal neoplasm in which blastemic, stromal, and epithelial cell types are present. Renal involvement is usually unilateral but may be bilateral (5% of cases).

II. **Clinical presentation.** Palpable abdominal mass extending from beneath the costal margin is the usual mode of presentation.

III. **Risk factors** include aniridia, hemihypertrophy, certain genitourinary anomalies, and a family history of nephroblastoma.

IV. **Diagnosis**
   A. **Laboratory studies.** There is no tumor marker for Wilms' tumor
   B. **Radiologic studies.** Ultrasonography is followed by IVP or CT scan, or both, which reveal intrinsic distortion of the calyceal system of the involved kidney. The possibility of tumor thrombus in the renal vein and inferior vena cava should be evaluated by ultrasonography and venography, if necessary.

V. **Management**
   A. **Unilateral renal involvement.** Nephrectomy is the first step in treatment. Surgical staging determines the administration of radiotherapy and chemotherapy; both are very effective.
   B. **Bilateral renal involvement.** Treatment of bilateral Wilms' tumor is highly individualized.

TERATOMA

I. **Definition.** Teratoma is a neoplasm containing elements derived from all 3 germ-cell layers: endoderm, mesoderm, and ectoderm. Teratomas in the neonate are sacrococcygeal in location and are believed to represent a type of abortive caudal twinning.

II. **Clinical presentation.** This tumor is usually grossly evident as a large exter-

nal mass in the sacrococcygeal area. Occasionally, however, it may be presacral and retroperitoneal in location, and it may present as an abdominal mass.
III. **Diagnosis.** See II, above. **Digital rectal examination** of the presacral space is important.
IV. **Management.** Because the incidence of malignancy in these tumors increases with age, **prompt surgical excision** is required.

ABDOMINAL WALL DEFECTS

GASTROSCHISIS

I. **Definition.** Gastroschisis is a centrally located, full-thickness abdominal wall defect with 2 distinctive anatomic features.
   A. **The extruded intestine never has a protective sac covering it.**
   B. **The umbilical cord is an intact structure at the level of the abdominal skin, just to the left of the defect.** Typically, the opening in the abdominal wall is 2–4 cm in diameter, and the solid organs (liver and spleen) reside in the peritoneal cavity.
II. **Pathophysiology.** Exposure of unprotected intestine to irritating amniotic fluid in utero results in its edematous, indurated, foreshortened appearance. Because of these intestinal abnormalities, development of appropriate peristalsis and effective absorption is significantly delayed, usually by several weeks. Fortunately, associated congenital anomalies are rare in patients with gastroschisis.
III. **Clinical presentation.** See I and II, above.
IV. **Diagnosis.** The key differential diagnosis is ruptured omphalocele, although the **diagnosis is readily apparent in most cases.** Increasingly, **prenatal ultrasonography** identifies gastroschisis.
V. **Management**
   A. **General considerations.** All agree that infants with gastroschisis should be delivered at a neonatal center equipped and staffed to provide definitive care. Less certain is the recommended mode of delivery. Some have argued that abdominal wall defect is an indication for cesarean section. However, recent articles note that in the absence of other factors, vaginal delivery does not increase the mortality, morbidity, or length of hospital stay for newborns with gastroschisis.
   B. **Specific measures**
      1. **Temperature regulation.** Immediate attention should be directed toward maintenance of normal body temperature. The tremendous intestinal surface area exposed to the environment puts these infants at great risk of hypothermia.
      2. **Protective covering.** It is best not to keep replacing moist, saline-soaked gauze over the exposed intestine, because doing so promotes evaporative heat loss. It is better to **apply a dry (or moist) protective dressing and then wrap the abdomen in layers of cellophane.** A warm, controlled environment should be provided.
      3. **Nasogastric decompression** is helpful.
      4. **Broad-spectrum antibiotic coverage** is appropriate, given the unavoidable contamination.
      5. **Total parenteral nutrition (TPN).** A protracted ileus is to be expected, and appropriate intravenous nutritional support must be provided.
      6. **Surgical correction.** As soon as the infant's condition permits, operative correction should be undertaken. Complete reduction of herniated intestine, with primary closure of the abdominal wall, or placement of unreduced intestine in a protective prosthetic silo, with subsequent staged reduction over 7–14 days, is usually performed.

OMPHALOCELE

I. **Definition.** An omphalocele is a herniation of abdominal contents into the base of the umbilical cord. The gross appearance of omphalocele differs from that of gastroschisis in 2 important respects.
   A. **A protective membrane encloses the malplaced abdominal contents** (unless rupture has occurred, eg, during the birth process).
   B. **Elements of the umbilical cord course individually over the sac and come together at its apex to form a normal-appearing umbilical cord.**
II. **Associated anomalies.** Significant associated congenital anomalies occur in about 25–40% of infants with omphalocele. Problems include chromosomal abnormalities, congenital diaphragmatic hernia, and a variety of cardiac defects.
III. **Clinical presentation.** There are different sizes of omphaloceles. The smaller ones typically contain only intestine; large or giant omphaloceles contain liver and spleen as well as the gastrointestinal tract. The peritoneal cavity in infants with large or giant omphaloceles is very small, as growth has proceeded without the solid organs in proper position.
IV. **Diagnosis.** The anomaly is **usually apparent.** Ruptured omphalocele may be confused with gastroschisis; both defects are characterized by exposed intestine, but infants with omphalocele do not possess an intact umbilical cord at the level of the abdominal wall, to the left of the defect. Careful studies to identify associated congenital anomalies should be carried out.
V. **Management.** Reduction, even in stages over a lengthy period of time, may be very difficult to achieve. Therapeutically, infants with omphalocele fall into 2 main groups.
   A. **Ruptured sac.** Infants with ruptured sacs resemble those with gastroschisis. The unprotected intestine should be cared for as described for gastroschisis (see p 450, **B.2**) and the problem should be corrected surgically on an emergent basis.
   B. **Intact sac.** Intact omphalocele is a less urgent surgical problem. The protective membrane conserves heat and in most cases allows effective peristalsis. This sac should be carefully protected. Some surgeons favor daily dressing changes with gauze pads impregnated with povidone iodine until the sac toughens and desiccates. The timing of surgery is influenced by a number of factors, including the dimensions of the defect, the size of the infant, and the presence of other anomalies.

EXSTROPHY OF THE BLADDER

I. **Definition.** Exstrophy of the bladder is a congenital malformation of the lower anterior abdominal wall. In this defect, the internal surface of the posterior wall of the urinary bladder extrudes through the abdominal wall defect. The problem occurs in varying degrees of severity, ranging from epispadias to complete extroversion of the bladder, with exposure of the ureteral orifices.
II. **Clinical presentation.** The lower abdominal wall defect is obvious; exposed bladder mucosa is markedly edematous and friable.
III. **Diagnosis.** Diagnosis is by **inspection. Radiologic evaluation of the proximal urinary tract** is advisable.
IV. **Management**
   A. **Protective covering.** The bladder should be carefully protected with **Vaseline gauze or cellophane wrap.** Attention should also be paid to protection of the surrounding skin.
   B. **Surgical repair.** In most centers, primary closure of the bladder is attempted within the first 48–72 hours of life, while the sacroiliac joints are still pliable and the pelvis can be "molded" to allow better approximation of the pubic rami.

CLOACAL EXSTROPHY

I. **Definition.** Cloacal exstrophy is a rare but devastating complex of anomalies, including imperforate anus, exstrophy of the bladder, omphalocele, and vesicointestinal fistula, frequently with prolapse of bowel through the fistula onto the bladder mucosa.

II. **Clinial presentation.** See I, above.

III. **Diagnosis.** Diagnosis is by **inspection.** Evaluation of the genitourinary system and gastrointestinal tract is appropriate.

IV. **Management**
   A. **Protective covering.** Exposed mucosa, both bladder and intestine, should be protected with **Vaseline gauze or cellophane wrap.** Ointments should be applied to the surrounding skin to prevent maceration.
   B. **Surgical care.** Prompt operation to separate the fecal and urinary streams is imperative.

MISCELLANEOUS SURGICAL CONDITIONS

NECROTIZING ENTEROCOLITIS

In most centers, necrotizing enterocolitis (NEC) is the most common indication for operation in neonates (see also Chap 66). Abdominal exploration is usually reserved for infants with full-thickness necrosis of the intestine, usually manifested by pneumoperitoneum (best identified by serial left lateral decubitus x-ray films). Other less common indications for surgery include cellulitis and induration of the abdominal wall and an unchanging abdominal mass. Delayed stricture formation, which is most common on the left side of the colon, complicates NEC in 15–25% of cases.

HYPOSPADIAS

I. **Definition.** Hypospadias is a developmental anomaly in which the external opening of the urethra is present on the underside of the penis or on the perineum rather than in its normal position at the end of the penile shaft.

II. **Clinical presentation.** There are different anatomic classifications, depending on the location of the meatal opening and on the degree of chordee (curvature of the penis). There is a high incidence of associated **cryptorchidism** in the patients. Severe cases of hypospadias may be confused with ambiguous genitalia.

III. **Diagnosis.** The anomaly is **readily apparent** (see I and II, above). **Radiologic evaluation of the urinary system** is appropriate.

IV. **Management.** Surgical correction should usually not be attempted in the newborn. Because foreskin tissue may be needed for later surgical correction, **circumcision must be avoided** in infants with hypospadias.

HERNIA AND HYDROCELE

I. **Definition.** Persistence of a patent processus vaginalis (related to testicular descent) is responsible for inguinal hernia-hydrocele in the neonate.
   A. **Inguinal hernia.** The opening of the patent processus at the internal ring is large enough to allow a loop of intestine to extrude from the abdominal cavity with an increase in intra-abdominal pressure.
   B. **Hydrocele.** The patent processus is too narrow to permit egress of intestine; peritoneal fluid drips down along the course of the narrow patent processus and accumulates in the scrotum.

II. **Diagnosis**
   A. **Inguinal hernias** tend to present as lumps or bulges that come and go at the pubic tubercle. Less commonly, they descend into the scrotum.

    B. **Hydroceles** are typically scrotal in location, are transilluminate, and are not reducible.
III. **Management**
    A. **Inguinal hernia** carries a 15–20% risk of incarceration during the first year of life. Accordingly, they are usually surgically repaired when the infant's general medical condition permits.
    B. **Hydrocele** frequently resolves without specific treatment, as the obliteration of the narrow patent processus continues after birth. Persistence of hydrocele for 6–12 months is an indication for surgical repair.

UNDESCENDED TESTICLES (CRYPTORCHIDISM)

Undescended testicles occur in about 33% of premature and 3% of term male infants. Many undescended testes will descend in the first few months after birth. Unless there is an associated inguinal hernia, surgical correction is usually not performed until the infant is 18 months to 2 years of age, although some surgeons favor earlier correction.

POSTERIOR URETHRAL VALVES

  I. **Definition.** Posterior urethral valves are abnormal valves in the urethra at the verumontanum. They represent the most common cause of congenital obstructive uropathy in males.
  II. **Pathophysiology.** The high degree of bladder outlet obstruction caused by posterior urethral valves results in proximal dilatation. The urinary bladder enlarges, the ureters become dilated and tortuous, and back pressure in the collecting systems compromises developing renal parenchyma.
 III. **Clinical presentation**
    A. **Prenatal ultrasonography** is currently identifying many infants with posterior urethral valves.
    B. **After birth, neonates** with this anomaly present with bilateral flank masses, distended bladder, and poor urinary stream (with dribbling).
 IV. **Diagnosis. Voiding cystourethrography** documents the abnormal valves.
  V. **Management.** The goal of therapy is preservation of renal function and avoidance of renal failure.
    A. **Evaluation of renal function and the infant's general status** should be carried out.
    B. **Stabilization, rehydration, correction of electrolyte abnormalities, and treatment of urinary tract infection** should be accompanied by transurethral drainage of the bladder, using a 5F infant feeding tube.
    C. **Surgical therapy**
      1. **Ablation of valves** is the initial operative procedure favored by most pediatric urologists.
      2. **Urinary diversion** may be indicated.

REFERENCES

Bethel CAI, Szashore JH, Touloukian RJ: Caesarean section does not improve outcome in gastroschisis. *J Pediatr Surg* 1989;**24**:1.

King LR (editor): *Urologic Surgery in Neonates and Young Infants.* Saunders, 1988.

Pierro A et al: Preoperative chemotherapy in "unresectable" hepatoblastoma. *J Pediatr Surg* 1989;**24**:24.

Powell DM, Othersen HB, Smith CD: Malrotation of the intestine in children: Effect of age on presentation and therapy. *J Pediatr Surg* 1989;**24**:777.

Welch J et al (editors): *Pediatric Surgery,* 4th ed. Year Book, 1986.

74 Thyroid Disorders

HYPOTHYROIDISM

I. **Definition.** Congenital hypothyroidism is a deficiency of thyroid function present at or before birth. Detection of thyroid deficiency in the neonatal period is critical, because delay will lead to irreversible brain damage.

II. **Incidence.** The incidence is about 1:4000 (boys 1:6650, girls 1:2750).

III. **Pathophysiology.** Hypothyroidism may be primary or secondary. **Primary hypothyroidism** may be due to many causes, including agenesis or dysgenesis of the thyroid gland, defects of hormone syntheses, or maternal ingestion of antithyroid drugs. **Secondary hypothyroidism** may be caused by a defect in thyroid-stimulating hormone (TSH) or thyrotropin-releasing hormone (TRH).

IV. **Risk factors.** Maternal ingestion of antithyroid drugs and maternal autoimmune thyroid disorders are risk factors for neonatal hypothyroidism.

V. **Clinical presentation**
   A. **Early.** Congenital hypothyroidism is usually not apparent at birth, but symptoms during the first 2 weeks of life may include hypotonia, lethargy, large anterior or posterior fontanelles, feeding difficulties (especially the infant's falling asleep during feedings), constipation, pallor, hypothermia, persistent neonatal jaundice, hoarse cry.
   B. **Late.** After 6 weeks, classic facial features may appear (puffy eyelids, coarse hair, large tongue, thick, dry skin). Other signs are umbilical hernia, abdominal distention, hyporeflexia, hypotension, anemia, and patent cranial sutures.

VI. **Diagnosis**
   A. **Routine screening by filter paper spot-testing** (dried drop of blood collected on Guthrie cards for thyroxine testing) is required at birth in most states. If the results are low, serum TSH and T_4 should be measured (normal serum T_4 is 5–11 μg/dL; normal serum TSH is < 2.5 μu/mL).
   B. **Low T_4, high TSH** confirms primary hypothyroidism.
   C. **Low T_4, normal TSH** may be seen in premature infants. However, infants with hypothyroidism have normal free thyroxine levels, resulting from low thyroid hormone–binding globulin (TBG) levels.
   D. **Thyroid scan** to differentiate athyreosis, ectopic thyroid, dyshormonogenesis, and goiter.
   E. **Measurements of TSH-blocking antibodies** to diagnose congenital transient hypothyroidism secondary to transplacental thyrotropin-blocking antibodies.
   F. **TRH stimulation test** to differentiate thyroid, pituitary, and hypothalamic defects.

VII. **Management.** It is **essential to treat congenital hypothyroidism as soon as possible after birth to prevent irreversible brain damage.** Consultation with a pediatric endocrinologist is recommended.
   A. **Drug therapy.** The drug of choice is **levothyroxine,** starting with 10 μg/kg/d and increasing gradually as needed based on T_4 and TSH levels. Therapeutic goals are to keep T_4 in normal range and TSH suppressed.
   B. **Laboratory follow-up.** TSH and T_4 are followed on an ongoing basis.

VIII. Prognosis. If thyroxine supplementation began in the first 6 weeks of life, the infant may have normal intelligence.

HYPERTHYROIDISM

I. **Definition.** Congenital hyperthyroidism is caused by excess thyroid hormone present at birth. Many affected infants (50%) are born to mothers with Graves' disease during pregnancy.

II. **Incidence.** The disorder occurs at random in genetically predisposed population.

III. **Pathophysiology and risk factors.** Congenital hyperthyroidism is almost invariably caused by transplacental passage of long-acting thyroid-stimulating immunoglobulins (TSIs) from mothers with Graves' disease.

IV. **Clinical presentation.** Signs of hyperthyroidism may be present in the first 24 hours of life unless the mother was receiving antithyroid medications, in which case the presentation may be delayed. Signs include increased appetite, irritability, microcephaly, weight loss, tachycardia, and hyperthermia. A goiter may be small and go undetected, or it may be large enough to cause tracheal compression.

V. **Diagnosis**
   A. **History.** A maternal history of Graves' disease is usually present.
   B. **Laboratory studies.** Confirmation is based on elevated T_3 and T_4, and normal free T_4.

VI. **Management**
   A. Because congenital hyperthyroidism is most often due to maternal Graves' disease, the disorder is **usually self-limited;** the infant's acquired TSI will usually decrease over a period of 3–12 weeks after delivery. Consultation with a pediatric endocrinologist is recommended.
   B. **If hyperthyroidism persists,** one of the following antithyroid medications should be administered.
      1. **Propylthiouracil (PTU),** 10 mg/kg/d orally in divided doses every 8 hours.
      2. **Lugol's iodine,** 1 drop orally 3 times daily.
      3. **Methimazole,** 1 mg/kg/d orally every 8 hours.

VII. **Prognosis.** Neonatal hyperthyroidism is self-limited in many instances and no sequelae have been recognized. However, it has a mortality rate of about 15% if not diagnosed and treated.

REFERENCES

Bernstein RE: Congenital hypothyroidism: Clinical pathological aspects and biochemical screening. *S Afr Med J* 1981;**59:**710.

Fisher DA, Klein AH: Thyroid development and disorders of thyroid function in the newborn. *N Engl J Med* 1981;**304:**702.

Graudal et al: Congenital hypothyroidism. *J Fam Pract* 1989;**29(1):**47.

Horlick M et al: Role of imaging in neonatal hypothyroidism, *Am J Dis Child* 1988;**142(11):**1139.

75 Commonly Used Medications

Acetaminophen (APAP, Liquiprin, Panadol, Tempra, Tylenol)

Indications and use: Analgesic-antipyretic in presence of aspirin allergy, hemostatic disturbances and upper GI disease.

Actions: Mechanism of analgesic effect is unclear. Reduction of fever is produced by direct action on the hypothalamic heat-regulating center.

Supplied: Suppositories, chewable tablets, elixir, liquid, drops, wafers.

Route: PO, PR.

Dosage: 5–10 mg/kg/dose q4h.

Adverse effects: Hepatic necrosis with overdosage; rash, fever, blood dyscrasias (neutropenia, pancytopenia, leukopenia, thrombocytopenia). May be hepatotoxic with chronic use.

Acetazolamide (Diamox)

Indications and use: For use as a mild diuretic or as an anticonvulsant in refractory neonatal seizures. To decrease CSF production in posthemorrhagic hydrocephalus; also used in the treatment of renal tubular acidosis.

Actions: Carbonic anhydrase inhibitor. Appears to retard abnormal discharge from CNS neurons. Beneficial effects may be related to direct inhibition of carbonic anhydrase or may be due to the acidosis produced. Also produces urinary alkalosis useful in the treatment of renal tubular acidosis.

Supplied: Injection, tablets.

Route: IV, PO.

Dosage:

- Diuretic: 5 mg/kg/dose qd–qod.
- Anticonvulsant: 8–30 mg/kg/24h PO divided q6–8h.
- Alkalinize urine: 5 mg/kg/dose 2 to 3 times over 24 hours.
- Decrease CSF production: 50–100 mg/kg/24h divided q6–8h.

Elimination: Unchanged in urine; half-life is 4–10 hours.

Adverse effects: Gastrointestinal irritation, anorexia, transient hypokalemia, drowsiness, paresthesias.

Comments: Limited clinical experience in neonates. Used as an adjunct to other medications in refractory seizures. Tolerance to diuretic effect with long-term use.

Albumin, Human (various)

Indications and use: Plasma volume expander. Treatment of hypoproteinemia.

Actions: Maintains plasma colloid oncotic pressure. Intravenous administration causes a shift of fluid from the interstitial spaces into the circulation. Serves as a carrier for many substances such as bilirubin. Limited nutritional value.

Supplied: Injection, 50 mg/mL (5%), 250 mg/mL (25%) (contains 130–160 meq/L sodium).

Route: IV.

Dosage: 0.5–1.0 g/kg IV (or 10–20 mL/kg IV bolus) repeated as necessary. Maximum 6 g/kg/d.

Adverse effects: Infrequent. Rapid infusion may cause vascular overload and precipitation of congestive heart failure. Hypersensitivity reactions may include chills, fever, nausea, and urticaria.

Comments: More purified than plasma protein fraction and thus less likely to cause hypotension. Very expensive.

Alprostadil (Prostaglandin E₁, Prostin VR)

Indications and use: Any state in which blood flow must be maintained through the ductus arteriosus to sustain either pulmonary or systemic circulation until corrective or palliative surgery can be performed. Examples are pulmonary atresia, pulmonary stenosis, tricuspid atresia, transposition of the great arteries, aortic arch interruption, coarctation of the aorta, and severe tetralogy of Fallot.

Actions: Vasodilator, platelet aggregation inhibitor. Smooth muscle of the ductus arteriosus is especially sensitive to its effects, responding to the drug with marked dilatation. Decreased response after 96 hours of infusion. Maximal improvement in PaO_2, usually within 30 minutes in cyanotic infants, 1.5–3.0 hours in acyanotic infants.

Supplied: Injection.

Route: IV.

Dosage: 0.05 µg/kg/min. Decrease to lowest rate that will maintain response.

Adverse effects: Cutaneous vasodilation, seizure-like activity, jitteriness, temperature elevation, hypocalcemia, apnea, thrombocytopenia, hypotension.

Comments: Use cautiously in infants with bleeding tendencies.

Atropine Sulfate

Indications and use: Sinus bradycardia, cardiopulmonary resuscitation, reversal of neuromuscular blockade. Used preoperatively to inhibit salivation and reduce excessive secretions of the respiratory tract.

Actions: A competitive antagonist of acetylcholine at smooth muscle, cardiac muscle, and various glandular cells, leading to increased heart rate, reduced gastrointestinal motility and tone, urinary retention, cycloplegia, and decreased salivation and sweating.

Supplied: Injection, tablets, soluble tablets, ophthalmic ointment, ophthalmic solution.

Route: IV, IM, SC, PO, ET.

Dosage:

- Bradycardia in infants and children: 0.02–0.03 mg/kg/dose q2–3min prn.
- Preanesthetic: < 5 kg, 0.04 mg/kg/dose; > 5 kg, 0.03 mg/kg/dose.

Adverse effects: Xerostomia, blurred vision, mydriasis, tachycardia, palpitations, constipation, urinary retention, ataxia, tremor, hyperthermia. Toxic effects especially likely in children receiving low doses.

Comments: Contraindicated in thyrotoxicosis, tachycardia secondary to cardiac insufficiency, and obstructive gastrointestinal disease. In low doses, may cause paradoxical bradycardia secondary to its central actions.

Bumetanide (Bumex)

Indications and use: Management of edema associated with congenital heart disease, congestive heart failure, hepatic or renal disease.

Actions: Inhibition of the active chloride and, possibly, sodium transport systems of the loop of Henle. Urinary excretion of sodium, chloride, potassium, hydrogen, calcium, magnesium, ammonium, phosphate, and bicarbonate increases with bumetanide-induced diuresis. Renal blood flow increases substantially due to renovascular dilation.

Supplied: Tablets, 0.5 mg, 1 mg, 2 mg; injection, 0.25 mg/mL.

Route: PO, IV, IM.

Dosage: 0.015 mg/kg/dose up to 0.1 mg/kg daily.

Adverse effects: Hypokalemia, hypochloremia, hyponatremia, metabolic alkalosis, hypotension.

Comments: Patients refractory to furosemide may respond to bumetanide for diuretic therapy. Although patient may respond differently, bumetanide is approximately 40 times more potent on a milligram per milligram basis than furosemide.

Caffeine Citrate

Indications and use: Apnea of prematurity.

Actions: Similar to those of other methylxanthine drugs (theobromine and theophylline). Caffeine appears to be more active on and less toxic to the CNS and the respiratory system. Proposed mechanisms of action include increased production of cAMP and alterations of intracellular calcium concentrations. Stimulates the CNS and exerts a positive inotropic effect on the myocardium. Stimulates voluntary skeletal muscle and gastric acid secretion. Increases renal blood flow and GFR. Stimulates glycogenolysis and lipolysis.

Supplied: Injection (investigational), tablets, capsules.

Route: IV (not IM), PO.

Dosage:

- Loading dose: 20 mg caffeine citrate (10 mg caffeine base) IV or PO.
- Maintenance dose (caffeine base): 2.5–5.0 mg/kg/d.

Adverse effects: Nausea, vomiting, gastric irritation, agitation, tachycardia, and diuresis. Symptoms of overdosage include arrhythmias and tonic-clonic seizures.

Comments: Contraindicated in hypersensitivity to the drug. Therapeutic levels are 5–20 µg/mL; severe toxicity is associated with levels > 50 µg/mL. Initial half-life in neonates is 90–100 hours, decreasing to 6 hours at approximately 60 weeks postconceptual age. Serum levels should be monitored.

Calcium Chloride

Indications and use: Symptomatic hypocalcemia such as neonatal tetany. Last-resort agent in cardiac arrest when other agents have failed to improve myocardial contraction. Overdose of calcium channel blocker.

Actions: Calcium is essential for the functional integrity of the nervous, muscular, skeletal, and cardiac systems and for clotting function.

Supplied: Injection, 100 mg/mL (10%, 10 mL) contains 27 mg (1.35 meq) elemental calcium and 1.35 meq chloride ion per milliliter.

Route: IV, PO.

Dosage:

- Cardiac arrest (as last resort): 0.2–0.3 mL/kg/dose (10% solution IV every 10 minutes prn).
- Maintenance in infants: 70 mg/kg/24h IV divided q6h, or as infusion; or 200 mg/kg/24h PO (as 2% solution) divided q6h.

Adverse effects: Arrhythmias (eg, bradycardia) and deterioration of cardiovascular function. Extravasation may cause skin sloughing. May potentiate digitalis-related arrhythmias.

Comments: Contraindicated in ventricular fibrillation or hypercalcemia. Use with caution in digitalized patients. Chloride form is preferred to gluconate form (see below) during cardiac arrest because the calcium in the chloride is already ionized and the gluconate requires metabolism to release the calcium ion. Do not mix with sodium bicarbonate.

Calcium Gluconate

Indications and use: Treatment of asymptomatic hypocalcemia, prevention of hypocalcemia in susceptible neonates, and prevention of hypocalcemia during exchange transfusion.

Actions: See Calcium Chloride. Calcium gluconate must be metabolized to release calcium ion.

Supplied: Injection, 100 mg/mL (9 mg {0.45 meq} elemental calcium per milliliter); tablets, 500 mg (45 mg calcium), 650 mg (58.5 mg calcium), 1 g (90 mg calcium).

Dosage:

- Maintenance IV: 200–500 mg/kg/24h divided q6h, or as infusion; maximum rate = 200 mg/kg over 10 minutes.
- Maintenance PO: 400–800 mg/kg/24h divided q6h.
- Exchange transfusion: 0.45 meq (1 mL 10%)/dL of citrated blood.

Adverse effects and comments: See Calcium Chloride. Oral form may cause constipation.

Captopril (Capoten)

Indications and use: Congestive heart failure and hypertension.

Actions: Competitive inhibitor of angiotensin-converting enzyme; causes fall in angiotensin II and aldosterone levels, decrease in systemic vascular resistance, and augmentation of cardiac output.

Supplied: Tablets.

Route: PO.

Dosage: Neonates: 0.1–0.4 mg/kg/dose, 1 to 4 times daily. Infants: 0.5–6.0 mg/kg/d divided q6–24h.

Adverse effects: Hypotension, rash, fever, eosinophilia, neutropenia, gastrointestinal disturbances.

Comments: Use with caution in patients with low renal perfusion pressure. Reduce dose with renal impairment. Tablets can be dissolved in water and administered orally within 1 hour.

Chloral Hydrate (Aquachloral Supprettes, Noctec)

Indications and use: Sedation.

Actions: CNS depressant. Mechanism of action not completely understood. Usual doses produce mild CNS depression and quiet, deep sleep; higher doses can result in general anesthesia with concurrent respiratory depression. Minimal analgesic effect.

Supplied: Capsules, syrup, suppositories.

Route: PO, PR.

Dosage: 20–30 mg/kg/dose PO or rectally divided q6–8h prn. Maximum dose is 50 mg/kg/dose.

Adverse effects: Gastrointestinal irritation resulting in nausea, vomiting, and diarrhea. Delirium, excitement, hallucinations, and dizziness. Respiratory depression, particularly if administered with opiates and barbiturates.

Comments: Contraindicated with marked renal or hepatic impairment.

Chlorothiazide (Diachlor, Diuril, Sodium Diuril)

Indications and use: Fluid overload, pulmonary edema, and hypertension.

Actions: The thiazide diuretics enhance the excretion of sodium chloride and water by interfacing with transport of sodium ions across the renal tubular epithelium in the cortical nephron. Potassium, bicarbonate, magnesium, phosphate, and iodide excretion are also enhanced, whereas calcium excretion is decreased. Duration of action of chlorothiazide and hydrochlorothiazide is 6–12 hours; onset of action is within 2 hours, and peak action is at 3–6 hours.

Supplied: Suspension; tablets; powder for injection, 500 mg (as sodium) per 20-mL vial.

Route: PO, IV.

Dosage: 20–40 mg/kg/d divided q12h.

Adverse effects: Hypokalemia, hypochloremic alkalosis, prerenal azotemia, hyperuricemia, hyperglycemia, hypermagnesemia, volume depletion, and dilutional hyponatremia may occur in situations of excessive fluid intake.

Comments: Do not use in patients with anuria or hepatic dysfunction.

Cholestryamine Resin (Questran)

Classification: Resin-binding agent.

Indications and use: For use as a resin-binding agent in patients with chronic diarrhea and short gut syndrome to decrease fecal output.

Action: Cholestyramine resin releases chloride ion and absorbs bile acid in the intestine, forming a nonabsorbable complex preventing enterohepatic recirculation of bile salts.

Supplied: Powder.

Route: PO.

Dosage: 1–2 g twice daily or 2.35 g/M^2 3 times daily.

Elimination: Not absorbed, excreted in the feces.

Adverse effects: Constipation. High doses can cause hyperchloremic acidosis and increased urinary calcium excretion.

Comments: May bind many other administered oral medications.

Cimetidine (Tagamet)

Indications and use: Duodenal and gastric ulcers, hypersecretory conditions (eg, Zollinger-Ellison syndrome).

Actions: A histamine (H_2) receptor antagonist; it competitively inhibits the action of histamine on the parietal cells, decreasing gastric acid.

Supplied: Tablets, liquid, injection.

Route: IV, PO.

Dosage: 20 mg/kg/d IV of PO divided q6h.

Comments: Limited use in neonates. Reduce theophylline dose 50% if used concurrently. May be useful to prevent stress ulceration.

Cosyntropin (Cortrosyn)

Indications and use: Aid in diagnosis of adrenocortical insufficiency.

Actions: Stimulates the adrenal cortex to secrete cortisol (hydrocortisone) and other substances.

Supplied: Injection, 0.25 mg/vial; dilution = 0.25 mg/mL. (0.25 mg is equivalent to 25 USP units of corticotropin.)

Route: IM, IV.

Dosage: 0.015 mg/kg as a single dose; infuse initial dilution over 2 minutes.

Adverse effects: Hypersensitivity (very rare).

Comments: For rapid diagnostic screening of adrenocortical insufficiency, plasma cortisol concentrations should be measured prior to and 60 minutes after administration of cosyntropin.

Curare: See Tubocurarine.

Dexamethasone (Decadron, others)

Indications and use: Resistant neonatal hypoglycemia, airway edema. Used chiefly as an anti-inflammatory or immunosuppressive agent. Because of its minimal mineralocorticoid activity, dexamethasone is not indicated for replacement therapy in adrenocortical insufficiency. Used investigationally in weaning infants with bronchopulmonary dysplasia (BPD) from the ventilator.

Actions: A potent long-acting glucocorticoid lacking sodium-retaining activity with low to moderate doses. Increases urinary calcium excretion.

Supplied: Tablets, 0.25, 0.5, 0.75, 1, 1.5, 2, 4, and 6 mg; oral solution, 0.5 mg/ 5 mL; elixir, 0.5 mg/5 mL; injection (acetate form not for IV use), 8 and 16 mg/ mL; injection (sodium phosphate form for IM or IV use), 4, 10, and 20 mg/mL; injection (sodium phosphate form for IV use only), 24 mg/mL; aerosol, 0.01 and 0.04%.

Route: IV, IM, PO, inhalation.

Dosage:

- BPD: (Dosage not well established) 0.5 mg/kg/d IV divided q12h for 3 days; then 0.3 mg/kg/d divided q12h for 3 days; then decrease dose by 0.1 mg/ kg/d q72h until 0.1 mg/kg/d is reached; then give on alternate days for 1 week and discontinue.
- Neonatal hypoglycemia: (Dosage not well established.) 0.25 mg/kg/dose IV or PO repeated q12h prn.
- Airway edema: 0.25 mg/kg/dose q12h, generally beginning 24 hours before planned extubation and continued for 2–4 doses afterward.

Adverse effects: Significant side effects with all corticosteroids, including increased susceptibility to infection, osteoporosis, growth retardation, hyperglycemia, fluid and electrolyte disturbances, cataracts, myopathy, and acute adrenal insufficiency.

Diazepam (Valium)

Indications and use: Status epilepticus, convulsions refractory to other combined anticonvulsant agents; hyperglycinemia, sedation, and muscle relaxant.

Actions: Exact mechanism is not known (see Lorazepam). Diazepam appears to act at the CNS level to produce sedative, hypnotic, skeletal muscle relaxant, and anticonvulsant effects.

Supplied: Tablets, 2, 5, and 10 mg; injections, 5 mg/mL; oral solution, 1 and 5 mg/mL.

Route: PO, IV (not to exceed 2 mg/min).

Dosage:

- Status epilepticus: 0.1–0.3 mg/kg/dose IV q15–30 min to maximum total dose of 2–5 mg, or 0.3–0.5 mg/kg/dose per rectum × 1 dose.
- Continuous refractory convulsions: 0.1–0.3 mg/kg/dose IV as bolus injec-

tion followed by 0.3 mg/kg/h as continuous IV infusion (dilute in saline to 0.1 mg/mL).

- Hyperglycinemia: 1.5–3.0 mg/kg/d PO divided q6–8h (in combination with sodium benzoate, 125–200 mg/kg/d PO divided q6–8h).
- Drug withdrawal; see p 299, Table 59–4.

Adverse effects: May cause drowsiness, ataxia, rash, vasodilation, respiratory arrest, and hypotension.

Comments: Observe for and be prepared to manage respiratory arrest.

Diazoxide (Hyperstat IV, Proglycem)

Indications and use: Hypertension and persistent neonatal hypoglycemia.

Actions: Nondiuretic thiazide with antihypertensive and hyperglycemic effects. Reduces total peripheral vascular resistance by direct relaxation of arteriolar smooth muscle. Inhibits pancreatic insulin release.

Supplied: Capsules, 50 mg; oral suspension, 50 mg/mL; injection, 300 mg/20 mL.

Route: IV, PO.

Dosage:

- PO: 8–15 mg/kg/d in 2 or 3 divided doses q8–12h.
- IV: 3–5 mg/kg/dose; repeat in 20 minutes if no effect.

Adverse effects: When given for short periods, adverse effects rare. May cause bilirubin displacement from albumin, hypotension, hyperglycemia, hyperuricemia, rash, fever, leukopenia, thrombocytopenia, and ketosis.

Digoxin (Lanoxin)

Indications and use: Congestive heart failure, atrial fibrillation or flutter, and paroxysmal AV nodal tachycardia.

Actions: Digoxin exerts a positive inotropic effect on the myocardium. Antiarrhythmic actions are due to an increase in AV nodal refractory period produced by increased vagal activity and by a sympatholytic effect.

Supplied: Pediatric injection, 100 µg/mL; tablets, 125, 250, and 500 µg; pediatric elixir, 50 µg/mL, capsules, 50, 100, 200 mg (Lanoxicaps).

Route: IV, PO, IM.

Dosage:

- (TDD = total digitalizing dose, to be divided $\frac{1}{2}, \frac{1}{4}, \frac{1}{4}$ q8h.) (*Note:* Oral doses (elixir) are approximately 20% higher than IV doses listed below.)
- Premature infants (up to 2.5 kg): TTD = 10–20 µg/kg IV; maintenance = 4 µg/kg/d q12h IV.
- Term infants: TDD = 30 µg/kg IV; maintenance = 4–5 µg/kg/d q12h IV.
- Infants 1–12 months: TDD = 35 µg/kg IV; maintenance = 5–10 µg/kg/d q12h IV.

Therapeutic levels: 0.5–2.0 ng/mL, up to 4 ng/mL in infants. Considerable overlap exists between toxic and therapeutic serum levels.

Adverse effects: Persistent vomiting is usually the most common sign of digitalis toxicity in infants. Other adverse effects are anorexia, nausea, dysrhythmias (paroxysmal ventricular contractions, blocks, tachycardia, other), and delirium. Toxicity is markedly enhanced by hypokalemia.

Management of toxicity: Give Fab fraction of specific digoxin antibody (digoxin immune fab [ovine] *[Digibind]*) intravenously in equimolar amounts (ie,

60 mg Fab/1 mg digoxin). Use is investigational in pediatrics. Give potassium chloride if hypokalemic.

Comments: Digitalis is contraindicated in second- and third-degree block, idiopathic hypertrophic subaortic stenosis (IHSS), and atrial flutter or fibrillation with slow ventricular rates.

Dobutamine (Dobutrex)

Indications and use: To increase cardiac output during states of depressed contractility such as septic shock, organic heart disease, or cardiac surgical procedures.

Actions: A direct beta-1 agonist; actions on beta$_2$- and alpha-adrenergic receptors are much less marked than those of dopamine. Unlike dopamine, dobutamine does not cause release of endogenous norepinephrine nor does it have any effect on dopaminergic receptors.

Supplied: Injection, 250 mg/20 mL.

Route: IV.

Dosage: 2–10 µg/kg/min by continuous infusion. Maximum dosage is 40 µg/kg/min.

Adverse effects: Generally dose-related. Chiefly ectopic heart beats, increased heart rate, and blood pressure elevations.

Comments: Contraindicated in idiopathic subaortic stenosis and atrial fibrillation.

Dopamine (Dopastat, Intropin)

Indications and use: To increase tissue perfusion after adequate fluid volume replacement in septic states; improve cardiac output and stroke volume with severe congestive heart failure refractory to digitalis and diuretics; and increase cardiac output, blood pressure, and urine flow in patients in shock.

Actions: Actions are dose-dependent. Low doses act directly on dopaminergic receptors to produce renal and mesenteric vasodilation; in moderate doses, beta$_1$-adrenergic effects become prominent, resulting in a positive inotropic effect on the myocardium; high doses stimulate alpha-adrenergic receptors, producing increased peripheral resistance and renal vasoconstriction.

Supplied: Injection, 40, 80, 160 mg/mL.

Route: IV by continuous infusion.

Dosage: (**Note:** Dose-effect relationship is speculative in neonates. Investigationally, doses of up to 100 µg/kg/min have not been shown to decrease urine output or to cause unacceptable alpha-adrenergic effects.)

- Low dose: 0.5–5.0 µg/kg/min causes increased renal perfusion.
- Moderate dose: 5–10 µg/kg/min causes increased cardiac output.
- High dose: 10–40 µg/kg/min causes systemic vasoconstriction.
- Suggested drip administration:

$$\frac{(6 \times \text{Infant's weight [kg]} \times \text{Desired dose } [\mu g/kg/min])}{\text{Desired amount of fluid mL/h}}$$

$$= \text{mg dopamine per 100 mL of solution}$$

Adverse effects: Dopamine may cause ectopic heart beats, tachycardia, hypotension, hypertension, and excessive diuresis. Gangrene of the extremities has occurred with high doses over prolonged periods. Extravasation may cause tissue necrosis and sloughing of surrounding tissues; if this occurs, inject phentolamine, 5 mg in 0.9% sodium chloride, throughout the affected area.

Comments: Administration of phenytoin intravenously to patients receiving dopamine may result in severe hypotension and bradycardia; therefore, use with extreme caution.

Doxapram (Dopram)

Indications and use: Apnea of prematurity resistant to methylxanthine therapy (investigational).

Actions: Analeptic agent with potent respiratory and CNS stimulant properties.

Supplied: Injection, 20 mg/mL.

Route: IV.

Dosage: 1–3 mg/kg/h by continuous IV infusion; decrease the infusion rate when control of apnea is achieved.

Therapeutic range: < 5 µg/mL. At a dose of 1.5 mg/kg/h, the mean serum concentration reported was 3.2 µg/mL.

Adverse effects: Increase in blood pressure, heart rate, cardiac output, and skeletal muscle hyperactivity may occur. Abdominal distention, increased gastric residuals, vomiting, jitteriness, hyperglycemia, glycosuria, and seizures have been reported in neonates.

Comments: Efficacy of doxapram in premature neonates with severe idiopathic apnea resistant to theophylline has been documented. Use cautiously because of its side effects. Should not be given during the first few days of life, when hypertensive episodes may be associated with an increased risk of intraventricular hemorrhage. Doxapram has a narrow therapeutic range, and its use warrants serum drug level monitoring. It is contraindicated in cardiovascular and seizure disorders. Benzyl alcohol is contained in the formulation, which may accumulate to toxic levels after prolonged use.

Epinephrine

Indications and use: Bradycardia, cardiac arrest, cardiogenic shock, anaphylactic reactions, bronchospasm.

Actions: Acts directly on both alpha- and beta-adrenergic receptors, with beta$_2$ effects predominating at lower doses. Exerts both positive chronotropic and inotropic effects on the heart and relaxes bronchial smooth muscle. Alpha-adrenergic stimulation produces an increase in systolic blood pressure and constriction of renal blood vessels.

Supplied: Solution for injection, 0.1 mg/mL (1:10,000) and 1 mg/mL (1:1000).

Route: IV or ET.

Dosage: (1:10,000 used IV)

- IV bolus: 0.1–0.3 mL/kg/dose q5min prn.
- IV infusion: Start with 0.1 µg/kg/min. Maximum dose is 1.5 µg/kg/min (titrate).
- Endotracheal: 0.1–0.3 mL/kg/dose diluted 1:1 with normal saline.

Adverse effects: Hypertension, tachycardia, nausea, pallor, tremor, cardiac arrhythmias, increased myocardial oxygen consumption, and decreased renal and splanchnic blood flow.

Epinephrine Hydrochloride (Susphrine)

Indications and use: Relaxation of bronchial smooth muscle, cardiac stimulation, and dilation of skeletal muscle vasculature.

Actions: Direct action on both alpha-adrenergic and beta-adrenergic receptors. Alpha-adrenergic effects are thought to occur from production of cAMP, whereas beta-adrenergic effects result from inhibition of adenyl cyclase activity.

Supplied: (Suspension 1:2000) 0.5 mL.

Route: SC.

Dosage: Suspension (1:2000) give 0.005 mL/kg/dose to a maximum of 0.15 mL q8–12h.

Adverse effects: Tremor, tachycardia, hypertension, increased myocardial oxygen consumption, decreased renal and splanchnic blood flow, and cardiac arrhythmias.

Comments: Longer-acting form of epinephrine useful in patients who require chronic therapy such as those with bronchopulmonary dysplasia (BPD).

Fentanyl Citrate (Sublimaze)

Indications and use: Analgesia, anesthesia, sedation.

Actions: A synthetic opiate agonist. Acts similarly to morphine and meperidine but without cardiovascular effects of those drugs and with shorter-lasting respiratory depressant effects.

Supplied: Injection, 50 µg/mL.

Route: IV.

Dosage:

- Analgesia: 2 µg/kg/dose q2–4h prn or by continuous infusion at 0.1–3 µg/kg/h.
- Anesthesia: Major surgery, 30–50 µg/kg/dose; minor surgery, 2–10 µg/kg/dose.
- Sedation: 2 µg/kg/dose q2–4h prn or by continuous infusion of 0.5–1.0 µg/kg/h (titrate).

Adverse effects: Bradycardia, muscular rigidity with reduced pulmonary compliance or apnea, bronchoconstriction, laryngospasm.

Comments: Limited experience in neonates, 100 µg of fentanyl is equivalent to 10 mg of morphine or 76 mg of meperidine. Concurrent ventilatory assistance is suggested with its use. Tachyphylaxis occurs after several days of therapy. Adheres to ECHO filter membranes; may have to adjust dose.

Ferrous Sulfate (20% Elemental Iron) (various)

Indications and use: Treatment and prevention of iron deficiency anemia.

Actions: Iron is needed for the production of heme proteins. The use of iron-fortified formulas during the first year of life will usually prevent iron deficiency anemia in both the preterm and term infant. Iron-fortified formulas can be fed safely to preterm infants. Of the ferrous salts available (sulfate, fumarate, gluconate), sulfate is preferred.

Supplied: Drops, 75 mg/0.6 mL (15 mg elemental iron); elixir, 220 mg/5 mL (44 mg elemental iron); syrup, 90 mg/5mL (18 mg elemental iron).

Route: PO.

Dosage: (Recommendations of the American Academy of Pediatrics; dosages are for elemental iron.)

- Term infants: 1 mg/kg/d starting no later than 2 months of age.
- Preterm infants: 2 mg/kg/d starting no later than 2 months of age.
- Iron deficiency anemia: 6 mg/kg/d in 4 divided doses.

Adverse effects: GI irritation (vomiting, diarrhea, constipation, darkens stool color).

Comments: Accidental iron poisoning in children is secondary in frequency only to aspirin poisoning. Antidote is chelation with deferoxamine. Gastric lavage with 1–5% sodium bicarbonate or sodium phosphate solution will prevent further absorption of iron.

Furosemide (Lasix)

Indications and use: Fluid overload, pulmonary edema, congestive heart failure, hypertension.

Actions: Inhibits active chloride transport in the ascending limb of the loop of Henle. Furosemide-induced diuresis results in enhanced excretion of sodium chloride, potassium, calcium, magnesium, bicarbonate, ammonium, hydrogen, and possibly phosphate. Intravenous administration increases venous capacitance independently of its diuretic effect, resulting in rapid improvement of pulmonary edema.

Supplied: Tablets, 20, 40, and 80 mg; oral solution, 10 mg/mL; injection, 10 mg/mL.

Route: PO, IV, IM.

Dosage:

- PO: 1–2 mg/kg/dose q12h as initial dose and increase slowly if needed, since more may be required due to highly variable bioavailability.
- IV or IM: 1 mg/kg/dose q12–24h slowly; may increase but not > 6 mg/kg/dose.
  If there is not an increase in urine output, double the above doses and repeat.

Adverse effects: Hypokalemia, hypocalcemia, hyponatremia. With prolonged use, nephrocalcinosis, hypochloremic metabolic alkalosis.

Gamma Globulin Intravenous (IV IgG) (Gamimune N, Sandoglobulin, Gammagard)

Indications and use: Immunodeficiency syndromes, suspected sepsis (*controversial*). Sandoglobulin is also indicated for treatment of idiopathic thrombocytopenic purpura (ITP).

Actions: Establishes immediate (passive) IgG antibody serum levels.

Supplied: Injection, 0.5 mg/mL (Gamimune 10, 50 and 100 mL) or powder for injection (Sandoglobulin 1, 3, and 6 g/vial)

Route: IV only.

Dosage:

- Suspected sepsis: IV IgG 400 mg/kg/dose × 1 dose; repeat weekly.
- Immunodeficiency syndrome:
  Sandoglobulin: 200 mg/kg (as initial dilution at rate of 0.5–1.0 mL/min once per month. If desired clinical response or level of IgG insufficient then increase dose to 300 mg/kg or repeat dose more frequently.

  Gamimune N: 100 mg/kg or 2 mL/kg (at initial flow rate of 0.01–0.02 mL/kg/min for 30 minutes, may dilute in 5% dextrose) once per month. If no adverse effects observed, then increase rate to 0.02–0.04 mL/kg/min. If desired clinical response not achieved or level of IgG insufficient, increase dose to 200 mg/kg (4 mL/kg) or repeat dose more frequently than once per month.

  Gammagard: 100 mg/kg once per month (initial rate of 0.5 mL/kg/h). If desired clinical response not achieved or level of IgG insufficient, increase dose to 200–400 mg/kg to maintain serum IgG level > 500 mg/dL.
- Idiopathic thrombocytopenia purpura:

Sandoglobulin: 0.4 g/kg/d for 5 consecutive days. (See above administration rate for immunodeficiency syndrome.)

Adverse effects: Hypotension and anaphylaxis. If either occurs, the rate of infusion should be decreased or stopped until resolved, then resumed at a slower rate as tolerated. Preparations contain antibodies to group B streptococcus and *E coli.* Substantial variation among lots and manufacturers.

Glucagon

Indications and use: Hypoglycemia as seen in infants of diabetic mothers (IDM); hypoglycemia due to other causes unresponsive to routine treatment. Bowel spasm during barium enema.

Actions: Glucagon, a hormone produced by the alpha cells of the pancreas, causes increased breakdown of glycogen to form glucose and inhibition of glycogen synthetase. Blood glucose elevation occurs. Produces relaxation of the smooth muscle in the gastrointestinal tract when the drug is administered parenterally.

Supplied: Injected, 1-mg (1-unit) vials.

Route: SC, IM, IV.

Dosage: 0.025–0.3 mg/kg/dose; may repeat in 20 minutes prn. (**Note:** In the IDM, give 0.3 mg/kg/dose up to 1 mg total as standard dose.)

Adverse effects: Hypersensitivity, nausea, and vomiting.

Comments: Incompatible with electrolyte-containing solutions; compatible with dextrose solutions. *Caution:* Do not delay initiation of glucose infusion while observing for glucagon effect.

Heparin Sodium (various)

Indications and use: Primary role is as an anticoagulant. Used to diagnose and treat disseminated intravascular coagulation (DIC) and to maintain patency of arterial or venous lines.

Actions: In combination with antithrombin III (heparin cofactor), heparin inactivates coagulation factors IX, X, XI, XII, and thrombin, inhibiting conversion of fibrinogen to fibrin.

Supplied: Injection, 10, 100, 1000, 5000 units/mL.

Route: SC, IV.

Dosage:

- Loading dose: 50 units/kg as IV bolus.
- Maintenance dosage: 10–20 units/kg/h as continuous infusion.
- To maintain line patency: 0.5–1.0 unit/mL of fluid q8h.
- Antidote: Protamine sulfate, 1 mg for each 100 units of heparin given in the preceding 3–4 hours up to a maximum dose of 50 mg.

Hepatitis B Immune Globulin (H-BIG, others)

Indications and use: Prophylaxis of hepatitis B exposure.

Actions: Passive immunization agent. Immune serum provides protection against the hepatitis B virus by directly providing specific antibody to hepatitis B surface antigen (HBsAg). The immunity is transient, usually lasting about 30 days.

Supplied: Injection, 1-, 4-, and 5-mL vials.

Route: IM only.

Dosage: 0.5 mL/kg administered within 12 hours after delivery. (Repeat at 3 months and 6 months if vaccine was not given.)

Adverse reactions: Swelling, warmth, erythema, and soreness at injection site. Rarely, rash, fever, and urticaria.

Comments: Do not use in IgA deficiency, thrombocytopenia, coagulopathy. Administer into gluteal or deltoid muscle region. Do not administer intravenously.

Hepatitis B Vaccine (Heptavax-B, Recombivax HB, Engerix B)

Indications and use: Prophylaxis for infants at increased risk for hepatitis B.

Actions: Induces protective antibody formation to hepatitis B virus (anti-HBs).

Supplied: Injection: Recombivax 10 μg/mL, Heptavax 20 μg/mL, Engerix 20 μg/mL and 10 μg/0.5 mL.

Route: IM only.

Dosage: 0.5 mL IM (equivalent to Recombivax 2.5 μg, Heptavax 10 μg, Engerix B 10 μg).

Adverse effects: Swelling, warmth, erythema, and soreness at injection site. Rarely, vomiting, rash, low-grade fever.

Comments: Do not give intravenously or intradermally. A single booster may be needed in 5 years. Administer in anterolateral thigh.

Hydralazine

Indications and use: For hypertension and as an afterload reducing agent to treat congestive heart failure.

Actions: Direct-acting vasodilator that reduces peripheral resistance and blood pressure and relaxes venous capacitance vessels. Reflex increase in heart rate, cardiac output, and stroke volume is probably produced in response to the decrease in peripheral vascular resistance.

Supplied: Tablets, 10, 25, 50, and 100 mg; injection, 20 mg/mL.

Route: IM, IV, PO.

Dosage:

- IV or IM: 0.1–0.5 mg/kg/dose q6h (maximum of 2 mg/kg/dose).
- PO: 0.5–7.0 mg/kg/d divided q6–8h.

Adverse effects: Most frequent are headache, palpitations, and tachycardia; most serious is a reversible lupuslike syndrome. Tachyphylaxis often occurs on chronic therapy.

Comments: Contraindicated in mitral valve rheumatic heart disease.

Hydrochlorothiazide (various)

Indications and use: Hypertension, pulmonary edema.

Actions: See Chlorothiazide.

Supplied: Tablets, 25, 50, and 100 mg; solution 50 mg/5 mL and 100 mg/mL.

Route: PO.

Dosage: Up to 3.3 mg/kg/d divided in 2 doses q12h.

Adverse effects and comments: See Chlorothiazide.

Hydrocortisone

Indications and use: Acute adrenal insufficiency, congenital adrenal hyperplasia, shock, allergic reactions.

Actions: Hydrocortisone is a steroid possessing glucocorticoid activity with some mineralocorticoid effects; most effects probably result from modification of enzyme activity, thus affecting almost all body systems. It promotes protein catabolism, gluconeogenesis, renal excretion of calcium, capillary-wall permeability and stability, and red cell production; suppresses immune and inflammatory responses.

Supplied: Injection (acetate sodium phosphate, sodium succinate), tablets, oral suspension (cypionate), topical ointment and cream (acetate).

Route: PO, IV, IM, topical.

Dosage:

- Acute adrenal insufficiency: 1–2 mg/kg/dose IV bolus; then 25–150 mg q24h divided q6h.
- Congenital adrenal hyperplasia: Initial dose, 0.5–0.7 mg/kg/q24h divided $\frac{1}{4}$ in AM, $\frac{1}{4}$ at noon, and $\frac{1}{2}$ at night; maintenance dose, 0.3–0.4 mg/kg/q24h divided as above.
- Shock: Initial dose, 35–50 mg/kg IV; then 50–150 mg/kg/q24h IV divided q6h for 48–72 hours.
- Topical (0.5%) apply to area 3 times daily.

Adverse effects and comments: See Dexamethasone. Application to large body surface areas may produce absorption with systemic effects. Avoid facial application.

Indomethacin (Indocin, Indocin IV; others)

Indications and use: Pharmacologic closure of patent ductus arteriosus.

Actions: Nonsteroidal anti-inflammatory drug (NSAID) with analgesic and anti-pyretic properties. Action is principally by inhibition of prostaglandin synthesis, thus inhibiting cyclo-oxygenase, an enzyme that catalyzes the formation of prostaglandin precursors (endoperoxides) from arachidonic acid.

Supplied: Powder for injection, 1-mg vials.

Route: IV.

Dosage: IV at 12–24h intervals. Indocin should be given q12h unless the patient has decreased urinary output.

- Initial dose: 0.2 mg/kg.
- Second dose: < 48 hours, 0.1 mg/kg; 2–7 days, 0.2 mg/kg; > 8 days, 0.25 mg/kg.
- Third dose: < 48 hours, 0.1 mg/kg; 2–7 days, 0.2 mg/kg; > 8 days, 0.25 mg/kg.

Adverse effects: May cause decreased platelet aggregation, transient oliguria (decreased GFR), hyponatremia, hyperkalemia, hypoglycemia. May increase indirect bilirubin levels.

Comments: Contraindicated in NEC or when stool Hematest > 3+, serum bilirubin > 10 mg/dL, BUN > 30 mg/dL, serum creatinine > 1.8 mg/dL, urine output ≤ 0.6 mL/kg/h for the preceding 8 hours, in thrombocytopenia (< 60,000/mm³), with active bleeding, or if there has been intraventricular bleeding within the preceding 7 days (*controversial*).

Insulin, Regular

Indications and use: Hyperglycemia, diabetes mellitus not controlled by diet alone, emergency treatment of diabetic ketoacidosis, hyperkalemia. Used investigationally to increase caloric intake when usual means are inadequate.

Actions: Hormone derived from the B cells of the pancreas and the principal hormone required for glucose utilization. In skeletal and cardiac muscle and adipose tissue, insulin facilitates transport of glucose into these cells. Stimulates lipogenesis and protein synthesis and inhibits lipolysis and release of free fatty acids from adipose cells. Promotes intracellular shift of potassium and magnesium.

Supplied: Injection, 40 and 100 units/mL. (Iletin I [beef and pork], Beef Regular Iletin II [purified beef], Humulin R [human insulin, recombinant DNA origin], Actrapid [purified pork], Pork Regular Iletin II [purified pork], Velosulin [purified pork]).

Route: IV, SC.

Dosage:

- Hyperglycemia: Loading dose, 0.1 unit/kg/dose infused IV over 15–20 minutes (dilute initial concentration to 0.1–1.0 unit/mL in 0.9% or 0.45% sodium chloride); maintenance dose, 0.02–0.1 unit/kg/h by continuous IV infusion (titrate with hourly determinations of blood glucose) (dilute insulin as above). Infuse for 2–24 hours, then reassess.
- Hyperkalemia: Give calcium gluconate, 50 mg/kg/dose IV, and sodium bicarbonate IV, 1 meq/kg/dose IV, first; then give dextrose, 250–500 mg/kg/dose, and insulin, 0.2 unit/kg/dose IV or unit for every 8–10 mL of dextrose given.
- Increase caloric intake (investigational): 0.02–0.4 unit/h IV as continuous infusion with hourly serum glucose determinations.

Adverse effects: Hypoglycemia (may cause coma, severe CNS injury), hyperglycemic rebound (Somogyi effect), urticaria, anaphylaxis.

Comments: Treat allergic reactions symptomatically with antihistamines. Human insulin is less antigenic than pork-derived insulin, which is less antigenic than beef-derived insulin. Insulin adsorbs to all plastic surfaces of IV systems. In concentrations of 10 units/L, approximately 50% of the insulin binds to the tubing. At greater concentrations approximately 5 units/L binds to the IV tubing. May have to adjust dose accordingly. Experience with continuous infusions is limited, but investigational use is increasing.

Isoproterenol (Isuprel, others)

Indications and use: Shock, cardiac arrest, Adams-Stokes syndrome, ventricular arrhythmias due to AV block, bronchospasm.

Actions: Acts on both beta$_1$- and beta$_2$-adrenergic receptors with minimal or no effect on alpha receptors in therapeutic doses. Relaxes bronchial smooth muscle, cardiac stimulation (inotropic and chronotropic), and peripheral vasodilation (reduces cardiac afterload).

Supplied: Injection (1:5000), 0.2 mg/mL; solution for nebulization, aerosol (various strengths).

Route: IV, inhalation.

Dosage: IV: 0.05–0.5 μg/kg/min (titrate). Inhalation/nebulization: 0.1 mL to max of 0.5 mL/dose. Dilute with 2 mL normal saline, given q4h prn.

Adverse effects: Tremor, vomiting, hypertension, tachycardia, cardiac arrhythmias.

Comments: Contraindicated in hypertension, degenerative heart disease, hyperthyroidism, tachycardia caused by digitalis toxicity, and preexisting cardiac arrhythmias. Increases cardiac oxygen consumption out of proportion to increase in cardiac oxygen output. Not considered an inotropic agent of choice.

Lidocaine (Xylocaine, others)

Indications and use: Intravenous lidocaine is used almost exclusively for the short-term control of ventricular arrhythmias (premature beats, tachycardia, and fibrillation) or for prophylactic treatment of such arrhythmias. Skin infiltration as a local anesthesic.

Actions: Type I antiarrhythmic agent, with most activity related to blockade of the fast sodium channels in Purkinje fibers. Also a CNS depressant with sedative, analgesic, and anticonvulsant properties.

Supplied: IV forms: Injection (pre-mixed) in D5W, 2 mg/mL (500 mL), 4 mg/mL (250, 500, and 1000 mL), 8 mg/mL (250 and 500 mL). Injection (for IV bolus) 10 mg/mL (5 mL) and 20 mg/mL (5 and 10 mL). Injection (for IV mixture) 40 mg/mL (25 and 50 mL). 100 mg/mL (10 mL) and 200 mg/mL (5 and 10 mL) 1% and 2% solution for local anesthesia.

Route: IV, SC, or ET.

Dosage: 1 mg/kg/dose as IV bolus q5min to maximum total dose of 5 mg/kg followed by IV infusion of 10–50 µg/kg/min to maximum of 4 mg/min.

Adverse effects: Adverse effects generally involve the CNS: drowsiness, dizziness, tremulousness, and paresthesias. Muscle twitching, seizures, coma, respiratory depression, and respiratory arrest may also occur.

Comments: Primarily metabolized by the liver; dosage adjustment is necessary in liver failure. Contraindicated in SA or AV nodal block.

Therapeutic levels: 1–5 µg/mL. Toxicity associated with levels > 5 µg/mL.

Lorazepam (Alzapam, Ativan)

Indications and use: In neonates, for the treatment of status epilepticus resistant to conventional anticonvulsant therapy (ie, phenobarbital, phenytoin).

Actions: A benzodiazepine; facilitates gamma aminobutyric acid (GABA) which mediates transmission and mimics the actions of glycine at its receptor sites. Penetrates the blood-brain barrier more slowly than diazepam; however the duration of action of lorazepam in the control of seizure activity in children studied was at least 3 hours in 83% of cases and 24 hours or longer in nearly 59% of cases. Median onset of seizure control is 10 minutes.

Supplied: Tablets, 0.5, 1, and 2 mg; injection, 2 and 4 mg/mL.

Route: PO, IM, IV.

Dosage: Status epilepticus:

- Initial dosage: 0.05 mg/kg/dose IV. If no response after 15 minutes, repeat initial dose. May dilute with an equal volume of sterile water, normal saline, or 5% dextrose in water. Infuse dose over 1–2 minutes.
- Maintenance dosage: Undetermined. Suggest 0.05 mg/kg/dose IV q6–24h prn.

Adverse effects: May cause respiratory depression, confusion, and syncope. Paradoxic CNS stimulation may occur, usually early in therapy; the drug should be discontinued if this effect occurs. Parenteral administration may produce apnea, hypotension, bradycardia, or cardiac arrest.

Magnesium Sulfate

Indications and use: Hypomagnesemia and refractory hypocalcemia.

Actions: May depress CNS and peripheral neuromuscular transmission by decreasing acetylcholine release. Acts on cardiac muscle to slow SA nodal impulse formation and prolong conduction time.

Supplied: Injection, oral.

Route: IM, IV, or PO.

Dosage: Hypomagnesemia or refractory hypocalcemia:

- Initial dosage: 0.2 meq/kg/dose IV or IM q6h until serum Mg level is normal or symptoms resolve or 0.8–1.6 meq/kg/dose PO 4 times daily.
- Maintenance dosage: 0.25–0.5 meq/24h IV (add to infusion or give IV) maximum of 1000 mg of salt q24h.

Adverse effects: Hypotension, flushing, depression of reflexes, depressed cardiac function, CNS and respiratory depression.

Comments: Contraindicated in renal failure. Monitor serum magnesium, calcium, and phosphate levels.

Meperidine (Demerol, others)

Indications and use: Preoperative medication and for relief of moderate to severe pain.

Actions: Stimulates opiate receptors in CNS. Meperidine produces respiratory depression proportionate to drug dose. Duration of respiratory depression can extend several hours beyond the plasma half-life.

Supplied: Injection 25, 50, 75, 100 mg/mL; tablets 50, 100 mg; syrup 50 mg/mL.

Route: PO, IM, IV, SC.

Dosage: 0.5–1.5 mg/kg. Maximum of 2 mg/kg/dose IV, IM, SC, and 4 mg/kg/dose PO.

Adverse effects: Normeperidine (active metabolite) has excitant effects that may precipitate tremors, myoclonus, or seizures. Other side effects include respiratory and circulatory depression, nausea, vomiting, constipation, and sedation.

Comments: Effects can be reversed by naloxone.

Methyldopa (Aldomet)

Indications and use: Hypertension.

Actions: Mechanism of action is not fully understood. Metabolized to alpha-methylnorepinephrine in the CNS, where it lowers arterial pressure by stimulation of central alpha-adrenergic receptors. Reduction of plasma renin may also play a role in its antihypertensive effect.

Supplied: Injection, tablets, suspension.

Route: IV, PO.

Dosage: 5–40 mg/kg/d divided q6–8h.

Adverse effects: Most common adverse effect is drowsiness, which occurs within the first 48–72 hours and may cause marked depression, orthostatic hypotension, sodium retention, edema, a positive direct Coombs test reaction in 10–20% of patients (reversible), and drug fever. Causes fluid and sodium retention and should be given with a diuretic.

Comments: Preferred route of administration is oral, but absorption from the gastrointestinal tract is unpredictable (10–15%). Contraindicated with active hepatic disease.

Metoclopramide (Reglan, others)

Indications and use: Used in a variety of gastrointestinal disorders. In neonates and infants, the drug has been used investigationally for feeding intolerance and gastroesophageal reflux.

Actions: Dopamine antagonist acting on the CNS and on other organs. Gastrointestinal smooth muscle stimulant. Increases the resting tone of the esophageal sphincter. In neonates, metoclopramide resulted in a significant decrease in gastric aspirate, increased weight gain, shortened GI transit time, and increased food intake.

Supplied: Syrup, tablets, injection.

Route: IM, IV, PO.

Dosage: 0.1 mg/kg/d divided q8h.

Adverse effects: CNS effects include restlessness, drowsiness, and fatigue. Extrapyramidal reactions may occur but usually subside 24 hours after discontinuance of the drug, and most patients will respond rapidly to diphenhydramine.

Comments: Contraindicated with bowel obstruction and seizure disorders.

Morphine Sulfate (various)

Indications and use: Analgesia, preoperative sedation, supplement to anesthesia, acute pulmonary edema.

Actions: CNS opiate receptor agonist resulting in analgesia, drowsiness, and alterations in mood and pain perception. Vasodilatory (especially coronary vessels).

Supplied: Injection, oral solution, tablets.

Route: IM, IV, SC.

Dosage: 0.1–0.2 mg/kg/dose q2–4h or continuous administration of 0.01–0.1 mg/kg/h.

Adverse effects: Dose-dependent side effects include miosis, respiratory depression, drowsiness, bradycardia, and hypotension. Constipation, sedation, dizziness, nausea, vomiting, and sweating occur frequently.

Naloxone (Narcan)

Indications and use: Narcotic reversal and investigationally for the treatment of septic shock.

Actions: A pure opiate antagonist with little or no agonistic activity. It has minimal or no pharmacologic effect, even in high doses, in patients who have not received opiates. Onset of action is within 1–2 minutes after intravenous injection and 2–5 minutes following subcutaneous or intramuscular injection. Duration of action is generally 45 minutes to 4 hours.

Supplied: Injection 0.4 mg/mL, 1.0 mg/mL.

Route: IV, IM, SC, IT.

Dosage: 0.1 mg/kg. May repeat in 5 minutes.

Comments: Contraindicated in infants of narcotic-addicted mothers because it precipitates acute withdrawal syndrome. Infant must be monitored for reappearance of respiratory depression and need for repeated doses.

Neostigmine Methylsulfate (Prostigmin)

Indications and use: Improvement of muscle strength in the treatment of myasthenia gravis. Reversal of nondepolarizing neuromuscular blocking agents (turbocurarine, pancuronium) and occasionally for postoperative distention and urinary retention.

Actions: Neostigmine inhibits hydrolysis of acetylcholine and thus produces generalized cholinergic responses.

Supplied: Injection 0.25 mg/mL, 0.5 mg/mL: and 1 mg/mL, tablets 15 mg (as bromide).

Route: IM, IV, SC, or PO.

Dosage:

- Myasthenia gravis:
  Diagnosis: 0.04 mg/kg/dose IM × 1 or 0.02 mg/kg/dose IV × 1.
  Treatment: 0.01–0.04 mg/kg/dose IM, IV, or SC q2–3h prn.
- Reversal of nondepolarizing neuromuscular blocking agents:

Infants: 0.025–0.1 mg/kg/dose. (Use with atropine: Dose 0.01–0.04 mg/kg; or 0.4 mg atropine for each mg of neostigmine.)

Adverse effects: Cholinergic crisis, which may include bronchospasm, increased bronchial secretions, vomiting, diarrhea, bradycardia, respiratory depression, seizures, and coma.

Comments: Antidote is atropine 0.01–0.04 mg/kg/dose. Reversal of blocking agent should not be attempted for at least 30 minutes after a dose of pancuronium or tubocurarine.

Nitroprusside (Nipride, Nitropress)

Indications and use: Severe hypertension and hypertension crisis, congestive heart failure, congenital heart lesions that have resulted in pulmonary hypertension with increased pulmonary vascular resistance.

Actions: Direct-acting vasodilator (arterial and venous) that reduces peripheral vascular resistance (afterload). Venous return is reduced (preload). Acts within seconds to lower blood pressure; when discontinued, the effect dissipates within minutes. Rapidly metabolized to thiocyanate, which is eliminated by the kidneys.

Supplied: Injection.

Route: Continuous IV infusion.

Dosage: 0.5–8.0 µg/kg/min (titrate to desired response) by IV infusion.

Adverse effects: Generally related to too-rapid reduction in blood pressure. Thiocyanate may accumulate, especially in patients receiving high doses or those who have impaired renal function. Cyanide toxicity can develop abruptly if large doses are administered rapidly. Cyanide causes early persistent acidosis. Thiocyanate toxicity appears at plasma levels of approximately 5–10 mg/dL; levels of 20 mg/dL have been associated with death. Thiocyanate levels should be monitored in any patient receiving 5 µg/kg/min or more of nitroprusside, especially patients with renal impairment. Toxicity is treated with 20% sodium thiosulfate (10 mg/kg/min for 15 minutes).

Comments: Contraindicated with increased intracranial pressure, hypertension secondary to arteriovenous shunts, or coarctation of the aorta. Reconstitute contents of 50-mg vial in 2–3 mL D5W, then further dilute in D5W for infusion. Protect from light.

Norepinephrine Bitartrate (Levarterenol, Levophen)

Indications and use: Vasoconstriction and cardiac stimulation as adjunctive therapy to correct shock after fluid volume replacement. Prolongation of local anesthetics by decreasing vascular absorption.

Actions: Direct effect on alpha-adrenergic receptors and beta-adrenergic receptors of the heart ($beta_1$) but not those of the bronchi or peripheral blood vessels ($beta_2$). Norepinephrine has less effect on $beta_1$ receptors than does epinephrine or isoproterenol.

Supplied: Injection.

Route: IV infusion.

Dosage: 0.02–0.1 µg/kg/min initially, titrated to attain desired perfusion. Concentration and infusion rate may be calculated by the following formulas. Dilute 0.3 mg × weight (kg) to 50 mL in D5W or 1.5 mg × weight (kg) to 250 mL in D5W.
Infusion rate in µg/kg/min = 0.1 × infusion rate in milliliters per hour.

Adverse effects: Respiratory distress, arrhythmias, bradycardia or tachycardia, hypertension, and vomiting.

Comments: In case of extravasation, use phentolamine 0.1–0.2 mg/kg SC up to 10 mg maximum, infiltrated into the area of extravasation within 12 hours.

Pancuronium Bromide (Pavulon)

Indications and use: To increase pulmonary compliance in an uncooperative neonate during mechanical ventilation. To produce skeletal muscle relaxation during surgery.

Actions: Nondepolarizing neuromuscular blocking agent that produces skeletal muscle paralysis mainly by causing a decreased response to acetylcholine at the myoneural junction. Pancuronium may cause an increase in heart rate. The onset of action is generally 30–60 seconds, with a duration of action of about 40–60 minutes, but it may be much longer in neonates.

Supplied: Injection 1 mg/mL, 2 mg/mL.

Route: IV.

Dosage:

- Initial dosage: 0.03 mg/kg IV; repeat prn.
- Maintenance dosage: 0.03–0.09 mg/kg IV q1–4h prn to maintain paralysis.

Adverse effects: Tachycardia may occur.

Comments: Neonates are particularly sensitive to the actions of pancuronium; prolonged paralysis may be noted. Ventilation must be supported during neuromuscular blockade. Many centers place a sign over patient's bedside to alert all medical personnel that the infant is paralyzed. Neostigmine and atropine (see dose p 474) are used for reversal.

Papaverine Hydrochloride (various)

Indications and use: Peripheral arterial spasms.

Actions: Directly relaxes vascular smooth muscle and results in vasodilation.

Supplied: Injection, tablets.

Route: PO, IM, IV (infuse over 1–2 minutes).

Dosage: 6 mg/kg/24h in 4 divided doses.

Comments: Intravenous infusion should be performed under a physician's supervision, since arrhythmias and fatal apnea may result from rapid injection. *Note:* Limited experience in neonates.

Paraldehyde (Paral)

Indications and use: Status epilepticus resistant to conventional therapy (ie, phenobarbital, phenytoin, diazepam, lorazepam).

Actions: A rapid-acting hypnotic agent effective against all types of seizures when administered in large doses. Precise mechanism of action is unknown.

Supplied: Oral solution, rectal liquid.

Route: PO, PR.

Dosage:

- Rectal: 0.3 mL/kg/dose q4–6h. Dilute in equal volume of cottonseed oil or olive oil. Maximum 10 g/dose (10 mL of undiluted paraldehyde/dose) per rectum.

Adverse effects: Side effects severely limit use. May cause pulmonary edema and hemorrhage, severe coughing, irritation to gastrointestinal mucosa, and thrombophlebitis. Overdose may cause cardiac and respiratory depression. Intramuscular injection may cause sterile abscess at injection site. Rectal administration may cause proctitis.

Comments: Routine use in infants is discouraged. Contraindicated in pulmonary or hepatic disease.

Note: Paraldehyde dissolves plastic and reacts with rubber stoppers in bottles and syringes. Do not use plastic equipment for administration. For rectal administration, use glass syringes.

Phenobarbital

Indications and use: Tonic-clonic and partial seizures, neonatal withdrawal syndrome, and neonatal jaundice.

Actions: Anticonvulsant that limits the spread of seizure activity and increases the threshold for electrical stimulation of the motor cortex. In neonates, the initial half-life is 100–120 hours or longer, gradually declining to 60–70 hours at about 3–4 weeks of age. Reduction in serum bilirubin levels is attributed to increased levels of glycuronyl transferase and intracellular Y-binding protein. More effective in reducing bilirubin levels in full-term infants than in premature infants and must be administered at least 2 or 3 days before detectable reductions can be observed. Phenobarbital is effective in controlling symptoms of neonatal withdrawal syndrome with the exception of vomiting and diarrhea.

Supplied: Oral elixir, tablets, injection.

Route: IV, IM, PO.

Dosage:

- Seizures:
  Loading dose: 20–30 mg/kg IV or IM over 15–30 minutes.
  Maintenance dose: 2.5–4.0 mg/kg/d as single dose. For neonates < 30 weeks start 1–3 mg/kg/d.
- Hyperbilirubinemia: Dose not clearly established. Generally 4–5 mg/kg/d for the first 4 days.
- Neonatal withdrawal syndrome: 5–20 mg/kg/d in 4 divided doses.

Adverse effects: Sedation, lethargy, paradoxical excitement, gastrointestinal distress, ataxia, and rash.

Comments: Contraindicated in porphyria. Monitor serum levels and adjust dosage to maintain between 15 and 40 µg/mL for anticonvulsant activity.

Phenytoin (Dilantin)

Indications and use: Seizures unresponsive to phenobarbital.

Actions: Raises seizure threshold of the motor cortex to electrical or chemical stimuli. Precise mechanism of anticonvulsant activity has not been determined. Bilirubin displaces phenytoin from albumin-binding sites, increasing the percentage of unbound drug; this may complicate the interpretation of serum levels. Follows zero-order pharmacokinetics, where small dosage adjustments may result in large changes in serum drug concentrations. Neonates and other infants absorb phenytoin poorly from the gastrointestinal tract. Use in the long-term management of seizures in neonates is questionable owing to the difficulty in appropriate dosing.

Supplied: Capsules, chewable tablets, oral suspension, injection.

Route: PO, IV.

Dosage:

- IV: 15–20 mg/kg as loading dose at a rate not greater than 0.5 mg/kg/min, followed by maintenance dose of 5–8 mg/kg/d divided q12–24h.
- PO: Highly variable—from 5–8 mg/kg/d up to 8 mg/kg/dose q12h.

Adverse effects: Few reports of toxicity in neonates, probably because of the difficulty of physically assessing the common toxic manifestations. In adults and children, adverse effects include nystagmus, ataxia, lethargy, slurred speech, diplopia, headache, hirsutism, behavioral changes, and gum hyperplasia. Hypotension occurs with rapid IV administration.

Comments: Therapeutic levels between 10 and 20 mg/mL. Multiple drug interactions.

Prazosin (Minipress)

Indications and use: Hypertension and congestive heart failure. Experimental in infants and should be used only when traditional therapy has failed.

Actions: Postsynaptic alpha-adrenergic blocking agent that reduces peripheral vascular resistance and blood pressure.

Supplied: Capsules 1, 2, 5 mg.

Route: PO.

Dosage:

- Test dose 5–10 µg/kg PO.
- Maintenance dosage: Up to 25 µg/kg/dose q6h.

Adverse effects: Dizziness, weakness, fatigue, palpitations, headache, and nausea can be seen. The most severe adverse effect in adults is the "first-dose phenomenon" in which severe orthostatic hypotension develops in the patient.

Procainamide Hydrochloride (various)

Indications and use: As prophylaxis to maintain normal sinus rhythm in paroxysmal atrial tachycardia, atrial fibrillation, premature atrial and ventricular contractions, and ventricular tachycardia.

Actions: Class I antiarrhythmic agent similar to quinidine. Partially metabolized by the liver to the active metabolite *N*-acetylprocainamide (NAPA).

Supplied: Capsules, tablets, sustained release tablets, injection.

Route: PO, IM, IV.

Dosage:

- IV (monitor ECG and blood pressure): 1.5–2.0 mg/kg (dilute to 10 mg/mL) over 10–30 minutes. Repeat as needed to maximum dose of 10–15 mg/kg; then continuous infusion of 20–60 mg/kg/min.
- PO: 5–15 mg/kg q4–6h.

Therapeutic levels: Procainamide: 3–10 µg/mL; toxicity associated with levels > 12 µg/mL. NAPA: 10–20 µg/mL; toxicity associated with levels over 30 µg/mL.

Adverse effects: Serious toxic effects if given rapidly IV, including asystole, myocardial depression, ventricular fibrillation, hypotension, reversible lupus-like syndrome. May cause nausea, vomiting, diarrhea, anorexia, skin rash, tachycardia, agranulocytosis, and hepatic toxicity.

Comments: Contraindicated in second- or third-degree heart block, bundle branch block, digitalis intoxication, and allergy to procaine. Do not use in atrial fibrillation or flutter until ventricular rate is adequately controlled, to avoid a possible paradoxic increase in ventricular rate. **Quinidine** (see p 479) is generally used for long-term therapy because it has less associated toxicity. Phenylephrine should be available to treat severe hypotension caused by IV procainamide, QRS or QT prolongation greater than 35% of baseline is an indication to withhold further doses of procainamide.

Propranolol (Inderal, others)

Indications and use: Hypertension, supraventricular tachycardia, premature ventricular contractions, tachycardia, and tetralogy spells.

Actions: Nonselective beta-adrenergic blocking agent. Inhibits adrenergic stimuli by competitively blocking beta-adrenergic receptors within the myocardium and bronchial and vascular smooth muscle. Decreases heart rate, myocardial contractility, and cardiac output.

Supplied: Tablets, sustained release capsules, injection.

Route: PO, IV.

Dosage:

- Arrhythmias:
  IV: 0.025–0.15 mg/kg/dose to a maximum of 1 mg/dose as slow push.
  PO: 0.5–2 mg/kg/d q6–8h. May increase to 1 mg/kg q6h or more as tolerated.
- Hypertension: 0.5–2.0 mg/kg/d PO q6–12h. May increase as tolerated.
- Tetralogy spells: 0.15–0.25 mg/kg/dose IV. May repeat q15min prn.

Adverse effects: Generally dose-related hypotension, nausea, vomiting, bronchospasm, heart block, depression, hypoglycemia, and depressed myocardial contractility.

Comments: Contraindicated in obstructive pulmonary disease, asthma, heart failure, shock, second- or third-degree heart block, hypoglycemia. Use with caution in renal or hepatic failure.

Prostaglandin E$_1$: See Alprostadil.

Protamine Sulfate (various)

Indications and use: Reversal of heparin; heparin overdose.

Actions: Combines with heparin, forming a stable salt complex. Devoid of anticoagulant activity. Effect on heparin is almost immediate and persists for approximately 2 hours.

Supplied: Injection.

Route: IV.

Dosage: For every 100 units of heparin estimated to remain in patient, give 1 mg by slow infusion over 1–3 minutes or not greater than 5 mg/min. Maximum dose of 50 mg.

Adverse effects: May cause fall in blood pressure, bradycardia, dyspnea, anaphylaxis. Excessive administration beyond that needed to reverse heparin effect may have anticoagulant effect.

Pyridoxine (vitamin B$_6$) (Hexalpha-Betalin, others)

Indications and use: For treatment of pyridoxine-dependent seizures and to prevent or treat vitamin B$_6$ deficiency.

Actions: Vitamin B$_6$ is essential in the synthesis of GABA, an inhibitory neurotransmitter in the CNS; GABA increases the seizure threshold. Vitamin B$_6$ is also required for heme synthesis and amino acid, carbohydrate, and lipid metabolism.

Supplied: Tablets, injection.

Route: PO, IM, IV.

Dosage: For vitamin B$_6$-dependent seizures, give 100 mg IV as a single test dose, followed by a 30-minute observation period. If a definite response is seen, begin maintenance of 50–100 mg PO daily.

Quinidine Sulfate (various)

Indications and use: Restoration of normal sinus rhythm in atrial flutter or fibrillation once the ventricular rate is controlled by digoxin. Prevention of atrial and ventricular arrhythmias.

Actions: Group I antiarrhythmic agent with cardiac effects similar to those of procainamide. Direct depressant effect on myocardial contractility, conduction velocity, and excitability. Causes increase in PR, QRS, and QT intervals.

Supplied: Capsules, tablets, sustained-release tablets, injection.

Route: PO, IM (quinidine gluconate, polygalaturonate) (IV not recommended).

Dosage: 5–15 mg/kg q6h PO or 2–4 mg/kg q2–4h IM. Total daily dose 10–30 mg/kg.

Therapeutic levels: 3–7 mg/mL.

Adverse effects: Severe hypotension with IV use. Adverse reactions in about 30% of patients include nausea, vomiting, diarrhea, blood dyscrasias, and drug fever. Overdose may cause cinchonism or respiratory depression.

Comments: Contraindicated with AV nodal block.

Ranitidine (Zantac)

Indications and use: Duodenal and gastric ulcers, gastroesophageal reflux, and hypersecretory conditions (eg, Zollinger-Ellison syndrome).

Actions: Histamine (H_2) receptor antagonist; competitively inhibits the action of histamine on the parietal cells, decreasing gastric acid.

Route: PO, IV.

Dosage: 0.1–0.8 mg/kg/dose IV q6h; 1–2 mg/kg/dose PO q12h.

Adverse effects: Constipation, diarrhea, sedation, tachycardia rarely.

Notes: Does not interact with other drugs. Injection contains 0.5% phenol. No short-term toxicity noted.

Sodium Bicarbonate (various)

Indications and use: Metabolic acidosis, cardiopulmonary resuscitation. Treatment of certain intoxications (eg, salicylates, phenothiazines) and renal tubular acidosis. Adjunctive treatment of hyperkalemia.

Actions: Alkalinizing agent that dissociates to provide bicarbonate ion.

Supplied: Oral tablets and powder, injection.

Route: PO, IV.

Dosage:

- Cardiac arrest:
  Initial dose: 2 meq/kg IV slowly over 2 minutes.
  Subsequent doses: Number of meq = 0.3 × wt (kg) × base deficit or 2–3 meq/kg q10min.
- Renal tubular acidosis:
  Distal: 2–3 meq/kg/d.
  Proximal: 5–10 meq/kg/d as initial dose; adjust prn for maintenance.

Adverse effects: Rapid correction of metabolic acidosis with sodium bicarbonate can lead to intraventricular hemorrhage, hyperosmolality, metabolic alkalosis, hypernatremia, and hypokalemia.

Comments: Use with close monitoring of arterial blood pH.

Sodium Polystyrene Sulfonate (Kayexalate)

Indications and use: Treatment of hyperkalemia.

Actions: Cation exchange resin that releases sodium in exchange for other cations such as potassium. Each gram of resin exchanges 1 meq sodium for each meq potassium removed. Other cations such as calcium, magnesium, and iron are also bound.

Supplied: Powder for suspension, suspension (in 33% sorbitol) (1.25 g/5mL, containing 4.1 meq sodium ion per gram).

Route: PO, PR (prepare in 20–25% sorbitol solution).

Dosage: 1 g resin will exchange 1 meq potassium. Usual dose is 1 g/kg/dose PO q6h or q2–6h PR.

Adverse effects: Large doses may cause fecal impaction. Hypokalemia, hypocalcemia, hypomagnesemia, and sodium retention may occur.

Spironolactone (Aldactone)

Indications and use: Primarily used in conjunction with a thiazide diuretic in the treatment of hypertension, congestive heart failure, and edema when prolonged diuresis is desirable.

Actions: Mild diuretic with potassium-sparing effects. Competitive antagonist of aldosterone.

Supplied: Tablets 25, 50, 100 mg.

Route: PO.

Dosage: 1.5–3.0 mg/kg/d divided q12h.

Adverse effects: Hyperkalemia, dehydration, hyponatremia, and gynecomastia (usually reversible).

Comments: Contraindicated in hyperkalemia, anuria, and rapidly deteriorating renal function. Monitor potassium closely when giving potassium supplements. More expensive but more effective than potassium supplements. Extemporaneous preparation of 1.25–5.0 mg/mL usually given.

Streptokinase (Kabikinase, Streptase)

Indications and use: Deep venous thrombosis and femoral artery thrombosis following cardiac catheterization.

Actions: Thrombolytic enzyme that converts plasminogen to the enzyme plasmin (fibrinolysin). Plasmin degrades fibrin, fibrinogen, and other plasma procoagulant proteins.

Supplied: Powder for injection.

Route: IV.

Dosage:

- Loading dose: 1500-2000 IU/kg infused over 30–60 minutes.
- Maintenance dosage: 1000 IU/kg/h as continuous infusion for 24–72 hours. Titrate dose to maintain thrombin time at 2–5 times normal control value.

Adverse effects: May cause severe spontaneous bleeding, hypersensitivity and anaphylactic reactions, fever (common), and chills.

Comments: Before starting therapy, obtain baseline for thrombin time, activated partial thromboplastin time, prothrombin time, hematocrit, and platelet count; repeat all tests every 12 hours. It is desired to maintain thrombin time at 2–5 times normal and prothrombin time and activated partial thromboplastin time as 1.5–2.0 times normal. Prepare final infusion solution to concentration of 1000 IU/mL in 5% dextrose in water. At the end of streptokinase therapy, begin IV heparin. ***Antidote:*** Aminocaproic acid, loading dose 200 mg/kg IV or PO stat followed by maintenance dose of 100 mg/kg/dose IV or PO q6h for up to 10 days after the procedure.

Note: Limited experience in neonates.

Surfactant (Exosurf Neonatal)

Indications and use: Surfactant therapy is indicated for the prophylactic treatment of infants with a birth weight < 1350 g who are at risk for the development of any type of respiratory distress syndrome (RDS), or for infants with a birth weight > 1350 g with coexisting, proven pulmonary immaturity and/or compromise. Exosurf Neonatal® is also indicated for neonates with established surfactant deficiency syndrome.

Actions: Surfactant acts to decrease the work of breathing, increase lung compliance, and increase alveolar expansion and stability by decreasing surface tension preventing atelectasis at end expiration. As a result, surfactant directly acts to reverse surfactant deficiency syndrome, prevent or reduce the development of pulmonary interstitial edema (PIE), which may progress to other forms of RDS, and reduce oxygen positive pressure mechanical ventilation requirements. The pharmacologic activity of commercial surfactant results from the combined action of three synthetic components: dipalmitoyl-phosphatidylcholine (DPPC), cetyl alcohol and tyloxapol. DPPC, the major component of natural surfactant rapidly and efficiently acts to dramatically decrease alveolar surface tension. Cetyl alcohol facilitates the dispersion and adsorption of DPPC onto the air:liquid interface of the alveoli. Cetyl alcohol modulates this physiologically essential function without the increased risk or immunogenicity of infectious potential associated with foreign protein substances. Tyloxapol provides the product with a hydrophillic agent that allows for reconsition of the lyophylized powder. Tyloxapol also plays a minor role in distribution of the active components into the smaller airways.

Supplied: Exosurf Neonatal is supplied in a kit containing a 10-mL vial containing DPPC 108 mg, cetyl alcohol 12 mg, tyloxapol 8 mg and NaCl 46.75 mg (tonicity agent), a 10-mL vial of sterile water for injection and endotracheal tube adaptors of varying sizes. Prior to reconstitution, the drug requires no special storage requirements. Once reconstituted using exactly 8 mL sterile water, the milky white suspension is stable for up to 12 hours either at room temperature or under refrigeration.

Route: Surfactant can only be administered endotracheally using a special ET tube adaptor supplied with the drug kit, without the interruption of mechanical ventilation and after radiographic confirmation of the location of the endotracheal tube (ET) tip in the trachea unless impractical due to time restraints.

Dosage and administration: Prior to administration of surfactant, the infant should be well suctioned, and suctioning should be withheld for 2 hours following the dose unless clinically necessary. Prophylactic surfactant is administered as a single 5 mL/kg dose as soon as RDS is clinically confirmed after birth. Second and third doses may be subsequently administered if necessary while the infant remains mechanically ventilated and under respiratory distress. Rescue treatment for infants who acutely develop RDS is administered as two 5 mL/kg doses, with the first dose given at the time of diagnosis, and the second 12–24 hours later.

Administration of the dose requires intubation and should be given in half doses with the first half given over 1–2 minutes using the appropriately sized ET adaptor with the infant positioned at the midline position. The adaptor fits into the ventilator line and has a Leur lock syringe port through which the drug is administered while maintaining the closed system of the respirator. The infant's head and torso are then rotated 45 degrees to the right and held in that position for 30 seconds. The infant is then returned to midline and the remaining drug administered in the same manner with the head and torso rotated to the left for 30 seconds.

Adverse effects: Significant adverse effects associated with Exosurf Neonatal during clinical use to this point include increased incidence of pulmonary hemorrhage, apnea and methylxanthine dosage requirements. Other adverse effects associated with the use of the drug involve increased risk of patent ductus arteriosus (PDA), thrombocytopenia, and acute changes in respiratory status; the latter of which may be a direct result of the pharmocologic activity of the drug and require rapid adjustment of mechanical ventilatory parameters.

Comments: Administration of surfactant requires close and continuous monitoring during and 30 minutes after administration of the dose to ensure maximum safety, efficacy, and benefit. This should include blood gas monitoring, adjustments of mechanical ventilatory parameters, and monitoring of changes in clinical signs and symptoms consistent with changes in oxygenation and pulmonary function.

Theophylline (various)

Indications and use: Apnea of prematurity. There is evidence that theophylline can improve lung compliance and aid in weaning infants from respiratory support in diseases such as bronchopulmonary dysplasia.

Actions: A methylxanthine. Theophylline probably acts by virtue of adenosine antagonism. Neonates have the unique ability to convert theophylline to caffeine in a ratio of 1.0:0.3, respectively, and caffeine may approach 50% of theophylline serum levels. Thus, it is impossible to distinguish the pharmacodynamic effects of theophylline from those of caffeine in the neonate. Theophylline produces excitation throughout all levels of the CNS; produces modest decreases in peripheral vascular resistance, and increases cardiac output; relaxes pulmonary airway smooth muscle, with resultant increase in vital capacity; decreases diaphragmatic fatigue; and may cause marked increases in cerebrovascular resistance, resulting in decreased cerebral blood flow. In premature infants at risk for ventricular hemorrhage, the latter effect may be deleterious.

Supplied: Oral elixirs and solutions, injection.

Route: IV, PO.

Dosage:

- Apnea of prematurity: 5–6 mg/kg PO or IV (infused over 15–20 minutes) as loading dose, followed by maintenance dose of 2 mg/kg q12h starting 12 hours after loading dose.
- Ventilator weaning: 6.5 mg/kg PO or IV as loading dose, followed by maintenance dose of 3–4 mg/kg q12h.

Adverse effects: Side effects and toxicity include hyperglycemia, diuresis, dehydration, feeding intolerance, tachycardia and other arrhythmias, hyperreflexia, jitteriness, and seizures.

Comments: Levels for apnea are 4–12 µg/mL. Toxicity is associated with levels greater than 15–20 µg/mL. Monitor serum levels on day 4 of therapy: peak level 1 hour after an IV dose is completed or 2 hours after an oral dose, and trough level 30 minutes before next dose. Levels of caffeine and theophylline should ideally be monitored—in neonates especially—any time toxicity is suspected or when apnea spells appear to be increasing in frequency.

Tolazoline (Priscoline)

Indications and use: Hypoxia caused by persistent pulmonary hypertension (PPH).

Actions: Alpha-adrenergic blocking agent with histaminergic properties. Results in pulmonary and systemic vasodilator effects. Histaminic effects stimulate gastric secretion and peripheral vasodilatation and increase salivary, lacrimal, respiratory tract, and pancreatic secretions. Response to tolazoline is marked by cutaneous flushing following by increased Pao_2.

Supplied: Injection.

Route: IV, IM.

Dosage: 1–2 mg/kg IV as initial dose (infused over 5–10 minutes) followed by a continuous infusion of 1–2 mg/kg/h. Some infants respond rapidly; others may require 30 minutes or more.

Adverse effects: Tachycardia, nausea, vomiting, diarrhea, gastrointestinal bleeding, increased gastrointestinal secretions, increased pilomotor activity, sweating, thrombocytopenia, agranulocytosis, and hypotension.

Comments: Contraindicated in renal failure, hypotension shock, and intraventricular hemorrhage. Dopamine and dobutamine are often used to support systemic pressure in neonates with PPH; both drugs may have adverse effects on peripheral vascular resistance, especially at higher dosages. For severe hypotension use ephedrine (0.2 mg/kg/dose) to increase peripheral vascular resistance or dopamine (< 10 µg/kg/min) to improve cardiac output. Epinephrine administered with tolazoline may cause a paradoxical reduction in blood pressure followed by an exaggerated rebound blood pressure elevation.

Tromethamine (THAM)

Indications and use: Metabolic acidosis when sodium bicarbonate is contraindicated because of elevated serum sodium (eg, metabolic acidosis in persistent fetal circulation treated with multiple doses of sodium bicarbonate).

Actions: Alkalinizing agent that acts as a proton (hydrogen ion) acceptor; combines with hydrogen ions and their associated anions of acids (lactic, pyruvic, carbonic, and other metabolic acids). The resulting salts are then renally excreted.

Supplied: Injection, 0.3M solution (36 mg/mL).

Route: IV.

Dosage:

- Loading dose: 3–5 mL/kg of undiluted solution infused over 5 minutes, or dose = wt in kg × 1.1 × base deficit in meq/L.
- Maintenance dosage: 3–16 mL/kg/h (undiluted solution) as continuous infusion, or prepare a 10–50% v/v dilution in 5% dextrose in water for continuous infusion. Titrate dose to desired response via frequent blood gas monitoring.

Adverse effects: Respiratory depression, thrombophlebitis, venospasm, alkalosis, transient hypocalcemia or hypoglycemia, and hyperkalemia. Extravasation may cause sloughing of the skin.

Comments: Contraindicated in anuria, uremia, and chronic respiratory acidosis. Do not administer for periods longer than 24 hours. Hyperkalemia is a problem especially with decreased renal function. If infiltration occurs, discontinue infusion immediately, inject 1% procaine (to which 75 units of hyaluronidase has been added) into the affected area, and infuse 0.1 mg/kg of phentolamine mesylate into the vasospastic area.

Tubocurarine (Curare)

Indications and use: To improve oxygenation in the uncooperative neonate during mechanical ventilation. To provide muscle relaxation during general anesthesia.

Actions: Nondepolarizing (competitive) neuromuscular blocking agent. Rapid IV administration may cause hypotension, bradycardia, and possibly circulatory collapse. Atropine is an effective prophylactic agent. Onset of paralysis is generally 1–2 minutes after IV administration. Duration of paralysis depends on the number of doses and the total dosage delivered and may persist for 20–90 minutes.

Supplied: Injection 3 mg/mL.

Route: IV; IM only if IV access is not available.

Dosage: Infuse undiluted over 1 minute to minimize cardiovascular effects.

- Initial dosage: 0.25–0.5 mg/kg IV.
- Maintenance dosage: 0.15 mg/kg/dose IV prn.

Adverse effects: Hypotension, bradycardia, possibly circulatory collapse and allergic reactions.

Comments: For reversal, give neostigmine, with atropine, IV. See dose p 474.

Varicella-Zoster Immune Globulin (VZIG)

Indications and use: For protection of infants of mothers with varicella-zoster infections (chickenpox) within 5 days before or 48 hours after delivery; of post-natally exposed preterm infants under 1000 g or under 28 weeks regardless of maternal history; and of postnatally exposed premature infants whose maternal history is negative for varicella.

Actions: Passive immunity through infusion of IgG antibody. Protection lasts 1 month or longer. VZIG does not reduce the incidence but acts to decrease the risk of complications.

Supplied: Injection, 125 units/1.25 mL.

Route: IM only.

Dosage: 0–10 kg: 125 units IM as a single dose injected at one site.

Adverse effects: Pain, erythema, swelling, and rash at the site of injection; rarely, anaphylaxis.

Comments: Best results are achieved if VZIG is given within 96 hours after exposure. It is obtained through the American Red Cross Blood Services. *Note:* Do not give IV.

Vecuronium Bromide (Vecuronium)

Indications and use: Skeletal muscle relaxation and paralysis in infants requiring mechanical ventilation.

Actions: Nondepolarizing muscle relaxant that competitively antagonizes autonomic cholinergic receptors. Onset of action is 1–2 minutes with a duration that varies with dose and age.

Supplied: Powder for injection.

Route: IV.

Dosage: 0.03–0.15 mg/kg IV push q1–2h to maintain paralysis.

Adverse effects: May cause hypoxemia.

Comments: Less tachycardia and hypotension when compared to pancuronium bromide. When used with narcotics, decreases in heart rate and blood pressure have been observed.

Verapamil (Calan, Isoptin)

Indications and use: To control supraventricular tachycardia (SVT). **Recent evidence puts in question the safey of using verapamil in infants (Till JA, Shinebourne EA: *Arch Dis Child* 1991;66:647). Some clinicians no longer use the drug because of possible irreversible side effects (profound bradycardia and hypotension).**

Actions: Calcium channel-blocking agent. Afterload reduction and decreased myocardial contractility.

Supplied: Injection, tablets, sustained release tablets.

Route: IV, PO.

Dosage:

- IV: 0.1–0.3 mg/kg over 1 minute. Repeat in 30 minutes if needed.
- PO: 3 mg/kg/dose q8h.

Adverse effects: May cause hypotension, bradycardia, asystole, heart block, dizziness, constipation. Some authors have reported an unacceptably high complication rate. May increase serum digoxin concentrations with the use of verapamil in neonates.

Comments: Do not use in shock, hypotension, second- or third-degree AV nodal block, sick sinus syndrome, or congestive heart failure unless due to supraventricular tachycardia. Do not use concomitantly with a beta blocker.

Vitamin D$_2$ (Ergocalciferol, Calciferol, Drisdol)

Indications and use: To prevent or treat rickets and to manage hypocalcemia due to vitamin D deficiency.

Actions: Regulation of plasma calcium and phosphate, supporting normal mineralization of bone.

Supplied: Capsules, solution, tablets, injection (1 mg = 40,000 IU; 1 µg = 40 IU).

Route: PO, IM, IV with intravenous multivitamin preparations.

Dosage: 400–800 IU/d.

Comments: Excessive doses may lead to hypervitaminosis D, manifested by hypercalcemia and its associated complications.

Vitamin E (Di-alpha-tocopherol Acetate, Aquasol E, others)

Indications and use: Investigational for treatment or prevention of anemia of prematurity, retinopathy of prematurity, bronchopulmonary dysplasia, and intraventricular hemorrhage.

Actions: A potent free radical scavenger. An antioxidant to prevent destruction of unsaturated fatty acids and cell membranes by uncontrolled free radicals. At birth, tissue stores of alpha-tocopherol (active form) are low.

Supplied: Capsules, drops, tablets.

Route: PO, IV (with intravenous multivitamin preparations).

Dosage:

- Requirements: The following recommendations are currently followed in infant formulas.
  Full-term infants: 0.3 IU/100 kcal or 0.7 IU/g linoleic acid.
  Premature infants: 1 IU/g of linoleic acid.
- Anemia of prematurity: Prevention or treatment requires only adequate nutritional intake of vitamin E.
- Alternative: Prophylaxis: 25–50 IU/d PO until 2–3 months of age. Treatment: 50–200 PO IU/d for 2 weeks.

Comments: Physiologic serum levels for premature infants are 1–3 mg/dL. Serum levels should be monitored when pharmacologic doses of vitamin E are administered. Liquid preparation is very hypersomolar (3000 mosm) and should be diluted at least 1:4 with sterile water. 1 mg of di-alpha-tocopheryl acetate = 1 IU.

Vitamin K₁ (Phytonadione, AquaMephyton, Mephyton)

Indications and use: Prevention and treatment of hemorrhagic disease of the newborn, vitamin K deficiency.

Actions: Required for the synthesis of blood coagulation factors II, VII, IX, and X. Because vitamin K_1 may require 3 hours or more to stop active bleeding, fresh-frozen plasma, 10 mL/kg, may be necessary when bleeding is severe. The drug has no antagonistic effects against heparin.

Supplied: Tablets, injection.

Route: PO, IM, IV. (For IV use, dilute in 5% dextrose in water and infuse slowly, not faster than 1 mg/min.)

Dosage:

- Neonatal hemorrhagic disease:
  Prevention: 1 mg IM at birth; if infant < 1500 g, give 0.5 mg IM at birth.
  Treatment: 1 mg as single dose IV.
- Deficiency state: 1 mg/dose PO, IM, or slowly IV.
- Oral anticoagulant overdose: 1–2 mg/dose IV q4–8h prn. (Follow serial prothrombin time and partial thromboplastin time for response.)

Adverse effects: Relatively nontoxic. Hemolytic anemia and kernicterus have been reported in neonates given menadiol sodium diphosphate (vitamin K_3; Synkayvite); however, vitamin K_1 has not been associated with toxic symptoms or hypersensitivity.

76 Commonly Used Antibiotics, Antivirals, and Antifungals

Acyclovir (Zovirax)

Classification: Antiviral agent.

Action and spectrum: Indicated in herpes simplex and varicella-zoster viral infections. Virostatic. Activated in virally infected cells, inhibits viral DNA polymerase, and is a viral chain terminator. Good activity against herpes simplex (types 1 and 2) and varicella-zoster viruses. Poor activity against Epstein-Barr virus and cytomegalovirus. CSF concentrations are 50% those of plasma.

Supplied: Injection, topical, capsules.

Route: Topical, IV, PO.

Dosage:

- Topical: Apply sufficient amount to cover lesion q3h.
- IV: 30–40 mg/kg/d divided q8h for 10–14 days (dilute to final concentration of 7 mg/mL and infuse over 60 minutes).

Adverse effects: Transient elevation of serum creatinine, thrombocytosis, jitters, rash, hives.

Comments: Drug of choice for documented or suspected herpes encephalitis (suggest 40 mg/kg/d IV in divided doses for 14 days).

Amikacin Sulfate (Amikin)

Classification: Aminoglycoside.

Action and spectrum: Primarily bactericidal against gram-negative organisms by inhibiting protein synthesis. Active against gram-negative bacteria, including most *Pseudomonas* and *Serratia.* No activity against anaerobic organisms.

Supplied: Injection.

Route: IM or IV (infuse over 30 minutes).

Dosage: Dosage should always be monitored and adjusted by use of pharmacokinetics. Initial empiric dosing based on body weight:

- < 1500 g: 10 mg/kg/d q24h.
- > 1500 g < 2500 g: 10 mg/kg/d divided q12h.
- > 2500 g: 20 mg/kg/d divided q12h.

Elimination: Renal (glomerular filtration); half-life is 4–8 hours; volume of distribution is 0.6 L/kg.

Comments: Lowest overall resistance of all the aminoglycosides and thus should be reserved for infections with organisms resistant to other aminoglycosides. Adjust dosage according to serum peak and trough levels. Draw serum levels at about the fourth maintenance dose (draw serum trough sample 30 minutes to just before dose and serum peak sample 30 minutes after infusion is complete). Therapeutic peak level 25–35 μg/mL and trough level 10 μg/mL. Nephrotoxicity associated with serum trough concentrations > 10 μg/mL;

ototoxicity with serum peak concentrations > 35–40 μg/mL (more cochlear damage than vestibular).

Amphotericin B (Fungizone)

Classification: Antifungal agent.

Action and spectrum: Acts by binding to sterols and disrupting the fungal cell membranes. Broad spectrum of activity against *Candida* and other fungi.

Supplied: Injection.

Route: IV.

Dosage:

- Initially: Test dose of 0.25 mg/kg IV over 2–4 hours, then infusion of 0.1 mg/mL concentration in 5% dextrose *only*.
- Increment: Increase daily dosage by 0.125–0.25 mg/kg/24h qd–qod as tolerated to maximum daily or alternate-day dosage of 0.75–1 mg/kg. A total dosage of 30–35 mg/kg should be given over 6 weeks or longer, though a lower dose may suffice. In general, infusions should be given over 2–4 hours, though infusion over 1–2 hours may be used if tolerated.
- *Intrathecal or intraventricular:* Reconstitute with sterile water at 0.25 mg/mL; Dilute with CSF fluid and reinfuse. Usual dose: 0.25–0.5 mg.

Elimination and metabolism: Slow renal excretion.

Adverse effects: Few adverse effects in neonates as opposed to adults. May cause fever, chills, vomiting, thrombophlebitis at injection sites, renal tubular acidosis, renal failure, hypomagnesemia, hypokalemia, bone marrow suppression with reversible decline in hematocrit, hypotension, hypertension, wheezing, and hypoxemia.

Comments: Irritation at infusion site may be reduced by addition of heparin (1 unit/mL) and hydrocortisone (2.5 mg/mg of amphotericin B). Protect solution from light. Monitor serum potassium, magnesium, urea nitrogen, creatinine, alkaline phosphatase, and AST (SGOT) qd–qod until the dosage is stabilized, then every week. Monitor CBC every week. Discontinue if BUN > 40 mg/dL or if serum creatinine > 3 mg/dL or if liver function tests are abnormal.

Ampicillin (Polycillin, others)

Classification: Semisynthetic penicillinase-sensitive penicillin.

Action and spectrum: The penicillins are bactericidal and act by inhibiting the late stages of cell wall synthesis. Ampicillin is as effective as penicillin G in pneumococcal, streptococcal, and meningococcal infections and is active also against many strains of *Salmonella, Shigella, Proteus mirabilis, Escherichia coli, Listeria,* and most strains of *Haemophilus influenzae.* It is inactivated by staphylococcal and *H influenzae* β-lactamases.

Supplied: Powder to make pediatric drops, oral suspension, and injection.

Route: PO, IM, IV.

Dosage:

- Meningitis:
  Age 0–7 days: 100–200 mg/kg/d IV or IM divided q12h.
  Age > 7 days: 200–300 mg/kg/d IV or IM divided q6–8h: maximum dose 400 mg/kg/d.
- Other indications:
  Age 0–7 days: 50 mg/kg/d PO, IV, or IM divided q12h.
  Age > 7 days: 75 mg/kg/d PO, IV, or IM divided q12h.

Elimination and metabolism: 90% excreted unchanged in urine. Half-life in neonates is 2 hours.

Adverse effects: Hypersensitivity (including anaphylactic reaction), rubella-like rash, abdominal discomfort, nausea, vomiting, diarrhea, eosinophilia. Very large doses may cause CNS excitation or convulsions.

Comments: Ampicillin is the penicillin of choice in combination with an amino-glycoside in the prophylaxis and treatment of infections with group B strepto-cocci, group D streptococci (enterococci), and *Listeria monocytogenes.* Contains 3 meq of sodium per gram.

Ampicillin/Sulbactam (Unasyn)

Classification: Combination β-lactamase inhibitor and β-lactam agent.

Action and spectrum: The bactericidal spectrum of ampicillin is extended by the addition of sulbactam, a β-lactamase inhibitor, to include β-lactamase-pro-ducing strains of *S aureus, S epidermidis,* enterococcus, *H influenzae, B catarrhalis,* and *Klebsiella* spp, including *K pneumoniae.* Also has good activity against *B fragilis,* making it a suitable choice for single drug treatment of intra-abdominal and pelvic infections cause by susceptible organisms.

Supplied: Injection.

Route: IV or IM.

Dosage:

> Age 0–7 days: 50 mg/kg/d IV or IM q12h.
> Age > 7 days: 75 mg/kg/d IV or IM q12h.
> - Meningitis:
> Age 0–7 days: 100–200 mg/kg/d IV q12h.
> Age > 7 days: 200–300 mg/kg/d IV or IM q6–8h.
> Maximum dose 400 mg/kg/d.

Elimination: See Ampicillin, above.

Adverse effects: See Ampicillin, above.

Comments: See Ampicillin, above.

Aztreonam (Azactam)

Classification: Monobactam antibiotic.

Action and spectrum: Antibacterial activity due to inhibition of mucopeptide synthesis in cell wall. Bactericidal against most *Enterobacteriaceae* and *Pseudomonas aeruginosa* but little or no activity against gram-positive aerobic bacteria or anaerobic bacteria.

Supplied: Injection.

Route: IV.

Dosage:

- Premature infants: 50 mg/kg/dose q12h.
- Term infants: 50 mg/kg/dose q8h.

Elimination: Renal (glomerular filtration and secretion). Half-life is approximately 6–10 hours. Volume of distribution 0.26–0.36 L/kg.

Adverse effects: Diarrhea, nausea, vomiting, rash irritation at infusion site, increased prothrombin time, transient eosinophilia.

Comments: Used primarily for *Pseudomonas* infections.

Carbenicillin Disodium (Geopen, Pyopen)

Classification: Semisynthetic penicillinase-sensitive penicillin.

Action and spectrum: Mechanism of action is identical to that of ampicillin. Increased activity against gram-negative organisms, including indole-positive *Proteus* sp, *Enterobacter, Serratia,* and *Pseudomonas aeruginosa. Klebsiella* sp are generally resistant. Carbenicillin is ordinarily not used alone to treat systemic infections and is synergistic when used in combination with amino-glycosides against most gram-negative organisms, including *Pseudomonas.*

Supplied: Injection.

Route: IM, IV.

Dosage:

- Age 0–7 days: 200 mg/kg/d divided q12h.
- Age > 7 days: 300–400 mg/kg/d divided q12h.

Elimination and metabolism: Excreted unchanged in the urine.

Adverse effects: Anaphylaxis, platelet dysfunction, hypokalemia, hyperna-tremia, asymptomatic rises in serum transaminases.

Comments: Rarely used, since ticarcillin is more active against *Pseudomonas* in a lower total dose. Contains 5.2–6.5 meq sodium per gram.

Cefazolin Sodium (Ancef, Kefzol)

Classification: First-generation cephalosporin.

Action and spectrum: A broad-spectrum semisynthetic β-lactam antibiotic bac-tericidal by virtue of its inhibition of cell wall synthesis. Good activity against gram-positive cocci (except enterococci), including penicillinase-producing staphylococci. Gram-negative coverage includes *E coli,* most *Klebsiella,* many *Haemophilus influenzae,* and indole-positive *Proteus.* Organism resistance is primarily due to elaboration of β-lactamases, which inactivate the antibiotic through hydrolysis.

Supplied: Injection.

Route: IM or IV (infuse over 20–30 minutes).

Dosage:

- Newborn and premature infants:
  < 2000 g: 40 mg/kg/d divided q12h.
  > 2000 g and age > 7 days: 60 mg/kg/d divided q12h.
- Age 1 month and older: 25–100 mg/kg/d divided q6–8h.

Elimination and metabolism: 100% excreted unchanged in urine. Half-life is 1.5–4 hours.

Adverse effects: Infrequent except for allergic reactions, including fever, rash, and urticaria. May cause leukopenia, thrombocytopenia, and a positive Coombs test reaction. Excessive dosage (especially in renal impairment) may result in CNS irritation with delirium or seizure activity.

Comments: Use with caution in patients with a history of severe allergic reac-tions to penicillins. Dosage reduction is required in moderate to severe renal failure. Contains 2 meq sodium per gram.

Cefotaxime Sodium (Claforan)

Classification: Third-generation cephalosporin.

Action and spectrum: Mechanism of action is identical to that of other β-lac-tam antibiotics and is bactericidal. Active chiefly against gram-negative orga-nisms (except *Pseudomonas* sp), including *E coli, Enterobacter* sp, *Klebsiella* sp, *Haemophilus influenzae* (including ampicillin-resistant strains), *Proteus mirabilis* and indole-positive *Proteus, Serratia marcescens, Neisseria gonor-*

rhoeae, and *Neisseria meningitidis.* Generally poor activity against gram-positive aerobic organisms.

Supplied: Injection.

Route: IM or IV (infuse over 30 minutes).

Dosage:

- ≤ 7 days old: 100 mg/kg/d divided q12h.
- > 7 days old: 150 mg/kg/d divided q8h.
- Meningitis: 200 mg/kg/d divided q6h.

Elimination and metabolism: Excreted principally unchanged in the urine. Half-life in neonates is 1–4 hours.

Adverse effects: Hypersensitivity reactions (rarely anaphylactic), thrombophlebitis, serum sickness-like reaction with prolonged administration, diarrhea, and, rarely, blood dyscrasias, hepatic dysfunction, or renal damage.

Comments: Cefotaxime should be reserved for suspected or documented gram-negative meningitis or sepsis. When used as empiric therapy, should combine with ampicillin or aqueous penicillin G to provide gram-positive coverage (ie, group B streptococci, pneumococci, *Listeria monocytogenes*). High degree of stability to β-lactamases. Third-generation cephalosporins have been proved to induce the emergence of multi-drug-resistant bacteria when used excessively and without proper clinical indications. Contains 2.2 meq sodium per gram.

Ceftazidime (Fortaz, Tazidime)

Classification: Third-generation cephalosporin.

Action and spectrum: A broad-spectrum gram-negative semisynthetic β-lactam antibiotic bactericidal by virtue of its inhibition of cell wall synthesis. Poor gram-positive activity as compared to first-generation cephalosporins but has good activity against gram-negative aerobic bacteria including *Neisseria meningitidis, Haemophilus influenzae,* and most of the *Enterobacteriacea.* It has excellent activity against *Pseudomonas aeruginosa* (the best of all third-generation cephalosporins). Ceftazidime has little activity against *Listeria monocytogenes* and enterococcus.

Supplied: IV.

Route: IM, IV over 20–30 minutes.

Dosage:

- < 2000 g < 7 days 30 mg/kg IV q12h.
- > 2000 g < 7 days 30 mg/kg IV q8h.
- > 2000 g > 7 days 30 mg/kg IV q8h.

Elimination: Renal (glomerular filtration) 100% excreted unchanged; half-life 2.2–4.7 hours.

Adverse effects: Infrequent except for allergic reactions including fever, rash and urticaria. May cause transient leukopenia, neutropenia, and thrombocytopenia, direct positive Coombs' test, and transient elevation in liver function test.

Comments: Penetrates well into CSF; concentrations approximate 25–50% of serum concentrations. Ceftazidime in combination with ampicillin (for *Listeria*) can be used to treat suspected gram-negative meningitis in the neonate. It is also an alternative to aminoglycosides for *P aeruginosa* therapy, particularly in patients with renal failure.

Ceftriaxone Sodium (Rocephin)

Classification: Third-generation cephalosporin.

Action and spectrum: Mechanism of action identical to that of other β-lactam antibiotics. High degree of stability to β-lactamases and good activity against both gram-negative and gram-positive organisms except for *Pseudomonas* sp, enterococci, methicillin-resistant staphylococci, and *Listeria monocytogenes.* Has longest serum half-life of all currently available cephalosporins.

Supplied: Injection.

Route: IM or IV (infuse over 30 minutes).

Dosage:

- Meningitis: 100 mg/kg/d divided q12h.
- Other infections: 50 mg/kg/d divided q12–24h.

Elimination and metabolism: Both biliary and renal excretion. Half-life is 5.2–8.4 hours.

Adverse effects: Mild diarrhea and eosinophilia are most common. May also cause neutropenia, rash, thrombophlebitis, and bacterial (gastrointestinal) or fungal overgrowth. Rare reports of increased prothrombin times.

Comments: Many clinical studies support once-a-day dosing. Do not use as sole drug in infections due to staphylococci or pseudomonal organisms. Combine with ampicillin for initial empirical therapy of meningitis (Ceftriaxone has poor activity against *Listeria*). Generally no dosage reduction is required in renal or hepatic dysfunction. Contains 2.4 meq sodium per gram.

Note: Ceftriaxone has been reported to increase free and erythrocyte-bound bilirubin in premature infants with hyperbilirubinemia. Therefore, extreme care should be taken with neonates with elevated bilirubin concentrations to avoid this.

Cefuroxime (Kefurox, Zinacef)

Classification: Second-generation cephalosporin.

Action and spectrum: Mechanism of action identical to that of other β-lactam antibiotics. Active against both gram-positive and gram-negative organisms, including streptococci (except enterococci), both penicillinase-producing and non-penicillinase-producing staphylococci (not including methicillin-resistant staphylococci), *Escherichia coli, Haemophilus influenzae* (including ampicillin-resistant strains), *Klebsiella* sp, *Neisseria gonorrhoeae* and *N meningitidis, Proteus mirabilis, Salmonella* sp, *Shigella* sp, and *Enterobacter* sp.

Supplied: Injection.

Route: IM or IV (IV preferred; infuse over 30 minutes).

Dosage:

- 100 mg/kg/d divided q12h.

Elimination and metabolism: Primarily excreted unchanged in the urine. Half-life is 5–8 hours in infants < 4 days and 1.6–3.8 hours in infants > 8 days.

Adverse effects: Generally free of adverse effects but may cause hypersensitivity reactions, thrombophlebitis, elevated serum transaminases, mildly elevated BUN, diarrhea, and, rarely, blood dyscrasias (transient neutropenia, leukopenia, thrombocytopenia).

Comments: Cefuroxime is the only first- or second-generation cephalosporin that crosses the blood-brain barrier and is therefore indicated in the treatment of bacterial meningitis. However, because it provides no activity against *Listeria,* ampicillin should be added in initial empirical therapy. Cefuroxime has added gram-negative coverage over first-generation cephalosporins while retaining very good gram-positive coverage. Decrease dosage in renal failure. Contains 2.4 meq sodium per gram.

Note: Limited experience reported in neonates. No current FDA approval for neonatal use.

Cephalothin Sodium (Keflin)

Classification: First-generation cephalosporin.

Action and spectrum: Mechanism of action identical to that of other β-lactam antibiotics. Active against both gram-positive and gram-negative organisms, including streptococci (except enterococci), both penicillinase-producing and non-penicillinase-producing staphylococci (but not methicillin-resistant staphylococci), *Escherichia coli, Proteus mirabilis, Klebsiella* sp, *Haemophilus influenzae, Salmonella* sp, and *Shigella* sp.

Supplied: Injection.

Route: IV (infuse over 30 minutes).

Dosage:

- < 2000 g and 0–7 days old: 40 mg/kg/d divided q12h.
- < 2000 g and > 7 days old: 60 mg/kg/d divided q8h.
- > 2000 g and 0–7 days old: 60 mg/kg/d divided q8h.
- > 2000 g and > 7 days old: 80 mg/kg/d divided q6h.

Elimination and metabolism: 75% excreted unchanged in the urine.

Adverse effects: Hypersensitivity reactions, thrombophlebitis, serum sickness-like reaction with prolonged use, diarrhea, neutropenia, leukopenia, transient elevation of AST (SGOT). May falsely elevate serum creatinine.

Comments: Generally better activity against gram-positive organisms than second-or third-generation drugs. Dosage adjustment required in renal failure. Contains 2.8 meq sodium per gram.

Chloramphenicol (Chloromycetin)

Action and spectrum: A broad-spectrum agent. Interferes with or inhibits protein synthesis. Bactericidal for *Haemophilus influenzae* and *Neisseria meningitis;* bacteriostatic for *Escherichia coli, Klebsiella, Serratia, Enterobacter, Salmonella, Shigella, Neisseria gonorrhoeae,* staphylococci, *Rickettsia rickettsii, Streptococcus pneumoniae,* and groups A, B, C, nonenterococcal D, and G streptococci. Drug of choice for *Salmonella typhi* infection.

Supplied: Injection, oral suspension, ophthalmic solution.

Route: PO, IM, or IV (infuse over 5–15 minutes).

Dosage:

- < 2000 g and 0–7 days old: 25 mg/kg/d q24h.
- < 2000 g and > 7 days old: 25 mg/kg/d q24h.
- > 2000 g and 0–7 days old: 25 mg/kg/d q24h.
- > 2000 g and > 7 days old: 50 mg/kg/d divided q12h.
- Ophthalmic solution: 1 drop OU q6–12h.

Elimination and metabolism: Metabolized by the liver. Half-life is 9–27 hours.

Adverse effects: Idiosyncratic reactions result in aplastic anemia (irreversible and rare), reversible bone marrow suppression (dose-related), allergy (rash, fever), diarrhea, vomiting, stomatitis, glossitis, *Candida* superinfection, "gray baby" syndrome (early signs are hyperammonemia and unexplained metabolic acidosis; other signs are abdominal distention, hypotonia, gray skin color, cardiorespiratory collapse).

Comments: Avoid use where possible. Must monitor serum levels. Desired peak is 10–25 µg/mL; levels > 50 µg/mL are strongly associated with "gray baby" syndrome. Monitor CBC with differential, platelet count, and reticulocyte count every 3 days.

Clindamycin (Cleocin)

Action and spectrum: Bactericidal activity by inhibiting protein synthesis. Active against both aerobic and anaerobic streptococci (except enterococci), most staphylococci (except methicillin-resistant strains), *Bacteroides* sp (except *B melaninogenicus*), *Fusobacterium varium, Actinomyces israelii, Clostridium perfringens,* and *Clostridium tetani.* It is chiefly used against the above anaerobes. Not effective against gram-negatives or many clostridial species.

Supplied: Injection, oral solution, capsules.

Route: PO, IM, or IV (infuse over 10–20 minutes).

Dosage:

- < 2000 g and 0–7 days old: 15 mg/kg/d divided q8h.
- < 2000 g and > 7 days old: 15 mg/kg/d divided q8h.
- > 2000 g and 0–7 days old: 15 mg/kg/d divided q8h.
- > 2000 g and > 7 days old: 20 mg/kg/d divided q6h.

Elimination and metabolism: Primarily hepatic metabolism.

Adverse effects: Sterile abscess formation at IM injection site. Vomiting and diarrhea occur frequently. Pseudomembranous colitis due to suppression of normal flora and overgrowth of *Clostridium difficile* is uncommon but potentially fatal (treated with oral vancomycin or metronidazole). Rash, glossitis, and pruritus occur occasionally. Serum sickness, anaphylaxis, hematologic (granulocytopenia, thrombocytopenia), and hepatic abnormalities occur rarely.

Comments: Does not cross the blood-brain barrier; therefore, do not use to treat meningitis.

Erythromycin (Ilosone, others)

Classification: Macrolide antibiotic.

Action and spectrum: Acts by suppression of protein synthesis. Action may be bactericidal or bacteriostatic at normal therapeutic concentrations. Spectrum of activity is broad and includes the streptococci (except enterococci), *Staphylococcus aureus, Clostridia, Corynebacterium diphtheriae, Listeria monocytogenes, Haemophilus influenzae, Bordetella pertussis, Brucella, Campylobacter fetus, Branhamella catarrhalis, Neisseria gonorrhoeae, Legionella micdadei* and *Legionella pneumophila, Rickettsia, Mycoplasma pneumoniae, Chlamydia trachomatis, Treponema pallidum,* and some *Bacteroides* sp. Ophthalmic form is routinely instilled into the eyes of newborn infants as prophylaxis against ophthalmia neonatorum.

Supplied: Oral suspension, oral drops, tablets, capsules, erythromycin base (Ilotycin Ophthalmic) ointment, injection.

Route: PO, IV over 60 minutes, ophthalmic.

Dosage:

- 0–7 days old: 20 mg/kg/d divided q12h.
- > 7 days old: 30 mg/kg/d divided q8h.
- > 2000 g: 30–40 mg/kg/d divided q8h.
- Ophthalmic as prophylaxis: $\frac{1}{2}$ inch OU once.
- Ophthalmic for acute infection: $\frac{1}{2}$ inch OU qid.

Elimination and metabolism: Hepatic metabolism, excreted via the bile and kidneys. Half-life is 1.5–3 hours (prolonged in renal failure).

Adverse effects: Stomatitis, epigastric distress, oral or perianal candidiasis. Transient cholestatic hepatitis and allergic reactions occur rarely. May cause increased serum levels of theophylline, digoxin, and carbamazepine.

Comments: Generally used in penicillin-allergic patients. Parenteral forms are painful and irritative. Do not use IM. Lactobionate formulation contains 180 mg of benzyl alcohol per gram of erythromycin.

Flucytosine

Classification: Antifungal agent.

Action and spectrum: Flucytosine penetrates fungal cells, where it acts as antimetabolite, ultimately interfering with protein synthesis. It is active in vivo against some strains of *Cryptococcus* and *Candida.* May be synergistic with amphotericin B.

Supplied: Capsules.

Route: Oral.

Dosage: 50–100 mg/kg/d divided q6h.

Dosage in renal impairment: For patients with renal impairment the dosage's frequency of administration must be changed to 12.5–25 mg/kg/d divided as follows:

- q12h for creatinine clearance of 20–40 mL/min.
- q24h for creatinine clearance of 10–20 mL/min.
- q24–48h for creatinine clearance of < 10 mL/min.

Serum concentrations: 24–120 μg/mL.

Pharmacokinetics: Volume of distribution—0.68 L/kg; half-life, 3 to 5 hours; renal elimination.

Adverse effects: Vomiting, diarrhea, rash, anemia, leukopenia, thrombocytopenia, elevated liver function tests, increased BUN and creatinine, CNS disturbances.

Gentamicin Sulfate (Garamycin, others)

Classification: Aminoglycoside.

Action and spectrum: Bactericidal activity by inhibition of bacterial protein synthesis. Active chiefly against gram-negative aerobic bacteria, including most *Pseudomonas, Proteus* sp, and *Serratia.* Some activity against coagulase-positive staphylococci but ineffective against anaerobes and streptococci. Provides some synergistic effect against group D streptococci (enterococci) when used in combination with a penicillin.

Supplied: Injection, intrathecal injection, ophthalmic solution.

Route: IM, IV (infuse over 30 minutes), IT.

Dosage: Dosage should always be monitored and adjusted by use of pharmacokinetics. Initial empirical dose can be based on body weight.

- Intravenous:
  < 1500 g: 3 mg/kg/d q24h.
  1500–2500 g: 3 mg/kg/d divided q12h.
  > 2500 g: 5 mg/kg/d divided q8h.
- Intrathecal or intraventricular: 1–2 mg qd.
- Ophthalmic solution: 1 drop OU q4–12h.

Elimination and metabolism: Renal excretion by glomerular filtration. Half-life is 4–8 hours initially.

Adverse effects: Irreversible vestibular injury, proteinuria, uremia, oliguria, macular rash.

Comments: Desired serum peak is 5–10 μg/mL (sample obtained 30 minutes after infusion completed) and desired serum trough is < 2 μg/mL (sample obtained 30 minutes to just prior to next dose). In general, a set of peak and trough levels should be obtained at about the fourth maintenance dose. Adjust dosage pharmacokinetically. Monitor serum creatinine every 3–4 days. Excessive serum peak levels are associated with ototoxicity and excessive trough levels with nephrotoxicity. May give orally in nursery epidemics of enteropathogenic *E coli* or NEC.

Note: The aminoglycosides should never be used alone against gram-positive pathogens.

Isoniazid (Laniazid, Nydrazid)

Classification: Antituberculous agent.

Action and spectrum: Bactericidal effect on growing tubercle bacilli by interfering with lipid and protein synthesis. Spectrum includes *Mycobacterium* spp (*M tuberculosis, M kansasii, M avium*).

Supplied: Injection, tablets.

Route: PO, IM.

Dosage:

- Primary tuberculosis: 10–15 mg/kg/d divided q12–24h with rifampin for 9–12 months.
- Skin test conversion: 10–15 mg/kg/24h PO q24h for 9 months.

Adverse effects: Peripheral neuropathy, seizures, encephalopathy, blood dyscrasias, allergy, reddish discoloration of all body secretions.

Comments: Concurrent administration of pyridoxine, 1–2 mg/kg/d, is recommended.

Kanamycin Sulfate (Kantrex)

Classification: Aminoglycoside.

Action and spectrum: Mechanism of action is identical to that of gentamicin. Active primarily against gram-negative aerobic bacteria, including *Escherichia coli, Klebsiella, Enterobacter, Serratia, Proteus,* and some *Pseudomonas* sp. Some activity against staphylococci and mycobacteria. Not active against other gram-positive organisms or anaerobes.

Supplied: Injection.

Route: IM or IV (infuse over 30 minutes).

Dosage: Dosage should always be monitored and adjusted by use of pharmacokinetics. Initial empirical dose can be based on body weight.

- < 1500 g: 10 mg/kg/d q24h.
- 1500–2500 g: 10 mg/kg/d divided q12h.
- > 2500 g: 20 mg/kg/d divided q12h.

Elimination and metabolism: Primarily renally excreted by glomerular filtration. Half-life is 4–8 hours.

Adverse effects: See Gentamicin.

Comments: See Gentamicin. Desired serum peak is 25–35 μg/mL (sample obtained 30 minutes after infusion complete) and serum trough is < 10 μg/mL (sample obtained 30 minutes to just prior to next dose). In general, a set of serum peak and trough levels should be obtained at about the fourth maintenance dose. Monitor serum creatinine every 3–4 days. Excessive serum peak levels are associated with ototoxicity and excessive trough levels with nephrotoxicity.

Ketoconazole (Nizoral)

Classification: Antifungal agent.

Action and spectrum: A broad-spectrum antifungal agent that acts by disrupting cell membranes. Fungicidal against *Blastomyces dermatitidis, Candida* sp, *Coccidioides immitis, Histoplasma capsulatum, Paracoccidioides brasiliensis,* and *Phialophora* sp. Development of resistance is rare.

Supplied: Oral suspension, tablets.

Route: PO.

Dosage: 2.5–5 mg/kg/d q24h.

Elimination and metabolism: Hepatic metabolism.

Adverse effects: Gastric distress is the most common side effect. Hepatic damage is rare.

Comments: Penetration into CSF is poor, which means that ketoconazole should not be used in the treatment of fungal meningitis. Minimum period of treatment for candidiasis is 1–2 weeks, but duration should be based on clinical response. Monitor liver function tests.

Note: Limited experience in neonates.

Methicillin Sodium (Staphcillin)

Classification: Penicillinase-resistant penicillin.

Action and spectrum: Mechanism of action identical to that of other β-lactam antibiotics. Active chiefly against penicillinase-positive and penicillinase-negative staphylococci. Less effective than penicillin G against other gram-positive cocci. No activity against enterococci.

Supplied: Injection.

Route: IM or IV (infuse over 20 minutes).

Dosage:

- Meningitis:
  < 2000 g and 0–7 days old: 100 mg/kg/d divided q12h.
  < 2000 g and > 7 days old: 150 mg/kg/d divided q8h.
  > 2000 g and 0–7 days old: 150 mg/kg/d divided q8h.
  > 2000 g and > 7 days old: 200 mg/kg/d divided q6h.
- Other diseases:
  < 2000 g and 0–7 days old: 50 mg/kg/d divided q12h.
  < 2000 g and > 7 days old: 75 mg/kg/d divided q8h.
  > 2000 g and 0–7 days old: 75 mg/kg/d divided q8h.
  > 2000 g and > 7 days old: 100 mg/kg/d divided q6h.

Elimination and metabolism: Renal. Half-life variable (60–120 minutes or longer).

Adverse effects: Nephrotoxicity (interstitial nephritis) occurs more often with methicillin than with other penicillins. May cause hypersensitivity reactions, anemia, leukopenia, thrombocytopenia, phlebitis at infusion site, and hemorrhagic cystitis (in poorly hydrated patients).

Comments: In cases of methicillin resistance, vancomycin becomes the antistaphylococcal drug of choice. Dosage adjustment necessary in renal impairment. Monitor serum urea nitrogen and creatinine. Contains 2.9 meq sodium per gram.

Metronidazole (Flagyl, others)

Classification: Bactericidal antibiotic.

Action and spectrum: The mechanism of action is not established. Good activity against anaerobic protozoa, including *Trichomonas vaginalis, Entamoeba histolytica, Giardia lamblia,* and *Balantidium coli.* Good activity also against gram-positive bacteria (*Clostridium* spp, *Peptococcus, Peptostreptococcus,* and *Veillonella* spp) and anaerobic gram-negative bacteria (*Bacteroides* spp and *Fusobacterium* spp). Nonsporulating gram-positive bacilli are often resistant (eg, *Propionibacterium* spp, *Actinomyces*), and the drug has minimal activity against aerobic and facultative anaerobic bacteria.

Supplied: Tablets, injection.

Route: PO or IV (infuse commercial dilution over 1 hour).

Dosage:

- < 2000 g: 15 mg/kg/d divided q12h.
- > 2000 g and 0–7 days old: 15 mg/kg/d divided q12h.
- > 2000 g and > 7 days old: 30 mg/kg/d divided q12h.

Elimination and metabolism: Hepatic metabolism with final excretion via the urine and feces. Large volume of distribution (penetrates into all body tissues and fluids).

Adverse effects: Occasional vomiting, diarrhea, insomnia, weakness, rash, phlebitis at injection site. Rarely, ataxia and leukopenia. Disulfiram-like reaction occurs with alcohol ingestion. Mutagenicity and carcinogenicity may occur, but not established in humans.

Comments: Some texts recommend an initial loading dose of 15 mg/kg, with the first maintenance dose either 48 hours later (for premature infants < 2000 g) or 24 hours later (for the infant > 2000 g at birth). Effectively penetrates into the CSF and therefore indicated for meningitis due to susceptible anaerobic pathogens.

Note: Some centers use empiric coverage with ampicillin and gentamicin for NEC. The use of metronidazole in NEC remains controversial.

Mezlocillin Sodium (Mezlin)

Classification: Semisynthetic extended-spectrum penicillin.

Action and spectrum: Mechanism of action identical to that of other β-lactam antibiotics. Effective principally against gram-negative organisms, including *Haemophilus influenzae, Klebsiella pneumoniae, Proteus mirabilis, Escherichia coli, Pseudomonas aeruginosa,* and some *Serratia* spp. Active also against many anaerobes, including *Peptococcus* spp, *Peptostreptococcus* spp, and *Bacteroides* spp (eg, *Bacteroides fragilis*).

Supplied: Injection.

Route: IM or IV (infuse over 30 minutes).

Dosage:

- 0–7 days: 150 mg/kg/d divided q12h.
- > 7 days: 225 mg/kg/d divided q8h.

Elimination and metabolism: Excreted primarily unchanged with urine; less than 10% hepatically metabolized.

Adverse effects: See Carbenicillin and Penicillin G (Aqueous), Parenteral.

Comments: Does not cause platelet dysfunction. Avoid IM use if possible. Adjust dosage in renal impairment. Mezlocillin contains 1.85 meq sodium per gram.

Note: Limited experience in neonates.

Nafcillin Sodium (Unipen)

Classification: Semisynthetic penicillinase-resistant penicillin.

Action and spectrum: Mechanism of action identical to that of other β-lactam antibiotics. Spectrum identical to that of methicillin (ie, primarily antistaphylococcal).

Supplied: Injection.

Route: IM or IV (infuse over 30 minutes).

Dosage:

- < 2000 g and 0–7 days old: 50 mg/kg/d divided q12h.
- < 2000 g and > 7 days old: 75 mg/kg/d divided q8h.
- > 2000 g and 0–7 days old: 50 mg/kg/d divided q8h.
- > 2000 g and > 7 days old: 75 mg/kg/d divided q6h.

Elimination and metabolism: Hepatic metabolism; concentrated in bile.

Adverse effects: Thrombophlebitis, hypersensitivity, and leukopenia.

Comments: Avoid IM use. Contains 2.9 meq sodium per gram.

Neomycin Sulfate (Mycifradin, others)

Classification: Aminoglycoside.

Action and spectrum: Mechanism of action identical to that of gentamicin. Indicated in the treatment of diarrhea due to enteropathogenic *Escherichia coli* and as preoperative prophylaxis before intestinal surgery.

Supplied: Tablets, oral solution. (125 mg/5 mL).

Route: PO.

Dosage: 50–100 mg/kg/d divided q4–6h.

Elimination and metabolism: Renal excretion if systemic absorption occurs; otherwise fecally excreted.

Adverse effects: Sensitization with allergic reaction.

Comments: Poorly absorbed from gastrointestinal tract. Inactive against anaerobic organisms.

Netilmicin Sulfate (Netromycin)

Classification: Aminoglycoside.

Action and spectrum: See Gentamicin.

Supplied: Injection.

Route: IM or IV (infuse over 30 minutes).

Dosage: Monitor and adjust by pharmacokinetics. Initial empirical dosing based on body weight:

- < 1500 g: 3 mg/kg/d divided q12h.
- 1500–2500 g: 3 mg/kg/d divided q12h.
- > 2500 g: 5 mg/kg/d divided q12h.

Elimination and metabolism: Renal excretion. Half-life is 4–8 hours.

Adverse effects: Ototoxicity associated with serum peak concentrations greater than 12 μg/mL; nephrotoxicity associated with serum trough concentrations greater than 4 μg/mL.

Comments: Monitor and adjust pharmacokinetically to maintain serum peak concentrations between 6 and 10 μg/mL (sample obtained 30 minutes after infusion completed) and serum trough concentrations below 3 μg/mL (sample obtained 30 minutes to just before next dose). Obtain initial set of serum peak and trough levels at about the fourth maintenance dose. Monitor serum creatinine every 3–4 days. Other comments: see Gentamicin.

Note: Limited experience in neonates.

Nystatin (Mycostatin, Nilstat)

Action and spectrum: Fungistatic and fungicidal in vitro against a wide variety of yeasts and yeastlike fungi. Acts by disrupting cell membranes. Neonatal indications include oral candidiasis (thrush), *Candida* diaper rash, and benign mucocutaneous candidiasis.

Supplied: Oral suspension, 100,000 units/mL; topical cream, powder, and ointment, 100,000 units/g.

Route: PO, topical.

Dosage:

- Oral thrush: 0.5–1 mL to each side of the mouth tid–qid after feedings for 7–10 days.
- Diaper rash: Topical cream applied tid–qid for 7–10 days.

Elimination and metabolism: Poorly absorbed. Most is passed unchanged in the stool.

Adverse effects: Side effects uncommon.

Comments: Owing to the drying effect, the cream form is preferred if the diaper rash area is weeping.

Oxacillin Sodium (Bactocill, Prostaphlin)

Classification: Semisynthetic penicillinase-resistant penicillin.

Action and spectrum: Mechanism of action is identical to that of other β-lactam antibiotics. Spectrum of activity is identical to that of nafcillin and methicillin. Primary use is as a surgical prophylactic agent.

Supplied: Injection.

Route: IM or IV (infuse over 30 minutes).

Dosage:

- < 2000 g and 0–7 days old: 50 mg/kg/d divided q12h.
- < 2000 g and > 7 days old: 100 mg/kg/d divided q8h.
- > 2000 g and 0–7 days old: 75 mg/kg/d divided q8h.
- > 2000 g and > 7 days old: 150 mg/kg/d divided q6h.

Elimination and metabolism: Metabolized chiefly in the liver and excreted in bile. Renal excretion is substantial but requires no adjustment in renal failure.

Adverse effects: Hypersensitivity reactions (rash), thrombophlebitis, mild leukopenia, elevation in AST (SGOT).

Comments: Avoid IM injection of oxacillin. This drug contains 2.8 meq sodium per gram.

Penicillin G (Aqueous), Parenteral

Action and spectrum: Mechanism of action is identical to that of other β-lactam antibiotics. Effective mainly against streptococci, some community-acquired staphylococci (except methicillin-resistant and penicillinase-producing strains), *Neisseria gonorrhoeae, Neisseria meningitidis, Bacillus anthracis, Clostridium tetani, Clostridium perfringens, Bacteroides* (oropharyngeal strains), *Leptospira,* and *Treponema pallidum.*

Supplied: Injection, potassium (Pfizerpen) or sodium.

Route: IM or IV (infuse over 20 minutes).

Dosage:

- Meningitis:
  < 2000 g and 0–7 days old: 100,000 units/kg/d divided q12h.
  < 2000 g and > 7 days old: 150,000 units/kg/d divided q8h.
  > 2000 g and 0–7 days old: 150,000 units/kg/d divided q8h.
  > 2000 g and > 7 days old: 200,000 units/kg/d divided q6h.
- Other diseases:
  < 2000 g and 0–7 days old: 50,000 units/kg/d divided q12h.
  < 2000 g and > 7 days old: 75,000 units/kg/d divided q8h.
  > 2000 g and 0–7 days old: 50,000 units/kg/d divided q8h.
  > 2000 g and > 7 days old: 100,000 units/kg/d divided q6h.

Elimination and metabolism: Renal.

Adverse effects: Allergic reactions, rarely anaphylactic. Rash, fever, change in bowel flora, *Candida* superinfection, diarrhea, hemolytic anemia. Very large doses may cause seizures.

Comments: 1600 units = 1 mg. Some strains of group B streptococci are penicillinase producers, thus requiring the addition of an aminoglycoside antibiotic for synergistic bactericidal effect. Good activity against anaerobes. Drug of choice for tetanus neonatorum. Contains 1.7 meq of sodium or potassium per million units.

Penicillin G Benzathine (Bicillin L-A, Permapen)

Action and spectrum: See Penicillin G (Aqueous), Parenteral. A drug of choice in the treatment of asymptomatic congenital syphilis.

Supplied: Injection.

Route: IM only. (Viscosity requires ≥ 23-gauge needle.)

Dosage: 50,000 units/kg once.

Elimination and metabolism: Renally excreted over a prolonged interval owing to slow absorption from the injection site.

Adverse effects and comments: See Penicillin G (Aqueous), Parenteral. 1211 units = 1 mg. Not often used.

Penicillin G Procaine (Duracillin A.S., Wycillin)

Action and spectrum: See Penicillin G (Aqueous), Parenteral. A drug of choice in the treatment of symptomatic or asymptomatic congenital syphilis.

Supplied: Injection.

Route: IM only. (Viscosity requires ≥ 23-gauge needle.)

Dosage: 50,000 units/kg/dose q24h.

Elimination and metabolism: See Penicillin G (Aqueous), Parenteral.

Adverse effects: See Penicillin G (Aqueous), Parenteral. May also cause sterile abscess formation at injection site. Contains 120 mg procaine per 300,000 units, which may cause allergic reactions, myocardial depression, or systemic vasodilatation. There is cause for much greater concern about these effects in the neonate than in older patients.

Comments: 1000 units = 1 mg. Not often used.

Piperacillin Sodium (Pipracil)

Classification: Semisynthetic extended-spectrum penicillin.

Action and spectrum: See Mezlocillin. Good in vivo activity against *Pseudomonas aeruginosa.*

Supplied: Injection.

Route: IM or IV (infuse over 30 minutes).

Dosage:

- < 2000 g and 0–7 days old: 150 mg/kg/d divided q12h.
- < 2000 g and > 7 days old: 225 mg/kg/d divided q8h.
- > 2000 g and 0–7 days old: 225 mg/kg/d divided q8h.
- > 2000 g and > 7 days old: 300 mg/kg/d divided q6h.

Elimination and metabolism: Excreted unchanged in the urine.

Adverse effects: See Mezlocillin. Hypokalemia and leukopenia are less pronounced.

Comments: Avoid IM use where possible. Should be reserved for cases resistant to ticarcillin. Contains 1.85 meq (42.5 mg) sodium per gram.

Polymyxin B Sulfate (Aerosporin)

Action and spectrum: Acts by disrupting the integrity of the bacterial cell wall. Bactericidal against most aerobic gram-negative bacilli. Chiefly useful against *Pseudomonas.* Effective also against *Escherichia coli, Enterobacter,* and *Klebsiella.* Not active against *Proteus.*

Supplied: Injection.

Route: PO, IV (dilute to final concentration of 1000–2000 units/mL in 5% dextrose and infuse over 1–2 hours).

Dosage:

- IV: 30,000–40,000 units/kg/d divided q8h.
- PO: 10–20 mg/kg/d divided q6–8h for up to 5 days.

Elimination and metabolism: Slow renal excretion.

Adverse effects: May cause reversible renal injury (proteinuria, hematuria, azotemia), rash, fever, neuromuscular blockade (rare), thrombophlebitis at injection site.

Comments: Poor tissue penetration. Does not cross blood-brain barrier. Not absorbed orally. Not often used.

Pyrimethamine (Daraprim)

Action and spectrum: Folic acid antagonist selective for plasmodial dihydrofolate reductase. Activity highly selective for plasmodia (cidal) and *Toxoplasma gondii.*

Supplied: Tablets.

Route: PO.

Dosage: For toxoplasmosis, give 1 mg/kg/d divided q12h for 4 weeks. Combine with sulfadiazine.

Elimination and metabolism: Hepatic metabolism.

Adverse effects: Anorexia, vomiting, megaloblastic anemia, leukopenia, thrombocytopenia, pancytopenia, atrophic glossitis, rash, seizures, shock.

Comments: Give folinic acid (leucovorin), 1 mg orally daily or 3 mg twice weekly, if leukopenia or thrombocytopenia occurs. Administer with feedings if vomiting persists. Give sulfadiazine alone in empirical therapy of toxoplasmosis until the diagnosis is ruled out. Reduced dosage in hepatic dysfunction.

Rifampin (Rifadin, Rimactane)

Action and spectrum: A broad-spectrum antibiotic that exerts its bacteriostatic action by inhibiting DNA-dependent RNA polymerase activity. Effective against mycobacteria, *Neisseria,* and gram-positive cocci (eg, staphylococci). Resistance develops rapidly, so the drug should always be used in combination with other agents for synergistic effect.

Supplied: Capsules. (10 mg/mL extemporaneous preparation available.)

Route: PO, IV.

Dosage: 10–20 mg/kg/d divided q12h.

Elimination and metabolism: Hepatic. Half-life is about 3 hours.

Adverse effects: Gastrointestinal irritation (anorexia, vomiting, diarrhea), hypersensitivity (rash, pruritus, eosinophilia), drowsiness, ataxia, blood dyscrasias (leukopenia, thrombocytopenia, hemolytic anemia), hepatitis (rare), elevation of serum urea nitrogen and uric acid levels. Causes pink to red discoloration of urine.

Comments: Crosses into CSF. When rifampin is used, it should always be added to other agents to provide synergistic effect (eg, vancomycin plus gentamicin with or without rifampin for infection with vancomycin-resistant or tolerant staphylococci).

Note: Rifampin is a potent enzyme inducer of hepatic metabolism. Patients receiving phenytoin, phenobarbital, or theophylline preparation may have a substantial decrease in serum concentration of these drugs after starting rifampin. Careful monitoring of serum drug concentrations is necessary.

Sulfacetamide Sodium (Isopto Cetamide, Sodium Sulamyd, others)

Action and spectrum: Mechanism, see sulfadiazine. Indicated in acute conjunctivitis. Spectrum includes *Staphylococcus aureus, Streptococcus pneumoniae, Haemophilus influenzae* and *Moraxella* spp.

Supplied: Ophthalmic solution (10%), ointment.

Route: Topical.

Dosage: 1–2 gtts ou q2h initially, then increase time interval as condition responds or $\frac{1}{4}$ inch ointment ou q4–6h for 7–10 days.

Comments: See sulfadiazine for adverse effects. May cause local irritation. Ophthalmic solution preferred over neomycin-containing ophthalmic preparation because of decreased incidence of local irritation and allergic response.

Sulfadiazine

Action and spectrum: Acts via competitive antagonism of *p*-aminobenzoic acid, an essential factor in folic acid synthesis. Spectrum of action includes both gram-positive and gram-negative organisms. In neonatology, used chiefly against *Toxoplasma gondii* in combination with pyrimethamine.

Supplied: Tablets.

Route: PO.

Dosage: For toxoplasmosis, give 120 mg/kg/d divided q6h for 4 weeks. Combine with pyrimethamine.

Elimination and metabolism: Rapid renal excretion.

Adverse effects: Hypersensitivity (fever, rash, hepatitis, vasculitis, lupuslike syndrome), neutropenia, agranulocytosis, thrombocytopenia, aplastic anemia, Stevens-Johnson syndrome, crystalluria (keep urine alkaline and output high). Kernicterus may occur.

Comments: Avoid use in neonates except for treatment of congenital toxoplasmosis. See comments under pyrimethamine regarding folinic acid use.

Ticarcillin Disodium (Ticar)

Classification: Semisynthetic extended-spectrum penicillin.

Action and spectrum: See Mezlocillin.

Supplied: Injection.

Route: IM or IV (infuse over 30 minutes).

Dosage:

- < 2000 g and 0–7 days old: 150 mg/kg/d divided q12h.
- < 2000 g and > 7 days old: 225 mg/kg/d divided q8h.
- > 2000 g and 0–7 days old: 225 mg/kg/d divided q8h.
- > 2000 g and > 7 days old: 300 mg/kg/d divided q6h.

Elimination and metabolism: Renally excreted.

Adverse effects: See Mezlocillin. Hypokalemia pronounced.

Comments: Drug of first choice when considering an extended-spectrum penicillin. Avoid IM use if possible. Contains 5.2 meq sodium per gram.

Ticarcillin Disodium and Clavulanate Potassium (Timentin)

Classification: Combination antibiotic of ticarcillin (a carboxypenicillin) and clavulanic acid (β-lactamase inhibitor).

Spectrum: Good antipseudomonal activity similar to ticarcillin except additional coverage of lactamase-producing species, particularly gram-positive cocci (eg, *Staphylococcus aureus*, *Streptococcus pneumoniae* and group B streptococcus). Good coverage against gram-negative organisms, including *E coli*, *Klebsiella*, and *Proteus*. Also demonstrated activity against anaerobes like *Clostridium* and *Peptostreptococcus*.

Supplied: Injection.

Route: IV.

Dosage:

- < 2000 g and 0–7 days old: 150 mg/kg/d divided q12h.
- < 2000 g and > 7 days old: 225 mg/kg/d divided q8h.
- > 2000 g and 0–7 days old: 225 mg/kg/d divided q8h.
- > 2000 g and > 7 days old: 300 mg/kg/d divided q6h.

Elimination: Ticarcillin, renal (tubular secretion); clavulanic acid, hepatic and renal.

Adverse effects: See Ticarcillin.

Tobramycin Sulfate (Nebcin)

Classification: Aminoglycoside.

Action and spectrum: Mechanism of action and spectrum identical to those of gentamicin.

Supplied: Injection, ophthalmic drops, ophthalmic ointment.

Route: IM or IV (infuse over 30 minutes), topical (ophthalmic).

Dosage:

- IM or IV: Monitor and adjust by pharmacokinetics. Initial empirical dosing based on body weight:

    < 1500 g: 3 mg/kg/d q24h.

1500–2500 g: 3 mg/kg/d divided q12h.
> 2500 g: 5 mg/kg/d divided q8h.
- Ophthalmic: Instill 1 or 2 drops OU 2–6 times a day or more often as needed; or apply a small amount of ointment OU q3–4h until improvement occurs. Reduce treatment prior to discontinuance.

Elimination and metabolism: Renal.

Adverse effects: See Gentamicin.

Comments: Reserve for cases resistant to gentamicin. Obtain serum peak and trough concentrations at about the fourth maintenance dose. Desired serum peak concentration is 5–10 μg/mL (sample obtained 30 minutes after infusion complete); desired serum trough concentration is < 2 μg/mL (sample obtained 30 minutes to just before the next dose).

Vancomycin Hydrochloride (Vancocin, others)

Action and spectrum: Bactericidal action by interference with bacterial cell wall synthesis. Active against most gram-positive cocci and bacilli, including streptococci, staphylococci (including methicillin-resistant staphylococci), clostridia (including *Clostridium difficile*), *Corynebacterium,* and *Listeria monocytogenes.* Bacteriostatic against enterococci. No cross-resistance between vancomycin and other antibiotics has been reported. The drug of choice against methicillin-resistant staphylococci and *C difficile.*

Supplied: Injection, oral solution.

Route: IV, PO.

Dosage:

- IV: Monitor and adjust by pharmacokinetics. Initial empirical dosing based on body weight:

	CNS Infections	Other Infections
< 800 g and < 27 weeks old:	35 mg/kg/dose q36h	27 mg/kg/dose q36h
800–1200 g and 27–30 weeks old:	32 mg/kg/dose q36h	24 mg/kg/dose q24h
1200–2000 g and 31–36 weeks old:	35 mg/kg/dose q18h	27 mg/kg/dose q18h
	or	or
	24 mg/kg/dose q12h	18 mg/kg/dose q12h
> 2000 g and > 36 weeks old but < 7 days old:	30 mg/kg/dose q12h	22.5 mg/kg/dose q12h
>2000 g and > 7 days old:	20 mg/kg/dose q8h	15 mg/kg/dose q8h

- PO: To treat pseudomembranous colitis due to *C difficile* or staphylococcal enterocolitis, give 20–40 mg/kg/d divided q6h for 5–7 days.

Elimination and metabolism: Renally excreted. Half-life 7–9 hours.

Adverse effects: Allergy (rash, fever, anaphylaxis), ototoxicity (with serum peak levels > 40 μg/mL), nephrotoxicity (serum trough levels > 10 μg/mL), thrombophlebitis at site of injection. Too rapid infusion may cause rash, chills, and fever (red-man syndrome) mimicking anaphylactic reaction. Rapid infusion may cause apnea and bradycardia without other signs of "red-man syndrome." Infuse dose over at least 60 minutes.

Comments: Monitor and adjust dose pharmacokinetically to maintain serum peak levels of 20–40 μg/mL (sample drawn 30 minutes after infusion complete) and serum trough levels of 5–10 μg/mL (sample drawn 30 minutes to just before next dose). In general, draw serum peak and trough levels at about the fourth maintenance dose. Monitor serum creatinine. If staphylococci exhibit vancomycin tolerance, combine vancomycin and an aminoglycoside with or without rifampin. Oral doses are poorly absorbed. Powder for injection, diluted and flavored, is the most economical means of oral dosing.

Vidarabine (Vira-A)

Action and spectrum: Antiviral agent for treatment of herpes encephalitis. Inhibits viral DNA formation. Good activity against herpes simplex type 1, poor activity against adenoviruses or RNA viruses. Activity against varicella-zoster virus unconfirmed.

Supplied: Injection (monohydrate), 200 mg/mL, equivalent to 187.4 mg vidarabine; ophthalmic ointment, 3%.

Route: Ophthalmic, IV (dilute to 1 mg/2.2 mL and infuse over 12–24 hours).

Dosage:

- Ophthalmic: Apply a small amount OU q3h.
- IV:
  - < 1 month: 30 mg/kg q18–24h.
  - > 1 month: 15 mg/kg/d.

Adverse effects: Rash, pain at injection site. Decreased reticulocyte count, white cell count, and platelet count. Elevated total bilirubin and AST (SGOT).

Comments: Rarely used. Volume necessary for IV infusion may cause fluid overload. Acyclovir is usual agent of choice. Must filter final solution (use 0.45-micron filter).

77 Effects of Drugs and Substances on Lactation and Breast-Feeding

The drugs and substances listed below are those for which reliable data on their effect during lactation have been compiled. This listing is undoubtedly incomplete as it is impossible to list every possible medication. Clinical judgment about the possible effects of maternal drug intake while nursing must always be exercised.

Drug or Substance	Compatability with Breast-Feeding, Effect on Lactation and Adverse Effects on Infant
Acetaminophen	Generally compatible with breast-feeding.
Albuterol	Generally compatible with breast-feeding. Monitor for agitation and spitting up. Use inhaled form to decrease maternal absorption.
Alcohol	Generally compatible with breast-feeding. Monitor for drowsiness, diaphoresis, weakness, and failure to thrive. Intake of 1 g/kg/d may decrease maternal milk ejection reflex.
Amantadine	Contraindicated. Causes release of levodopa in central nervous system.
Amikacin	Generally compatible with breast-feeding. Low concentrations in breast milk because of poor oral absorption.
Aminoglycosides	Generally compatible with breast-feeding. All antibiotics are excreted in breast milk in limited amounts. Apparently safe, not absorbed in newborn gastrointestinal tract. Monitor for diarrhea.
Aminophylline	Generally compatible with breast-feeding. Monitor for irritability.
Amiodarone	Breast-feeding is not recommended because of iodine contained in each dose and possible accumulation of amiodarone in the infant.
Amitriptyline	Generally compatible with breast-feeding.
Amoxapine	Generally compatible with breast-feeding.
Amoxicillin	Generally compatible with breast-feeding. Monitor for diarrhea.
Amphetamine	Generally compatible with breast-feeding. Monitor for irritability, poor sleeping patterns.
Ampicillin	Generally compatible with breast-feeding. Monitor for diarrhea.
Aspartame	Generally compatible with breast-feeding. Use cautiously in carrier of phenylketonuria.
Aspirin	Generally compatible with breast-feeding. Monitor for spitting up or bleeding. Increased risk with high doses used for rheumatoid arthritis (3–5 g/d).
Atenolol	Generally compatible with breast-feeding.

Drug or Substance	Compatability with Breast-Feeding, Effect on Lactation and Adverse Effects on Infant
Atropine	Generally compatible with breast-feeding. No adverse effects reported.
Bethanechol	Generally compatible with breast-feeding. May cause abdominal pain and diarrhea.
Bromides	Breast-feeding not recommended because of possible drowsiness and rash.
Bromocriptine	Contraindicated. Suppresses lactation.
Brompheniramine	Generally compatible with breast-feeding. Monitor for agitation, poor sleeping pattern, feeding problems.
Butorphanol	Generally compatible with breast-feeding.
Caffeine	Generally compatible with breast-feeding. Monitor for irritability, poor sleeping patterns.
Calcitonin	May inhibit lactation.
Captopril	Generally compatible with breast-feeding.
Carbamazepine	Generally compatible with breast-feeding. Risk of bone marrow suppression if taken chronically.
Carbimazole	Generally compatible with breast-feeding. Monitor for goiter.
Cascara sagrada	Generally compatible with breast-feeding. Monitor for diarrhea.
Cefaclor	Generally compatible with breast-feeding. Monitor for diarrhea.
Cefadroxil	Generally compatible with breast-feeding. Monitor for diarrhea.
Cefamandole	Generally compatible with breast-feeding. Monitor for diarrhea.
Cefazolin	Generally compatible with breast-feeding. Monitor for diarrhea.
Cefonicid	Generally compatible with breast-feeding. Monitor for diarrhea.
Cefoperazone	Generally compatible with breast-feeding. Monitor for diarrhea.
Ceforanide	Generally compatible with breast-feeding. Monitor for diarrhea.
Cefotaxime	Generally compatible with breast-feeding. Monitor for diarrhea.
Ceftizoxime	Generally compatible with breast-feeding. Monitor for diarrhea.
Ceftrlaxone	Generally compatible with breast-feeding. Monitor for diarrhea.
Cefuroxime	Generally compatible with breast-feeding. Monitor for diarrhea.
Cephalexin	Generally compatible with breast-feeding. Monitor for diarrhea.
Cephalosporins	Generally compatible with breast-feeding. All antibiotics are excreted in breast milk in limited amounts. Monitor for rash; sensitization possible.
Cephalothin	Generally compatible with breast-feeding. Monitor for diarrhea.
Cephapirin	Generally compatible with breast-feeding. Monitor for diarrhea.
Cephradine	Generally compatible with breast-feeding. Monitor for diarrhea.

Drug or Substance	Compatability with Breast-Feeding, Effect on Lactation and Adverse Effects on Infant
Chloral hydrate	Generally compatible with breast-feeding. Monitor for sedation, rash.
Chloramphenicol	Discontinue during breast-feeding. Risk of bone marrow toxicity. Nurse after 24 hours off the drug.
Chloroform	Generally compatible with breast-feeding.
Chloroquine	Generally compatible with breast-feeding.
Chlorothiazide	Generally compatible with breast-feeding but may suppress lactation, especially in first month of lactation. Adverse effects have not been reported, but infant's electrolytes and platelets should be monitored.
Chlorpheniramine	Generally compatible with breast-feeding. Monitor for agitation, poor sleeping pattern, feeding problems.
Chlorpromazine	Generally compatible with breast-feeding. Monitor for sedation.
Chlorpropamide	Contraindicated. Excreted in breast milk and may cause hypoglycemia.
Chlortetracycline	Generally compatible with breast-feeding. Monitor for diarrhea.
Chocolate	Generally compatible with breast-feeding. Irritability or increased bowel activity if mother consumes excessive amounts (> 16 oz/d).
Cimetidine	Contraindicated. May suppress gastric acidity in infant, inhibit drug metabolism, and cause CNS stimulation.
Clindamycin	Discontinue during breast-feeding. Risk of gastrointestinal bleeding. Nurse after 24 hours off the drug.
Clonazepam	Generally compatible with breast-feeding. Monitor for respiratory and CNS depression.
Clonidine	Contraindicated. Excreted in breast milk.
Cloxacillin	Generally compatible with breast-feeding. Monitor for diarrhea.
Cocaine	Contraindicated. Causes cocaine intoxication in infant from maternal intranasal use (hypertension, tachycardia, mydriasis, apnea) and from topical use on mother's nipples (apnea and seizures).
Codeine	Generally compatible with breast-feeding. Monitor for sedation. Milk ejection reflex (letdown) may be inhibited.
Contraceptives, oral	Contraindicated. Can cause breast enlargement and proliferation of vaginal epithelium in infants.
Coumadin (warfarin, dicumarol)	Generally compatible with breast-feeding.
Cyclophosphamide	Contraindicated. Possible immune suppression. Unknown effect on growth or association with carcinogenesis.
Cyproheptadine	Generally compatible with breast-feeding. Monitor for agitation, poor sleeping pattern, feeding problems.
Desipramine	Generally compatible with breast-feeding.
Dextroamphetamine	Contraindicated. May cause infant stimulation.
Diazepam	Contraindicated. May cause infant sedation.

Drug or Substance	Compatability with Breast-Feeding, Effect on Lactation and Adverse Effects on Infant
Diazoxide	Contraindicated. May case hyperglycemia.
Dicumarol	See Coumadin.
Digoxin	Generally compatible with breast-feeding. Monitor for spitting up, diarrhea, heart rate changes.
Diphenhydramine	Generally compatible with breast-feeding. Monitor for agitation, poor sleeping pattern, feeding problems.
Dipyridamole	Generally compatible with breast-feeding.
Disopyramide	Generally compatible with breast-feeding.
Ephedrine	Generally compatible with breast-feeding. Monitor for agitation.
Ergotamine	Contraindicated. Causes vomiting, diarrhea, convulsions.
Erythromycin	Generally compatible with breast-feeding. Monitor for diarrhea.
Ethambutol	Generally compatible with breast-feeding.
Ethanol	See Alcohol.
Ethosuximide	Generally compatible with breast-feeding. Rare occurrence of bone marrow suppression and gastrointestinal upset.
Fava beans	Generally compatible with breast-feeding. Hemolysis in patients with G6PD deficiency.
Fenoprofen	Excreted in breast milk in small quantities.
Folic acid	Generally compatible with breast-feeding.
Gallium-69	Discontinue during breast-feeding. Radioactivity can remain in breast milk for 2 weeks.
Gentamicin	Generally compatible with breast-feeding. Monitor for diarrhea, bloody stools.
Gold salts	Contraindicated. May cause rash, inflammation of kidney and liver.
Guanethidine	Generally compatible with breast-feeding.
Haloperidol	Generally compatible with breast-feeding.
Halothane	Generally compatible with breast-feeding.
Heparin	Generally compatible with breast-feeding.
Heroin	Generally compatible with breast-feeding. Monitor for depression, withdrawal.
Hydralazine	Generally compatible with breast-feeding.
Hydromorphone	Generally compatible with breast-feeding. Monitor for sedation. Milk ejection reflex (letdown) may be inhibited.
Ibuprofen	Generally compatible with breast-feeding. Effects unknown.
Imipramine	Generally compatible with breast-feeding.
Insulin	Generally compatible with breast-feeding.
Iodine-125	Contraindicated. Risk of thyroid cancer. Radioactivity present in milk for 12 days.
Iodine-131	Contraindicated. Radioactivity in milk for 2–14 days.
Isoniazid	Generally compatible with breast-feeding. Monitor for rash, diarrhea, constipation.
Isoproterenol	Generally compatible with breast-feeding. Monitor for agitation, spitting up. Use aerosol form to decrease maternal absorption.
Isotretinoin	Contraindicated.
Kanamycin	Generally compatible with breast-feeding. Low concen-

Drug or Substance	Compatability with Breast-Feeding, Effect on Lactation and Adverse Effects on Infant
	trations in breast milk due to poor oral absorption. Monitor for diarrhea.
Labetalol	Generally compatible with breast-feeding. Monitor for hypotension, bradycardia.
Levodopa	Contraindicated. Inhibitory effect on prolactin release.
Levothyroxine (T₄)	Generally compatible with breast-feeding. Probably does not interfere with neonatal thyroid screening.
Liothyronine (T₃)	Generally compatible with breast-feeding. Probably does not interfere with neonatal thyroid screening.
Lithium	Probably compatible with breast-feeding; however, infant should be monitored for cyanosis, hypotonia, bradycardia, and other lithium toxicities, even though these have not been reported.
Lorazepam	Generally compatible with breast-feeding. Monitor for sedation.
Magnesium sulfate	Generally compatible with breast-feeding.
Meperidine	Generally compatible with breast-feeding. Monitor for sedation. Milk ejection reflex (letdown) may be inhibited.
Mepindolol	Generally compatible with breast-feeding. Monitor for hypotension, bradycardia.
Meprobamate	Generally compatible with breast-feeding but excreted in milk in high amounts. Monitor for sedation.
Metaproterenol	Generally compatible with breast-feeding. Monitor for agitation, spitting up. Use aerosol form to decrease maternal absorption.
Methadone	Generally compatible with breast-feeding. Monitor for sedation, depression, withdrawal on cessation of methadone treatment.
Methimazole	Contraindicated. Potential for interfering with thyroid function.
Methotrexate	Contraindicated. Possible immune suppression. Its effect on growth and association with carcinogenesis are unknown.
Methyldopa	Generally compatible with breast-feeding. Risk of hemolysis, increased liver enzymes.
Methyprylon	Generally compatible with breast-feeding. Monitor for drowsiness.
Metoclopramide	Generally compatible with breast-feeding. Increases milk production.
Metoprolol	Generally compatible with breast-feeding.
Metronidazole	Discontinue during breast-feeding. Do not nurse until 12–24 hours after discontinuing to allow excretion of drug.
Minoxidil	Generally compatible with breast-feeding. Monitor for hypotension.
Monosodium glutamate	Generally compatible with breast-feeding.
Morphine	Generally compatible with breast-feeding. Monitor for sedation. Milk ejection reflex (letdown) may be inhibited.
Nadolol	Generally compatible with breast-feeding.
Naproxen	Generally compatible with breast-feeding. Adverse ef-

Drug or Substance	Compatability with Breast-Feeding, Effect on Lactation and Adverse Effects on Infant
	fects unknown.
Nicotine	Generally compatible with breast-feeding. Excessive amounts may cause diarrhea, vomiting, tachycardia, irritability, and decreased milk production.
Nitrofurantoin	Generally compatible with breast-feeding. Excreted in milk in small amounts. Monitor infants with G6PD deficiency for hemolytic anemia.
Oral contraceptives	See Contraceptives, oral.
Oxacillin	Generally compatible with breast-feeding. Monitor for diarrhea.
Oxazepam	Generally compatible with breast-feeding. Monitor for sedation, depression.
Oxprenolol	Generally compatible with breast-feeding. Monitor for hypotension, bradycardia.
Oxycodone (Percodan, Percocet)	Generally compatible with breast-feeding. Monitor for drowsiness.
Penicillins	Generally compatible with breast-feeding. All antibiotics are excreted in breast milk in limited amounts. Monitor for rash, diarrhea, spitting up.
Phencyclidine	Contraindicated. Excreted in high amounts in breast milk.
Phenindione	Contraindicated. Causes hemorrhage in infants.
Phenobarbital	Generally compatible with breast-feeding. Monitor for sucking problems, sedation, rashes.
Phenylbutazone	Generally compatible with breast-feeding.
Phenylpropanolamine	Generally compatible with breast-feeding. Monitor for agitation.
Phenytoin	Generally compatible with breast-feeding. Monitor for methemoglobinuria (rare).
Pindolol	Generally compatible with breast-feeding. Monitor for hypotension, bradycardia.
Potassium iodide	Contraindicated. Goiter and allergic reactions may be seen.
Prednisone	Generally compatible with breast-feeding. Safety of long-term therapy has not been established. If maternal dose is more than 2 times physiologic, avoid breast-feeding.
Primidone	Generally compatible with breast-feeding. Monitor for irritability.
Prochlorperazine	Generally compatible with breast-feeding.
Propoxyphene	Generally compatible with breast-feeding. Monitor for withdrawal after long-term high-dose maternal use.
Propranolol	Generally compatible with breast-feeding. Monitor for hypotension, bradycardia.
Propylthiouracil	Generally compatible with breast-feeding.
Pseudoephedrine	Generally compatible with breast-feeding. Monitor for agitation.
Pyridoxine	Generally compatible with breast-feeding.
Pyrimethamine	Generally compatible with breast-feeding.
Quinidine	Generally compatible with breast-feeding. Monitor for rash, anemia, arrhythmias. Risk of optic neuritis with chronic use.

Drug or Substance	Compatability with Breast-Feeding, Effect on Lactation and Adverse Effects on Infant
Radiopharmaceuticals (generally)	Discontinue during breast-feeding. Consult nuclear medicine physician for selection of radionuclide with shortest excretion time.
Ranitidine	Contraindicated. May decrease infants gastric acidity.
Reserpine	Generally compatible with breast-feeding. Monitor for infantile galactorrhea.
Riboflavin	Generally compatible with breast-feeding.
Rifampin	Generally compatible with breast-feeding.
Saccharin	Generally compatible with breast-feeding.
Secobarbital	Generally compatible with breast-feeding.
Sulfamethoxazole, sulfonamide	Contraindicated. Highly bound drugs can displace bilirubin from protein, increasing risk of kernicterus, without effect on serum bilirubin.
Technitium-99m	Contraindicated. Radioactivity present in breast milk for 15 hours to 3 days.
Terbutaline	Generally compatible with breast-feeding. Monitor for agitation and spitting up. Use inhaled form to decrease maternal absorption if available.
Tetracyclines	Contraindicated. Causes staining of teeth and growth inhibition.
Theophylline	Generally compatible with breast-feeding. Monitor for irritability.
Thiamine	Generally compatible with breast-feeding.
Thioridazine	Generally compatible with breast-feeding.
Thiouracil	Contraindicated. Causes decreased thyroid function. (Does not apply to propylthiouracil.)
Ticarcillin	Generally compatible with breast-feeding. Monitor for diarrhea.
Timolol	Generally compatible with breast-feeding. Monitor for hypotension, bradycardia.
Tobramycin	Generally compatible with breast-feeding. Poor oral absorption. Monitor for diarrhea.
Tolbutamide	Generally compatible with breast-feeding. Monitor for jaundice.
Trifluoperazine	Generally compatible with breast-feeding.
Trimethoprim	Generally compatible with breast-feeding.
Valproic acid	Generally compatible with breast-feeding but carries risk of hepatitis, hemorrhagic pancreatitis.
Vegetarian diet	Generally compatible with breast-feeding. Monitor for vitamin B_{12} deficiency (failure to thrive, psychomotor retardation, megaloblastic anemia).
Vitamin B_{12}	Generally compatible with breast-feeding.
Vitamin D	Generally compatible with breast-feeding. Monitor for increased calcium levels.
Vitamin K	Generally compatible with breast-feeding.
Warfarin	See Coumadin.

78 Effects of Drugs and Substances Taken During Pregnancy

The drugs listed below include a fetal-risk category to indicate a systemically absorbed drug's potential for causing birth defects or neonatal disorders. Regardless of the designated risk category or presumed safety, no drug or substance should be used during pregnancy unless it is clearly needed. Please refer to the manufacturer's product literature or reference listed at the end of the chapter for further information.

FDA Fetal-Risk Categories

Category A	Adequate studies in pregnant women have not demonstrated a risk to the fetus in the first trimester of pregnancy; there is no evidence of risk in the last 2 trimesters.
Category B	Animal studies have not demonstrated a risk to the fetus, but there are no adequate studies in pregnant women.
	or
	Animal studies have shown an adverse effect, but adequate studies in pregnant women have not demonstrated a risk to the fetus during the first trimester of pregnancy and there is no evidence of risk in the last 2 trimesters.
Category C	Animal studies have shown an adverse effect on the fetus, but there are no adequate studies in humans. The benefits from the use of the drug in pregnant women may be acceptable despite its potential risks.
	or
	There are no animal reproduction studies and no adequate studies in humans.
Category D	There is evidence of human fetal risk, but the potential benefits from the use of the drug in pregnant women may be acceptable despite its potential risks.
Category X	Studies in animals or humans or adverse reaction reports, or both, have demonstrated fetal abnormalities. The risk of use in pregnant women clearly outweighs any possible benefit.

Drug or Substance	FDA Fetal Risk Category, Adverse Effects, and Clinical Comments
Acebutolol	Category B. May cause bradycardia and hypotension in infants exposed near term. Carefully monitor blood pressure and heart rate.

Drug or Substance	FDA Fetal Risk Category, Adverse Effects, and Clinical Comments
Acetaminophen	Category B. Safe for short-term use in therapeutic doses. If medication is required to treat fever or pain, use acetaminophen rather than aspirin.
Acetazolamide	Category C. No reports of fetal risk available.
Acetohexamide	Category D. Pregnant diabetics should be managed with insulin, not oral hypoglycemics. Causes symptomatic hypoglycemia due to hyperinsulinemia in the newborn. Monitor infant's serum glucose for 5 days after birth. (See Chap 41 for treatment of hypoglycemia.)
Acetophenazine	Category C. No reports of fetal risk available.
Acetylcholine	Category C. No reports of fetal risk available.
Acyclovir	Category C. Report of 2 infants exposed in utero exhibited no toxicity.
Albumin	Category C. No known problems associated with its use in pregnancy.
Albuterol	Category C. Used to prevent premature labor, as is terbutaline and ritodrine. May cause fetal tachycardia ($>$ 160 beats/min) and hypoglycemia in the newborn. Decreases incidence of neonatal respiratory distress syndrome.
Alcohol	Category D or X if used excessively. Causes multiple congenital anomalies. Causes fetal alcohol syndrome (prenatal and postnatal growth deficiency, facial dysmorphogenesis, CNS abnormalities, impairment in mental and motor functioning), spontaneous abortion, renal anomalies, alcohol withdrawal syndrome, and other abnormalities.
Alteplase (TPA tissue-type plasminogen activator)	Category C. No information available.
Amantadine	Category C. Teratogenic in animals in high doses. In one reported case, exposure to amantidine in the first trimester may have caused a single ventricle with pulmonary atresia.
Ambenonium	Category C. No reports of fetal risk available. Intravenous anticholinesterases could potentially induce premature labor.
Amikacin	Category C. No reports of adverse effects in the fetus. Testing for ototoxicity is recommended because other aminoglycosides, kanamycin and streptomycin, have been associated with eighth cranial nerve damage.
Amiloride	Category B. No reports of fetal risk available.
Aminocaproic acid	Category C. No reports of fetal risk available.
Aminoglutethimide	Category D. Possible virilization when given throughout pregnancy.
Aminophylline	Category C. At birth, transient tachycardia, irritability, and vomiting may occur, especially if mother's serum concentrations are above the therapeutic range. No congenital defects have been reported.

Drug or Substance	FDA Fetal Risk Category, Adverse Effects, and Clinical Comments
Aminopterin	Category X. Several reports have described fetal malformations when the drug has been used unsuccessfully to induce abortion in the first trimester.
Para-amino-salicylic acid (PAS)	Category C. In one study, congenital defects were found in 5 infants; other studies have reported no fetal risk.
Amiodarone	Category C. Transient bradycardia reported in one newborn. Since this drug contains iodine, there is potential concern regarding the fetal thyroid gland. Thyroid function testing of newborns of mothers who have taken the drug during pregnancy is recommended.
Amitriptyline	Category D. Malformations, neonatal withdrawal, and urinary retention in the neonate are potential problems.
Ammonium chloride	Category B. Three possible malformations (inguinal hernia if the drug was taken during the first trimester, cataracts, and benign tumors) have been reported. Acidoses may occur in the mother and fetus when the drug is taken near term.
Amobarbital	Category D. Increased incidence of congenital defects reported. May cause withdrawal syndrome.
Amoxapine	Category C. No reports of fetal risk available.
Amoxicillin	Category B. No evidence of fetal or neonatal risk.
Amphetamines	Category D. With amphetamine abuse, there is an increased incidence of preterm labor, placental abruption, fetal distress, postpartum hemorrhage, intrauterine growth retardation, feeding difficulty, drowsiness, and lassitude that may last several months.
Amphotericin B	Category B. No reports of fetal risk available.
Ampicillin	Category B. No reports of fetal risk available.
Amyl nitrite	Category C. Insufficient data to draw conclusions regarding the safety of this agent during pregnancy.
Anileridine	Category B. Potential risk of withdrawal syndrome and respiratory depression from maternal use of this narcotic analgesic.
Anisindione	Category D. This drug is a coumadin (warfarin) derivative; there is significant risk of congenital defects. May cause the fetal warfarin syndrome (nasal hypoplasia with a flattened, upturned appearance, stippled epiphyses, and possibly other features such as low birth weight, eye defects, developmental retardation, congenital heart disease, and death). May also cause hemorrhage. If anticoagulation is required during pregnancy, heparin is a safer choice.
Antacids	Category C. No teratogenic effects reported. Avoid chronic use of high doses.
Antazoline	Category C. No data available for this antihistamine.
Aspirin	Category C. May cause increased risk of hemorrhage, closure of the ductus arteriosus, and prolonged labor. First-trimester use does not increase risk of congenital heart defects. Risk is greatest in the last 3 months of pregnancy. High doses may cause increased perinatal mortality and intrauterine growth

Drug or Substance	FDA Fetal Risk Category, Adverse Effects, and Clinical Comments
	retardation. If medication is required to treat fever or pain, use acetaminophen rather than aspirin.
Atenolol	Category C. May cause bradycardia and hypotension in infants exposed near term. Monitor blood pressure and heart rate carefully.
Atropine	Category C. No reports of fetal risk available.
Aurothioglucose	Category C. No reports of fetal risk available; however, experience with its use during pregnancy limited.
Azathioprine	Category D. Most investigators have found azathioprine to be relatively safe. In a few cases, however, abnormalities have been reported, including leukopenia and thrombocytopenia, immunosuppression, transient chromosomal aberrations, and congenital defects. Interferes with effectiveness of an intrauterine contraceptive device.
Bacampicillin	Category B. No reports of fetal risk available.
Bacitracin	Category C. No reports of fetal risk available.
BCG vaccine	Category C. Animal studies have not been done. If possible, avoid use in pregnancy.
Belladonna	Category C. Associated with fetal malformations of varying severity in general and with minor malformations when used in the first trimester.
Benzocaine	Category C. No adverse effects reported.
Benzoyl peroxide	Category C. No adverse effects reported.
Benzthiazide	Category D. Thiazide-related diuretics may cause increased risk of congenital defects if taken during the first trimester. May also cause hypoglycemia, thrombocytopenia, hyponatremia, hypokalemia, and death. May inhibit labor. Use during pregnancy only if required for patients with heart disease. Carefully monitor infant's electrolytes, platelet count, and serum glucose after birth.
Benztropine	Category C. May cause decreased intestinal motility in the infant.
Beta carotene.	Category C. No reports of fetal risk available.
Betamethasone	Category C. Stimulates fetal lung maturation, thus reducing incidence and severity of respiratory distress syndrome. No reports of congenital defects associated with human use of corticosteroids in pregnancy.
Bethanechol	Category C. No reports of fetal risk available, but data limited.
Biperiden	Category C. No reports of fetal risk available.
Bisacodyl	Category C. Bulk-forming (methylcellulose) or surfactant (docusate) laxatives preferred for use in pregnancy over this stimulant laxative.
Bismuth subsalicylate (Pepto-Bismol)	Contains salicylates. See Aspirin.
Bleomycin	Category C. If possible, avoid during pregnancy. Two normal infants were born to mothers receiving bleomycin and other antineoplastic agents in the 2nd and 3rd trimesters.

Drug or Substance	FDA Fetal Risk Category, Adverse Effects, and Clinical Comments
Bretylium	Category C. No reports of fetal risk available; however, may cause maternal hypotension, with potential risk to the fetus from reduced uterine blood flow and hypoxia.
Bromides	Category D. Possible association with polydactyly, GI malformations, clubfoot, and congenital dislocation of hip. May cause neonatal bromism (poor suck, diminished Moro's reflex, hypotonia). Monitor serum bromide concentrations in the newborn.
Bromocriptine	Category C. Does not pose significant risk to the fetus.
Brompheniramine	Category C. Increased risk of fetal malformations if taken during the first trimester.
Buclizine	Category C. Possible increased risk of fetal malformations.
Busulfan	Category D. Use during pregnancy associated with fetal malformations and low birth weight.
Butalbital	Category C. No association with fetal malformations reported. However, withdrawal syndrome may occur; observe infant for 48 hours after birth.
Butorphanol	Category B. No association with fetal malformations reported; however, respiratory depression and withdrawal syndrome may occur.
Caffeine	Category B. Moderate consumption of caffeine probably does not pose a risk to the fetus; even so, it is prudent to avoid or limit its consumption. Consumption of 6–8 cups of coffee per day may be associated with decreased fertility, spontaneous abortion, and low birth weight.
Calcifediol	Category A for RDA amounts; category D for therapeutic and higher doses. Calcifediol is a vitamin D analog. High doses of vitamin D are teratogenic in animals but not in humans. Because vitamin D raises calcium levels, it may be associated with supravalvular aortic stenosis syndrome, which is often associated with hypercalcemia of infancy.
Calcitonin	Category B. No reports of fetal risk available.
Calcitriol	Category A for RDA amounts; category D for therapeutic and higher doses. High doses of vitamin D are teratogenic in animals but not in humans. Because vitamin D raises calcium levels, it may be associated with supravalvular aortic stenosis syndrome, which is often associated with hypercalcemia of infancy.
Camphor	Category C. No reports of fetal risk with topical application available. May cause fetal death and respiratory failure with maternal ingestion.
Captopril	Category C. Fetal malformations and intrauterine growth retardation have been associated with the use of captopril during pregnancy in 2 cases. Is embryocidal in animals. Data are limited, but it is recommended that this drug be avoided during pregnancy.
Carbachol	Category C. No reports of fetal risk available.

Drug or Substance	FDA Fetal Risk Category, Adverse Effects, and Clinical Comments
Carbamazepine	Category C. May case craniofacial defects, fingernail hypoplasia, developmental delay (similar to fetal hydantoin syndrome).
Carbarsone	Category D. Contains arsenic, which has been associated with lesions of the CNS. If possible, avoid during pregnancy.
Carbenicillin	Category B. This drug has been used in a large number of pregnancies; no malformations have been associated with its use.
Carbimazole	Category D. May cause aplasia cutis (scalp defects). For the treatment of hyperthyroidism during pregnancy, use propylthiouracil rather than carbimazole or methimazole.
Carbinoxamine	Category C. No reports of fetal risk available, but data limited.
Carphenazine	Category C. No reports of fetal risk available, but data limited.
Casanthranol	Category C. No reports of fetal anomalies reported in 109 infants exposed to this drug during pregnancy.
Cascara Sagrada	Category C. Higher than expected risk for benign tumors in one study, but confirmation needed.
Castor oil	Category C. May cause premature labor.
Cefaclor	Category B. No reports of fetal risk available.
Cefadroxil	Category B. No reports of fetal risk available.
Cefamandole	Category B. Data are limited, but no abnormalities noted in one infant exposed to this drug in the first trimester.
Cefazolin	Category B. No reports of fetal risk available.
Cefonicid	Category B. No reports of fetal risk available.
Cefoperazone	Category B. No adverse newborn effects noted when administered to the mother at term.
Ceforanide	Category B. No reports of fetal risk available.
Cefotaxime	Category B. No reports of fetal risk available.
Cefoxitin	Category B. No adverse newborn effects noted when administered to the mother at term.
Ceftizoxime	Category B. No adverse newborn effects noted when administered to the mother at term.
Ceftriaxone	Category B. No adverse newborn effects noted when administered to the mother at term.
Cefuroxime	Category B. No adverse newborn effects noted.
Cephalexin	Category B. No adverse newborn effects noted.
Cephalothin	Category B. No adverse newborn effects noted.
Cephapirin	Category B. No data available.
Cephradine	Category B. No adverse newborn effects noted.
Chloral hydrate	Category C. No adverse effects reported.
Chlorambucil	Category D. Reports of unilateral agenesis of kidney and ureter, cardiovascular anomalies. May cause low birth weight.
Chloramphenicol	Category C. No congenital defects reported. Avoid at term because of the risk for gray syndrome (cardiovascular collapse).
Chlordiazepoxide	Category D. Some studies have found increased risk of fetal malformations; however, others have not confirmed this. When given at term, neonatal depression

Drug or Substance	FDA Fetal Risk Category, Adverse Effects, and Clinical Comments
	with hypotonia persisting for up to a week has been reported. Neonatal withdrawal syndrome may occur.
Chloroquine	Category C. Generally considered safe, but there may be a small increased risk of birth defects.
Chlorothiazide	Category D. Thiazide-related diuretics may cause increased risk of congenital defects if taken during the first trimester. May also cause hypoglycemia, thrombocytopenia, hyponatremia, hypokalemia, and death. May inhibit labor. Use in pregnancy only if required for patients with heart disease. Monitor infant's electrolytes, platelet count, and serum glucose carefully after birth.
Chlorpheniramine	Category B. Possible association with fetal malformations reported, but statistical significance unknown.
Chlorpromazine	Category C. Probably safe and effective for treatment of vomiting and nausea of pregnancy when used occasionally at low doses. Avoid administration at term because it may cause hypotension. May cause extrapyramidal syndrome (tremors, increased muscle tone) in the infant when administered near term.
Chlorpropamide	Category D. Pregnant diabetics should be managed with insulin, not oral hypoglycemics. Causes symptomatic hypoglycemia due to hyperinsulinism in the newborn. Monitor the infant's serum glucose for 5 days after birth (see p 211 for treatment of hypoglycemia).
Chlortetracycline	Category D. Tetracyclines should be avoided during pregnancy because they may cause adverse effects, including yellow staining of teeth, inhibition of bone growth, maternal liver toxicity, and congenital defects.
Chlorthalidone	Category D. Thiazide-related diuretics may cause increased risk of congenital defects if taken during the first trimester. May also cause hypoglycemia, thrombocytopenia, hyponatremia, hypokalemia, and death. May inhibit labor. Use in pregnancy only if required for patients with heart disease. Carefully monitor infant's electrolytes, platelet count, and serum glucose after birth.
Cholecalciferol	Category A for RDA amounts; category D for therapeutic and higher doses. Calcifediol is a vitamin D analog. High doses of vitamin D are teratogenic in animals but not in humans. Because vitamin D raises calcium levels, it may be associated with supravalvular aortic stenosis syndrome, which is often associated with hypercalcemia of infancy.
Cholera vaccine	Category C. Inactivated bacterial vaccine. May be given in pregnancy to meet travel requirements.
Cholestyramine	Category C. Not systemically absorbed but may bind fat-soluble vitamins in GI tract and cause vitamin deficiency in the fetus, although this effect has not been reported.
Ciclopirox	Category B. No adverse effects reported.

Drug or Substance	FDA Fetal Risk Category, Adverse Effects, and Clinical Comments
Cimetidine	Category B. One report of transient liver impairment in the newborn has not been confirmed by other investigators.
Cisplatin	Category D. Data limited to one case report in which no adverse effects to the fetus were reported.
Citrate and citric acid (Shohl's, Bicitra, Polycitra)	Category C. Avoid sodium citrate in toxemic patients (contains 1 mEq/mL sodium).
Clemastine	Category C. No data available.
Clindamycin	Category B. No adverse effects reported.
Clofibrate	Category C. No adverse effects reported; however, data limited. Avoid administration near term, especially in preterm infants, because of their limited capacity for glucuronidation of this compound.
Clomiphene	Category X. May cause neural tube defects and other fetal malformations.
Clomipramine	Category D. Three cases of infant lethargy, hypotonia, cyanosis, jitteriness, irregular respirations, respiratory acidosis, and hypothermia have been reported.
Clonazepam	Category C. May cause apnea.
Clonidine	Category C. Data limited; however, no adverse effects reported.
Clotrimazole	Category B. No adverse effects reported.
Cloxacillin	Category B. No adverse effects reported.
Coal tar	Category C. No adverse effects reported.
Cocaine	Category C. May cause withdrawal syndrome, multisystem abnormalities due to the vasoconstrictive properties of the drug including urogenital anomalies, prematurity, spontaneous abortions, fetal growth retardation, neurobehavioral deficits, EEG abnormalities, cerebral infarctions, cardiorespiratory pattern abnormalities, and abruptio placentae.
Codeine	Category C. May cause malformations, respiratory depression, and withdrawal syndrome.
Colchicine	Category C. Use by the father prior to conception associated with atypical Down's syndrome; however, not confirmed by other investigators.
Colestipol	Category C. Not systemically absorbed but may bind fat-soluble vitamins in GI tract and cause vitamin deficiency in the fetus, although this effect has not been reported.
Colistimethate	Category B. No adverse effects reported.
Contraceptives, oral	Category X. May affect development of sexual organs and may cause hyperbilirubinemia in the newborn.
Corticotropin	Category C. No adverse effects reported.
Cortisone	Category D. No association with congenital malformations found in one large study; however, other studies reported abnormalities including cataracts, cyclopia, interventricular septal defect, gastroschisis, and other abnormalities.
Coumadin	Category D. Significant risk of congenital defects. May cause fetal warfarin syndrome (hypoplastic, flattened nasal bridge, stippled epiphyses, and possibly

Drug or Substance	FDA Fetal Risk Category, Adverse Effects, and Clinical Comments
	other features such as low birth weight, eye defects, development retardation, congenital heart disease, and death). May also cause hemorrhage. If anticoagulation is required during pregnancy, heparin given at the lowest effective dose is probably a safer choice.
Crotamiton	Category C. No adverse effects reported. It is one of the preferred drugs for treatment of scabies in pregnant women.
Cyclacillin	Category B. Has been used in a large number of pregnancies and has not been associated with malformations.
Cyclamate	Category C. No adverse effects reported.
Cyclizine	Category B. Teratogenic in animals but not in humans.
Cyclophosphamide	Category D. May cause fetal malformations from first-trimester exposure, possible pancytopenia, low birth weight. Paternal use of the drug prior to conception may cause malformations in the infant.
Cyproheptadine	Category B. No adverse effects reported.
Cytarabine	Category D. May cause chromosomal abnormalities and congenital anomalies with maternal or paternal use prior to conception, and low birth weight; however, normal infants have been delivered.
Dacarbazine	Category C. No information available.
Dactinomycin	Category C. Stillbirth and low birth weight may occur; however, normal infants have been delivered.
Danthron	Category C. One study reported a higher than expected risk of benign tumors, but confirmation of this is needed.
Daunorubicin	Category D. Successful pregnancies with normal infants reported; however, abnormalities such as low birth weight, anemia, hypoglycemia, intrauterine death, and myocardial necrosis may occur. Paternal use may result in congenital defects in the infant.
Deferoxamine	Category C. No abnormalities reported.
Demeclocycline	Category D. Tetracyclines should be avoided during pregnancy because they may cause adverse effects, including yellow staining of teeth, inhibition of bone growth, maternal liver toxicity, and congenital defects.
Desipramine	Category C. Withdrawal syndrome reported.
Desmopressin	Category B. No adverse effects reported.
Dexamethasone	Category C. No known congenital defects reported. Given in premature labor to stimulate fetal lung maturation.
Dextroamphetamine	Category D. May cause congenital defects such as cardiac abnormalities, biliary atresia, and eye defects; may cause withdrawal syndrome.
Diatrizoate	Category D. Monitor thyroid function because this drug may suppress the fetal thyroid gland when administered by intra-amniotic injection.
Diazepam	Category D. May cause hypotonia, lethargy, sucking difficulties, and withdrawal syndrome. May also cause craniofacial abnormalities, sullen and expression-

Drug or Substance	FDA Fetal Risk Category, Adverse Effects, and Clinical Comments
	less face, low Apgar scores, apneic spells, delayed motor development, and hypotonia.
Diazoxide	Category C. May cause transient fetal bradycardia and hyperglycemia.
Dicloxacillin	Category B. No adverse effects reported.
Dicumarol	Category D. This drug is a coumadin (warfarin) derivative; there is significant risk of congenital defects. May cause fetal warfarin syndrome (hypoplastic, flattened nasal bridge, stippled epiphyses, and possibly other features such as low birth weight, eye defects, developmental retardation, congenital heart disease, and death). May also cause hemorrhage. If anticoagulation is required during pregnancy, heparin given at the lowest effective dose is probably a safer choice.
Dienestrol	Category X. Contraindicated during pregnancy. May lead to high estrogen concentrations in the blood leading to fetal malformations.
Diethylstilbestrol	Category X. May result in complications of the reproductive system, including carcinoma of the cervix and vagina. Hirsutism and irregular menses may result, but this is controversial. GU abnormalities, including neoplasms, may also occur in male offspring.
Digitalis	Category C. No congenital defects reported. Neonatal death has resulted from maternal overdose.
Digitoxin	Category C. No congenital defects reported.
Digoxin	Category C. No congenital defects reported.
Dihydrotachysterol	Category A for RDA amounts; category D for therapeutic and higher doses. Calcifediol is a vitamin D analog. High doses of vitamin D are teratogenic in animals but not in humans. Because vitamin D raises calcium levels, it may be associated with supravalvular aortic stenosis syndrome, which is often associated with hypercalcemia of infancy.
Dimenhydrinate	Category B. Has not been associated with major or minor fetal malformations. May have oxytocic effect.
Diphenhydramine	Category C. May be associated with fetal malformations such as GU malformations, inguinal hernia, club foot, ventricular septal defect, and other abnormalities such as oral clefts and withdrawal syndrome.
Diphenoxylate (combined with atropine, Lomotil)	Category C. No abnormalities reported.
Diphtheria and tetanus toxoids	Category C. No data available on safety of diphtheria toxoid; therefore, the manufacturer does not recommend use of the combination product in pregnancy.
Dipyridamole	Category C. No abnormalities reported.
Disopyramide	Category C. No abnormalities reported.
Disulfiram	Category X. Causes fetal malformations and spontaneous abortion.
Dobutamine	Category C. No adverse effects reported, but data limited.

Drug or Substance	FDA Fetal Risk Category, Adverse Effects, and Clinical Comments
Docusate	Category C. No fetal malformations reported. Possible hypomagnesemia with use throughout pregnancy.
Dopamine	Category C. No adverse effects reported.
Doxepin	Category C. Possible decrease in GI motility if given at term.
Doxorubicin	Category D. Normal pregnancies have occurred in mothers treated with this drug; however, fetal malformations have also been reported.
Doxycycline	Category D. Tetracyclines should be avoided during pregnancy because they may cause adverse effects, including yellow staining of teeth, inhibition of bone growth, maternal liver toxicity, and congenital defects.
Doxylamine	Category B. Probably not associated with malformations.
Droperidol	Category C. No adverse effects reported.
Echothiophate	Category C. No information available, but transplacental passage not likely due to its chemical structure.
Edrophonium	Category C. No adverse effects reported. May cause premature labor.
Ephedrine	Category C. Minor fetal malformations may possibly be associated with its use during the first trimester. May cause fetal tachycardia.
Epinephrine	Category C. May cause fetal malformations with first-trimester use and inguinal hernia with use anytime during pregnancy.
Ergocalciferol	Category A for RDA amounts; category D for therapeutic and higher doses. Calcifediol is a vitamin D analog. High doses of vitamin D are teratogenic in animals but not in humans. Because vitamin D raises calcium levels, it may be associated with supravalvular aortic stenosis syndrome, which is often associated with hypercalcemia of infancy.
Ergotamine derivatives	Category X. May cause intrauterine fetal death from drug-induced increased in uterine motility and placental vasoconstriction.
Erythromycin	Category B. No abnormalities reported.
Estradiol	Category X. Estrogenic hormones contraindicated during pregnancy. In utero exposure may cause developmental changes in psychosexual performance of boys, less heterosexual experience, and fewer masculine interests.
Estrogens (conjugated)	Category X. Estrogenic hormones contraindicated during pregnancy. May cause fetal malformations.
Ethacrynic acid	Category D. May decrease placental perfusion, ototoxicity. Not recommended for use in pregnancy.
Ethambutol	Category B. No abnormalities reported.
Ethinyl estradiol	Category X. Use of estrogenic hormones during pregnancy contraindicated. In utero exposure may cause developmental changes in psychosexual performance of boys, less heterosexual experience, and fewer masculine interests.
Ethiodized oil	Category D. May cause neonatal hypothyroidism.
Ethisterone	Category D. Possible association with congenital anomalies.

Drug or Substance	FDA Fetal Risk Category, Adverse Effects, and Clinical Comments
Ethosuximide	Category C. May cause congenital anomalies, spontaneous hemorrhage in the neonate.
Ethynodiol	Category D. May cause modified development of sexual organs and hyperbilirubinemia of the newborn.
Famotidine	Category B. No adverse effects reported, but data limited.
Fenoprofen	Category B; category D if used near term. No congenital malformations reported. May cause constriction of ductus arteriosus in utero, persistent pulmonary hypertension of the newborn, and inhibition of labor.
Fenoterol	Category B. No malformations reported. Inhibits uterine activity at term.
Fentanyl	Category B; category D with prolonged high doses. No malformations reported. May cause respiratory depression and withdrawal syndrome.
Ferrous sulfate	Category B. No adverse effects reported.
Flucytosine	Category C. No defects reported, although its metabolite (fluorouracil) may produce fetal malformations.
Fludrocortisone (Florinef)	Category C. Observe infant for signs of adrenocortical insufficiency and treat if required.
Fluoride	Category C. Crosses the placenta. No information available on fetal effects.
Fluorouracil	Category D. May cause fetal malformations (first-trimester use), cyanosis and jerking extremities (third-trimester use), and low birth weight (used at any time during pregnancy).
Fluphenazine	Category C. Extrapyramidal effects; possible congenital malformations in one infant.
Folic acid	Category A. Folate deficiency may result in congenital anomalies.
Formaldehyde	No FDA fetal risk category established. Increased risk of spontaneous abortion and small-for-gestational-age infants.
Furazolidone	Category C. No congenital defects reported.
Furosemide	Category C. No congenital defects reported. Generally not indicated in pregnancy except in patients with cardiovascular disorders.
Gentamicin	Category C. No congenital defects reported. Potentiation of magnesium sulfate-induced neuromuscular weakness. Monitor infant for ototoxicity as this has occurred with other aminoglycosides (kanamycin and streptomycin).
Gentian violet	Category C. Fetal malformations may possibly occur, but confirmation needed.
Glycopyrrolate	Category B. Minor fetal malformations may possibly occur but are unlikely.
Gold sodium thiomalate	Category C. Probably no risk to the fetus, but experience limited.
Griseofulvin	Category C. Teratogenic in animals, but no data available for humans.
Guaifenesin	Category C. May cause inguinal hernias with first-trimester use.
Haloperidol	Category C. Limb reductions reported in 2 reports, but other studies have not confirmed this.

Drug or Substance	FDA Fetal Risk Category, Adverse Effects, and Clinical Comments
Heparin	Category C. No reports of congenital defects reported. Heparin preferred over oral anticoagulants during pregnancy.
Hepatitis B immune globulin (HBIG)	Category B. No adverse effects reported.
Hepatitis B vaccine	Category C. No adverse effects reported.
Heroin	Category B; category D with prolonged high-dose use. May cause congenital malformations, jaundice, respiratory distress syndrome, low Apgar scores, withdrawal, low birth weight, and increased perinatal mortality.
Hexachlorophene	Category C. Increased risk of anomalies with excessive first-trimester use.
Hexamethonium	Category C. No congenital abnormalities reported.
Homatropine	Category C. Possible association with minor malformations.
Hyaluronidase	Category C. No adverse effects reported.
Hydralazine	Category C. No congenital abnormalities reported.
Hydrocodone	Category B; category D with prolonged high-dose use. No malformations reported; however, respiratory depression or withdrawal syndrome may occur.
Hydromorphone	Category B; category D with prolonged high-dose use. No malformations reported; however, respiratory depression or withdrawal syndrome may occur.
Hydroxy-progesterone	Category D. May cause ambiguous genitalia. In males, may cause less heterosexual experience and fewer masculine interests.
Hydroxyzine	Category C. Possible relation between fetal malformations and use during first trimester, but statistical significance not known.
Ibuprofen	Category B; category D in third trimester. No congenital anomalies reported. May cause closing of the ductus arteriosus in utero, persistent pulmonary hypertension of the newborn, and inhibition of labor.
Idoxuridine	Category C. No data available on use in human pregnancy.
Imipramine	Category D. May cause fetal malformations, withdrawal syndrome, and urine retention.
Indomethacin	Category B; category D if taken in third trimester. May cause delayed labor, premature closure of the ductus arteriosus, persistent pulmonary hypertension of the newborn, and death.
Insulin	Category B. Insulin rather than oral hypoglycemics should be used to control diabetes. Poorly controlled diabetes associated with an increased risk of congenital defects.
Intravenous fat emulsion	Category C. No adverse effects reported.
Iodine	Category D. Topical use may result in significant absorption of iodine, resulting in transient hypothyroidism in the newborn. See also Povidone iodine and Potassium iodide.

Drug or Substance	FDA Fetal Risk Category, Adverse Effects, and Clinical Comments
Iron (ferrous sulfate)	Category B. No adverse effects reported.
Isocarboxazid	Category C. Increased risk of fetal malformations.
Isoetharine	Category C. Use in the first-trimester associated with a possible increased risk of minor fetal malformations.
Isoniazid	Category C. Increased risk of fetal malformations found in one study but not confirmed by other studies.
Isoproterenol	Category C. Use in the first-trimester associated with a possible increased risk of minor fetal malformations.
Isosorbide dinitrate	Category C. Possible association of fetal malformation with first-trimester exposure to vasodilators.
Isotretinoin (Accutane, retinoic acid)	Category X. With first-trimester use, causes severe birth defects including external ear, CNS, craniofacial, cardiac, and thymic anomalies. Prevent pregnancy during use and discontinue the drug 1 month prior to conception.
Isoxuprine	Category C. No congenital defects reported; however, fetal tachycardia and neonatal ileus may occur, and infants with cord levels exceeding 10 ng/mL may have respiratory distress syndrome, hypotension, hypocalcemia, and death.
Kanamycin	Category D. May cause eighth cranial nerve damage.
Labetalol	Category C. May cause hypotension and bradycardia. Monitor infant for 48 hours after birth.
Lactulose	Category B. No information available.
Laetrile	Category C. Theoretical risk of cyanide poisoning.
Levallorphan	Category D. May cause neonatal respiratory depression.
Levarterenol	Category D. No fetal malformations reported but may cause reduction of uterine blood flow.
Levorphanol	Category B with therapeutic doses; category D if used at high doses for prolonged periods of time. May cause respiratory depression and withdrawal syndrome.
Levothyroxine	Category A. First-trimester use possibly associated with cardiovascular anomalies, Down's syndrome and polydactyly, but confirmation needed.
Lincomycin	Category B. No congenital anomalies or other problems reported.
Lindane (Kwell)	Category C. May cause neurotoxicity and aplastic anemia. Use pyrethrins with piperonyl butoxide rather than lindane to treat lice during pregnancy.
Liothyronine	Category A. No adverse effects reported.
Liotrix	Category A. First-trimester use possibly associated with cardiovascular anomalies, Down's syndrome, and polydactyly, but confirmation needed.
Lithium	Category D. May cause cardiac congenital defects when used in the first trimester and toxicity in the newborn (cyanosis, hypotonia, bradycardia, nephrogenic diabetes insipidis, and other disorders) when used near term. Reduce risk by using lowest dose

Drug or Substance	FDA Fetal Risk Category, Adverse Effects, and Clinical Comments
	possible, monitoring serum concentrations, and avoiding sodium-restricted diets and sodium-wasting diuretics.
Loperamide	Category B. No adverse effects reported.
Lorazepam	Category C. May cause neonatal respiratory depression and hypotonia.
LSD	Category X. Causes chromosomal breakage.
Lynestrenol	Category D. Use of progestogens not recommended during pregnancy.
Lypressin	Category B. No adverse effects reported.
Magnesium salts	Category B. May cause neonatal respiratory depression and muscle weakness if used just prior to delivery and congenital rickets with prolonged infusion. Possible respiratory arrest when gentamicin given to newborns with high magnesium levels. Inhibits indomethacin effect for ductal closure.
Mandelic acid	Category C. Possible association with fetal malformations, but confirmation needed.
Mannitol	Category C. No adverse effects reported.
Maprotiline	Category B. No adverse effects reported.
Marijuana	Category not established. May cause impaired fetal growth.
Measles vaccine	Category X. Not for use during pregnancy because of risk of fetal malformations.
Mechlorethamine	Category D. Possible fetal malformations with first-trimester use and low birth weight with use any time during pregnancy.
Meclizine	Category B. Possible fetal malformations reported, but confirmation needed.
Meclofenamate	Category B; category D if taken in third trimester. May cause delayed labor, premature closure of the ductus arteriosus, and persistent pulmonary hypertension of the newborn.
Medroxy-progesterone	Category D. Not recommended for use in pregnancy because of risk of fetal malformations associated with use of female sex hormones.
Melphalan	Category D. May cause low birth weight.
Menadione	Category C; category X if given at term. May cause hyperbilirubinemia with increased risk of kernicterus if given at term. Use phytonadione (vitamin K_1), not menadione or menadiol (Synkayvite), at birth for prevention of hemorrhagic disease of the newborn.
Meperidine	Category B; category D with prolonged use of high doses. May cause respiratory depression and withdrawal syndrome. First-trimester use possibly associated with inguinal hernia, but confirmation needed.
Mephentermine	Category C. No adverse effects reported.
Mephenytoin	Category C. No adverse effects reported.
Mephobarbital	Category D. May cause withdrawal and hemorrhagic disease of the newborn.
Mepindolol	Category C. May cause bradycardia and hypotension in infants exposed near term. Carefully monitor blood pressure and heart rate.

Drug or Substance	FDA Fetal Risk Category, Adverse Effects, and Clinical Comments
Meprobamate	Category D. May be associated with fetal malformations when used in the first trimester. Avoid during pregnancy.
Mercaptopurine	Category D. May cause fetal malformations, pancytopenia, and low birth weight.
Mercury	Category not established. May be associated with increased risk of cerebral palsy.
Mesoridazine	Category C. No adverse effects reported.
Mestranol	Category X. May cause fetal malformations. Avoid estrogenic hormones during pregnancy.
Metaproterenol	Category C. Prevents premature labor. May cause fetal tachycardia and neonatal hypoglycemia.
Metaraminol	Category D. May reduce uterine blood flow.
Methadone	Category B; category D with prolonged use of high doses. May cause withdrawal syndrome, low birth weight, and death.
Methamphetamine	Category D. With amphetamine abuse, there is an increased incidence of preterm labor, placental abruption, fetal distress, postpartum hemorrhage, intrauterine growth retardation, feeding difficulty, drowsiness, and lassitude that may last several months.
Methantheline	Category C. Possibly associated with minor fetal malformations.
Methaqualone	Category D. Possible fetal malformations reported.
Methenamine	Category C. Associated with fetal malformations, but confirmation needed.
Methicillin	Category B. No adverse effects reported.
Methimazole	Category D. May cause aplasia cutis (scalp defects). Use propylthiouracil rather than carbimazole or methimazole to treat hyperthyroidism during pregnancy.
Methotrexate	Category D. Associated with fetal malformations and low birth weight.
Methsuximide	Category C. No adverse effects reported.
Methyldopa	Category C. Probably not associated with fetal malformations. Monitor neonate for hypotension for 48 hours after delivery.
Methylene Blue	Category C. Possibly associated with fetal malformations, but confirmation needed. May cause hemolytic anemia, hyperbilirubinemia, and methemoglobinemia with intra-amniotic injection of large doses.
Methylergonovine	Category C. Stimulates contractions of uterus. Indicated only for postpartum use and in the second stage of labor.
Methylphenidate	Category C. No adverse effects reported.
Methysergide	Category not established. Do not use in pregnancy due to oxytocic properties.
Metoclopramide	Category B. No adverse effects reported, but data limited.
Metolazone	Category D. Thiazide-related diuretics may cause increased risk of congenital defects if taken during the first trimester. May also cause hypoglycemia, thrombocytopenia, hyponatremia, hypokalemia,

Drug or Substance	FDA Fetal Risk Category, Adverse Effects, and Clinical Comments
	and death, and may inhibit labor. Use during pregnancy only If required for patients with heart disease. Carefully monitor infant's electrolytes, platelet count, and serum glucose after birth.
Metoprolol	Category B. Hypotension and bradycardia may occur. Monitor infant for 48 hours after birth.
Metrizamide	Category D. Monitor the infant's thyroid function at birth (see p 454, Thyroid Diseases). A related drug, diatrizoate, has suppressed the fetal thyroid gland when administered by intra-amniotic injection.
Metronidazole	Category B. Possible fetal malformations with first-trimester use.
Miconazole	Category B. No adverse effects reported.
Mineral Oil	Category C. No adverse effects reported, but many inhibit maternal absorption of fat-soluble vitamins (ADEK).
Minocycline	Category D. Tetracyclines should be avoided during pregnancy because they may cause adverse effects, including yellow staining of teeth, inhibition of bone growth, maternal liver toxicity, and congenital defects.
Minoxidil	Category C. No adverse effects reported.
Mithramycin (Plicamycin)	Category X. May cause fetal harm. Avoid during pregnancy.
Molindone	Category C. No adverse effects reported.
Morphine	Category B; category D with prolonged use of high doses. May cause respiratory depression and withdrawal syndrome. First-trimester use possibly associated with inguinal hernia, but confirmation needed.
Moxalactam	Category C. No adverse effects reported.
Mumps virus vaccine	Category X. Not for use in pregnancy because of risk of malformations.
Nadolol	Category C. May cause bradycardia and hypotension in infants exposed near term. Carefully monitor blood pressure and heart rate.
Nafcillin	Category B. No adverse effects reported.
Nalbuphine	Category B. May cause respiratory depression and withdrawal syndrome.
Naldixic acid	Category B. No adverse effects reported.
Naloxone	Category B. No adverse effects reported.
Naproxen	Category B; category D if given near term. May cause closure of the ductus arteriosus, with resulting pulmonary hypertension of the newborn. Avoid use near term.
Neomycin	Category C. No fetal malformations reported. May cause ototoxicity, which has been reported with use of other aminoglycosides.
Neostigmine	Category C. No fetal malformations reported.
Niacin/niacinamide	Category A for RDA doses; category C with excessive intake. No adverse effects reported.
Nicotine	Category X. May cause dose-related low birth weight, decreased placental blood flow, increased risk of stillborn or neonatal death, and sudden infant death syndrome (SIDS).

Drug or Substance	FDA Fetal Risk Category, Adverse Effects, and Clinical Comments
Nifedipine	Category C. No adverse effects reported, but experience limited.
Nitrofurantoin	Category B. No adverse effects reported. May theoretically cause hemolysis if given near term in patients with glucose-6-phosphate dehydrogenase (G6PD) deficiency.
Nitroglycerin	Category C. No adverse effects reported; however, fetal malformations have been reported with first-trimester use of other vasodilators.
Nitroprusside	Category C. May cause fetal bradycardia.
Norethindrone	Category D. May cause masculinization of female infants.
Norethynodrel	Category D. May cause masculinization of female infants.
Nortriptyline	Category D. May possibly cause fetal malformations, but confirmation needed. May cause urine retention in the newborn.
Novobiocin	Category C. No adverse effects reported, but may cause hyperbilirubinemia if used near term.
Nystatin	Category B. No adverse effects reported.
Oleandomycin	Category C. No adverse effects reported.
Opium	Category B for therapeutic doses; category D for prolonged use of high doses. May cause respiratory depression and withdrawal syndrome. May also cause inguinal hernia, but confirmation needed.
Oral contraceptives	See Contraceptives, oral.
Oxacillin	Category B. No adverse effects reported.
Oxazepam	Category C. No adverse effects reported.
Oxprenolol	Category C. May cause bradycardia and hypotension in infants exposed near term. Carefully monitor blood pressure and heart rate.
Oxtriphylline	Category C. No adverse effects reported.
Oxycodone	Category B for therapeutic doses; category D for prolonged use of high doses. May cause withdrawal syndrome and respiratory depression. No congenital malformations reported.
Oxymorphone	Category B for therapeutic doses; category D for prolonged use of high doses. May cause withdrawal syndrome and respiratory depression. No congenital malformations reported.
Oxytetracycline	Category D. Tetracyclines should be avoided during pregnancy because they may cause adverse effects, including yellow staining of teeth, inhibition of bone growth, maternal liver toxicity, and congenital defects.
Pantothenic acid	Category A for RDA doses; category C for excessive doses. No adverse effects reported.
Paraldehyde	Category C. Easily diffuses across placenta and may cause neonatal respiratory depression when used at term.
Paramethadione	Category D. Increased risk of spontaneous abortion and other abnormalities, including tetralogy of Fallot, mental retardation, and failure to thrive.

Drug or Substance	FDA Fetal Risk Category, Adverse Effects, and Clinical Comments
Paregoric	Category B for therapeutic doses; category D for prolonged use of high doses. May cause withdrawal syndrome and respiratory depression. No congenital malformations reported.
Parenteral nutrition (TPN)	Category C. No adverse effects reported.
Penicillamine	Category D. May cause connective tissue abnormalities (cutis laxa).
Penicillin G/Penicillin G, benzathine/ Penicillin V	Category B. Association with adverse effects very unlikely.
Penicillin G, Procaine	Category B. Association with congenital malformations unlikely.
Pentazocine	Category B for therapeutic doses; category D for prolonged use of high doses. May cause withdrawal syndrome and respiratory depression. No congenital malformations reported.
Pentobarbital	Category D. May cause withdrawal syndrome and hemorrhage in the newborn.
Perphenazine	Category C. No adverse effects reported.
Phenacetin	Category B. May cause fetal malformations (musculoskeletal malformations, kidney and adrenal anomalies), but confirmation needed.
Phenazopyridine	Category B. No adverse effects reported.
Phencyclidine (PCP)	Category X. May cause dysmorphic features, nystagmus, hypertonicity, respiratory distress, and withdrawal syndrome.
Phenelzine	Category C. May cause fetal malformations.
Phenindione	Category D. There is significant risk of congenital defects. If anticoagulation is required during pregnancy, heparin is a safer drug choice.
Pheniramine	Category C. First-trimester use possibly associated with fetal malformations.
Phenobarbital	Category D. May cause withdrawal syndrome, hemorrhagic disease in the newborn, and minor fetal malformations.
Phenylephrine	Category C. Fetal malformations reported, but confirmation needed. May cause constriction of uterine vessels.
Phenylpropanolamine	Category C. May cause constriction of uterine vessels. May also cause malformations, but confirmation needed.
Phenytoin	Category D. May cause fetal hydantoin syndrome (craniofacial—broad nasal bridge, low set hairline, short neck, microcephaly; limbs—hypoplasia of nails and distal phalanges; impaired growth; and many other abnormalities). May also cause tumors and hemorrhage in the newborn at delivery.
Phytonadione	Category C. No adverse effects reported.
Pilocarpine	Category C. No adverse effects reported.
Pindolol	Category B. May cause bradycardia and hypotension in infants exposed near term. Carefully monitor blood pressure and heart rate.

Drug or Substance	FDA Fetal Risk Category, Adverse Effects, and Clinical Comments
Piperazine	Category B. No adverse effects reported.
Pneumococcal vaccine	Category C. No adverse effects reported; however, use during pregnancy for high-risk patients only.
Poliovirus vaccine, inactivated (Salk, injection, IPV) and Poliovirus vaccine (live, oral, OPV)	Category C. No adverse effects reported; however, use during pregnancy for patients with high risk of exposure only. IPV is preferred over OPV except for patients who need immediate protection.
Polymyxin B	Category B. No adverse effects reported.
Potassium chloride/potassium citrate/ potassium acetate/potassium gluconate	Category A. No adverse effects reported.
Potassium iodide	Category D. May cause hypothyroidism and goiter with prolonged use; however, the 10-day preparation for thyroid surgery is safe.
Povidone-iodine	Category D. Topical use may result in significant absorption of iodine, resulting in transient hypothyroidism with goiter in the newborn.
Prazosin	Category C. No adverse effects reported.
Prednisone/ prednisolone	Category B. May possibly cause immunosuppression and cataracts; carries a small risk of fetal malformations.
Primaquine	Category C. No adverse effects reported. May theoretically cause hemolysis if given near term in patients with glucose-6-phosphate dehydrogenase (G6PD) deficiency.
Primidone	Category D. Possible risk of fetal malformations similar to those associated with phenytoin and of tumors and hemorrhage of the newborn at birth.
Probenecid	Category B. No adverse effects reported.
Procarbazine	Category D. May cause fetal malformations and low birth weight.
Prochlorperazine	Category C. Fetal malformations reported rarely.
Promazine	Category C. Fetal malformations reported rarely.
Promethazine	Category C. Not a teratogen; however, may cause respiratory depression when given at term.
Propantheline	Category C. No adverse effects reported.
Propoxyphene	Category C. May possibly cause fetal malformations and has caused neonatal withdrawal syndrome.
Propranolol	Category C. May cause low birth weight, fetal depression at birth, prolonged labor, neonatal hypoglycemia, hypotension, and bradycardia. Carefully monitor blood pressure, respirations, and heart rate in infants exposed near term.
Propylthiouracil	Category D. Fetal malformations reported, but association with this drug unclear. May cause reversible hypothyroidism and goiter in the infant. Drug of choice to use to treat hypothyroidism during pregnancy.
Protamine	Category C. No adverse effects reported.

Drug or Substance	FDA Fetal Risk Category, Adverse Effects, and Clinical Comments
Pseudoephedrine	Category C. May cause minor fetal malformations with first-trimester use.
Psyllium (Metamucil)	Category B. Psyllium or another bulk-producing laxative is preferred if a laxative is needed during pregnancy.
Pyrantel pamoate	Category C. No adverse effects reported.
Pyrethrins with piperonyl butoxide	Category C. No adverse effects reported.
Pyridostigmine	Category C. May cause premature labor when given near term.
Pyridoxine	Category A. Probably does not cause fetal malformations.
Pyrilamine	Category C. May cause fetal malformations and benign tumors.
Pyrimethamine	Category C. Probably does not cause birth defects. Administer with folinic acid supplementation.
Pyrvinium pamoate	Category C. No adverse effects reported.
Quinacrine	Category C. May cause fetal malformations with first-trimester use.
Quinidine	Category C. May cause neonatal thrombocytopenia.
Quinine	Category X. Has caused malformations of the limbs, CNS, heart, and GI tract as well as deafness, and other abnormalities.
Rabies immune globulin	Category B. No adverse effects reported.
Ranitidine	Category B. No adverse effects reported, but data limited.
Reserpine	Category C. May cause fetal malformations, increased respiratory secretions, cyanosis, hypothermia, lethargy, and anorexia.
Rifampin	Category C. Probably not a teratogen. May cause hemorrhagic disease of the newborn; prevent with vitamin K administration.
Rubella vaccine	Category X. This live virus vaccine should not be used during pregnancy because of risk of congenital rubella syndrome.
Scopolamine	Category C. May cause tachycardia, fever, and lethargy.
Secobarbital	Category D. May cause hemorrhagic disease of the newborn. Prevent with vitamin K administration.
Selenium sulfide	Category C. No adverse effects reported.
Simethicone	Category C. No adverse effects reported.
Sodium iodide (1 131)	Category X. Has caused fetal malformations, damage to fetal thyroid gland, and hypothyroidism.
Sodium polystyrene sulfonate (Kayexalate)	Category C. No adverse effects reported.
Spectinomycin	Category B. No adverse effects reported.
Spironolactone	Category D. No adverse effects reported; however, there is a potential risk of antiandrogenic effects.
Streptokinase	Category C. No adverse effects reported.
Streptomycin	Category D. May cause eighth cranial nerve damage.

Drug or Substance	FDA Fetal Risk Category, Adverse Effects, and Clinical Comments
Sucralfate	Category B. No adverse effects reported.
Sulfasalazine	Category B. May increase risk of kernicterus when given near term.
Sulfonamides	Category B. May increase risk of kernicterus when given near term.
Sulindac	Category B; category D if used during last trimester. No congenital anomalies reported. May cause closing of the ductus arteriosus in utero, persistent pulmonary hypertension of the newborn, and inhibition of labor.
Terbutaline	Category B. May cause fetal tachycardia and neonatal hypoglycemia.
Tetanus immune globulin	Category B. No adverse effects reported.
Tetanus toxoid	Category C. No adverse effects reported.
Tetracycline	Category D. Tetracyclines should be avoided during pregnancy because they may cause adverse effects, including yellow staining of teeth, inhibition of bone growth, maternal liver toxicity, and congenital defects.
Theophylline	Category C. May cause transient tachycardia, irritability, and vomiting at birth, especially if mother's serum concentrations are above the therapeutic range. No congenital defects reported.
Thiabendazole	Category C. No adverse effects reported, but data limited.
Thiethylperazine	Category C. Do not use during pregnancy because of risk of fetal malformations.
Thioguanine	Category D. May cause fetal malformations and chromosomal abnormalities.
Thioridazine	Category C. Probably safe for use in pregnancy.
Thiotepa	Category D. No adverse effects reported, but data limited.
Thiothixene	Category C. No information available.
Thyroid	Category A. Probably safe for use in pregnancy.
Ticarcillin	Category B. No adverse effects reported.
Timolol	Category C. May cause bradycardia and hypotension in infants exposed near term. Carefully monitor blood pressure and heart rate.
Tobacco	Category X. Dose-related risk of low birth weight, decreased placental blood flow, decreased fetal breathing movements, stillbirth, neonatal death, and sudden infant death syndrome (SIDS).
Tobramycin	Category D. No congenital defects have been reported. Potentiation of magnesium sulfate-induced neuromuscular weakness. Monitor infant for ototoxicity, as it has occurred with other aminoglycosides (eg, kanamycin and streptomycin).
Tolazamide	Category C. May cause prolonged neonatal hypoglycemia when given near term.
Tolazoline	Category C. May cause fetal malformations.
Tolbutamide	Category C. May cause prolonged neonatal hypoglycemia when given near term.
Tolmetin	Category B; category D if given near term. No congeni-

Drug or Substance	FDA Fetal Risk Category, Adverse Effects, and Clinical Comments
	tal anomalies reported. May cause closing of the ductus arteriosus in utero, persistent pulmonary hypertension of the newborn, and inhibition of labor.
Tolnaftate (Tinactin)	Category C. No information available.
Tranylcypromine	Category C. May cause fetal malformations.
Triamterine	Category D. No adverse effects reported.
Trifluoperazine	Category C. Probably safe for use in pregnancy.
Trihexyphenidyl	Category C. May cause congenital defects.
Trimeprazine	Category C. Has been associated with congenital defects, but confirmation needed.
Trimethadione	Category D. Causes adverse effects on the fetus, including intrauterine growth retardation, mental and physical retardation, impaired hearing, cardiac defects, abnormally set ears, oral clefts, fetal demise, urogenital malformations, skeletal abnormalities, and other abnormalities.
Trimethapan	Category C. No adverse effects reported.
Trimethobenzamide	Category C. May cause congenital defects and extrapyramidal dysfunction in the neonate.
Trimethoprim	Category C. This drug is a folate antagonist so there is a risk of fetal malformations; however, none attributable directly to trimethoprim have been reported.
Tripelennamine	Category B. No adverse effects reported.
Triprolidine	Category C. No adverse effects reported.
Tromethamine	Category C. No information available.
Urokinase	Category B. No adverse effects reported.
Valproic acid	Category D. Increases risk of spina bifida and fetal malformations similar to those caused by phenytoin.
Vancomycin	Category C. May cause hypotension if given near term. Infuse over 1 hour and monitor blood pressure.
Vasopressin	Category B. No fetal malformations reported. May cause uterine contractions.
Verapamil	Category C. May cause decreased urine blood flow, hypotension, and fetal bradycardia.
Vidarabine	Category C. Insufficient data available.
Vincristine	Category D. Congenital defects such as atrial septal defect, kidney malformation, pancytopenia, and low birth weight have been reported.
Vitamin A	Category A. Probably safe for use in pregnancy when used at the RDA dose, but congenital defects have been reported with excessive doses.
Vitamin B$_{12}$	Category A. No adverse effects reported.
Vitamin C	Category A. No reports directly linking this vitamin to congenital defects in humans. May cause scurvy in infants if it is used at high doses during pregnancy.
Vitamin D	Category A for RDA dose; category D for therapeutic and higher doses. High doses of vitamin D are teratogenic in animals but not in humans. Because vitamin D raises calcium levels, it may be associated with supravalvular aortic stenosis syndrome, which is often associated with hypercalcemia of infancy.
Vitamin E	Category A. No adverse effects reported.
Vitamin K	See Phytonadione; Menadione.

Warfarin — Category D. There is significant risk of congenital defects. May cause fetal warfarin syndrome (hypoplastic, flattened nasal bridge, stippled epiphyses; and other features such as low birth weight, eye defects, development retardation, congenital heart disease, and death). May also cause hemorrhage. If anticoagulation is required during pregnancy, heparin given at the lowest effective dose is probably a safer choice.

Zinc sulfate — Category C. No information available. Manufacturer recommends that supplementation not be given during pregnancy.

REFERENCES

Briggs GG, Freeman RK, Yaffe SJ: *Drugs in Pregnancy and Lactation,* 2nd ed. Williams & Wilkins, 1986.

Manufacturer's product information for medication listed.

Appendices

APPENDIX A. ABBREVIATIONS USED IN NEONATOLOGY

AFP. Alpha-fetoprotein

AGA. Appropriate for gestational age

ARC. AIDS-related complex

ASD. Atrial septal defect

ATN. Acute tubular necrosis

BG. Babygram (x-ray that includes the chest and abdomen)

BPD. Biparietal diameter
Bronchopulmonary dysplasia

BW. Birth weight
Body weight

CBG. Capillary blood gases

CDH. Congenital diaphragmatic hernia

CHD. Congenital hip dislocation
Congenital heart disease

CID. Cytomegalovirus inclusion disease

CLD. Chronic lung disease

CPIP. Chronic pulmonary insufficiency of prematurity

CST. Contraction stress test

DDST. Denver Developmental Screening Test

ECMO. Extracorporeal membrane oxygenator

EDC. Estimated date of confinement

FBS. Fasting blood sugar
Fetal blood sample

FHR. Fetal heart rate

FHT. Fetal heart tones

GA. Gestational age
General anesthesia

GDM. Gestational diabetes mellitus

$G_xP_xAb_xLC_x$. Shorthand for gravida/para/abortion/living children

G$_x$P$_x$0000. First zero, full term; second zero, premature; third zero, abortion; fourth zero, living children

HC. Head circumference

HCM. Health care maintenance

HDON. Hemolytic disease of the newborn

HLHS. Hypoplastic left heart syndrome

HMD. Hyaline membrane disease

IDAM. Infant of a drug-addicted mother

INF. Intravenous nutritional feedings

IODAM. Infant of a drug-addicted mother

IODM. Infant of a diabetic mother

IUGR. Intrauterine growth retardation

IVH. Intraventricular hemorrhage

LBW. Low birth weight

LBWL. Low birth weight "lytes"

LGA. Large for gestational age

L/S ratio. Lecithin:sphingomyelin ratio

MAS. Meconium aspiration syndrome

MCA. Multiple congenital abnormalities

MCT. Medium-chain triglycerides

MSUD. Maple syrup urine disease

NEC. Necrotizing enterocolitis

NICU. Neonatal intensive care unit

NST. Nonstress test

OCT. Oxytocin challenge test

OFC. Occipital frontal circumference

P&PD. Percussion and postural drainage

PBLC. Premature birth, living child

PDA. Patent ductus arteriosus

PFC. Persistent fetal circulation

PIE. Pulmonary interstitial emphysema

PLAST. Percussion, lavage, suction, turn

PPH. Persistent pulmonary hypertension

PROM. Premature rupture of membranes

RDS. Respiratory distress syndrome

RLF. Retrolental fibroplasia

ROM. Range of motion
Rupture of membranes

ROP. Retinopathy of prematurity

RT. Rubella titer

RVH. Right ventricular hypertrophy

Sao$_2$. Oxygen saturation of arterial blood

SEH. Subependymal hemorrhage

SGA. Small for gestational age

SIDS. Sudden infant death syndrome

SVD. Spontaneous vaginal delivery

TAR. Thrombocytopenia-absent radii (a syndrome)

TBLC. Term birth, living child

TEF. Tracheoesophageal fistula

THAM. Trishydroxymethylaminomethane (tromethamine)

THAN. Transient hyperammonemia of the newborn

TOF. Tetralogy of Fallot

TORCH. Toxoplasmosis, other, rubella, cytomegalovirus, herpes simplex

TORCHS. The same plus syphilis

TTN. Transient tachypnea of the newborn

UAC. Umbilical artery catheter

UVC. Umbilical vein catheter

VBG. Venous blood gas

VLBW. Very low birth weight

APPENDIX B. APGAR SCORING

Apgar scores are a numerical expression of the condition of a newborn infant on a scale of 0–10. The scores are usually recorded at 1 and 5 minutes after delivery and become a permanent part of the health record. They have clinical usefulness not only during the nursery stay but at later child health visits also, when clinical status at delivery may have a bearing on current diagnostic assessments. The system was originally described by Virginia Apgar, MD, an anesthesiologist, in 1953.

Sign	0	1	2
Appearance (color)	Blue or pale	Pink body with blue extremities	Completely pink
Pulse (heart rate)	Absent	Slow (< 100/min)	> 100/min
Grimace (reflex irritability)	No response	Grimace	Cough or sneeze
Activity (muscle tone)	Limp	Some flexion	Active movements
Respirations	Absent	Slow, irregular	Good, crying

APPENDIX C. BLOOD PRESSURE DETERMINATIONS

APPENDIX TABLE C-1. NORMAL BLOOD PRESSURE IN PREMATURE INFANTS[a]

| Day | 600–999g | | 1000–1249 g | |
---	Systolic (SD)[b]	Diastolic (SD)	Systolic (SD)	Diastolic (SD)
1	37.9 (17.4)	23.2 (10.3)	44 (22.8)	22.5 (13.5)
3	44.9 (15.7)	30.6 (12.3)	48 (15.4)	36.5 (9.6)
7	50.0 (14.8)	30.4 (12.4)	57 (14.0)	42.5 (16.5)
14	50.2 (14.8)	37.4 (12.0)	53 (30.0)	
28	61.0 (23.5)	45.8 (27.4)	57 (30.0)	

[a] Based on data from Ingelfinger JR, Powers L, and Epstein MF: Blood pressure norms in low birth weight infants: Birth through four weeks. *Pediatr Res* 1983;**17**:319A.
[b] SD = standard deviation (plus or minus).

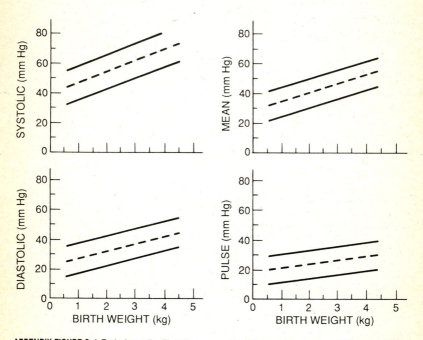

APPENDIX FIGURE C-1. Typical systolic, diastolic, mean aortic, and pulse pressure measured through umbilical artery catheters in healthy newborns up to 12 hours of age. (Reproduced, with permission, from Versmold HT et al: Aortic blood pressure during the first 12 hours of life in infants with birth weight from 610 to 4220 grams. *Pediatrics* 1981;**67**:611.)

APPENDIX D. CEREBROSPINAL FLUID NORMAL VALUES

OPENING PRESSURE
Newborn	80–110 mm water
Infant	< 200 mm water

Glucose
Premature	24–63 mg/dL (CSF:blood ratio 55–105%)
Term	44–128 mg/dL (CSF:blood ratio 44–128%)

PROTEIN
Premature	65–150 mg/dL
Term	20–170 mg/dL

WHITE CELL COUNT
Premature	0–25/mm^3 (57% PMNs)
Term	0–22/mm^3 (61% PMNs)

APPENDIX E. CHARTWORK

ADMISSION HISTORY

A. **Identification (ID).** State the name, age, sex, and weight of the infant. Include whether the patient or mother was transported from another facility or if he was born at home or within the hospital.
Infant James, a 3-hour-old 1800-gram white male, is an inborn patient from Baltimore, Maryland.

B. **Chief complaint (CC).** The major problems of the patient are usually listed in the order of severity of disease process or occurrence.
 1. *Respiratory distress syndrome.*
 2. *Suspected neonatal sepsis.*
 3. *Premature birth living child (PBLC).*

C. **Referring physician.** Include the name, address, and phone number of the referring physician.
Dr. Nick Pavona, Grove Lane Medical Center, Baltimore, Maryland telephone (301) 446-6631.

D. **History of present illness (HPI).** The history of the present illness is more helpful if it is divided into 4 separate paragraphs.

1. **Initial statement.** This part of the HPI includes the patient's name, gestational age, birth weight, sex, age of the mother, and the number of times she has been pregnant along with the number of living children she has.

2. **Prenatal history.** Discuss the maternal prenatal care and record the number of prenatal clinic visits. Include any medications the mother was taking, any pertinent prenatal tests done, and the results.

3. **Labor and delivery.** Include a detailed history of the labor and delivery: type of delivery, type of anesthesia, any medication used, and any fetal monitoring (including results).

4. **Infant history.** Discuss the initial condition of the infant and the need for resuscitation and write a detailed description of what occurred. Include the Apgar scores and discuss when the infant became symptomatic or when problems were first noted.
Infant James is a 1800-g white male delivered to a 19-year-old G2 now P2, LC2 married white female.
The mother had excellent prenatal care. She had her first prenatal visit at approximately 8-weeks' gestation and then saw her

obstetrician routinely. She was on no medications nor has any history of ethanol or cigarette abuse.

She had rupture of membranes (ROM) at 33 weeks with some mild contractions. At that time, she was seen by her obstetrician, who confirmed the premature rupture of the membranes. She was admitted to the hospital and started on IV ritodrine in an attempt to stop the labor. She was also closely observed for signs of infection. After 4 days of hospitalization, fever developed, with an increase in her white cell count. Because of suspicion of chorioamnionitis, ritodrine was stopped and pitocin was begun to induce labor. Ampicillin and gentamicin were started after cervical cultures were obtained; results are pending. External fetal monitoring had been normal until 4 hours after the pitocin induction, at which time it showed late decelerations. At this point, an emergency cesarean section was performed. General anesthesia was used, and the infant was delivered within 6 minutes.

The infant was delivered depressed at birth, with 1-minute Apgar of 4. He required bag-mask ventilation with 100% oxygen. No medications were needed. The 5-minute Apgar was 7. The infant appeared poorly perfused and had poor color without oxygen. He was stabilized and transported on 100% oxygen to the NICU.

E. **Family history (FH).** The family history should include any previous complicated births and their history, miscarriages, neonatal deaths, or premature births. Also include any major family medical problems (eg, hemophilia, sickle cell disease).

Mrs. James had one prior uncomplicated vaginal delivery that went to term. There is a history of myelodysplasia in infant James' maternal first cousin.

F. **Social history (SH).** In the social history, include a brief statement discussing the parent's age, marital status, siblings, occupation, and where they are from.

The parents are separated and both live in Baltimore. Mother is a 19-year-old factory worker and cares for their 2-year-old daughter; the father is 24 and works as a custodial engineer.

G. **Laboratory data.** List the admission laboratory and radiology results.

H. **Assessment.** State your evaluation of the infant's problems. It can include a list of suspected and potential problems, as well as a differential diagnosis.

1. *Respiratory distress syndrome: Since the infant is premature, hyaline membrane disease must be considered. Pneumonia is also a likely cause because of the maternal history of suspected chorioamnionitis.*

2. *Suspected neonatal sepsis: Because of the high suspicion of chorioamnionitis and the premature onset of labor, there is an increased septic risk in this infant. Certain pathogens need to be ruled out. Group B streptococcus is the most common pathogen in this age group, but Listeria monocytogenes and gram-negative pathogens should be considered.*

3. *Premature birth living child: The infant is a 33 weeks' gestation by Ballard examination.*

I. **Plan.** Include the therapeutic and diagnostic plans for the infant. (See section "Admission Orders," p 545.)

PROGRESS NOTES

The most commonly used format for daily progress notes is the *SOAP* method. *SOAP* is an acronym in which *S* = subjective, *O* = objective, *A* = assessment, and P = plan. Each problem should be discussed in this format. First, state the problems you are to discuss in the order of severity or occurrence and assign a number to them. Then discuss each problem in the *SOAP* format as outlined below.

A. **Subjective (S).** Include an overall subjective view of the patient by the physician.

B. **Objective (O).** Include data that can be objectively gathered, usually in 3 areas:
   1. Vital signs (temperature, respiratory rate, pulse, blood pressure).
   2. Pertinent physical examination.
   3. Laboratory data and other test results.

C. **Assessment (A).** Include evaluation of the above data.

D. **Plan (P).** Discuss the medication changes, laboratory orders, and any other new orders, as well as the treatment plan.

E. **Example.** Below is an example of part of a progress note using the *SOAP* format.

   Problem 1. Respiratory distress syndrome
   Problem 2. Suspected neonatal sepsis
   Problem 3. Premature birth living child (PBLC)

   Problem 1. Respiratory distress syndrome
   S Infant James is now 4 days old and doing much better. He has been able to wean down to 30% oxygen with good arterial gases.
   O Vital signs: temperature 98.7, respirations 52, pulse 140, blood pressure 55/35.
   Physical examination: The peripheral perfusion appears good with no obvious cyanosis. There is no grunting or nasal flaring, but the infant has mild substernal and intercostal retractions. The chest sounds slightly wet.
   Laboratory data and other test results: Arterial blood gases on 30% oxygen—pH 7.32, CO_2 48, O_2 67, 97% saturation. Chest x-ray shows mild haziness in both lung fields.
   A Infant James has resolving mild hyaline membrane disease.
   P The plan is to wean the oxygen as long as his arterial Pao_2 is greater than 55.

ADMISSION ORDERS

The following format is useful for writing admission orders. It involves the mneumonic *A.D.C. VAN DISSEL.* This stands for Admit, Diagnosis, Condition, Vital signs, Activity, Nursing procedures, Diet, Input and Output, Specific drugs, Symptomatic drugs, Extras, and Laboratory data.

A. **Admit.** Specify the location of the patient (neonatal intensive care unit, newborn nursery) and the attending physician in charge and house officer along with their paging numbers.

B. **Diagnosis.** List the admitting diagnoses.
   1. *Respiratory distress syndrome.*
   2. *Suspected neonatal sepsis.*
   3. *Premature birth living child.*

C. **Condition.** Note if the patient is in stable or critical condition.

D. **Vital signs.** State the desired frequency of monitoring of vital signs. Specify rectal or axillary temperature. Rectal temperature is usually done initially to obtain a core temperature and also to rule out imperforate anus. Then, follow axillary temperature. Other parameters include blood pressure, pulse, respiratory rate. Weight, length, and head circumference should also be obtained on admission.

E. **Activity.** All are at bed rest but one can specify "minimal stress or hands-off protocol" here. This notation is used for infants who react poorly to stress by dropping their oxygenation as in patients with persistent pulmonary hypertension. At most centers, it means handle the infant as little as possible and record all vital signs off the monitor.

F. **Nursing procedure.** Respiratory care (ventilator settings, chest percussion and postural drainage orders, endotracheal suctioning with frequency). Also require that a daily weight and head circumference be recorded. The frequency of Dextrostix (or Chemstrip-bG) testing is included in this section, since it is a bedside procedure.

G. **Diet.** All infants admitted to the neonatal intensive care unit are usually made NPO (nothing by mouth) for at least 6 to 24 hours until they are accessed and stabilized. When appropriate, write specific diet orders.

H. **Input and output (I and O).** Request that the nursing staff record accurate input and output of each baby. This record is especially important for infants on intravenous fluids and those just starting oral feedings. Specify how often you want the urine tested for specific gravity and glucose.

I. **Specific drugs.** State drugs to be administered, giving specific dosages and routes of administration. It is useful to also include the milligrams-per-kilogram-per-day dose of the drug to allow cross-checking and verification of the dose ordered. An example is:

Ampicillin 150 mg IV q12h (300 mg/kg/d divided q12h).

For all infants, order the following medications at the time of admission.

1. Vitamin K (see Chap 75) is given to prevent hemorrhagic disease of the newborn.

2. Erythromycin eye ointment (see Chap 76) is given to prevent gonococcal ophthalmia.

J. **Symptomatic drugs.** These drugs are not routinely used in a neonatal intensive care unit and would include such items as pain and sleep medications.

K. **Extras.** Any other orders required but not included above, such as roentgenograms, electrocardiography, and ultrasonography.

L. **Laboratory data.** Include laboratory data drawn on admission, plus routine laboratory orders with frequency (eg, arterial blood gases q2h, sodium and potassium bid).

DISCHARGE SUMMARY

The following information is written at the time of discharge and provides a summary of the infant's illness and hospital stay.

A. **Date of admission.**

B. **Date of discharge.**

C. **Admitting diagnosis.**

D. **Discharge diagnosis.** List in order of occurrence or severity.

E. **Attending physician and service caring for the patient.**

F. **Referring physician and address.**

G. **Procedures.** Include all invasive procedures.

H. **Brief history, physical examination, and laboratory data on admission.** Use the admission history, physical examination, and laboratory data as a guide.

I. **Hospital course.** The easiest way to approach this section of the discharge summary is to discuss each problem in paragraph form.

J. **Condition at discharge.** A complete physical examination is done at the time of discharge and is included in this section. It is important to include the discharge weight, head circumference, and length so that growth can be assessed at the time of the patient's initial checkup.

Also include the type and amount of formula the patient is on and any pertinent discharge laboratory values.
K. **Discharge medications.** Include the name(s) of medication(s), the dosage(s), and length of treatment. If the patient is being sent home on an apnea monitor, it is helpful to include the monitor settings and the planned course of treatment.
L. **Disposition.** Note where the patient is being sent (outside hospital, home, foster home).
M. **Discharge instructions and follow-up.** Include instructions to the parents on medications and when the patient is to return to clinic (and exact location). It is helpful to indicate tests that need to be done on follow-up and any results that need to be rechecked (eg, bilirubin, repeat phenylketonuria screen).
N. **Problem list.** Same list as the discharge diagnosis list.

APPENDIX F. EXCHANGE TRANSFUSION TABLE

The following table was developed at the University of Kentucky Medical Center to help with decisions about when to use exchange transfusion in a baby. The birth weight is plotted against the infant's age in days. If the indirect bilirubin, expressed in milligrams per deciliter (mg/dL), exceeds the number listed in the table, exchange transfusion should be considered. Clinical judgment should always be exercised when interpreting this table.

Birth Weight (g)	Days						
	1	2	3	4	5	6	7
< 1000	> 10	> 10	> 10	> 12	> 12	> 12	> 12
1000–1249	> 12	> 12	> 12	> 12	> 15	> 15	> 15
1250–1499	> 15	> 15	> 15	> 15	> 16	> 16	> 16
1500–1749	> 17	> 17	> 17	> 17	> 17	> 17	> 17
1750–1999	> 17	> 17	> 17	> 17	> 18	> 18	> 18
2000–2499	> 18	> 18	> 18	> 18	> 19	> 19	> 19
> 2500	> 20	> 20	> 20	> 20	> 20	> 20	> 20

APPENDIX G. GROWTH CHARTS

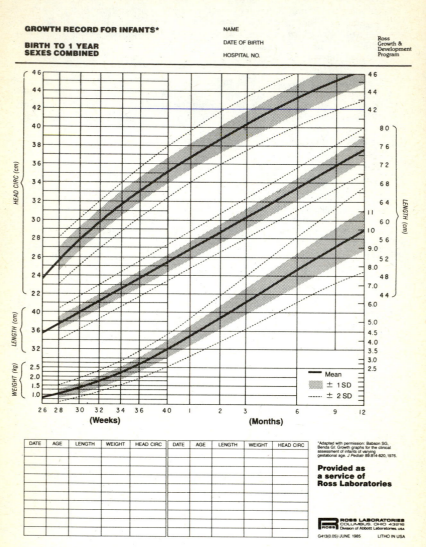

APPENDIX FIGURE G-1. Growth charts for infants. (Reprinted with the permission of Ross Laboratories.)

APPENDIX FIGURE G-2. Growth chart for girls; weight and length: birth to 36 months. (Reprinted with the permission of Ross Laboratories.)

GIRLS: BIRTH TO 36 MONTHS
PHYSICAL GROWTH
NCHS PERCENTILES*

NAME _____ RECORD # _____

*Adapted from: Hamill PVV, Drizd TA, Johnson CL, Reed RB, Roche AF, Moore WM: Physical growth: National Center for Health Statistics percentiles. AM J CLIN NUTR 32:607-629, 1979. Data from the Fels Research Institute, Wright State University School of Medicine, Yellow Springs, Ohio.

© 1982 Ross Laboratories

DATE	AGE	LENGTH	WEIGHT	HEAD CIRC.	COMMENT

in vivo performance . . .

SIMILAC® Infant Formula
Closest to mother's milk.

ISOMIL® Soy Protein Formula
When the baby can't take milk.

ADVANCE® Nutritional Beverage

ROSS LABORATORIES
COLUMBUS, OHIO 43216
DIVISION OF ABBOTT LABORATORIES, USA

G106 (0.05)/JUNE 1985   LITHO IN USA

APPENDIX FIGURE G-3. Growth chart for girls; head circumference and weight: birth to 36 months. (Reprinted with the permission of Ross Laboratories.)

BOYS: BIRTH TO 36 MONTHS
PHYSICAL GROWTH
NCHS PERCENTILES*

APPENDIX FIGURE G-4. Growth chart for boys; weight and length: birth to 36 months. (Reprinted with the permission of Ross Laboratories.)

APPENDIX FIGURE G-5. Growth chart for boys; head circumference and weight: birth to 36 months. (Reprinted with the permission of Ross Laboratories.)

APPENDIX H. ISOLATION GUIDELINES

ISOLATION PRECAUTIONS FOR PERINATAL PATIENTS

INFECTION/DISEASE		MATERNAL PRECAUTIONS	NEONATAL PRECAUTIONS	ROOM-IN*	MOTHER MAY VISIT IN NURSERY	BREAST-FEEDING	ADDITIONAL CONSIDERATIONS
AIDS	*Maternal*	Use gown and gloves when in contact with blood/body fluid.	Bathe immediately in delivery room unless unstable.	Yes	Yes	No	Stress handwashing instructions.
	Neonatal	Use gown and gloves when in contact with blood/body fluid.	Bathe as soon as possible when stable.	Yes	Yes	No	Prevent needle sharps injury. For blood spills, use sodium hypochlorite solution.
CHICKEN POX (See Varicella)							
CYTOMEGALOVIRUS (CMV) (*Acute illness only*)	*Maternal*	Isolation not required.	Bathe immediately in delivery room unless unstable.	Yes	Yes	Yes	Stress handwashing instructions.
	Neonatal		Use careful handwashing after contact with urine or respiratory secretions.	Yes	Yes	Yes	
CHLAMYDIA TRACHOMATIS *Genital*	*Maternal*	Wear gloves when touching genital discharge for duration of illness.		Yes	Yes	Yes	Prophylactic use of topical erythromycin at birth prevents inclusion conjunctivitis but not chlamydial pneumonia.
Conjunctivitis	*Neonatal*		Wear gloves when touching purulent exudate for duration of illness.	Yes	Yes	Yes	
Pneumonia	*Neonatal*		Wear gloves when touching respiratory secretions for duration of illness.	Yes	Yes	Yes	Stress handwashing.
DIARRHEA	*Maternal*	Use gown and gloves for possible contact with feces.	No rooming-in when mother is symptomatic.	Yes	Yes	Yes	Stress handwashing instructions
	Neonatal	None.	Place in separate room for close nursing observation. Use gown and gloves when in contact with feces.	No	Yes	Yes	

(continued)

INFECTION/DISEASE		MATERNAL PRECAUTIONS	NEONATAL PRECAUTIONS	ROOM-IN*	MOTHER MAY VISIT IN NURSERY	BREAST-FEEDING	ADDITIONAL CONSIDERATIONS
GONOCOCCUS	Maternal	Use gloves when in contact with genital discharge.	Bathe in delivery room as soon as possible.	Yes, after 24 hours of antibiotic therapy.	Yes, after 24 hours of antibiotic therapy.	Yes, after 24 hours of antibiotic therapy.	Stress handwashing instructions.
GONOCOCCAL OPTHALMIA NEONATORIUM		None.	Use gloves when handling infected material.	Yes, after 24 hours of maternal treatment with antibiotics.	Yes, after 24 hours of maternal treatment with antibiotics.	Yes, after 24 hours of maternal treatment with antibiotics.	
GROUP B STREPTOCOCCUS							
Genital Infection	Maternal	Private bathroom.	Baby may stay in well-baby nursery.	Yes	Yes	Yes	Stress handwashing instructions.
Pneumonia	Maternal		Mother should wear mask while newborn is in the room and should not kiss infant.	Yes, after 48 hours of appropriate antibiotics.	Yes, after 48 hours of appropriate antibiotics.	Yes, after 48 hours of appropriate antibiotics.	
	Neonatal		Special-care nursery.	No	Yes	Yes	
HEPATITIS-A		Private room if patient hygiene is poor. Use gown and gloves if contact with feces is likely. Continue isolation for 7 days from onset of jaundice.	Use gown and gloves until bathed. Bathe as soon as possible.	Yes	Yes	Yes	Stress handwashing instructions.
HEPATITIS-B		Use gown and gloves when in contact with blood/body fluids.	Use gown and gloves until bathed. Bathe as soon as possible in delivery room before injections. Admit sick neonates to special-care nursery in unit isolation.	Yes	Yes	Yes	For blood spills, use sodium hypochlorite solution.
HEPATITIS—NON A—NON B		Use gown and gloves when in contact with blood/body fluids.	Use gown and gloves until bathed. Bathe as soon as possible. Admit sick neonates to special-care nursery in unit isolation.	Yes	Yes	Yes	For blood spills, use sodium hypochlorite solution.

(continued)

INFECTION/DISEASE	MATERNAL PRECAUTIONS	NEONATAL PRECAUTIONS	ROOM-IN*	MOTHER MAY VISIT IN NURSERY	BREAST-FEEDING	ADDITIONAL CONSIDERATIONS
STAPHYLOCOCCUS AUREUS						
Maternal	See Medical Center Infection Control Manual, "Disease Specific Isolation Precautions" for details, which vary according to site of infection.		No	No	No	Two or more concurrent cases of impetigo related to a nursery or a single case of breast abscess in a nursing mother or infant is presumptive evidence of an epidemic; report immediately to attending physician and infection control.
Neonatal		Private room. Use of protective apparel depends on infected site. Refer to your specific medical center's infection control manual.	No	Yes	Yes	Stress handwashing instructions.
STREPTOCOCCUS-GROUP B (see Group B Streptococcus)						
SYPHILIS *Maternal*	Use gloves when handling secretions, blood, or moist, open lesions. Use gown if soiling is anticipated.	Use gown and gloves until bathed. Bathe in delivery room as soon as possible. Use gloves when handling secretions, discharge, blood, or moist, open lesions.	Yes, after 24 hours of treatment with antibiotics.		Yes, after 24 hours of treatment with antibiotics.	Precautions needed until 24 hours after treatment with antibiotics. Stress handwashing instructions.
Neonatal		(as above)	No	Yes	Yes	
TOXOPLASMOSIS	None	None	Yes	Yes	Yes	

(continued)

INFECTION/DISEASE	MATERNAL PRECAUTIONS	NEONATAL PRECAUTIONS	ROOM-IN*	MOTHER MAY VISIT IN NURSERY	BREAST-FEEDING	ADDITIONAL CONSIDERATIONS
TUBERCULOSIS						
1. Mother with positive PPD and no evidence of current disease.	None	None	Yes	Yes	Yes	Infant should be tested; PPD at 4–6 weeks of age, at 3–4 months of age, and at 12 months of age.
2. Mother with untreated (newly diagnosed) minimal disease, or disease has been treated for 2 or more weeks and is judged to be noncontagious at delivery.	None	None	Yes	Yes	Yes	Infant should have chest x-ray and PPD at 4–6 weeks of age; if negative, retest at 3–4 and 6 months of age.
3. Mother with current pulmonary TB. Suspected of being contagious at time of delivery.	Private room with special ventilation. Use mask if mother coughs and does not reliably cover mouth. Use gown if soiling of clothing is likely.	None	No contact until mother is judged non-contagious.	Yes, after lesions have crusted.	Not until mother is judged non-contagious.	
4. Mother has extrapulmonary spread of TB (miliary, bone, meningitis, etc.)	Use gown and gloves for possible contact with draining lesions.	None	No contact until mother is judged non-contagious.	Yes, after lesions have crusted.	Not until mother is judged non-contagious.	Infant should be given isoniazid (INH) until 6 months of age, then repeat PPD. If PPD positive, continue INH for a total of 12 months.
VARICELLA (CHICKEN POX) *Maternal/Neonatal*	Give labor and delivery and postpartum care in private room with special ventilation; keep door closed. Use gown, mask, and gloves. Continue precautions until all lesions are crusted.	Private room with special ventilation. keep door closed. Use gown, mask, and gloves. If infant must be hospitalized beyond 10 days of age, continue isolation precautions until 21 days of age.	Yes, after lesions have crusted.	Yes, after lesions have crusted.	Yes, after lesions have crusted.	May be contagious 1–2 days before the onset of rash. Persons who have had chicken pox do not need to wear masks. Hospitalized patients should be discharged prior to the 10th day following exposure, if possible, since onset may be as early as 11 days after contact. Exercise isolation precautions with exposed susceptible patients beginning 10 days after exposure and continuing until 21 days after last exposure.

INFECTION/DISEASE	MATERNAL PRECAUTIONS	NEONATAL PRECAUTIONS	ROOM-IN*	MOTHER MAY VISIT IN NURSERY	BREAST-FEEDING	ADDITIONAL CONSIDERATIONS
HERPES SIMPLEX *Genital* *Maternal* 1. Mother has active primary or recurrent sores or has had a positive culture during the 2 weeks prior to delivery.	Use gloves when in contact with lesion secretions until all lesions are crusted. If lesions are severe or primary, place in private room. Wear gown if soiling is likely. Use gloves for touching lesion secretions.	None				Scalp monitors should be avoided when possible for infants of women suspected to have genital herpes.
2. Mother's membranes intact at delivery.	(as above)	None	Yes	Yes	Yes	No need to postpone circumcision even if infant possibly exposed at birth
3. Mother's membranes ruptured more than 6 hours before delivery.	(as above)	Place in unit isolation if infant must return to nursery before rooming-in.	Yes	Yes	Yes, unless vesicular lesions involve breast.	
Labial Mother has oral blisters.	(as above)	None	Yes	Yes	Yes	Stress handwashing instructions.
Neonatal Infection or positive culture in absence of disease.	None	Use gown if soiling likely; use gloves when touching lesion secretions for duration of illness.	No	Yes	Yes	Culture obtained 24—48 hours or later after birth are more likely to identify neonatal infection. A positive culture obtained less than 24 hours after birth mandates immediate antibiotics, even in absence of symptoms.
LICE (see Pediculosis)						
LISTERIOSIS *Maternal*		May stay in well-baby nursery.	Yes	Yes	Yes	Stress handwashing instructions.

(continued)

INFECTION/DISEASE		MATERNAL PRECAUTIONS	NEONATAL PRECAUTIONS	ROOM-IN*	MOTHER MAY VISIT IN NURSERY	BREAST-FEEDING	ADDITIONAL CONSIDERATIONS
MEASLES (RUBEOLA)	*Maternal*	Use isolation room for labor and delivery and postpartum recovery. Use mask, gown, and gloves. See your specific medical center's infection control manual.	Isolation nursery or private room. Discharge prior to 17th day if possible.	No	No	No	Contagious during prodrome and up to 4 days of rash illness.
PEDICULOSIS (LICE)	*Maternal*	Private room if hygiene is poor. Use gown and gloves in close contact for 24 hours after start of effective therapy.	None	No contact until 24 hours after start of effective therapy, then may room-in or visit.	No	Not until 24 hours after start of effective therapy.	Contacts should be examined and treated if infected.
	Neonatal						
RUBELLA	*Maternal*	Private room. Use mask when in close contact.	Private room or discharge home. Use mask when in close contact. Wear gown and gloves if soiling with urine or respiratory secretions is likely.	No	No	No	Isolate for 7 days after onset of rash. Persons who have had rubella do not need to wear masks. Susceptible persons, stay out of room if possible.
RUBELLA	*Congenital*	None	Private room. Wear gown and gloves if soiling with urine and respiratory secretions is likely.	No	Yes	Yes	Rubella is contagious for a year; gloves and handwashing are necessary unless nasopharyngeal and urine cultures after 3 months of age are negative for rubella virus. Day-care providers should be aware of the potential hazard to susceptible pregnant contacts. Susceptible persons, stay out of room if possible.
SCABIES	*Maternal*	Private room if hygiene is poor. Use gown and gloves when in close contact for 24 hours after the start of effective therapy.	None	No contact until 24 hours after start of effective therapy then may room-in or visit in nursery.	No	Not until 24 hours after start of effective therapy.	Treatment of household contacts is recommended.

APPENDIX I. PHOTOTHERAPY TABLE

The following table was developed at the University of Kentucky Medical Center to help with decisions about when to begin patients on phototherapy. The birth weight is plotted against the age of the baby in days. If the indirect bilirubin level, expressed in milligrams per deciliter (mg/dL), exceeds the number listed in the table, then phototherapy should be seriously considered. Clinical judgment should always be exercised when interpreting this table.

Birth Weight (g)	Days						
	1	2	3	4	5	6	7
< 1000	> 3	> 3	> 3	> 5	> 5	> 7	> 7
1000–1249	> 5	> 5	> 5	> 7–8	> 8	> 10	> 12
1250–1499	> 8	> 8	> 8	> 10	> 12	> 12	> 12
1500–1749	> 10	> 10	> 10	> 12	> 12	> 13	> 13
1750–1999	> 10	> 10	> 12	> 13	> 13	> 13	> 13
2000–2499	> 10	> 12	> 12	> 15	> 15	> 15	> 15
> 2500	> 10	> 12	> 13	> 15	> 17	> 17	> 17

APPENDIX J. TEMPERATURE CONVERSION TABLE

Celcius	Fahrenheit	Celcius	Fahrenheit
34.0	93.2	37.6	99.6
34.2	93.6	37.8	100.0
34.4	93.9	38.0	100.4
34.6	94.3	38.2	100.7
34.8	94.6	38.4	101.1
35.0	95.0	38.6	101.4
35.2	95.4	38.8	101.8
35.4	95.7	39.0	102.2
35.6	96.1	39.2	102.5
35.8	96.4	39.4	102.9
36.0	96.8	39.6	103.2
36.2	97.1	39.8	103.6
36.4	97.5	40.0	104.0
36.6	97.8	40.2	104.3
36.8	98.2	40.4	104.7
37.0	98.6	40.6	105.1
37.2	98.9	40.8	105.4
37.4	99.3	41.0	105.8

Celsius = (Fahrenheit − 32) x 5/9
Fahrenheit = (Celsius x 9/5) + 32

APPENDIX K. UMBILICAL CATHETER MEASUREMENTS

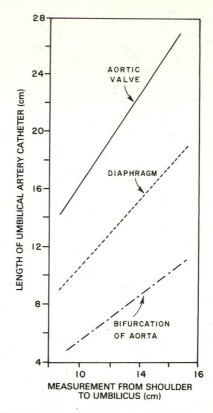

APPENDIX FIGURE K-1. The umbilical artery catheter can be placed in one of 2 positions. The "low" catheter is placed below the level of L3 to avoid the renal and mesenteric vessels. The "high" catheter is placed between the thoracic vertebrae from T6 to T9. The graph is used as a guide to help determine the catheter length for each position. The "low" line corresponds to the aortic bifurcation in the graph, whereas a "high" line corresponds to the diaphragm. To determine catheter length: Measure (in centimeters) a perpendicular line from the top of the shoulder to the umbilicus. This determines the shoulder-umbilical length. Plot this number on the graph to determine the proper catheter length for the umbilical artery catheter. It is helpful to add the length of the umbilical stump to the catheter length. (Data from Dunn PM: Localization of the umbilical catheter by post-mortem measurement. *Arch Dis Child* 1966;41:69.)

APPENDIX FIGURE K-2. The umbilical venous catheter is placed above the level of the diaphragm. Determine the shoulder-umbilical length as for the umbilical artery catheter. Use this number and determine the catheter length using the graph. Remember to add the length of the umbilical stump to the length of the catheter. (Data from Dunn PM: Localization of the umbilical catheter by post-mortem measurement. *Arch Dis Child* 1966;41:69.)

APPENDIX L. WEIGHT CONVERSION TABLE

Ounces	1 lb	2 lb	3 lb	4 lb	5 lb	6 lb	7 lb	8 lb
				Grams				
0	454	907	1361	1814	2268	2722	3175	3629
1	482	936	1389	1843	2296	2750	3204	3657
2	510	964	1418	1871	2325	2778	3232	3686
3	539	992	1446	1899	2353	2807	3260	3714
4	567	1021	1474	1928	2381	2835	3289	3742
5	595	1049	1503	1956	2410	2863	3317	3771
6	624	1077	1531	1985	2438	2892	3345	3799
7	652	1106	1559	2013	2466	2920	3374	3827
8	680	1134	1588	2041	2495	2948	3402	3856
9	709	1162	1616	2070	2523	2977	3430	3884
10	737	1191	1644	2098	2552	3005	3459	3912
11	765	1219	1673	2126	2580	3033	3487	3941
12	794	1247	1701	2155	2608	3062	3515	3969
13	822	1276	1729	2183	2637	3090	3544	3997
14	851	1304	1758	2211	2665	3119	3572	4026
15	879	1332	1786	2240	2693	3147	3600	4054

To convert from kilograms to pounds, multiply kg by 2.2.
To convert from pounds to grams, multiply lb by 454.

APPENDIX M. WHITE BLOOD COUNT GRAPH

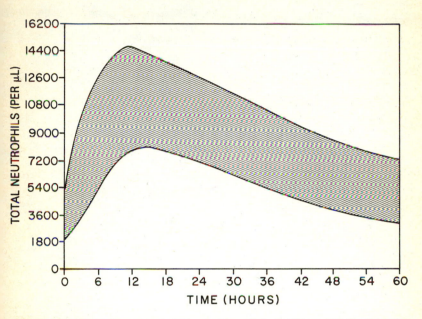

APPENDIX FIGURE M-1. Reference range for total neutrophil count in the first 60 hours of life. The total number of neutrophils is calculated as follows:

$$\frac{(\text{No. of segs} + \text{No. of stabs/bands}) \times \text{Total white blood cell count}}{100}$$

The heavy lines denote the range of neutrophil counts of normal healthy infants. A neutrophil count that falls below the curve suggests bacterial infection. A count that falls above the curve also suggests bacterial infection but less strongly. (After Manroe BL et al: The neonatal blood count in health and disease: I. Reference values for neutrophilic cells. *J Pediatr* 1979;**95**:89.)

APPENDIX FIGURE M-2. Reference range for immature neutrophils in the first 60 hours of life. An immature neutrophil count above the curve suggests bacterial infection. See also p 239. (After Manroe; see Fig M-1.)

APPENDIX FIGURE M-3. Reference range for the proportion of immature to total neutrophils (I:T) in the first 60 hours of life. An immature to total neutrophil (I:T) proportion above the curve suggests bacterial infection. See also p 239. (After Manroe; see Fig M-1.)

Index

high-frequency jet ventilation for, 122, 404
radiographic appearance of, 89–90, 93*i*
ventilator treatment plans in, 45
Pulmonary parenchymal insufficiency, in congenital diaphragmatic hernia, 447
Pulmonary stenosis
with intact ventricular septum, 30
peripheral, 29
radiographic appearance of, 94
Pulmonary toilet, in meconium aspiration, 419–420
Pulmonary vascular bed, decreased, in persistent pulmonary hypertension, 284
Pulmonary vasoconstriction, in persistent pulmonary hypertension, 284
Pulmonary vasodilators, in persistent pulmonary hypertension, 286
Pulmonary venous return, anomalous, 30
radiographic appearance of, 93
Pulse oximetry, 37–39
in extremely low birth weight infants, 110
skin care and, 111
Pulse rate, assessment of in newborn physical exam, 25
Pulses
assessment of in newborn physical exam, 30
bounding, in patent ductus arteriosus, 282
in cyanosis, 186
PVL. *See* Periventricular leukomalacia
Pyelography, intravenous
in hypertension, 207
in neuroblastoma, 449
in sepsis, 336
in Wilms' tumor, 449
Pyloric stenosis, unconjugated (indirect) hyperbilirubinemia and, 304
Pyopen. *See* Carbenicillin
Pyrantel pamoate, during pregnancy, 535
Pyridoxine dependence, seizures and, 245, 383
Pyridoxine (vitamin B₆), **479**
during breast-feeding and lactation, 513
in breast milk supplements, 74*t*
in infant formulas and breast milk, 64–69*t*
neonatal requirements for, for low birth weight infant, 61*t*
Pyrimethamine, **503–504**
during breast-feeding and lactation, 513
for toxoplasmosis, 341
Pyroglutamic acidemia
amino and organic acid analysis in, 325*t*
laboratory findings in, 319*t*
Pyruvate metabolism, disorders of, 317*t*, 319*t*

Questran. *See* **Cholestyramine**
Quinacrine, during pregnancy, 535
Quinidine, **479–480**
during breast-feeding and lactation, 513
during pregnancy, 535
toxicity caused by, arrhythmias and, 168, 169, 172
Quinine, during pregnancy, 535

Rabies immune globulin, during pregnancy, 535
Racemic epinephrine, 47
Radial artery
catheterization of, 133–134
puncture of, **131–132**

Radiant warmers
for extremely low birth weight infants, 105
fluid requirements and, 107
for hypothermia, 35
in extremely low birth weight infant, 35–36
Radiation, heat loss by, 34
Radiology, **81–96**
clinical pearls, 87–96
normal findings, 84–87
techniques in, 81–84
Radionuclide scanning, in acute renal failure, 426
Radiopharmaceuticals, during breast-feeding and lactation, 513–514
Ranitidine, **480**
during breast-feeding and lactation, 514
before cesarean delivery, neonate affected by, 10
during pregnancy, 535
for ulcers, 178–179
stress, 193, 196
Ranula, 28
Rapid antigen tests, in meningitis, 338
Rapid delivery room assessment, of gestational age, 20, 21*t*
Rapid plasma reagin test, 353
Rapid-rate ventilation, 287. *See also* Hyperventilation, for persistent pulmonary hypertension
Rashes, assessment of in newborn physical exam, 26
RDS. *See* Respiratory distress syndrome
Reactive nonstress test, 4
Recombivax HB. *See* Hepatitis B vaccine
Rectal biopsy, in distal intestinal obstruction, 443, 444
Rectal enemas, for distal intestinal obstruction, 444
Rectal examination, digital, in teratoma, 450
Rectal trauma, bloody stool caused by, 177, 178
Rectum, assessment of, in newborn physical exam, 31
Recurrent familial cholestasis, 311
Red cell aggregation, in polycythemia and hyperviscosity, 263
Red cell casts, in hematuria, 427
Red cell defects
hemolytic anemia caused by, 258
in polycythemia and hyperviscosity, 263
unconjugated (indirect) hyperbilirubinemia and, 303
Red cell hemolysis, in hyperkalemia, 204
Red cell studies, in anemia, 259
Red reflex, assessment of in newborn physical exam, 28
Reflexes. *See also specific type*
assessment of, in newborn physical exam, 32
in high-risk infants, 103
in perinatal asphyxia, 395
Reflux. *See also* Gastric aspirate
with digested formula, 191, 192, 194
with undigested formula, 191, 192, 193–194
Refractory hyperkalemia, management of, 205
Regional anesthesia, for cesarean delivery, 9, 10
vs general, 11–12
Reglan. *See* Metoclopramide
Remedication, after exchange transfusion, 151
Renal abnormalities